Users' Guides

—— to the ——

Medical

Literature

Notice

Users' Guides
—— to the ——
Medical
Literature

A MANUAL FOR
EVIDENCE-BASED CLINICAL PRACTICE
3rd EDITION

Editors

Gordon Guyatt, MD, MSc
Departments of Clinical Epidemiology
& Biostatistics and Medicine
Faculty of Health Sciences
McMaster University
Hamilton, Ontario, Canada

Drummond Rennie, MD
Former Deputy Editor, JAMA
Chicago, Illinois
Philip R. Lee Institute for Health Policy
Studies
University of California, San Francisco
San Francisco, California, USA

Maureen O. Meade, MD, FRCPC, MSc
Departments of Medicine and Clinical
Epidemiology & Biostatistics
Faculty of Health Sciences
McMaster University
Hamilton, Ontario, Canada

Deborah J. Cook, MD, MSc
Departments of Medicine and Clinical
Epidemiology & Biostatistics
Faculty of Health Sciences
McMaster University
Hamilton, Ontario, Canada

New York Chicago San Francisco Athens
London Madrid Mexico City
Milan New Delhi Singapore Sydney
Toronto

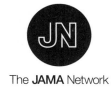

The **JAMA** Network

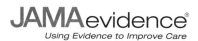

Using Evidence to Improve Care

The **JAMA** Network

2 3 4 5 6 7 8 9 0   DOC/DOC   18 17 16 15

ISBN 978-0-07-179071-0
MHID 0-07-179071-3

The JAMA Network Journals:
Editor in Chief: Howard Bauchner, MD
Executive Managing Editor: Annette Flanagin, RN, MA
Assistant Editor: Kate Pezalla, MA
Manuscript Editor: Laura King, MA, ELS
Cover Illustration: Cassio Lynm, MA, CMI, and Alison E. Burke, MA, CMI

McGraw-Hill Professional:
This book was set in Minion Pro, Regular, 10/12 pt by MPS Limited.
The editors were Sarah Henry and Robert Pancotti.
The production supervisor was Richard Ruzycka.
Project management was provided by Asheesh Ratra, MPS Limited.
The text designer was Eve Siegel; the cover art director was Anthony Landi.
RR Donnelley was the printer and binder.

This book is printed on acid-free paper.

Cover illustration: © 2014 Cassio Lynm and Alison E. Burke. The decision aid included in the illustration on the cover was developed within the MAGIC research and innovation program (http://www.magicproject.org/share-it) in collaboration with the DECIDE project (www.decide-consortium.eu).

Library of Congress Cataloging-in-Publication Data

Users' guides to the medical literature. A manual for evidence-based clinical practice / [edited by] Gordon Guyatt, Drummond Rennie, Maureen O. Meade, Deborah J. Cook.—Third edition.
      p. ; cm.—(JAMAevidence)
   Manual for evidence-based clinical practice
   Preceded by: Users' guides to the medical literature / the Evidence-Based Medicine Working Group ; editors, Gordon Guyatt ... [et al.]. 2nd ed. 2008.
   "The JAMA Network"
   Includes bibliographical references and index.
   ISBN 978-0-07-179071-0 (paperback : alk. paper) — ISBN 0-07-179071-3 (paperback : alk. paper)
   I. Guyatt, Gordon, editor. II. Rennie, Drummond, editor. III. Meade, Maureen, editor. IV. Cook, Deborah, editor. V. The JAMA Network.
VI. Title: Manual for evidence-based clinical practice. VII. Series: JAMAevidence.
   [DNLM: 1. Evidence-Based Medicine—Resource Guides. 2. Clinical Medicine—Resource Guides. 3. Decision Making—Resource Guides.
4. Review Literature as Topic—Resource Guides. WB 39]
   R723.7
   610—dc23
                                                                                                                      2014031343

McGraw-Hill Education books are available at special quantity discounts to use as premiums and sales promotions or for use in corporate training programs. To contact a representative, please visit the Contact Us pages at www.mhprofessional.com.

To our students, in many countries, whose interest, passion, and probing questions made possible the development of the methods we use to communicate the concepts of evidence-based medicine.

GG, MOM, and DJC

To Deb, who has watched over and tended me while I have watched over and tended this wonderful group, with gratitude for her love and her good humor.

DR

CONTENTS

The Foundations

Therapy

Harm (Observational Studies)

Diagnosis

Prognosis

Summarizing the Evidence

Moving From Evidence to Action

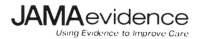

JAMAevidence: Using Evidence to Improve Care

Founded around the *Users' Guides to the Medical Literature*, *The Rational Clinical Examination: Evidence-Based Clinical Diagnosis*, and *Care at the Close of Life: Evidence and Experience*, JAMAevidence offers an invaluable online resource for learning, teaching, and practicing evidence-based medicine (EBM). Updated regularly, the site includes fully searchable content of the *Users' Guides to the Medical Literature*, *The Rational Clinical Examination*, and *Care at the Close of Life* and features podcasts from the leading minds in EBM, interactive worksheets, functional calculators, and a comprehensive collection of PowerPoint slides for educators and students.

www.JAMAevidence.com

Please visit www.JAMAevidence.com for subscription information.

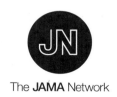

The **JAMA** Network

CONTRIBUTORS

Thomas Agoritsas, MD, Dr Med
Health Information Research Unit
Department of Clinical Epidemiology &
    Biostatistics
McMaster University
Hamilton, Ontario, Canada

Elie A. Akl, MD
Department of Medicine
American University of Beirut
Riad-El-Solh, Beirut, Lebanon

Ana C. Alba, MD, PhD
Toronto General Hospital
University Health Network
Toronto, Ontario, Canada

Paul Elias Alexander
Department of Clinical Epidemiology &
    Biostatistics
Health Research Methodology Graduate
    Program
McMaster University
Hamilton, Ontario, Canada

Waleed Alhazzani, MD, FRCPC, MSc
Departments of Medicine and Clinical
    Epidemiology & Biostatistics
McMaster University
Hamilton, Ontario, Canada

Pablo Alonso-Coello, MD
Hospital de la Santa Creu i Sant Pau
Barcelona, Spain

John Attia, MD, PhD
Department of Medicine and Clinical
    Epidemiology
University of Newcastle
Department of General Medicine
John Hunter Hospital
Clinical Research Design, IT and Statistical
    Support Unit
Hunter Medical Research Institute
Newcastle, New South Wales, Australia

Alexandra Barratt, MBBS, MPH, PhD, FAFPHM
Department of Public Health
Sydney Medical School
University of Sydney
Sydney, New South Wales, Australia

Dirk Bassler, MD, MSc
Department of Neonatology
University of Zurich
Zurich, Switzerland

Shannon M. Bates, MDCM, MSc, FRCP(c)
Department of Medicine
McMaster University
Hamilton, Ontario, Canada

Mohit Bhandari, MD, MSc, FRCSC
Departments of Surgery and Clinical
    Epidemiology & Biostatistics
McMaster University
Hamilton, Ontario, Canada

Linn Brandt, MD
Department of Medicine
Innlandet Hospital Trust
Gjøvik, Norway
Department of Medicine
University of Oslo
Oslo, Norway

Matthias Briel, MD, MSc
Department of Clinical Epidemiology & Biostatistics
McMaster University
Hamilton, Ontario, Canada
Basel Institute for Clinical Epidemiology
    and Biostatistics
University Hospital Basel
Basel, Switzerland

Romina Brignardello-Petersen, DDS, MSc
Evidence-Based Dentistry Unit
Universidad de Chile
Santiago, Chile
Institute of Health Policy, Management and Evaluation
University of Toronto
Toronto, Ontario, Canada

John Brodersen, MD, GP, PhD
Department of Public Health
University of Copenhagen
Copenhagen, Denmark

Jan Brożek, MD, PhD
Departments of Clinical Epidemiology &
 Biostatistics and Medicine
McMaster University
Hamilton, Ontario, Canada

Stirling Bryan, PhD
Centre for Clinical Epidemiology & Evaluation
University of British Columbia
Vancouver, British Columbia, Canada

Heiner C. Bucher, MPH
Basel Institute for Clinical Epidemiology
 and Biostatistics
University Hospital Basel
Basel, Switzerland

Jason W. Busse, DC, PhD
Departments of Anesthesia and Clinical
 Epidemiology & Biostatistics
McMaster University
Hamilton, Ontario, Canada

Daniel Capurro, MD, PhD
Department of Internal Medicine
School of Medicine
Pontificia Universidad Católica de Chile
Santiago, Chile
Department of Biomedical Informatics
 and Medical Education
School of Medicine
University of Washington
Seattle, Washington, USA

Alonso Carrasco-Labra, DDS, Msc, PhD(c)
Department of Clinical Epidemiology &
 Biostatistics
McMaster University
Hamilton, Ontario, Canada
Evidence-Based Dentistry Unit
Universidad de Chile
Santiago, Chile

Stacy M. Carter, MPH(Hons), PhD
Centre for Values, Ethics and the Law in Medicine
University of Sydney
Sydney, New South Wales, Australia

Jaime Cerda, MD
Department of Public Health
Pontificia Universidad Católica de Chile
Santiago, Chile

Lorena Cifuentes Aguila, MD
Department of Pediatrics
Pontificia Universidad Católica de Chile
Santiago, Chile

Juan Carlos Claro, MD
Department of Internal Medicine
Pontificia Universidad Católica de Chile
Santiago, Chile

Deborah J. Cook, MD, FRCPC, MSc, OC
Departments of Clinical Epidemiology &
 Biostatistics and Medicine
McMaster University
Hamilton, Ontario, Canada

Richard Cook, BSc, MMath, PhD
Department of Statistics and Actuarial Science
University of Waterloo
Waterloo, Ontario, Canada

Antonio L. Dans, MD, MSc
University of the Philippines
Manila, Philippines

Leonila F. Dans, MD, MSc
University of the Philippines
Manila, Philippines

PJ Devereaux, MD, PhD, FRCPC
Departments of Clinical Epidemiology &
 Biostatistics and Medicine
McMaster University
Hamilton, Ontario, Canada

Benjamin Djulbegovic, MD, PhD
Department of Internal Medicine
University of South Florida
H. Lee Moffitt Cancer Center & Research Institute
Tampa, Florida, USA

Michael F. Drummond, MCom, PhD
Centre for Health Economics
University of York,
Heslington, York, UK

Pierre Durieux, MD, MPH
Santé Publique et Informatique Médicale
Université Paris Descartes – Ecole de
    Médecine
Paris, France
Hôpital Européen Georges Pompidou
Paris, France

Shanil Ebrahim, PhD, MSc
Departments of Clinical Epidemiology &
    Biostatistics and Anesthesia
McMaster University
Hamilton, Ontario, Canada
Department of Medicine
Stanford Prevention Research Center
Stanford University
Stanford, California, USA

**Mahmoud Elbarbary, MD, PhD, MSc,
MBBCH, EDIC**
Department of Clinical Epidemiology &
    Biostatistics
McMaster University
Hamilton, Ontario, Canada
National & Gulf Center for Evidence-Based
    Health Practice
Riyadh, Saudi Arabia

Glyn Elwyn, MD, MSc, FRCGP, PhD
The Dartmouth Centre for Health Care
    Delivery Science
Hanover, New Hampshire, USA

Maicon Falavigna, MD, MSc, PhD
Department of Internal Medicine
Institute for Education
    and Research
Hospital Moinhos de Vento
Porto Alegre, Brazil
Department of Clinical Epidemiology &
    Biostatistics
McMaster University
Hamilton, Ontario, Canada

Eddy Fan, MD, PhD
Interdepartmental Division of Critical
    Care Medicine
University of Toronto
Toronto, Ontario, Canada

Ignacio Ferreira-González, MD, PhD
Cardiology Department
Vall d'Hebron Hospital
CIBER de Epidemiología y Salud Pública
    (CIBERESP)
Barcelona, Spain

Toshi A. Furukawa, MD, PhD
Departments of Health Promotion and Human
    Behavior and Clinical Epidemiology
Kyoto University Graduate School of
    Medicine
Kyoto, Japan

David Gardner, PharmD
College of Pharmacy
Dalhousie University
Halifax, Nova Scotia, Canada

Amit X. Garg, PhD
Department of Medicine
University of Western Ontario
London, Ontario, Canada

Mita Giacomini, MPH, MA, PhD
Department of Clinical Epidemiology &
    Biostatistics
McMaster University
Hamilton, Ontario, Canada

**Paul Glasziou, MBBS, PhD, FAFPHM,
FRACGP, MRCGP**
Department of Health Sciences
    and Medicine
Bond University
Robina, Queensland, Australia

Ron Goeree, MA
PATH Research Institute
St. Joseph's Healthcare
Department of Clinical Epidemiology &
    Biostatistics
Hamilton, Ontario, Canada

Jeremy Grimshaw, MBChB, PhD, FRCGP, FCAHS
Clinical Epidemiology Program
Centre for Practice-Changing Research
Ottawa Hospital Research Institute
The Ottawa Hospital
Ottawa, Ontario, Canada

Gordon Guyatt, MD, MSc, FRCPC, OC
Departments of Clinical Epidemiology &
    Biostatistics and Medicine
McMaster University
Hamilton, Ontario, Canada

**Alfred Theodore (Ted) Haines, MD, CCFP,
MSc, DOHS, FRCPC**
Departments of Clinical Epidemiology &
    Biostatistics and Family Medicine
McMaster University
Chedoke-McMaster Hospitals
LAMP Community Health Centre
Occupational Health Clinic for Ontario
    Workers
Hamilton, Ontario, Canada

Rose Hatala, MD, MSc
University of British Columbia
Vancouver, British Columbia, Canada

R. Brian Haynes, MD, PhD
Departments of Clinical Epidemiology &
    Biostatistics and Medicine
McMaster University
Hamilton, Ontario, Canada

Robert Hayward, MD
Owogo Inc.
Centre for Health Evidence
Department of Medicine
University of Alberta
Edmonton, Alberta, Canada

**Nicholas R. Hicks, MA, BM, BCh, FRCP,
MRCGP, FFPH**
COBIC
Oxfordshire, UK
Department of Primary Care Health
    Sciences
University of Oxford
Oxford, UK

Anne M. Holbrook, MD, PharmD, MSc, FRCPC
Department of Medicine
McMaster University
Hamilton, Ontario, Canada

Elizabeth G. Holliday, MSc, PhD
School of Medicine and Public Health
University of Newcastle
Clinical Research Design, IT and Statistical
    Support Unit
Hunter Medical Research Institute
Callaghan, New South Wales, Australia

Kirsten Howard, MPH, PhD
Department of Public Health
School of Public Health
University of Sydney
Sydney, New South Wales, Australia

Brian Hutton, PhD
Clinical Epidemiology Program
Ottawa Hospital Research Institute
Ottawa, Ontario, Canada

Claire Infante-Rivard, MD, PhD
Department of Epidemiology, Biostatistics
    and Occupational Health
McGill University
Montreal, Quebec, Canada

John P. A. Ioannidis, MD, DSc
Departments of Medicine, Health Research
    and Policy, and Statistics
Stanford Prevention Research Center
Meta-Research Innovation Center
Stanford University
Stanford, California, USA

Les Irwig, MBBCh, PhD, FFPHM
Department of Epidemiology
Screening and Test Evaluation Program
School of Public Health
University of Sydney
Sydney, New South Wales, Australia

**Cynthia A. Jackevicius, BScPhm, PharmD,
MSc, BCPS, FCSHP**
Western University of Health Sciences
Pomona, California, USA

Institute for Clinical Evaluative Sciences
Institute for Health Policy, Management
and Evaluation
University of Toronto
Toronto, Ontario, Canada
Veterans Affairs Greater Los Angeles
Healthcare System
Los Angeles, California, USA

**Gemma Louise Jacklyn, BAppSc,
MPH(Hons)**
School of Public Health
University of Sydney
Sydney, New South Wales, Australia

Roman Jaeschke, MD, MSc, FRCPC
Department of Medicine
St. Joseph's Healthcare
Hamilton, Ontario, Canada

Sheri A. Keitz, MD, PhD
University of Massachusetts Memorial
Medical Center
University of Massachusetts Medical School
Worcester, Massachusetts, USA

Deborah Korenstein, MD
Division of General Internal Medicine
Department of Medicine
Mount Sinai School of Medicine
New York, New York, USA

Regina Kunz, MD, MSc
Swiss Academy of Insurance Medicine
University Hospital Basel
Basel, Switzerland

Andreas Laupacis, MD, MSc, FRCPC
Health Policy and Citizen Engagement
Li Ka Shing Knowledge Institute
St. Michael's Hospital
University of Toronto
Toronto, Ontario, Canada

Luz Maria Letelier, MD
Internal Medicine Department and Evidence
Based Health Care Program
Pontificia Universidad Católica de Chile
Santiago, Chile

Mitchell Levine, MD, MSc
Department of Clinical Epidemiology & Biostatistics
McMaster University
Centre for Evaluation of Medicines
St. Joseph's Healthcare
Hamilton, Ontario, Canada

Braden Manns, MD
Departments of Medicine & Community
Health Sciences
University of Calgary
Calgary, Alberta, Canada

Kirsten Jo McCaffery, BSc, PhD
School of Public Health, Screening and Test
Evaluation Program
Centre for Medical Psychology & Evidence-based
Decision-making
University of Sydney
Sydney, New South Wales, Australia

Lauren McCullagh, MPH
North Shore LIJ Health System Office
Hofstra North Shore-LIJ Medical School
Manhasset, New York, USA

Mark McEvoy
Centre for Clinical Epidemiology and Biostatistics
School of Medicine and Public Health
Hunter Medical Research Institute
University of Newcastle
Newcastle, New South Wales, Australia

Thomas McGinn, MD, MPH
Medicine Service Line
North Shore-LIJ Health System Office
Hofstra North Shore-LIJ Medical School
Manhasset, New York, USA

K. Ann McKibbon, MLS, PhD, FMLA
Department of Clinical Epidemiology & Biostatistics
McMaster University
Hamilton, Ontario, Canada

Maureen O. Meade, MD, MSc, FRCPC
Departments of Clinical Epidemiology &
Biostatistics and Medicine
McMaster University
Hamilton, Ontario, Canada

Edward J. Mills, PhD, MSc, MSt
Global Evaluative Sciences
Vancouver, British Columbia, Canada

Cosetta Minelli, MD, PhD
Respiratory Epidemiology, Occupational
    Medicine and Public Health
National Heart and Lung Institute
Imperial College
London, UK

**Paul Moayyedi, BSc, MBChB, PhD, MPH,
FRCP, FRCPC**
Division of Gastroenterology
McMaster University
Hamilton, Ontario, Canada

Victor M. Montori, MD, MSc
Knowledge and Evaluation Research Unit
Mayo Clinic
Rochester, Minnesota, USA

Sohail M. Mulla, MSc
Department of Clinical Epidemiology &
    Biostatistics
Health Research Methodology Graduate Program
McMaster University
Hamilton, Ontario, Canada

M. Hassan Murad, MD, MPH
Division of Preventive Medicine
Mayo Clinic
Rochester, Minnesota, USA

Reem A. Mustafa, MD
Department of Medicine
University of Missouri-Kansas City
Overland Park, Kansas, USA

Dale M. Needham, FCPA, MD, PhD
Department of Physical Medicine
    and Rehabilitation
Johns Hopkins University
Baltimore, Maryland, USA

Ignacio Neumann, MD, MSc
Department of Internal Medicine
Pontificia Universidad Católica de Chile
Santiago, Chile
Department of Clinical Epidemiology &
    Biostatistics
McMaster University
Hamilton, Ontario, Canada

Thomas B. Newman, MD, MPH
Departments of Epidemiology & Biostatistics,
    Pediatrics and Laboratory Medicine
University of California, San Francisco
San Francisco, California, USA

Vlado Perkovic, MBBS, PhD, FASN, FRACP
George Institute for Global Health
    Australia, Medicine
University of Sydney
Sydney, New South Wales, Australia

Gaietà Permanyer-Miralda, MD, PhD
Epidemiology Unit and Cardiology Department
Hospital General Vall d'Hebron
Barcelona, Spain

Kameshwar Prasad, MD, DM, MMSc
Department of Neurology
Neurosciences Centre
All India Institute of Medical Sciences
New Delhi, India

Peter J. Pronovost, MD, PhD, FCCM
Departments of Anesthesiology and Critical Care
    Medicine and Surgery
Armstrong Institute for Patient Safety
    and Quality
Johns Hopkins University
Baltimore, Maryland, USA

Milo A. Puhan, MD, PhD
Department of Epidemiology and Public Health
Epidemiology, Biostatistics and Prevention
    Institute
University of Zurich
Zurich, Switzerland

Gabriel Rada, MD
Internal Medicine Department
Evidence-Based Healthcare Program
Pontificia Universidad Católica de Chile
Santiago, Chile

Adrienne G. Randolph, MD, MSc
Department of Anaesthesia
Harvard Medical School
Department of Anesthesia, Perioperative
  and Pain Medicine
Boston Children's Hospital
Boston, Massachusetts, USA

W. Scott Richardson, MD
Department of Medicine
Georgia Regents University-University
  of Georgia Medical Partnership
Athens, Georgia, USA

David M. Rind, MD
Department of Medicine
Harvard Medical School
Editorial and Evidence-Based Medicine, UpToDate
Wolters Kluwer Health
Waltham, Massachusetts, USA

Solange Rivera Mercado, MD
Department of Family Medicine
Pontificia Universidad Católica de Chile
Santiago, Chile

Bram Rochwerg, BSc, MD
Department of Medicine
McMaster University
Hamilton, Ontario, Canada

Nancy Santesso, BSc(Hon), MLIS, PhD(c)
Department of Clinical Epidemiology & Biostatistics
McMaster University
Hamilton, Ontario, Canada

Holger J. Schünemann, MD, PhD, MSc, FRCPC
Departments of Clinical Epidemiology &
  Biostatistics and Medicine
McMaster University
Hamilton, Ontario, Canada

Ian A. Scott, MBBS, FRACP, MHA, MEd
Department of Internal Medicine
  and Clinical Epidemiology
Princess Alexandra Hospital
Department of Medicine
University of Queensland
Brisbane, Queensland, Australia

**Rodney J. Scott, BSc(Hons), PhD, DSc,
FRCPath, FHGSA, FFSc(RCPA)**
Division of Molecular Medicine
Information Based Medicine Program
Hunter Medical Research Institute
University of Newcastle
Newcastle, New South Wales, Australia

Frederick Spencer, MD, FRCP(c)
Department of Medicine
Divisions of Cardiology and Hematology/
  Thrombosis
McMaster University
St. Joseph's Healthcare
Hamilton, Ontario, Canada

Sadeesh Srinathan, MD, MSc
University of Manitoba Health
  Sciences Centre
Winnipeg, Manitoba, Canada

Ian Stiell, MD, MSc, FRCP(c)
OHRI Chair of Emergency Medicine Research
Clinical Epidemiology, Ottawa Hospital
  Research Institute
Department of Emergency Medicine,
  University of Ottawa
Ottawa, Ontario, Canada

Sharon E. Straus, MSc, MD, FRCPC
Department of Medicine
Division of Geriatric Medicine
University of Toronto
Li Ka Shing Knowledge Institute
St. Michael's Hospital
Toronto, Ontario, Canada

Xin Sun, PhD
Chinese Evidence-based Medicine Center
West China Hospital
Sichuan University
Chengdu, Sichuan, China

Ammarin Thakkinstian, PhD
Section for Clinical Epidemiology
  and Biostatistics
Ramathibodi Hospital
Mahidol University
Rachatevee, Bangkok

John Thompson, PhD
Department of Health Sciences
University of Leicester
Leicester, UK

Kristian Thorlund, MSc, PhD
Department of Clinical Epidemiology &
  Biostatistics
McMaster University
Hamilton, Ontario, Canada

George Tomlinson, PhD
Department of Medicine
University Health Network and Mount
  Sinai Hospital
Dalla Lana School of Public Health,
  Institute of Health Policy Management
  and Evaluation
University of Toronto
Toronto, Ontario, Canada

Gerard Urrutia, MD, MS, PhD
Clinical Epidemiology
Hospital de la Santa Creu i Sant Pau
Barcelona, Spain

Per Olav Vandvik, MD, PhD
Department of Medicine
University of Oslo
Norwegian Knowledge Centre
  for the Health Services
Oslo, Norway

Michael Walsh, MD, PhD
Departments of Medicine and Clinical
  Epidemiology & Biostatistics
Population Health Research Institute

Hamilton Health Sciences and McMaster University
Division of Nephrology
St. Joseph's Hospital
Hamilton, Ontario, Canada

Stephen D. Walter, PhD, FRSC
Department of Clinical Epidemiology &
  Biostatistics
McMaster University
Hamilton, Ontario, Canada

Mark C. Wilson, MD, MPH
Department of Internal Medicine
Graduate Medical Education
Carver College of Medicine
University of Iowa Hospitals and Clinics
Iowa City, Iowa, USA

Juan Wisnivesky, MD PhD
Mount Sinai School of Medicine
New York, New York, USA

Peter Wyer, MD
Columbia University Medical Center
New York, New York, USA

John J. You, MD, MSc
Departments of Medicine and Clinical
  Epidemiology & Biostatistics
McMaster University
Hamilton, Ontario, Canada

Yuqing Zhang, MD, MSc
Department of Clinical Epidemiology &
  Biostatistics
McMaster University
Hamilton, Ontario, Canada

FOREWORD

When I was attending school in wartime Britain, staples of the curriculum, along with cold baths, mathematics, boiled cabbage, and long cross-country runs, were Latin and French. It was obvious that Latin was a theoretical exercise—the Romans were dead, after all. However, although France was clearly visible just across the Channel, for years it was either occupied or inaccessible, so learning the French language seemed just as impractical and theoretical an exercise. It was unthinkable to me and my teachers that I would ever put it to practical use—that French was a language to be spoken.

This is the relationship too many practitioners have with the medical literature—clearly visible but utterly inaccessible. We recognize that practice should be based on discoveries announced in the medical journals. But we also recognize that every few years the literature doubles in size, and every year we seem to have less time to weigh it,[1] so every day the task of taming the literature becomes more hopeless. The translation of those hundreds of thousands of articles into everyday practice appears to be an obscure task left to others, and as the literature becomes more inaccessible, so does the idea that the literature has any utility for a particular patient become more fanciful.

This book, now in its third edition, is intended to change all that. It is designed to make the clinician fluent in the language of the medical literature in all its forms. To free the clinician from practicing medicine by rote, by guesswork, and by their variably integrated experience. To put a stop to clinicians being ambushed by drug company representatives, or by their patients, telling them of new therapies the clinicians are unable to evaluate. To end their dependence on out-of-date authority. To enable the practitioner to work from the patient and use the literature as a tool to solve the patient's problems. To provide the clinician access to what is relevant and the ability to assess its validity and whether it applies to a specific patient. In other words, to put the clinician in charge of the single most powerful resource in medicine.

The Users' Guides Series in *JAMA*

I have left it to Gordon Guyatt, MD, MSc, the moving force, principal editor, and most prolific coauthor of the Users' Guides to the Medical Literature series in *JAMA*, to describe the history of this series and of this book in the accompanying preface. But where did *JAMA* come into this story?

In the late 1980s, at the invitation of my friend David Sackett, MD, I visited his department at McMaster University to discuss a venture with *JAMA*—a series that examined the evidence behind the clinical history and examination. After these discussions, a series of articles and systematic reviews was developed and, with the enthusiastic support of then *JAMA* Editor in Chief George Lundberg, MD, *JAMA* began publishing the Rational Clinical Examination series in 1992.[2] By that time, I had formed an excellent working relationship with the brilliant group at McMaster. Like their leader, Sackett, they tended to be iconoclastic, expert at working together and forming alliances with new and talented workers, and intellectually exacting. Like their leader, they delivered on their promises.

So, when I heard that they were thinking of updating the wonderful little series of Readers' Guides published in 1981 in the *Canadian Medical Association Journal* (*CMAJ*), I took advantage of this working relationship to urge them to update and expand the series for *JAMA*. Together with Sackett, and first with Andy Oxman, MD, and then with Gordon Guyatt taking the lead (when Oxman left to take a position in Oslo), the Users' Guides to the Medical Literature series was born. We began publishing articles in the series in *JAMA* in 1993.[3]

At the start, we thought we might have 8 or 10 articles, but the response from readers was so enthusiastic and the variety of types of article in the literature so great that ever since I have found myself receiving, sending for review, and editing new articles for the series. Just before the first edition of this book was published in 2002, Gordon Guyatt and I closed this series at 25, appearing as 33 separate journal articles.

The passage of years during the preparation of the original *JAMA* series and the publication of the first edition of this book had a particularly useful result. Some subjects that were scarcely discussed in the major medical journals in the early 1990s but that had burgeoned years later could receive the attention that had become their due. For instance, in 2000, *JAMA* published 2 Users' Guides[4,5] on how readers should approach reports of qualitative research in health care. To take another example, systematic reviews and meta-analyses, given a huge boost by the activities of the Cochrane Collaboration, had become prominent features of the literature, and as Gordon Guyatt points out in his preface, the change in emphasis in the Users' Guides to preappraised resources continues.

The Book

From the start, readers kept urging us to put the series together as a book. That had been our intention right from the start, but each new article delayed its implementation. How fortunate! When the original Readers' Guides appeared in the *CMAJ* in 1981, Gordon Guyatt's phrase "evidence-based medicine" had never been coined, and only a tiny proportion of health care workers possessed computers. The Internet did not exist and electronic publication was only a dream. In 1992, the Web—for practical purposes—had scarcely been invented, the dot-com bubble had not appeared, let alone burst, and the health care professions were only beginning to become computer literate. But at the end of the 1990s, when Guyatt and I approached my colleagues at *JAMA* with the idea of publishing not merely the standard printed book but also Web-based and CD-ROM formats of the book, they were immediately receptive. Putting the latter part into practice has been the notable achievement of Rob Hayward, MD, of the Centre for Health Evidence of the University of Alberta.

The science and art of evidence-based medicine, which this book does so much to reinforce, has developed remarkably during the past 25 years, and this is reflected in every page of this book. Encouraged by the immediate success of the first and second editions of the *Users' Guides to the Medical Literature*, Gordon Guyatt and the Evidence-Based Medicine Working Group have once again brought each chapter up to date for this third edition. They have also added 6 completely new chapters: Evidence-Based Medicine and the Theory of Knowledge, How to Use a Noninferiority Trial, How to Use an Article About Quality Improvement, How to Use an Article About Genetic Association, Understanding and Applying the Results of a Systematic Review and Meta-analysis, and Network Meta-analysis.

An updated Web version of the *Users' Guides to the Medical Literature* will accompany the new edition. As part of the online educational resource, JAMAevidence, the *Users' Guides to the Medical Literature* online is intertwined with the online edition of *The Rational Clinical Examination: Evidence-Based Clinical Diagnosis*. Together they serve as the cornerstones of a comprehensive online educational resource for teaching and learning evidence-based medicine. Interactive calculators and worksheets provide practical complements to the content, and downloadable PowerPoint presentations serve as invaluable resources for instructors. Finally, podcast presentations bring the foremost minds behind evidence-based medicine to medical students, residents, and faculty around the world.

Once again, I thank Gordon Guyatt for being an inspired author, a master organizer, and a wonderful teacher, colleague, and friend. I know personally and greatly admire a good number of his colleagues in the Evidence-Based Medicine Working Group, but it would be invidious to name them, given the huge collective effort this has entailed. This is an enterprise that came about only because of the strenuous efforts of many individuals. On the *JAMA* side, I must thank Annette Flanagin, RN, MA, a wonderfully efficient, creative, and diplomatic colleague at *JAMA*. All of this was coordinated and kept up to schedule by the energy and meticulous efficiency of Kate Pezalla, MA. My colleague, Edward Livingston, MD, a surgeon and a perceptive critic, is taking over the *Users' Guides to the Medical Literature* series at *JAMA*, and I am confident it will prosper in his hands. In addition, I acknowledge the efforts of our partners at McGraw-Hill Education—James Shanahan, Scott Grillo, Michael Crumsho, and Robert Pancotti.

Finally, I thank my friends Cathy DeAngelis, MD, MPH, and her successor, Howard Bauchner, MD, MPH, former and current Editors in Chief of The JAMA Network, for their strong backing of me, my colleagues, and this project. Howard inherited this project. Once I found out that his immediate and enthusiastic acceptance of it was based on his regular use of early articles in the Users' Guides series, any concern about its reception vanished. Indeed, Howard was the instigator of Evidence-Based Medicine—An Oral History,[2,3] a video series of personal views on the birth and early growth of evidence-based medicine that has helped put the Users' Guides into perspective. Howard's infectious good spirits and sharp intelligence bode well for further editions of this book.

Drummond Rennie, MD

University of California, San Francisco

References

1. Durack DT. The weight of medical knowledge. *N Engl J Med*. 1978;298(14):773-775.
2. Smith R, Rennie D. Evidence-based medicine—an oral history. *JAMA*. 2014;311(4):365-367.
3. Evidence-based medicine—an oral history website. http://ebm.jamanetwork.com. Accessed August 17, 2014.

PREFACE

Evidence-based medicine (EBM)—as a concept with that particular moniker—is now almost 25 years old. Looking back, periods of infancy, childhood, adolescence,[1] and now a mature adulthood are evident.[2] This third edition of the *Users' Guides to the Medical Literature* firmly establishes the maturity of the EBM movement.

The first articulation of the world view that was to become EBM appeared in 1981 when a group of clinical epidemiologists at McMaster University, led by David Sackett, MD, published the first of a series of articles that advised clinicians on how to read clinical journals.[3] Although a huge step forward, the series had its limitations. After teaching what they then called *critical appraisal* for a number of years, the group became increasingly aware of both the necessity and the challenges of going beyond reading the literature in a browsing mode and instead using research studies to solve patient management problems on a day-to-day basis.

In 1990, I assumed the position of residency director of the Internal Medicine Program at McMaster. Through Dave Sackett's leadership, critical appraisal had evolved into a philosophy of medical practice based on knowledge and understanding of the medical literature supporting each clinical decision. We believed that this represented a fundamentally different style of practice and required a term that would capture this difference.

My mission as residency director was to train physicians who would practice this new approach to medicine. In the spring of 1990, I presented our plans for changing the program to the members of the Department of Medicine, many of whom were unsympathetic. The term suggested to describe the new approach was *scientific medicine*. Those already hostile were incensed at the implication that they had previously been "unscientific." My second try at a name for our philosophy of medical practice, *evidence-based medicine*, became extremely popular in a very short time. To use the current vernacular, it went viral.[4]

After that fateful Department of Medicine meeting at McMaster, the term *EBM* first appeared in the autumn of 1990 in an information document for residents entering, or considering application to, the residency program. The relevant passage follows:

> Residents are taught to develop an attitude of "enlightened scepticism" towards the application of diagnostic, therapeutic, and prognostic technologies in their day-to-day management of patients. This approach . . . has been called "evidence-based medicine." . . . The goal is to be aware of the evidence on which one's practice is based, the soundness of the evidence, and the strength of inference the evidence permits. The strategy employed requires a clear delineation of the relevant question(s); a thorough search of the literature relating to the questions; a critical appraisal of the evidence and its applicability to the clinical situation; a balanced application of the conclusions to the clinical problem.

The first published appearance of the term was in the American College of Physicians' *Journal Club* in 1991.[5] Meanwhile, our group of enthusiastic evidence-based medical educators at McMaster were refining our practice and teaching of EBM. Believing that we were on to something important, we linked up with a larger group of academic physicians, largely from the United States, to form the first Evidence-Based Medicine Working Group and published an article in *JAMA* that defined and expanded on the description of EBM, labeling it as a "paradigm shift."[6]

This working group then addressed the task of producing a new set of articles, the successor to the Readers' Guides, to present a more practical approach to applying the medical literature to clinical practice. With the unflagging support and wise counsel of *JAMA* Deputy Editor Drummond Rennie, MD, the Evidence-Based Medicine Working Group created a 25-part series called the Users' Guides to the Medical Literature, published in *JAMA* between 1993 and 2000.[7] The series continues to be published in *JAMA*, with articles that address new concepts and applications.

The first edition of the *Users' Guides to the Medical Literature* was a direct descendant of the *JAMA* series. By the time of the book's publication in 2002, EBM had already undergone its first fundamental evolution, the realization that evidence was never sufficient for clinical decision making. Rather, management decisions always involve trade-offs between desirable and undesirable consequences and thus require value and preference judgments. Indeed, in the first edition of the *Users' Guide to the Medical Literature*, the first principle of EBM was presented as Clinical Decision Making: Evidence Is Never Enough, joining the previously articulated principle of a hierarchy of evidence.

It did not take long for people to realize that the principles of EBM were equally applicable for other health care workers, including nurses, dentists, orthodontists, physiotherapists, occupational therapists, chiropractors, and podiatrists. Thus, terms such as *evidence-based health care* and *evidence-based practice* are appropriate to cover the full range of clinical applications of the evidence-based approach to patient care. Because our Users' Guides are directed primarily at physicians, we have continued with the term *EBM*.

The second edition incorporated 2 new EBM developments in EBM thinking. First, we had realized that only a few clinicians would become skilled at critically appraising original journal articles and that preappraised evidence would be crucial for evidence-based clinical practice. Second, our knowledge of how best to ensure that clinical decisions were consistent with patient values and preferences was rudimentary and would require extensive study.

This third edition of the *Users' Guides to the Medical Literature* builds on these realizations, most substantially in the revised guide to finding the evidence. The emphasis is now on preappraised resources and particularly on the successor to medical texts: electronic publications that produce updated evidence summaries as the data appear and provide evidence-based recommendations for practice.

Awareness of the importance of preappraised evidence and evidence-based recommendations is reflected in other changes in the third edition. We have added a fundamental principle to the hierarchy of evidence and the necessity for value and preference judgments: that optimal clinical decision making requires systematic summaries of the best available evidence.

This principle has led to a fundamental revision of the Users' Guide to systematic reviews, which now explicitly includes the meta-analyses and acknowledges 2 core considerations. The first is how well the systematic review and meta-analysis were conducted. The second, inspired by the contributions of the GRADE (Grading of Recommendations Assessment, Development and Evaluation) Working Group,[8] demands an assessment of the confidence that one can place in the estimates of effect emerging from the review and meta-analysis. However well done the review, if the primary evidence on which it is based warrants little confidence, inferences from the review will inevitably be very limited.

The third edition of the *Users' Guides to the Medical Literature* incorporates the lessons we have learned in more than 20 years of teaching the concepts of EBM to students with a wide variety of backgrounds, prior preparation, clinical interest, and geographic location. Indeed, among our many blessings is the opportunity to travel the world, helping to teach at EBM workshops. Participating in workshops in Thailand, Saudi Arabia, Egypt, Pakistan, Oman, Kuwait, Singapore, the Philippines, Japan, India, Peru, Chile, Brazil, Germany, Spain, France, Belgium, Norway, the United States, Canada, and Switzerland—the list goes on—provides us with an opportunity to try out and refine our teaching approaches with students who have a tremendous heterogeneity of backgrounds and perspectives. At each of these workshops, the local EBM teachers share their own experiences, struggles, accomplishments, and EBM teaching tips that we can add to our repertoire.

We are grateful for the extraordinary privilege of sharing, in the form of the third edition of *Users' Guides to the Medical Literature*, what we have learned.

Gordon Guyatt, MD, MSc
McMaster University

References

1. Daly J. *Evidence-based Medicine and the Search for a Science of Clinical Care.* Berkeley, CA: Milbank Memorial Fund and University of California Press; 2005.

2. Smith R, Rennie D. Evidence-based medicine—an oral history. *JAMA.* 2014;311(4):365-367.

3. Department of Clinical Epidemiology & Biostatistics, McMaster University. How to read clinical journals, I: why to read them and how to start reading them critically. *Can Med Assoc J.* 1981;124(5):555-558.

4. Evidence-based medicine—an oral history website. http://ebm.jamanetwork.com. Accessed August 17, 2014.

5. Guyatt G. Evidence-based medicine. *ACP J Club (Ann Intern Med).* 1991;114(suppl 2):A-16.

6. Evidence-Based Medicine Working Group. Evidence-based medicine: a new approach to teaching the practice of medicine. *JAMA.* 1992;268(17):2420-2425.

7. Guyatt GH, Rennie D. Users' guides to the medical literature. *JAMA.* 1993;270(17):2096-2097.

8. Guyatt GH, Oxman AD, Vist GE, et al; GRADE Working Group. GRADE: an emerging consensus on rating quality of evidence and strength of recommendations. *BMJ.* 2008;336(7650):924-926.

Users' Guides

—— to the ——

Medical
Literature

THE FOUNDATIONS

1

How to Use the Medical Literature—and This Book—to Improve Your Patient Care

Gordon Guyatt and Maureen O. Meade

IN THIS CHAPTER

The objective of this book is to help you make efficient use of the published literature in guiding your patient care. What does the published literature comprise? Our definition is broad. You may find *evidence*[a] in a wide variety of sources, including original journal articles, *reviews* and *synopses* of *primary studies*, *clinical practice guidelines*, and traditional and innovative medical textbooks. Increasingly, clinicians can most easily access many of these sources through the Internet.

THE STRUCTURE OF THE *USERS' GUIDES TO THE MEDICAL LITERATURE*: THE FOUNDATIONS

This book is not like a novel that you read from beginning to end. Indeed, the *Users' Guides* are designed so that each part is largely self-contained. Thus, we anticipate that clinicians may be selective in their reading of the core content chapters and will certainly be selective when they move beyond the essentials. On the first reading, you may choose only a few advanced areas that interest you. If, as you use the medical literature, you find the need to expand your understanding of, for instance, studies addressing *screening* tests or the use of *surrogate outcomes*, you can consult the relevant chapters to familiarize or reacquaint yourself with the issues. You may also find the glossary a useful reminder of the formal definitions of terms used herein. Finally, we rely heavily on

examples to make our points. You will find examples identified by their blue background.

The book comprises 7 sections: The Foundations, Therapy, Harm, Diagnosis, Prognosis, Summarizing the Evidence, and Moving From Evidence to Action (Box 1-1).

The first section of this book introduces the foundations of *evidence-based practice*. Two chapters in this section, What Is Evidence-Based Medicine? and Evidence-Based Medicine and the Theory of Knowledge, present the 3 guiding principles of *evidence-based medicine* (EBM) and place EBM in the context of a humanistic approach to medical practice. The subsequent chapters in this section deal with defining your clinical question, locating the best evidence to address that question, and distinguishing *bias* from *random error* (a key principle of critical appraisal).

Clinicians are primarily interested in making accurate diagnoses and selecting optimal treatments for their patients. They also must avoid exposing patients to *harm* and offer patients prognostic information. Thus, chapters in 4 sections of this book (Therapy, Harm, Diagnosis, and Prognosis) begin by outlining what every medical student, intern and resident, and practicing physician and other clinicians will need to know to use articles that present primary data that address these 4 principal issues in providing patient care.

Increasingly, we have become aware that individual studies are often unrepresentative of all relevant studies (ie, showing larger or smaller *treatment effects* than *pooled estimates* of all relevant studies), imprecise, or limited in their applicability—so much so that, since the previous edition of this book, we have added the need for systematic summaries of all relevant studies as a core principle of EBM. This has major implications for clinicians looking to use the literature to provide optimal patient care. Efficient and optimally effective evidence-based practice dictates bypassing the critical assessment of primary studies and, if they are available, moving straight to the evaluation of rigorous *systematic reviews*. Even more efficient than using a systematic review is moving directly to an evidence-based recommendation. Ideally, management recommendations—summarized in clinical practice guidelines or *decision analyses*—will incorporate the best evidence and make explicit the value judgments

---

BOX 1-1
Sections of This Book
The Foundations
Therapy
Harm
Diagnosis
Prognosis
Summarizing the Evidence
Moving From Evidence to Action

---

[a]The italicization, here and in every other chapter, represents the first occurrence in the chapter of a word defined in the glossary.

used in moving from evidence to recommendations for action. Unfortunately, many clinical practice guidelines sometimes provide recommendations that are inconsistent with the best evidence or with typical patient *values and preferences*. The last 2 sections of the book, Summarizing the Evidence and Moving From Evidence to Action, provide clinicians with guides for using systematic reviews (with and without *meta-analyses*) and recommendations to optimize their patient care.

Our approach to addressing diagnosis, therapy, harm, and *prognosis* begins when the clinician faces a clinical question (Figure 1-1). Having identified the problem, the clinician then formulates a structured clinical question (the "Ask," Figure 1-1) (see Chapter 4, What Is the Question?) and continues with finding the best relevant evidence (the "Acquire," Figure 1-1) (see Chapter 5, Finding Current Best Evidence).

Many chapters of this book include an example of a search for the best evidence. These searches were accurate at the time they were done, but you are unlikely to get exactly the same results if you replicate the searches now. The reasons for this include additions to the literature and occasional structural changes in databases. Thus, you should view the searches as illustrations of searching principles, rather than as currently definitive searches that address the clinical question. Having identified the best evidence, the clinician then proceeds through the next 3 steps in evaluating that evidence: appraisal, considering how to apply the results, and acting (Figure 1-1). The appraisal includes 2 questions: "How serious is the *risk of bias*?" and "What are the results?" The first question, "How serious is the risk of bias?" deals with the extent to which the results represent an unbiased estimate of the truth. In the first 2 editions of this book, we referred to risk of bias as *validity* and used the question, "Are the results valid?" We have made this change because "risk of bias" is a more explicit and transparent term. In 3 chapters (Chapter 8, How to Use a Noninferiority Trial; Chapter 12.5, Measuring Patients' Experience; and Chapter 28.2, Economic Analysis), limitations of study design related to these topics include issues beyond risk of bias. Therefore, in these 3 chapters, we continue to use the term validity and the question "Are the results valid?" to capture the risk of bias and these additional issues.

FIGURE 1-1

Using the Medical Literature to Provide Optimal Patient Care

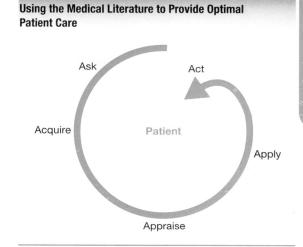

The second question in the appraisal step is, "What are the results?" For issues of therapy or harm, this will involve assessing the magnitude and precision of the impact of the intervention (a treatment or possible harmful exposure) (see Chapter 7, Therapy [Randomized Trials]; Chapter 8, How to Use a Noninferiority Trial; Chapter 9, Does Treatment Lower Risk? Understanding the Results; Chapter 10, Confidence Intervals: Was the Single Study or Meta-analysis Large Enough? and Chapter 14, Harm [Observational Studies]). For issues of diagnosis, this will involve generating *pretest probabilities* and then *posttest probabilities* on the basis of test results (see Chapter 16, The Process of Diagnosis; Chapter 17, Differential Diagnosis; and Chapter 18, Diagnostic Tests). For issues of prognosis, this will involve determining the likelihood of events occurring over time and the precision of those estimates (see Chapter 20, Prognosis).

Once we understand the results, we move to dealing with applicability (Figure 1-1) and ask ourselves the third question: "How can I apply these results to patient care?" This question has 2 parts. First, can you generalize (or, to put it another way, particularize) the results to your patient? For instance, your confidence in estimates of treatment effect decreases if your patient is too dissimilar from those who participated in the trial or trials. Second, what is the significance of the results for your patient? Have the investigators measured all *patient-important outcomes*? What is the tradeoff among the benefits, *risks*, and *burdens* of alternative management strategies?

Often, you will find a systematic review that, if it is done well and includes a meta-analysis (see Chapter 22, The Process of a Systematic Review and Meta-analysis), will have conducted the search and risk of bias appraisals and, further, summarized the results and suggested the confidence you can place in estimates (see Chapter 23, Understanding and Applying the Results of a Systematic Review and Meta-analysis). In addition, you often will find a recommendation that, if developed rigorously, is based on trustworthy systematic reviews of the evidence and explicitly considers patient values and preferences (see Chapter 26, How to Use a Patient Management Recommendation: Clinical Practice Guidelines and Decision Analyses) and provides guidance on the issue of applying the results to your patient. In our discussions of systematic reviews and guidelines, we introduce the *GRADE* (*Grading of Recommendations Assessment, Development and Evaluation*) approach to summarizing evidence and developing recommendations, an approach that we believe represents a major advance in EBM (see Chapter 23, Understanding and Applying the Results of a Systematic Review and Meta-analysis, and Chapter 28.1, Assessing the Strength of Recommendations: The GRADE Approach).

The final step in using the evidence is action (Figure 1-1). Often, this will involve shared decision making with your patients (see Chapter 27, Decision Making and the Patient), a key part of the EBM process.

We have kept the initial chapters of each part of this book simple and succinct. From an instructor's point of view, these core chapters constitute a curriculum for a short course in using the literature for medical students, resident physicians, or students of other health professions. They also are appropriate for a continuing education program for practicing physicians and other clinicians.

ADVANCED TOPICS

Moving beyond the foundations, the advanced topics in this book will interest clinicians who want to practice EBM at a more sophisticated level. They are organized according to the core issues addressed in the sections on Therapy, Harm, Diagnosis, and Prognosis. If you would like to gain a deeper understanding of a topic raised in a core chapter, an alert will often direct you to another relevant chapter. For instance, a comment regarding surrogate outcomes in the Therapy section, *spectrum bias* in the Diagnosis chapter, or *fixed-effects* and *random-effects models* in the second of the systematic review chapters may lead you to read the relevant advanced topic chapter (Chapter 13.4, Surrogate Outcomes; Chapter 19.1, Spectrum Bias; and Chapter 25.1, Fixed-Effects and Random-Effects Models, respectively).

The presentations of advanced topics will deepen your understanding of study methods, statistical issues, and use of the numbers that emerge from medical research. We wrote the advanced chapters mindful of an additional audience: those who teach evidence-based practice. Many advanced entries read like guidelines for an interactive discussion with a group of learners in a tutorial or on the ward. That is natural enough because the material was generated in such small-group settings. Indeed, the Evidence-Based Medicine Working Group has produced materials that specifically discuss the challenges that arise when these concepts are presented in small-group settings, including a series of 5 articles published in the *Canadian Medical Association Journal*[1] and another 5 articles in the *Journal of General Internal Medicine.*[2]

Experience on the wards and in outpatient clinics, and with the first 2 editions of the *Users' Guides to the Medical Literature*, has taught us that this approach is well suited to the needs of any clinician who is eager to achieve an evidence-based practice.

References

1. Wyer PC, Keitz S, Hatala R, et al. Tips for learning and teaching evidence-based medicine: introduction to the series. *CMAJ.* 2004;171(4):347-348.

2. Kennedy CC, Jaeschke R, Keitz S, et al. Evidence-Based Medicine Teaching Tips Working Group. Tips for teachers of evidence-based medicine: adjusting for prognostic imbalances (confounding variables) in studies on therapy or harm. *J Gen Intern Med.* 2008;23(3):337-343.

2

What Is Evidence-Based Medicine?

Gordon Guyatt, Roman Jaeschke, Mark C. Wilson,
Victor M. Montori, and W. Scott Richardson

IN THIS CHAPTER

Evidence-based medicine (EBM) involves conscientiously working with patients to help them resolve (sometimes) or cope with (often) problems related to their physical, mental, and social health. The EBM approach necessitates awareness and understanding of clinical research *evidence*. For those involved in making health care decisions, EBM encompasses creating implementation strategies to ensure practice evidence that is well grounded in best evidence research summaries.

At the core of EBM is a care and respect for patients who will suffer if clinicians fall prey to muddled clinical reasoning and to neglect or misunderstanding of research findings. Practitioners of EBM strive for a clear and comprehensive understanding of the evidence underlying their clinical care and work with each patient to ensure that chosen courses of action are in that patient's best interest. Practicing EBM requires clinicians to understand how uncertainty about clinical research evidence intersects with an individual patient's predicament and preferences. In this chapter, we outline how EBM proposes to achieve these goals and, in so doing, define the nature of EBM.

THREE FUNDAMENTAL PRINCIPLES OF EBM

Conceptually, EBM involves 3 fundamental principles. First, optimal clinical decision making requires awareness of the best available evidence, which ideally will come from systematic summaries of that evidence. Second, EBM provides guidance to decide whether evidence is more or less trustworthy—that is, how confident can we be of the properties of diagnostic tests, of our patients' *prognosis*, or of the impact of our therapeutic options? Third, evidence alone is never sufficient to make a clinical decision. Decision makers must always trade off the benefits and *risks, burden,* and costs associated with alternative management strategies and, in doing so, consider their patients' unique predicament and *values and preferences.*[1]

Best Evidence Summaries

In 1992, Antman et al[2] published an article that compared the recommendations of experts for management of patients with myocardial infarction

to the evidence that was available at the time the recommendations were made. Figures 2-1 and 2-2 summarize their results in *forest plots*. Both are cumulative *meta-analyses*: the first of thrombolytic therapy for myocardial infarction and the second for lidocaine antiarrhythmic therapy. In both cases, the line in the center represents an *odds ratio* of 1.0 (treatment is neither beneficial or harmful). As in any forest plot, the dots represent the best estimates of *treatment effect* (often from individual studies; in this case from the totality of accumulated evidence), and the associated lines represent the 95% *confidence intervals* (CIs).

The "Patients" column presents the total number of patients enrolled in all *randomized clinical trials* (RCTs) conducted to the date specified in the "Year" column—the reason we call it a cumulative meta-analysis. In both figures, early on, with relatively few patients, the CIs are wide, but they progressively narrow as new trials were reported.

For the thrombolytic example, by 10 trials and approximately 2500 patients, it appears that thrombolytic therapy reduces mortality, but the CIs are still wide enough to permit residual uncertainty. By 30 trials and more than 6000 patients, the reduction in odds of death of approximately 25% seems secure.

Despite this apparently definitive result, additional trials that enrolled 40 000 patients—half of whom did not receive the benefits of life-prolonging thrombolytic therapy—were conducted. Why was this necessary?

The right side of each figure, which presents the guidance expressed in then-current reviews and textbooks as the data were accumulating, provides the answer to this question. Until approximately a decade after the answer was in, there was considerable disagreement among experts, with many recommending against, or not mentioning, thrombolytic therapy. To the detriment of patients who did not receive thrombolytic therapy during this period, it took a decade for the experts to catch up with the evidence.

Figure 2-2 tells a perhaps even more disturbing story. This cumulative meta-analysis reveals that there was never any RCT evidence that suggested a lower mortality with prophylactic lidocaine after myocardial infarction—indeed, *point estimates* suggested an increase in death rate. Nevertheless, although we

FIGURE 2-1

Thrombolytic Therapy in Acute Myocardial Infarction

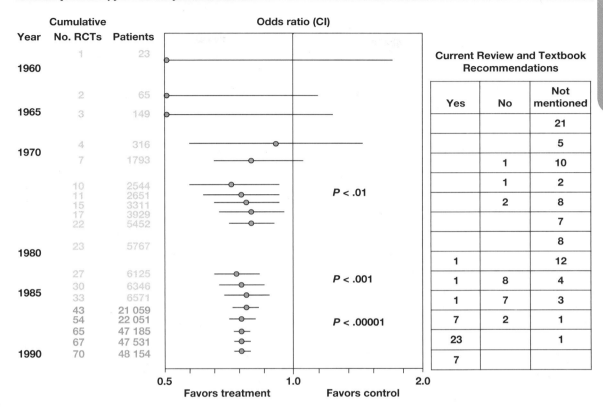

Abbreviation: CI, confidence interval; RCTs, randomized clinical trials.

This is a cumulative meta-analysis of thrombolytic therapy for myocardial infarction. The line down the center, the odds ratio, equals 1.0. The dots represent best estimates, and the lines around the dots are 95% CIs. The numbers on the left side of the figure are trials and patient totals across trials.

Early on, the CIs are very wide. By 10 trials, it appears therapy reduces mortality, but the effect is still uncertain. By 30 trials, the effect seems secure. However, 40 000 more patients were enrolled after the answer was in. Why?

The right side of the figure displays current reviews and textbook recommendations as data accumulated. Recommendations are in favor ("Yes"), against ("No"), or "Not mentioned." Two key points: (1) at the same time, experts disagreed, and (2) it took 10 years for experts to catch up with evidence.

Adapted from Antman et al.[2]

once again see widespread disagreement among the experts, most texts and reviews were recommending prophylactic lidocaine during the 2 decades during which the RCT evidence was accumulating.

Why the expert disagreement, the lag behind the evidence, and the recommendations inconsistent with the evidence? These stories come from the era before *systematic reviews* and meta-analyses were emerging in the late 1980s. If the evidence summaries presented in the forest plots had been available to the experts, they would have grasped the benefits of thrombolytic therapy far earlier than they did and abandoned prophylactic lidocaine far earlier. Indeed, following EBM principles that limit reliance on biologic rationale and place far more emphasis on empirical evidence (see Chapter 3, Evidence-Based Medicine and the Theory of Knowledge), the experts may never have started using lidocaine.

FIGURE 2-2

Prophylactic Lidocaine in Acute Myocardial Infarction

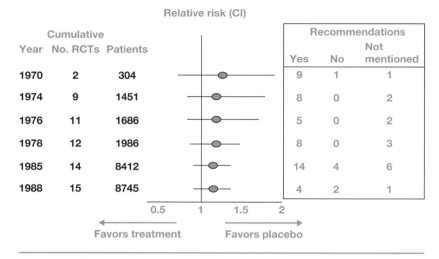

			Relative risk (CI)	Recommendations		
Year	Cumulative No. RCTs	Patients		Yes	No	Not mentioned
1970	2	304		9	1	1
1974	9	1451		8	0	2
1976	11	1686		5	0	2
1978	12	1986		8	0	3
1985	14	8412		14	4	6
1988	15	8745		4	2	1

0.5   1   1.5   2

←— Favors treatment   Favors placebo —→

Abbreviation: CI, confidence interval; RCTs, randomized clinical trials.

This slide shows a cumulative meta-analysis of the effect of prophylactic lidocaine in preventing death from myocardial infarction. In this case, there is never any evidence of benefit. Ultimately, harm is not proved, but there clearly is no benefit. Most experts, however, were recommending therapy despite RCT evidence. Also, as in Figure 2-1, there was a lot of disagreement among experts.

Adapted from Antman et al.[2]

Rational clinical decisions require systematic summaries of the best available evidence. Without such summaries, clinicians—expert or otherwise—will be unduly influenced by their own preconceptions and by unrepresentative and often lower-quality evidence. This, the first principle of EBM, immediately raises another question: "How does one recognize the best evidence?"

Guides to Confidence in Estimates

Summaries of the best evidence for diagnosis, prognosis, or treatment present evidence, respectively, for how to interpret test results, predict patients' likely fate, or understand the impact of alternative management strategies. Sometimes, such evidence is trustworthy—we have high confidence in estimates of test properties, patients' prognosis, or treatment effects. At other times, limitations in evidence leave us uncertain. Evidence-based medicine provides guidance to distinguish between these situations and the range of confidence between them.

Historically, EBM answered the question, "What is the best evidence?" with *hierarchies of evidence*, the most prominent of which was the hierarchy related to evidence that supported therapeutic interventions (Figure 2-3). Issues of diagnosis or prognosis require different hierarchies. For studies of the accuracy of diagnostic tests, the top of the hierarchy includes studies that enrolled patients about whom clinicians had diagnostic uncertainty and that undertook a *blind* comparison between the candidate test and a *criterion standard* (see Chapter 18, Diagnostic Tests, and Chapter 20, Prognosis). For prognosis, prospective *observational studies* accurately documenting *exposures* and outcomes and following up all patients during relevant periods would sit atop the hierarchy.

Returning to the hierarchy of therapy, noting the limitations of human intuition,[3] EBM places the unsystematic observations of individual clinicians lowest on the hierarchy. Noting that predictions based on physiologic experiments are often right but sometimes disastrously wrong, EBM places such experiments at the next step up in the hierarchy. Observational studies that measure the apparent impact on *patient-important outcomes* and RCTs constitute the next 2 steps up the hierarchy of evidence.

All of the sources of evidence mentioned thus far involve generalizations from groups of patients to an individual, and all are limited in this regard. The same strategies that minimize *bias* in conventional therapeutic trials that involve multiple patients, however, can guard against misleading results in studies that involve single patients.[4] In the *n-of-1 RCT*, a patient and clinician are blind to whether that patient is receiving active or *placebo* medication. The patient makes quantitative ratings of troublesome symptoms during each period, and the n-of-1 RCT continues until both the patient and the clinician conclude that the patient is or is not obtaining benefit from the target intervention. An n-of-1 RCT can provide definitive evidence of treatment effectiveness in individual patients[5,6] and is thus at the top of the evidence hierarchy. Unfortunately, n-of-1 RCTs are restricted to chronic conditions with treatments that act and cease acting quickly and are subject to considerable logistic challenges. We therefore must usually rely on studies of other patients to make inferences regarding our patient.

This hierarchy is far from absolute, and a more sophisticated framework has emerged for judging confidence in estimates of effect. Table 2-1 summarizes that framework, formulated by the *GRADE* (*Grading of Recommendations Assessment, Development and Evaluation*) Working Group, originally to provide an approach to the development of *clinical practice guidelines*.[7,8] The GRADE approach involves rating our confidence in estimates of the effects of health care interventions (also referred to as quality of evidence) as high, moderate, low, or very low. Consistent with the previous hierarchy approach, in the GRADE guidance, RCTs begin as high confidence and observational studies begin as low confidence. We lose confidence in a body of RCT evidence, however, if studies have major problems in design and execution (*risk of bias*); results are *imprecise*, *inconsistent*, or *indirect* (eg, the population of interest differs from the population studied—see Chapter 13.4, Surrogate Outcomes); or we have a high suspicion of *publication bias* (see Chapter 23, Understanding and Applying the Results of a

FIGURE 2-3

Hierarchy of Evidence

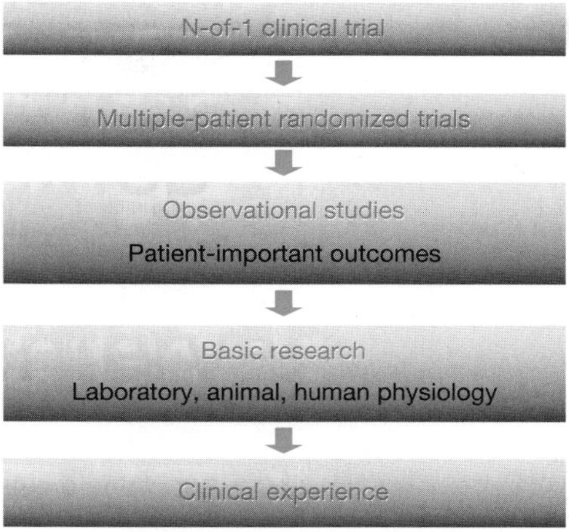

Because we would like to optimally individualize patient care, n-of-1 randomized clinical trials are at the top of the hierarchy of study designs, followed by conventional randomized trials. Next in the hierarchy are observational studies; we should try to find studies that focus on outcomes important to the patient. Next, if there are no clinical studies available, we may look at basic scientific research, although caution must be used in extrapolating the results to the clinical setting. Clinical experience is at the bottom of the hierarchy, either your own or that of colleagues or experts.

Systematic Review and Meta-analysis). When a body of RCT evidence suffers from a number of these limitations, the confidence in estimates may be low or even very low.

Similarly, if treatment effects are sufficiently large and consistent, the GRADE approach allows for moderate or even high confidence ratings from carefully conducted observational studies. For example, observational studies have allowed extremely strong inferences about the efficacy of insulin in diabetic ketoacidosis or that of hip replacement in patients with debilitating hip osteoarthritis.

The EBM approach implies a clear course of action for clinicians addressing patient problems. They should seek the highest-quality evidence available to guide their clinical decisions. This approach makes it clear that any claim that there is no evidence for the effect of a particular treatment is a non sequitur. The available evidence may warrant very low confidence—it may be the unsystematic observation of a single clinician or physiologic studies that point

Study Design	Confidence in Estimates	Lower If ...[a]	Higher If ...[a]
Randomized trial	High	Risk of bias −1 Serious −2 Very serious	
	Moderate	Inconsistency −1 Serious −2 Very serious	Large effect +1 Large +2 Very large
	Low	Indirectness −1 Serious −2 Very serious	
Observational study		Imprecision −1 Serious −2 Very serious	Dose response +1 Evidence of a gradient
	Very low	Publication bias −1 Likely −2 Very likely	

[a]Minus and plus signs refer, respectively, to rating down and rating up confidence in estimates. The 1 refers to rating down or up by 1 level (eg, from high to moderate or moderate to high), and the 2 refers to rating down or up by 2 levels (eg, high to low or low to high).

to mechanisms of action that are only indirectly related—but there is always evidence.

Evidence Is Never Enough to Drive Clinical Decision Making

First, picture a woman with chronic pain from terminal cancer. She has come to terms with her condition, resolved her affairs, said her good-byes, and wishes to receive only palliative care. She develops severe pneumococcal pneumonia. Evidence that antibiotic therapy reduces morbidity and mortality from pneumococcal pneumonia warrants high confidence. This evidence does not, however, dictate that this patient should receive antibiotics. Her values—emerging from her comorbidities, social setting, and beliefs—are such that she would prefer to forgo treatment.

Now picture a second patient, an 85-year-old man with severe dementia who is mute and incontinent, is without family or friends, and spends his days in apparent discomfort. This man develops pneumococcal pneumonia. Although many clinicians would argue that those responsible for his decision making should elect not to administer antibiotic therapy, others would suggest that they should. Again, evidence of treatment effectiveness does not automatically imply that treatment should be administered.

Finally, picture a third patient, a healthy 30-year-old mother of 2 children who develops pneumococcal pneumonia. No clinician would doubt the wisdom of administering antibiotic therapy to this patient. This does not mean, however, that an underlying value judgment has been unnecessary. Rather, our values are sufficiently concordant, and the benefits so overwhelm the risk of treatment that the underlying value judgment is unapparent.

By values and preferences, we mean the collection of goals, expectations, predispositions, and beliefs that individuals have for certain decisions and their potential outcomes. The explicit enumeration and balancing of benefits and risks that are central to EBM bring the underlying value judgments involved in making management decisions into bold relief.

Acknowledging that values play a role in every important patient care decision highlights our limited understanding of how to ensure that decisions are consistent with individual and, where appropriate, societal values. As we discuss further in the final section of this chapter, developing efficient processes for helping patients and clinicians work together toward optimal decisions consistent with patient values and preferences remains a frontier for EBM.

Next, we comment on additional skills that clinicians must master for optimal patient care and the relation of those skills to EBM.

CLINICAL SKILLS, HUMANISM, AND EBM

In summarizing the skills and attributes necessary for *evidence-based practice*, Box 2-1 highlights how EBM complements traditional aspects of clinical expertise. One of us, an intensive care specialist, developed a lesion on his lip shortly before an important presentation. He was concerned and, wondering whether he should take acyclovir, proceeded to spend the next 30 minutes searching for and evaluating the highest-quality evidence. When he began to discuss his remaining uncertainty with his partner, an experienced dentist, she cut short the discussion by exclaiming, "But, my dear, that isn't herpes!"

This story illustrates the necessity of obtaining the correct diagnosis before seeking and applying research evidence regarding optimal treatment. After making the diagnosis, the clinician relies on experience and background knowledge to define the relevant management options. Having identified those options, the clinician can search for, evaluate, and apply the best evidence regarding patient management.

In applying evidence, clinicians rely on their expertise to define features that affect the applicability of the results to the individual patient. The clinician must judge the extent to which differences in treatment (for instance, local surgical expertise or the possibility of patient *nonadherence*) or patient characteristics (such as age, comorbidity, or the patient's personal circumstances) may affect estimates of benefit and risk that come from the published literature.

BOX 2-1

Knowledge and Skills Necessary for Optimal Evidence-Based Practice

- Diagnostic expertise
- In-depth background knowledge
- Effective searching skills
- Effective critical appraisal skills
- Ability to define and understand benefits and risks of alternatives
- In-depth physiologic understanding that allows application of evidence to the individual
- Sensitivity and communication skills required for full understanding of patient context
- Ability to elicit and understand patient values and preferences and work with patients in shared decision making

---

We note that some of these skills—the sensitivity to the patient's unique predicament and the communication skills necessary for shared decision making—are often not typically associated with EBM. We believe they are, in fact, at the core of EBM. Understanding the patient's personal circumstances is of particular importance and requires advanced clinical skills, including listening skills and compassion. For some patients, incorporation of patient values for major decisions will mean a full enumeration of the possible benefits, risks, and inconveniences associated with alternative management strategies. For some patients and problems, this discussion should involve the patient's family. For other problems—the discussion of *screening* with prostate-specific antigen with older male patients, for instance—attempts to involve family members might violate cultural norms.

Some patients are uncomfortable with an explicit discussion of benefits and risk and object to clinicians placing what they perceive as excessive responsibility for decision making on their shoulders. In such cases, it is the physician's responsibility to develop insight to ensure that choices will be consistent with the patient's values and preferences while remaining sensitive to the patient's preferred role in decision making.

ADDITIONAL CHALLENGES FOR EBM

Busy clinicians—particularly those early in their development of the skills needed for evidence-based practice—will find that they often perceive time limitations as the biggest challenge to evidence-based practice. This perception may arise from having inadequate access to various evidence-based resources. Fortunately, a tremendous array of sophisticated evidence-based information is now available for clinicians working in high-income countries, and the pace of innovation remains extremely rapid (see Chapter 5, Finding Current Best Evidence).

Access to preprocessed information cannot, however, address other skills required for efficient evidence-based practice. These skills include formulating focused clinical questions, matching prioritized questions to the most appropriate resources, assessing confidence in estimates, and understanding how to apply results to clinical decision making. Although these skills take time to learn, the reward in terms of efficient and effective practice can more than compensate.

Another challenge for evidence-based practice is ensuring that management strategies are consistent with patients' values and preferences. In a time-constrained environment, how can we ensure that patients' involvement in decision making has the form and extent that they desire and that the outcome reflects their needs and desires? Evidence-based medicine leaders are now making progress in addressing these challenges.[9,10]

This book deals primarily with decision making at the level of the individual patient. Evidence-based approaches can also inform health care policy making, day-to-day decisions in public health, and systems-level decisions, such as those facing hospital managers. In each of these areas, EBM can support the appropriate goal of gaining the greatest health benefit from limited resources.

In the policy arena, dealing with differing values poses even more challenges than in the arena of individual patient care. Should we restrict ourselves to alternative resource allocation within a fixed pool of health care resources, or should we consider expanding health care services at the cost, for instance, of higher tax rates for individuals or corporations? How should we deal with the large body of observational studies that suggest that social and economic factors may have a larger influence on the health of populations than health care provision? How should we deal with the tension between what may be best for a person and what may be optimal for the society of which that person is a member? The debate about such issues is at the core of evidence-based policy making in health care; it also has implications for decision making at the individual patient level.

References

1. Napodano R. *Values in Medical Practice*. New York, NY: Humana Sciences Press; 1986.

2. Antman EM, Lau J, Kupelnick B, Mosteller F, Chalmers TC. A comparison of results of meta-analyses of randomized control trials and recommendations of clinical experts: treatments for myocardial infarction. *JAMA*. 1992;268(2):240-248.

3. Nisbett R, Ross L. *Human Inference*. Englewood Cliffs, NJ: Prentice-Hall; 1980.

4. Guyatt G, Sackett D, Taylor DW, Chong J, Roberts R, Pugsley S. Determining optimal therapy—randomized trials in individual patients. *N Engl J Med*. 1986;314(14):889-892.

5. Guyatt GH, Keller JL, Jaeschke R, Rosenbloom D, Adachi JD, Newhouse MT. The n-of-1 randomized controlled trial: clinical usefulness: our three-year experience. *Ann Intern Med*. 1990; 112(4):293-299.

6. Larson EB, Ellsworth AJ, Oas J. Randomized clinical trials in single patients during a 2-year period. *JAMA*. 1993;270(22): 2708-2712.

7. Guyatt GH, Oxman AD, Kunz R, Vist GE, Falck-Ytter Y, Schünemann HJ; GRADE Working Group. What is "quality of evidence" and why is it important to clinicians? *BMJ*. 2008; 336(7651):995-998.

8. Balshem H, Helfand M, Schünemann HJ, et al. GRADE guidelines, 3: rating the quality of evidence. *J Clin Epidemiol*. 2011;64(4):401-406.

9. Montori VM, Guyatt GH. Progress in evidence-based medicine. *JAMA*. 2008;300(15):1814-1816.

10. Stiggelbout AM, Van der Weijden T, De Wit MP, et al. Shared decision making: really putting patients at the centre of healthcare. *BMJ*. 2012;344:e256.

3

Evidence-Based Medicine and the Theory of Knowledge

Benjamin Djulbegovic and Gordon Guyatt

IN THIS CHAPTER

Approaches to scientific inquiry—including *evidence-based medicine* (EBM)—depend on how one views the nature of knowledge as evidence, how it should be acquired, and how it should be applied (epistemology). The goal of this chapter is to make the EBM perspective on this issue—seldom clearly articulated—clearer. In this discussion, we highlight the 3 key principles of EBM (see Chapter 2, What Is Evidence-Based Medicine?).

WHAT IS EVIDENCE?

Philosophers do not agree about the definition of evidence.[1] The concept is further complicated by language: different languages translate "evidence" in different ways. Some consider it synonymous with "proof," "fact," or "knowledge."

Many philosophers define evidence as "grounds for belief."[1] In this view, evidence provides support for a contention or belief.[1,2] Thus, evidence, which can constitute measurements of observable events or reports of sensory states (eg, pain, fatigue, and nausea), serves to enhance (or diminish) our confidence in some particular claim.[1,2] In this view, evidence is not tied to any specific theory of knowledge.[3] Rather, evidence represents the necessary basis for effective problem solving and decision making.

BOX 3-1

Epistemologic Principles of Evidence-Based Medicine

1. The pursuit of truth is best accomplished by examining the totality of evidence, rather than by selecting a limited sample of evidence, which is at risk of being unrepresentative and will certainly be less precise than the totality.

2. Not all evidence is equal, and a set of principles can identify more vs less trustworthy evidence.

3. Evidence is necessary but not sufficient. Clinical decision making requires the application of values and preferences.

Evidence-based medicine suggests a broad definition of evidence: any empirical observation or report of a symptom or mental state constitutes potential evidence, whether systematically collected or not. Thus, the unsystematic observations of individual clinicians constitute a source of evidence, a patient's report of feeling tiredness or pain would represent a second source of evidence, physiologic experiments constitute another source, and clinical trial results constitute a fourth.

CLAIMS SHOULD CONSIDER ALL OF THE MOST CREDIBLE EVIDENCE

Most philosophers contend that the concept of evidence is inseparable from the concept of justification (ie, what is justified or reasonable to believe depends entirely on the trustworthiness of one's evidence). This view is known as *evidentialism*.[4] Frequently, however, evidence is inconsistent (ie, points to different conclusions). Under these circumstances, people tend to select evidence that favors their particular views, which often vary, sometimes markedly.

Evidence-based medicine, while acknowledging that interpretation of evidence is inevitably subjective, is consistent with philosophical views that endorse a central role of evidence as the basis of generating agreement among rational observers.[1,2] Philosophers also have found that the pursuit of truth is best accomplished by examining the totality of evidence[5] rather than selecting evidence that favors a particular view.[6] This position is a core principle of EBM, denoted herein as the first principle of EBM (Box 3-1).[2] In practice, this means that our inferences (and decisions) are best informed by systematic reviews (ie, syntheses of the totality of relevant high-quality evidence) of the effects of health care interventions as epitomized by the work of the Cochrane Collaboration.[7]

Evidence-based medicine espouses the view that the extent to which we believe in a proposition should be directly related to the confidence we can place in the relevant evidence.[2] Evidence is more believable if it is generated by rigorous scientific studies. Thus, we should hold only those beliefs based on evidence obtained by credible processes,[8] a view known as reliabilism.[8]

This begs the question of how we recognize rigorous studies (ie, what determines the confidence we can place in the evidence). Evidence-based medicine has a detailed answer to this question and in supplying that answer assumes a link between evidence in which we can be confident and "truth."[2] This provides the philosophical basis for the second principle of EBM: not all evidence is equal (Box 3-1). In this book, we offer guidance for determining more vs less credible evidence (see Chapter 2, What Is Evidence-Based Medicine? and Chapter 23, Understanding and Applying the Results of a Systematic Review and Meta-analysis).

EMPIRICAL EVIDENCE VS THEORY

One of the central and recurring tensions in the theory of knowledge is whether science should permit only observations of the observable world or, in addition, place value on theoretical constructs. The prominence of EBM in contemporary clinical practice and education has been achieved by an insistence on adherence to standards of credible evidence.[2] The medical literature is replete with the disastrous consequences of acting on apparently compelling but in fact untrustworthy research findings (see Chapter 11.2, Surprising Results of Randomized Trials). The insistence in evidence-based medicine on obtaining rigorous observations in real-life clinical situations is consistent with the views of those who would ignore theory and attend solely to empirical observations.

This characterization is, however, an oversimplification. Evidence-based medicine makes use of theoretical constructs, but it demands rigorous testing of the proposed theories. That is, in EBM, the role of theory is not to describe the world but to accurately predict empirical observations.

Thus, EBM not only promotes skepticism of theoretical constructs but also encourages skepticism about the results of empirical observations with no plausible theoretical basis.[2] This book has many examples of situations in which, once robust and trustworthy evidence is available, the prevailing theory of the day is quickly discarded. For instance, compelling theory and observational studies suggested the benefits of antioxidant vitamins for

reducing the risk of both cancer and cardiovascular events—an idea appropriately discarded by most clinicians as soon as sufficiently large and rigorously conducted *randomized trials* showed no benefit. On the other hand, results from homeopathy trials are viewed with skepticism in part due to judgments regarding the implausibility of homeopathic theory, illustrating that theory has a role in EBM reasoning.[2]

These brief epistemologic considerations demonstrate that EBM draws on all major traditions of philosophical theories of scientific evidence.[2] Evidence-based medicine, however, is not a scientific or philosophical theory of knowledge. Rather, EBM is designed as a structure for optimal clinical practice. This brings us to the third EBM principle: to improve the process of problem solving and decision making for individual patients and for populations, evidence is necessary but not sufficient (Box 3-1).

EVIDENCE IS NECESSARY BUT NOT SUFFICIENT FOR CLINICAL DECISION MAKING

As highlighted above, EBM has emerged as a result of our hunger for evidence or information[9] to guide problem solving and decision making. Evidence-based medicine, however, distinguishes "conclusions" from "decisions."[10] Conclusions are judged by the truthfulness under formalized inferential assumptions, whereas decisions deal with consequences of specific actions in specific circumstances. Humans process the possible consequences of actions at the level of emotions and cognitive or analytical appraisal. Modern cognitive science proposes that our decision making is governed by dual processes that consist of type 1 processes (which are intuitive, automatic, fast, narrative, experiential, and affect based) and type 2 processes (which are analytical, slow, verbal, and deliberative and support formal logical and probabilistic analyses).[11]

Our ultimate choices depend on the interaction of type 1 and type 2 decision-making processes. This is the reason that, for example, 2 patients who develop severe pneumococcal pneumonia in the setting of terminal cancer dominated by chronic pain and low quality of life may make different health care decisions. Aware that evidence leaves us confident that treatment reduces morbidity and mortality from pneumococcal pneumonia, 1 patient may choose antibiotics. The other, however, may decide to forgo treatment because she has come to terms with her terminal condition, resolved her personal affairs, and wishes to receive palliative care. Both decisions are likely to require careful reflection, including discussion with loved ones.

CONCLUSIONS

Because EBM proposes specific associations among theory, evidence, and knowledge, the theoretical basis of EBM can be understood as a system of

acquiring and evaluating evidence to gain knowledge. Evidence-based medicine, however, does not propose a theory of medical knowledge or have a rigorous epistemologic stance. With these considerations in mind, EBM can be defined from an epistemologic point of view as a set of principles and methods to ensure that population-based policies and individual decisions are consistent with all the most credible evidence while relying on both type 1 and type 2 cognitive processes to weigh the trade-offs involved in alternative courses of action.

References

1. Kelly T. Evidence. In: Zalta E, ed. *The Stanford Encyclopedia of Philosophy*. Fall 2008 ed. http://plato.stanford.edu/archives/fall2008/entries/evidence. Accessed June 26, 2014.

2. Djulbegovic B, Guyatt GH, Ashcroft RE. Epistemologic inquiries in evidence-based medicine. *Cancer Control*. 2009;16(2): 158-168.

3. Dougherty T. Introduction. In: Dougherty T, ed. *Evidentialism and Its Discontents*. Oxford, UK: Oxford University Press; 2011:1-14.

4. Feldman R, Conee E. Evidentialism. *Philos Stud*. 1985;48:15-34.

5. Good IJ. On the principle of total evidence. *Br J Philos Sci*. 1967;17(4):319-321.

6. Wittgenstein L. *Tractatus Logico-Philosophicus*. London, England: Routledge Classic; 1922. (Reprinted in 1974.)

7. The Cochrane Collaboration. http://www.cochrane.org. Accessed June 26, 2014.

8. Goldman AI. Toward a synthesis of reliabilism and evidentialism? or: evidentialism's troubles, reliabialism's rescue package. In: Dougherty T, ed. *Evidentialism and Its Discontents*. Oxford, UK: Oxford University Press; 2011:254-280.

9. Pirolli P, Card S. Information foraging. *Psychol Rev*. 1999; 106(4):643-675.

10. Tukey J. Conclusions vs decisions. *Technometrics*. 1960; 2(4):423-433.

11. Stanovich KE. *Rationality and the Reflective Mind*. Oxford, UK: Oxford University Press; 2011.

4

What Is the Question?

Gordon Guyatt, Maureen O. Meade, Thomas Agoritsas,
W. Scott Richardson, and Roman Jaeschke

IN THIS CHAPTER

THREE WAYS TO USE THE MEDICAL LITERATURE

Consider a medical student, early in her training, seeing a patient with newly diagnosed type 2 diabetes mellitus. She will ask questions such as the following: "What is type 2 diabetes mellitus?" "Why does this patient have polyuria?" "Why does this patient have numbness and pain in his legs?" "What treatment options are available?" These questions address normal human physiology and the pathophysiology associated with a medical condition.

Traditional medical textbooks, whether in print or online, that describe underlying pathophysiology or epidemiology of a disorder provide an excellent resource for addressing these *background questions*. In contrast, the sorts of *foreground questions* that experienced clinicians usually ask require different resources. Formulating a question is a critical and generally unappreciated skill for *evidence-based practice*. The following ways to use the medical literature provide opportunities to practice that skill.

Staying Alert to Important New Evidence

A general internist is checking e-mails on a smartphone while riding public transit to work. While screening a weekly e-mail alert from EvidenceUpdates (http://plus.mcmaster.ca/EvidenceUpdates, Figure 4-1), the internist sees an article titled, Cardiovascular Effects of Intensive Lifestyle Intervention in Type 2 Diabetes,[1] recently published and rated by internist colleagues as newsworthy and highly relevant for practice.

This internist is in the process of addressing a question that clinicians at all stages of training and career development are constantly posing: "What important new evidence should I know to optimally treat patients?" Clinicians traditionally addressed this question by attending rounds and conferences and by subscribing to target medical journals in which articles relevant to their practice appear. They kept up-to-date by skimming the table of contents and reading relevant articles.

This traditional approach to what we might call the browsing mode of using the medical literature has major limitations of inefficiency and its resulting frustration. Many screened articles may prove of little relevance or newsworthiness or fail to meet the critical appraisal criteria that are presented in this book. To make matters worse, the volume of research is markedly increasing,[2] and relevant studies appear in a large variety of journals.[3] *Evidence-based medicine* offers solutions to these problems.

The most efficient strategy for ensuring you are aware of recent developments relevant to your practice is to subscribe to e-mail alerting systems, such as EvidenceUpdates, used by the internist in this example. This free service has research staff screening approximately 45 000 articles per year in more than 125 clinical journals for methodologic quality and a worldwide panel of practicing physicians rating them for clinical relevance and newsworthiness.[4] You can tailor alerting

FIGURE 4-1

Example of E-mail Alert From EvidenceUpdates

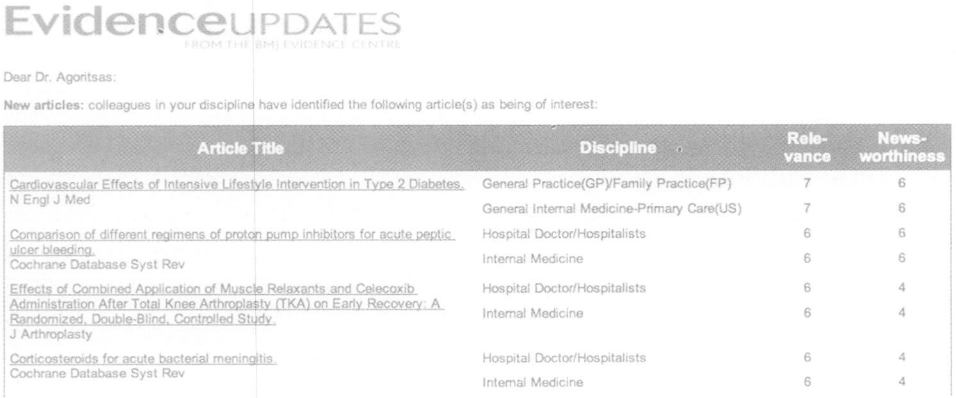

EvidenceUPDATES
FROM THE BMJ EVIDENCE CENTRE

Dear Dr. Agoritsas:

New articles: colleagues in your discipline have identified the following article(s) as being of interest:

Article Title	Discipline	Relevance	Newsworthiness
Cardiovascular Effects of Intensive Lifestyle Intervention in Type 2 Diabetes. N Engl J Med	General Practice(GP)/Family Practice(FP)	7	6
	General Internal Medicine-Primary Care(US)	7	6
Comparison of different regimens of proton pump inhibitors for acute peptic ulcer bleeding. Cochrane Database Syst Rev	Hospital Doctor/Hospitalists	6	6
	Internal Medicine	6	6
Effects of Combined Application of Muscle Relaxants and Celecoxib Administration After Total Knee Arthroplasty (TKA) on Early Recovery: A Randomized, Double-Blind, Controlled Study. J Arthroplasty	Hospital Doctor/Hospitalists	6	4
	Internal Medicine	6	4
Corticosteroids for acute bacterial meningitis. Cochrane Database Syst Rev	Hospital Doctor/Hospitalists	6	4
	Internal Medicine	6	4

systems to your information needs (clinical disciplines and frequency of alerts) and identify the 20 to 50 articles per year that will influence your practice.[5] Several other free or subscription-based alerting systems are available, both for a wide scope of disciplines (eg, NEJM Journal Watch, http://www.jwatch.org) and for specific subspecialties (eg, OrthoEvidence, http://www.myorthoevidence.com).

An alternative to alerting systems are *secondary evidence-based journals*. For example, in internal and general medicine, *ACP Journal Club* (http://acpjc.acponline.org) publishes *synopses* of articles that meet criteria of both high clinical relevance and methodologic quality. We describe such secondary journals in more detail in Chapter 5, Finding Current Best Evidence. If you prefer browsing to receiving alerts, such preappraised sources of *evidence* may increase your efficiency.

Some specialties (primary care and mental health care) and subspecialties (cardiology, oncology, and obstetrics and gynecology) already have specialty-devoted secondary journals; others do not. The New York Academy of Medicine keeps a current list of available secondary journals in many health care disciplines (http://www.nyam.org/fellows-members/ebhc/eb_publications.html). If your specialty does not yet have its own journal, you can apply your own relevance and methodologic screening criteria to articles in your target specialty or subspecialty journals. When you have learned the skills, you will be surprised at the small proportion of studies to which you need attend and the efficiency with which you can identify them.

Problem Solving

Experienced clinicians managing a patient with type 2 diabetes mellitus will ask questions such as "In patients with new-onset type 2 diabetes mellitus, which clinical features or test results predict the development of diabetic complications?" "In patients with type 2 diabetes mellitus requiring drug therapy, does starting with metformin treatment yield improved diabetes control and reduce long-term complications better than other initial treatments?" Here, clinicians are defining specific questions raised in caring for patients and then consulting the literature to resolve these questions.

Asking Background and Foreground Questions

One can think of the first set of questions, those of the medical student, as *background questions* and

FIGURE 4-2

Background and Foreground Questions

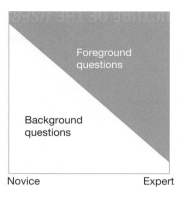

of the browsing and problem-solving sets as *foreground questions*. In most situations, you need to understand the background thoroughly before it makes sense to address foreground issues.

Experienced clinicians may occasionally require background information when a new condition or medical *syndrome* (eg, Middle East respiratory syndrome coronavirus), a new diagnostic test (eg, molecular diagnosis), or a new treatment modality (eg, dipeptidyl peptidase 4 inhibitors) appears in their clinical arena.

Figure 4-2 represents the evolution of the questions we ask as we progress from being novices posing background questions to experts posing foreground questions. This book explores how clinicians can use the medical literature to solve their foreground questions.

CLARIFYING YOUR QUESTION

The Structure: Patients, Exposures, Outcome

Clinical questions often spring to mind in a form that makes finding answers in the medical literature a challenge. Dissecting the question into its component parts to facilitate finding the best evidence is a fundamental skill. One can divide questions of therapy or *harm* into 4 parts following the *PICO* framework: patients or population, intervention(s) or exposure(s), comparator, and *outcome* (Box 4-1). For questions of prognosis, you can use 1 of 2 alternative structures. One has only 3 elements: patients, exposure (time), and outcome. An alternative focuses on patient-related factors, such as age and sex, that can modify prognosis: patients,

1. *Therapy:* determining the effect of interventions on *patient-important outcomes* (*symptoms*, function, morbidity, mortality, and costs)

2. *Harm:* ascertaining the effects of potentially harmful agents (including therapies from the first type of question) on patient-important outcomes

3. *Differential diagnosis:* in patients with a particular clinical presentation, establishing the frequency of the underlying disorders

4. *Diagnosis:* establishing the *power* of a test to differentiate between those with and without a *target condition* or disease

5. *Prognosis:* estimating a patient's future course

Finding a Suitably Designed Study for Your Question Type

You need to correctly identify the category of study because, to answer your question, you must find an appropriately designed study. If you look for a *randomized trial* to inform the properties of a diagnostic test, you will not find the answer you seek. We will now review the study designs associated with the 5 major types of questions.

To answer questions about a therapeutic issue, we seek studies in which a process analogous to flipping a coin determines participants' receipt of an *experimental treatment* or a control or standard treatment: a randomized trial (see Chapter 7, Therapy [Randomized Trials]). Once investigators allocate participants to treatment or *control groups*, they follow them forward in time to determine whether they have, for instance, a stroke or myocardial infarction—what we call the outcome of interest (Figure 4-3).

exposure (eg, older age or male), comparison (eg, younger age or female), and outcome. For diagnostic tests, the structure we suggest is patients, exposure (test), and outcome (criterion standard).[6]

Five Types of Foreground Clinical Questions

In addition to clarifying the population, intervention or exposure, and outcome, it is productive to label the nature of the question that you are asking. There are 5 fundamental types of clinical questions:

FIGURE 4-3

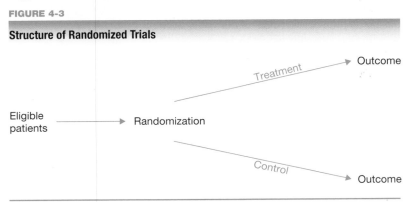

Structure of Randomized Trials

Eligible patients → Randomization

Treatment → Outcome

Control → Outcome

When randomized trials are not available, we look to *observational studies* in which—rather than randomization—clinician or patient preference, or happenstance, determines whether patients receive an intervention or alternative (see Chapter 6, Why Study Results Mislead: Bias and Random Error).

Ideally, we would also look to randomized trials to address issues of harm. For most potentially harmful exposures, however, randomly allocating patients is neither practical nor ethical. For instance, one cannot suggest to potential study participants that an investigator will decide by the flip of a coin whether or not they smoke during the next 20 years. For exposures such as smoking, the best one can do is identify observational studies (often subclassified as *cohort* or *case-control studies*) that provide less trustworthy evidence than randomized trials (see Chapter 14, Harm [Observational Studies]).

Figure 4-4 depicts a common observational study design in which patients with and without the exposures of interest are followed forward in time to determine whether they experience the outcome of interest. For smoking, an important outcome would likely be the development of cancer.

For sorting out differential diagnosis, we need a different study design (Figure 4-5). Here, investigators collect a group of patients with a similar presentation (eg, painless jaundice, syncope, or headache), conduct an extensive battery of tests, and, if necessary, follow patients forward in time. Ultimately, for each patient the investigators hope to establish the underlying cause of the symptoms and *signs* with which the patient presented.

Establishing the performance of a diagnostic test (ie, the test's properties or operating characteristics) requires a slightly different design (Figure 4-6). In diagnostic test studies, investigators identify a group of patients among whom they suspect a disease or condition of interest exists (such as tuberculosis, lung cancer, or iron-deficiency anemia), which we call the target condition. These patients undergo the new diagnostic test and a *reference standard* (also referred to as *gold standard* or *criterion standard*). Investigators evaluate the diagnostic test by comparing its classification of patients with that of the reference standard (Figure 4-6).

A final type of study examines a patient's prognosis and may identify factors that modify that prognosis. Here, investigators identify patients who

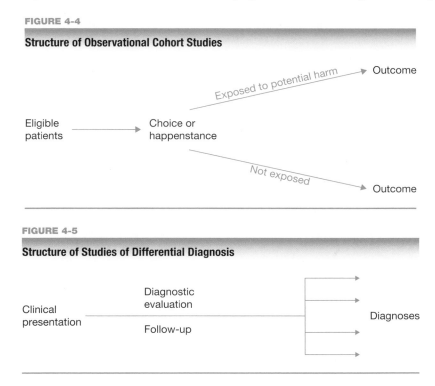

FIGURE 4-4

Structure of Observational Cohort Studies

Eligible patients → Choice or happenstance

Exposed to potential harm → Outcome

Not exposed → Outcome

FIGURE 4-5

Structure of Studies of Differential Diagnosis

Clinical presentation — Diagnostic evaluation / Follow-up → Diagnoses

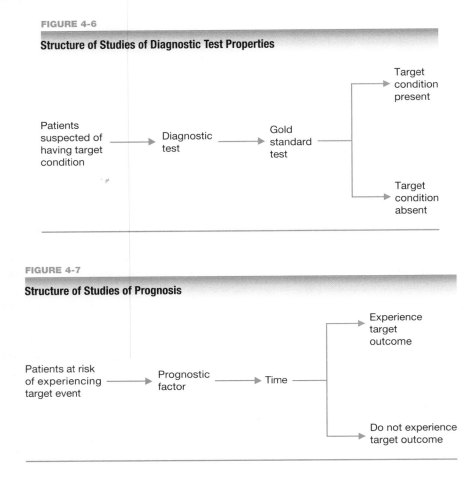

FIGURE 4-6

Structure of Studies of Diagnostic Test Properties

FIGURE 4-7

Structure of Studies of Prognosis

belong to a particular group (such as pregnant women, patients undergoing surgery, or patients with cancer) with or without factors that may modify their prognosis (such as age or *comorbidity*). The exposure here is time, and investigators follow up patients to determine whether they experience the *target outcome*, such as an adverse obstetric or neonatal event at the end of a pregnancy, a myocardial infarction after surgery, or survival in cancer (Figure 4-7).

Three Examples of Question Clarification

We will now provide examples of the transformation of unstructured clinical questions into the structured questions that facilitate the use of the medical literature.

Example 1: Diabetes and Target Blood Pressure

A 55-year-old white woman presents with type 2 diabetes mellitus and hypertension. Her glycemic control is excellent with metformin, and she has no history of complications. To manage her hypertension, she takes a small daily dose of a thiazide diuretic. During a 6-month period, her blood pressure is near 155/88 mm Hg.

Initial Question: When treating hypertension, at what target blood pressure should we aim?

Digging Deeper: One limitation of this formulation of the question is that it fails to specify the population in adequate detail. The benefits of tight control of blood pressure may differ among patients with diabetes vs those without diabetes, in type 1 vs type 2 diabetes, and among patients with and without diabetic complications.

The detail in which we specify the patient population is a double-edged sword. On the one hand, being very specific (middle-aged women with uncomplicated type 2 diabetes) will ensure that the answer we get is applicable to our patient. We may, however, fail to find any studies that restrict themselves to this population. The solution is to start with a specific patient population but be ready to remove specifications to find a relevant article. In this case, we may be ready to remove the "female," "middle-aged," "uncomplicated," and "type 2," in that order. If we suspect that the optimal target blood pressure may be similar among patients with and without diabetes, and if it proves absolutely necessary, we might remove "diabetes" from the question.

The order in which we remove the patient specifications depends on how likely it is that those characteristics will influence response to treatment. We suggest removing "female" first because we think it likely that optimal target blood pressure will be similar in men and women. Similarly, younger, middle-aged, and elderly individuals are likely to have the same optimal targets (although here we are not quite so sure). As our doubts about the same optimal targets across populations becomes progressively greater (uncomplicated vs complicated diabetes, type 1 vs type 2, or patients with diabetes vs those without), we become increasingly reluctant to remove the particular patient characteristic from the question.

We may wish to specify that we are interested in the addition of a specific antihypertensive agent. Alternatively, the intervention of interest may be any antihypertensive treatment. Furthermore, a key part of the intervention will be the target for blood pressure

control. For instance, we might be interested in knowing whether it makes any difference if our target diastolic blood pressure is less than 80 mm Hg vs less than 90 mm Hg. Another limitation of the initial question formulation is that it fails to specify the criteria (the outcomes of interest) by which we will judge the appropriate target for our hypertensive treatment.

Improved (Searchable) Question: A Question About Therapy

- *Patients:* Patients with hypertension and type 2 diabetes without diabetic complications.
- *Intervention/Exposure:* Any antihypertensive agent that aims at a target diastolic blood pressure of 90 mm Hg.
- *Comparator:* Target diastolic blood pressure of 80 mm Hg.
- *Outcomes:* Stroke, myocardial infarction, cardiovascular death, and total mortality.

Example 2: Transient Loss of Consciousness

A previously well, although a heavy drinker, 55-year-old man presents to the emergency department with an episode of transient loss of consciousness. On the evening of presentation, he had his usual 5 beers and started to climb the stairs at bedtime. The next thing he remembers is being woken by his son, who found him lying near the bottom of the stairs. The patient took about a minute to regain consciousness and remained confused for another 2 minutes. His son did not witness any shaking, and there had not been any incontinence. Physical examination findings were unremarkable; the electrocardiogram revealed a sinus rhythm with a rate of 80/min and no abnormalities. Glucose, sodium, and other laboratory results were normal, and a blood alcohol test result was negative.

Initial Question: How extensively should I investigate this patient?

Digging Deeper: The initial question gives us little idea of where to look in the literature for an answer. As it turns out, there are a host of questions that could be helpful in choosing an optimal investigational strategy. We could, for instance, pose a question of differential diagnosis: If we knew the distribution of ultimate diagnoses in such patients, we could choose to investigate the more common and omit investigations targeted at remote possibilities.

Other information that would help us would be the properties of individual diagnostic tests. If an electroencephalogram were extremely accurate for diagnosing a seizure or a 24-hour Holter monitor for diagnosing arrhythmia, we would be far more inclined to order these tests than if they missed patients with the underlying problems or falsely identified patients as not having the problems.

Alternatively, we could ask a question of prognosis. If patients had benign prognoses, we might be much less eager to investigate extensively than if patients tended to have poor outcomes. Finally, the ultimate answer to how intensively we should investigate might come from a randomized trial in which patients similar to this man were allocated to more vs less intensive investigation.

Improved (Searchable) Questions: A Question About Differential Diagnosis

- *Patients:* Middle-aged patients presenting with transient loss of consciousness.
- *Intervention/Exposure:* Thorough investigation and follow-up for common and less common diagnoses.
- *Comparator:* Minimal investigation and follow-up.
- *Outcomes:* Frequency of underlying disorders, such as vasovagal syncope, seizure, arrhythmia, and transient ischemic attack.

A Question About Diagnosis

- *Patients:* Middle-aged patients presenting with transient loss of consciousness.

- *Intervention/Exposure:* Electroencephalogram.
- *Outcomes:* Reference standard investigation (probably long-term follow-up).

A Question About Prognosis

- *Patients:* Middle-aged patients presenting with transient loss of consciousness.
- *Exposure/Comparison:* Time.
- *Outcomes:* Morbidity (complicated arrhythmias or seizures, strokes, or serious accidents) and mortality in the year after presentation.

A Question About Diagnostic Impact

You can think of this also as a question of therapy; the principles of critical appraisal are the same.

- *Patients:* Middle-aged patients presenting with loss of consciousness.
- *Intervention/Exposure:* Comprehensive investigation.
- *Comparator:* Minimal investigation.
- *Outcomes:* Morbidity and mortality in the year after presentation.

Example 3: Squamous Cell Carcinoma

A 60-year-old man with a 40-pack-year smoking history presents with hemoptysis. A chest radiograph shows a parenchymal mass with a normal mediastinum, and a fine-needle aspiration and biopsy of the mass reveals non–small cell carcinoma. Aside from hemoptysis, the patient is asymptomatic, and the physical examination results are normal.

Initial Question: What investigations should we undertake before deciding whether to offer this patient surgery?

Digging Deeper: The key defining features of this patient are his non–small cell carcinoma and the fact that his medical history, physical examination, and chest radiograph indicate no evidence of intrathoracic or extrathoracic metastatic disease. Alternative investigational strategies address 2 issues: Does the patient have occult mediastinal disease, and does he have occult extrathoracic metastatic disease? Investigational strategies for addressing the possibility of occult mediastinal disease include undertaking a mediastinoscopy or performing computed tomography (CT) of the chest and proceeding according to the results of this investigation. Investigational strategies for extrathoracic disease include brain and abdominal CT and bone scanning. Positron emission tomography–CT (PET-CT) represents an alternative approach for both intrathoracic and extrathoracic disease.

What outcomes are we trying to influence in our choice of investigational approach? We would like to prolong the patient's life, but the extent of his underlying tumor is likely to be the major determinant of survival, and our investigations cannot change that. We wish to detect occult mediastinal metastases if they are present because, if the cancer has spread, resectional surgery is unlikely to benefit the patient. Thus, in the presence of mediastinal metastatic disease, patients will usually receive palliative approaches and avoid an unnecessary thoracotomy.

We could frame our structured clinical question in 2 ways. One would be asking about the usefulness of the PET-CT scan for identifying metastatic disease. More definitive would be to ask a question of diagnostic impact, analogous to a therapy question: What investigational strategy would yield superior patient-important outcomes?

Improved (Searchable) Questions: A Question About Diagnosis

- *Patients:* Newly diagnosed non–small cell lung cancer with no evidence of extrapulmonary metastases.
- *Intervention:* PET-CT scan of the chest.
- *Outcome:* Mediastinal spread at mediastinoscopy.

A Question About Diagnostic Impact (Therapy)

- *Patients:* Newly diagnosed non–small cell lung cancer with no evidence of extrapulmonary metastases.
- *Intervention:* PET-CT.
- *Comparator:* Alternative diagnostic strategies.
- *Outcome:* Unnecessary thoracotomy.

CONCLUSION: DEFINING THE QUESTION

Constructing a searchable and answerable question that allows you to use the medical literature to solve problems is no simple matter. It requires a detailed understanding of the clinical issues involved in patient management. The 3 examples in this chapter illustrate that each patient encounter may trigger a number of clinical questions and that you must give careful thought to what you really want to know. Bearing the structure of the question in mind—patient or population, intervention or exposure, outcome, and, for therapy or harm questions, comparison—is helpful in arriving at an answerable question. Identifying the type of questions—therapy, harm, differential diagnosis, diagnosis, and prognosis—will not only ensure you choose the right question structure but also ensure that you are looking for a study with an appropriate design.

Careful definition of the question will provide another benefit: you will be less likely to be misled by a study that addresses a question related to that in which you are interested, but with 1 or more important differences. For instance, making sure that the study compares experimental treatment to current optimal care may highlight the limitations of trials that use a *placebo* comparator rather than an alternative active agent. Specifying that you are interested in patient-important outcomes (such as long bone fractures) identifies the limitations of studies that focus on *substitute* or *surrogate end points* (such as bone density). Specifying that you are primarily interested in avoiding progression to dialysis will make you appropriately wary of a *composite end point* of progression to dialysis or doubling of serum creatinine level. You will not reject such studies out of hand, but the careful definition of the question will help you to critically apply the results to your patient care.

A final crucial benefit from careful consideration of the question is that it sets the stage for efficient and effective literature searching to identify and retrieve the current best evidence (see Chapter 5, Finding Current Best Evidence). Specifying a structured question and identifying an appropriate study design to answer it will allow you to select and use searching resources efficiently and thus enhance your evidence-based practice.

References

1. Wing RR, Bolin P, Brancati FL, et al; Look AHEAD Research Group. Cardiovascular effects of intensive lifestyle intervention in type 2 diabetes. *N Engl J Med*. 2013;369(2):145-154.

2. Bastian H, Glasziou P, Chalmers I. Seventy-five trials and eleven systematic reviews a day: how will we ever keep up? *PLoS Med*. 2010;7(9):e1000326.

3. McKibbon KA, Wilczynski NL, Haynes RB. What do evidence-based secondary journals tell us about the publication of clinically important articles in primary healthcare journals? *BMC Med*. 2004;2:33.

4. Haynes RB, Cotoi C, Holland J, et al; McMaster Premium Literature Service (PLUS) Project. Second-order peer review of the medical literature for clinical practitioners. *JAMA*. 2006;295(15):1801-1808.

5. Haynes RB. ACP Journal Club: the best new evidence for patient care. *ACP J Club*. 2008;148(3):2.

6. Agoritsas T, Merglen A, Courvoisier DS, et al. Sensitivity and predictive value of 15 PubMed search strategies to answer clinical questions rated against full systematic reviews. *J Med Internet Res*. 2012;14(3):e85.

5

Finding Current Best Evidence

Thomas Agoritsas, Per Olav Vandvik, Ignacio Neumann,
Bram Rochwerg, Roman Jaeschke, Robert Hayward,
Gordon Guyatt, and K. Ann McKibbon

IN THIS CHAPTER

INTRODUCTION

Searching for Evidence: A Clinical Skill

Searching for current best evidence in the medical literature has become a central skill in clinical practice.[1,2] On average, clinicians have 5 to 8 questions about individual patients per daily shift[3-5] and regularly use online *evidence-based medicine* (EBM) resources to answer them.[6-9] Some now even consider that "the use of search engines is as essential as the stethoscope."[10]

However, because of the increasing volume of new literature and speed of new research, finding useful evidence efficiently remains challenging. Approximately 2000 new articles are indexed in PubMed every day,[10] and although few of them directly inform clinical practice, as many as 75 are *randomized clinical trials* and 11 are *systematic reviews*.[11] These numbers explain why searching in PubMed is not the most efficient way to look for evidence-based answers. For example, when typing "stroke prevention in atrial fibrillation" in PubMed, you will see that current best evidence is literally lost in an output of almost 4000 citations, with a mix of trials, reviews, guidelines, and editorials that are impossible to screen for relevance during your daily practice.

Fortunately, numerous EBM resources now provide shorter and more efficient paths. These resources select, process, and organize the evidence; some, however, are more trustworthy than others. This chapter will help you navigate through existing EBM resources, distinguish the trustworthy from the less trustworthy, and maximize your chances of quickly finding answers based on current best evidence.

Start by Clarifying the Question

As we have seen in Chapter 4, What Is the Question? framing the question appropriately is an important prerequisite to any search. An initial distinction to make is whether you are asking a *background question* (eg, definition or pathophysiology of a syndrome or mechanism of a treatment modality) or a *foreground question* (eg, targeted questions of therapy, *harm*, diagnosis, or *prognosis* that provide the evidentiary basis for decision making). Although some EBM resources also answer background questions, this chapter, and the *Users' Guides to the Medical Literature* overall, focuses on efficiently finding answers to foreground questions.

Foreground questions often arise in a form that does not facilitate finding an answer (see Chapter 4, What Is the Question?). A first step is to translate and structure the question into its components, using the *PICO* framework, which accounts for the patient or population, the intervention or exposure, the comparator, and the outcomes (see Chapter 4, Box 4-1). When framing your question, remember to consider all *patient-important outcomes*. Doing so will guide you in selecting the body of evidence that adequately addresses your patient's dilemma between benefits and harms that matter to your patient's decision.

Structuring the question will not only clarify what you are looking for but also help you formulate relevant search terms and combine them into search strategies, adapted to each type of EBM resource. We explore, toward the end of this chapter (see Translating a Question Into Search Terms), how the issues of question formulation and choice of search strategies become particularly crucial when evidence is harder to find using preappraised resources and you need to search in larger databases, such as PubMed. Finally, clarifying your question will help you search for appropriate study designs (see Chapter 4, What Is the Question?) and select corresponding search filters (eg, Clinical Queries) to reduce the number of citations in search outputs and enhance your chances of finding the best relevant evidence.

Searching the Medical Literature Is Sometimes Futile

Consider the following clinical question: "In patients with pulmonary embolism, to what extent do those with pulmonary infarction have a poorer *health outcome* than those without pulmonary infarction?"

Before beginning your search to answer this question, you should think about how investigators would differentiate between those with and without infarction. Because there is no definitive method, short of autopsy, to make this differentiation, our literature search is doomed before we begin.

This example illustrates that the medical literature will not help you when no feasible study design or measurement tools exist that investigators could use to resolve an issue. Your search also will be futile if no one has conducted and published the necessary study. Before embarking on a search, carefully consider whether the yield is likely to be worth the time expended.

HOW EVIDENCE IS PROCESSED AND ORGANIZED INTO EBM RESOURCES

Evidence-based medicine resources are rapidly evolving and provide innovative solutions to deal with the production, summary, and appraisal of the evidence.[1] Numerous EBM resources are currently available. To clearly see how to navigate across available resources, we offer 3 classification systems: (1) *hierarchy of evidence* in primary studies, (2) level of processing of the evidence, and (3) categories of EBM resources (Figure 5-1). Together, these 3 classification systems describe the flow of evidence from primary studies to existing EBM resources.

Hierarchy of Evidence

At the level of *primary studies*, our first classification relates to the hierarchy of evidence (Figure 5-1, left box). For each type of question, EBM suggests a hierarchy of research designs to minimize the *risk of bias*. For questions regarding therapy or harm, well-conducted randomized clinical trials are superior to *observational studies*, which are superior to unsystematic clinical observations. Questions of diagnostic test properties, *differential diagnosis*, or prognosis require different hierarchies of study design (see Chapter 2, What Is Evidence-Based Medicine?).

Furthermore, within each type of design, some studies provide evidence of higher quality than others. The ideal EBM resource should facilitate access to studies with the most appropriate design and lowest risk of bias.

Levels of Processing

A second classification refers to the level of processing of the evidence (Figure 5-1, middle box). Primary studies can stand alone or be processed into systematic reviews. On the basis of clear eligibility criteria, authors of a systematic review conduct a comprehensive search for all primary studies, critically appraise their quality, and, when it is considered appropriate, provide a summary estimate of effects across studies. Well-conducted systematic reviews are far more useful than single primary studies because they represent the entire body of relevant evidence (see Chapter 22, The Process of a Systematic Review and Meta-analysis). Searching for systematic reviews instead of primary studies will save you substantial time and effort.

A further level of processing is to move from evidence (ideally systematic reviews) to recommendations for practice, as in *clinical practice guidelines* (see Moving From Evidence to Action). Providing recommendations requires judging the relative desirability of alternative courses of action. Therefore, this level of processing requires looking at the entire body of evidence, integrating and

FIGURE 5-1

From Evidence to Evidence-Based Resources

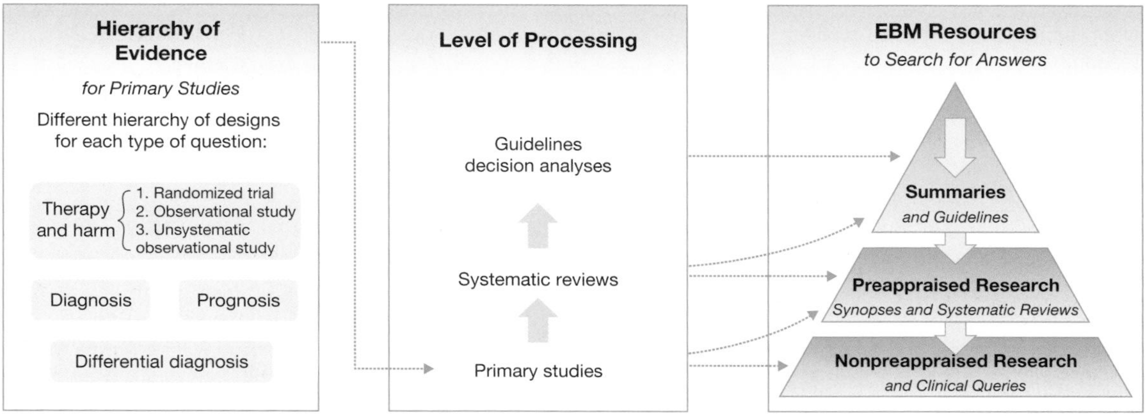

appraising the evidence from systematic reviews for each patient-important outcome, taking into account patient *values and preferences*, and being mindful of resource considerations. *Decision analyses* (see Chapter 26, How to Use a Patient Management Recommendation: Clinical Practice Guidelines and Decision Analyses) and health technology assessment reports also may provide a similar level of processing of the evidence. As for primary studies, some guidelines are more trustworthy than others, and

the ideal EBM resources should provide access to the more trustworthy ones.

Pyramid of EBM Resources

Although the 2 previous classifications—the hierarchy of evidence and level of processing—help you decide what type of evidence is likely to answer your question, they do not inform you of where to search for the evidence. For example, you may wonder where

TABLE 5-1

Categories of EBM Resources

Category	Layers[a]	Description	Examples
Summaries and guidelines	Online summary resources Databases of clinical practice guidelines	Summary of the body of evidence at a topic-level (not limited to a question, intervention, or outcome) Often with actionable recommendations for clinical decision making Regularly updated	UpToDate DynaMed Clinical Evidence Best Practice US National Guidelines Clearinghouse
Preappraised research	Synopses of systematic reviews Systematic reviews Synopses of studies	Structured abstracts or 1-page summaries of selected systematic reviews or studies Various degrees of preappraisal —Selection according to methodologic criteria —Clinicians' ratings —Clinicians' comments —Experts' structured appraisal Continuously updated Source of evidence alerts	ACP Journal Club McMaster *PLUS* DARE Cochrane Evidence Updates
Nonpreappraised research	Filtered studies	All primary studies with no preappraisal	PubMed (MEDLINE) CINAHL CENTRAL
	Unfiltered studies	Automatic filtering of databases for specific study designs or clinical content	Filters: Clinical Queries in PubMed
Federated searches	All layers of resources searched at once	Search engines that retrieve evidence from summaries and preappraised and nonpreappraised research, and organize the results accordingly	ACCESSSS Trip SumSearch Epistimonikos

Abbreviations: ACCESSSS, ACCess to Evidence-based Summaries, Synopses, Systematic Reviews and Studies; CENTRAL, Cochrane Central Register of Controlled Trials; CINAHL, Cumulative Index to Nursing and Allied Health Literature; DARE, Database of Abstracts of Reviews of Effects.

[a]These layers correspond to the 6-S pyramid from Haynes et al.[1,2]

to search for high-quality systematic reviews. Should you start your search in the Cochrane Library, use review filters in PubMed, or look in the reference list of an online summary such as UpToDate? To make that choice, you need to understand how evidence is organized into a third classification: the *pyramid of EBM resources* (Figure 5-1, right box). From a practical perspective, resources can be viewed in 3 broad categories: summaries and guidelines, preappraised research, and nonpreappraised research.

Table 5-1 outlines these categories of EBM resources. Box 5-1 and the subsequent paragraph provide a fuller description of each category with examples of resources.

BOX 5-1

Overview of EBM Resources

1. Summaries and guidelines.

Summaries are regularly updated online resources that aim to integrate the body of evidence at a topic level for several related questions. For example, a topic such as "treatment of type 2 diabetes mellitus in the elderly patient" will usually summarize evidence for drug therapy, strategies to control glycemic levels and avoid hypoglycemia, and lifestyle modification and the reduction of cardiovascular risk. These summaries often provide actionable recommendations for practice. Current examples widely used by clinicians include UpToDate (http://www.uptodate.com), DynaMed (https://dynamed.ebscohost.com), and Best Practice (http://bestpractice.bmj.com).

Guidelines follow a similar approach, usually focused on a specific topic or disease (eg, "antithrombotic therapy and prevention of thrombosis"[12]). Even more than summaries, guidelines are focused on providing recommendations for optimal patient management. Searching for available guidelines is more challenging because they are scattered across specialty journals and organization websites. A useful resource to search for guidelines is the US National Guideline Clearinghouse (http://www.guideline.gov), which includes guidelines from many countries.

2. Preappraised research.

When summaries or guidelines do not provide a satisfactory answer (eg, they provide an answer that is apparently not based on current best evidence or do not provide an answer at all), you must look directly at research findings, first from systematic reviews and then, if necessary, from primary studies. Many resources can prevent the unpleasant experience of searching the whole medical literature (at the risk of

getting lost) or having to screen and read articles as PDFs. These resources select only systematic reviews and studies that meet defined methodologic criteria and provide synopses—a 1-page structured abstract or description of reviews or studies. The degree and quality of preappraisal vary across resources. Some provide clinicians' ratings or short comments on relevance or newsworthiness, whereas others include a structured appraisal from experts. An example of the former is McMaster *PLUS* (Premium LiteratUre Service[13,14]; http://plus.mcmaster.ca/evidenceupdates), and examples of the latter are *ACP Journal Club* (http://acpjc.acponline.org) and DARE (Database of Abstracts of Reviews of Effects; www.crd.york.ac.uk/crdweb). You can access preappraised research in 2 complementary ways: by searching these specific databases for a given question and, for some of them, by subscribing to an e-mail alerting system. Personalized alerts are an efficient way to remain up-to-date on important new research in your area of interest (see, for example, BMJ EvidenceUpdates; http://plus.mcmaster.ca/evidenceupdates).

3. Nonpreappraised research.

Only when other sources have failed to provide an answer should you search for primary studies in the larger databases, such as MEDLINE (http://www.ncbi.nlm.nih.gov/pubmed) or CINAHL (http://www.cinahl.com). Because these databases include millions of articles, using them efficiently requires more advanced searching skills. Limiting your search with filters, such as Clinical Queries (http://www.ncbi.nlm.nih.gov/pubmed/clinical), provides a useful way to reduce the number of abstracts you need to review to identify the best evidence to address your clinical question.

You can navigate efficiently across these different types of resources, as well as search all 3 categories simultaneously, using *federated search engines,* such as ACCESSSS (http://plus.mcmaster.ca/accessss), Trip (http://www.tripdatabase.com), SumSearch (http://sumsearch.org), or Epistemonikos (http://www.epistemonikos.org). Before we describe these search engines in detail, we will look at general criteria that will help clinicians choose which EBM resources to select given their question and which to avoid.

To complement resources that help you answer clinical questions, additional resources can link the evidence with your daily practice, such as *clinical decision support systems*[15] or context-specific access to online resources within electronic medical records[16] (see Chapter 11.6, Clinical Decision Support Systems). However, although some clinical decision support systems have the potential to improve processes of care or patient outcomes,[17] most cover only a limited range of clinical problems, are not necessarily based on current best evidence, and are often "homebuilt" so that their use is questionable.[1]

THREE CRITERIA FOR CHOOSING AN EBM RESOURCE

All EBM resources are not equally trustworthy, and none provide answers to all questions. Efficient searching involves choosing the appropriate resources for your clinical question—in much the same way you choose diagnostic tests appropriate for your patient's symptoms. Table 5-2 offers an initial guideline for making resource choices.

Based on Current Best Evidence

Many online summaries and guideline websites promote themselves as "evidence-based," but few have explicit links to research findings. To judge the strength of the commitment to evidence to support inference, check whether you can distinguish statements that are based on high-quality vs low-quality evidence. If you cannot make this distinction, dismiss the resource altogether. Resources should provide citations to references to relevant research findings. Currency is important, and a simple way to judge whether the evidence is up-to-date is to look for the

date of the most recent reference cited: if it is more than 2 years old, it is possible that future studies lead to a different conclusion.[1,18,19] Generally, the process for keeping a resource up-to-date should be transparent and trustworthy. A date stamp should accompany each summarized topic or piece of evidence (eg, "This topic last updated: Sep 17, 2013"), along with access to the explicit mechanism used to screen for related new findings. An opaque process should raise a red flag that the evidence may be partial, biased, or already outdated.

A summary or guideline should use a rating system to assess the risk of bias of cited studies and the quality of reviews. Resources that provide recommendations should be based on the entire body of existing evidence, ideally summarized in systematic reviews, and provide the benefits and harms of available options. The resources also should use an appropriate system to grade strength of recommendations and provide explicit judgments concerning underlying values and preferences (see Moving From Evidence to Action). Finally, to be actionable, the recommendations should report numerical effect estimates for patient-important outcomes to support clinical judgment and shared decision making at the point of care. For example, the ninth edition of the Antithrombotic Therapy and Prevention of Thrombosis guideline issued a weak recommendation for aspirin for primary prevention of cardiovascular events in people older than 50 years, based on moderate confidence in estimates of effect (grade 2B).[20] The authors provide numerical estimates: for example, in people at moderate risk of cardiovascular events, prophylactic aspirin resulted in 19 fewer myocardial infarctions per 1000 (from 26 fewer to 12 fewer) but 16 more major extracranial bleeds per 1000 (from 7 more to 20 more).

Coverage and Specificity

An ideal resource will cover most of the questions relevant to your practice—and not much more. However, few, if any, resources are sufficient as such a one-stop shop for the evidence you need,[18] and resources from the 3 levels of the pyramid of EBM resources are often complementary. The higher you look in the pyramid, the more time it takes for the resource developers to process and summarize the evidence at a topic level, making these resources potentially out of date. To be

TABLE 5-2

Selection Criteria for Choosing or Evaluating EBM Resources

Criterion	Description of Criterion
On the basis of current best evidence	How strong is the commitment to evidence to support inference?
	Does it have citations to references to all evidence summaries and recommendations?
	Is the process for keeping it up-to-date transparent and trustworthy?
	Is the quality of the evidence assessed?
	Is the strength of recommendations reported?
	Are numerical effect estimates reported for patient important outcomes?
Coverage and specificity	Does the resource cover my discipline and specific area of practice adequately?
	Does it cover questions of the type I am asking (eg, therapy, diagnosis, prognosis, harm)?
Availability and access	Is it readily available in all locations in which I would use it?
	Can I easily afford it?

comprehensive in your searching, you will need to look for preappraised research for more recent evidence. Conversely, the lower you look in the pyramid, the larger, and often less specific, the resource. Thus, pre-appraised research limited to your area of practice, such as collections of synopses designed to help you keep up with information on the latest developments in a specific field or specialty—eg, *Evidence-Based Mental Health* (http://ebmh.bmj.com) or *Evidence-Based Nursing* (http://ebn.bmj.com)—may serve your needs efficiently.

The type of question also will affect your choice of a specific resource. For example, resources that focus on management issues informed mainly by randomized clinical trials, such as the Cochrane Database of Systematic Reviews, may not be ideal to answer questions of harm or rare adverse events. Similarly, background questions are more likely to be answered by summaries (eg, UpToDate or DynaMed) than preappraised research (eg, system-atic reviews or synopses). For example, if you have background questions about the Middle East respi-ratory syndrome coronavirus, both UpToDate and DynaMed have a dedicated entry on the topic that summarizes its case definition and the incidence of recent clusters.

Availability and Access

The most trustworthy and efficient resources are fre-quently expensive, particularly those at the top of the pyramid of EBM resources. For example, an individual subscription to an online summary often costs more than $250 annually. To establish your information resource regimen, you can map the EBM resources that are accessible to you through your university, school, or clinical institution and check whether they meet your information needs. Academic clinicians typically have access to the resources of their aca-demic institution or hospital libraries, including the full texts of many studies and reviews.

Clinicians in private practice in high-income countries may have access to some resources through their professional associations but otherwise may be burdened by the cost of subscriptions. Some coun-tries have national libraries that centralize access to many resources. Often, the institutional choice of resources is not made by practicing clinicians and may be guided by financial constraints. If an impor-tant resource is not available, make the case for it to your librarian (and suggest which other resources are less useful in practice).[1] If your institution is not will-ing to pay a license, consider subscribing individually.

Health professionals in lower-income countries may have institutional access to information resources through the World Health Organization's Health InterNetwork Access to Research Initiative (http://www.who.int/hinari/en) or other organizations but otherwise face even greater financial obstacles to information resources. Additional strategies include seeking open-access journals, writing to authors for a reprint or e-print of their article, and contacting colleagues in academic centers who have access to more extensive library facilities.

Preappraised resources are sometimes expensive as well, and therefore we further describe how searching federated search engines, such as ACCESSSS or Trip, can give you an overview of the clinical content of various resources to help you make subscription decisions.

Free e-mail systems, such as BMJ EvidenceUpdates (http://plus.mcmaster.ca/evidenceupdates), can alert you to important new findings, although access to full texts will vary according to your institutional or personal licenses. An increasing number of full-text articles are accessible through PubMed or Google Scholar or directly via open-access journals (eg, *CMAJ*, PLOS journals, and BioMed Central journals; see http://www.doaj.org for a directory of open-access journals). Many other journals provide free access to full-text articles 6 to 12 months after publication (eg, *BMJ*, *JAMA*, and *Mayo Clinic Proceedings*) or a portion of their content at the time of publication. However, focusing on free full-text articles and free Internet resources may give a partial and potentially biased view of current best evidence.[21]

Finally, ask your institution or professional organization how to access EBM resources at the point of care and obtain proxy server permission or remote access at home (eg, using a VPN connection). This will give you direct access to evidence on your smartphone and tablets and considerably enhance your *evidence-based practice*.

USING THE PYRAMID OF EBM RESOURCES TO ANSWER YOUR QUESTIONS

Numerous EBM resources are available, including many providers of summaries at the top level of the pyramid. Each has a different clinical scope, as well as different methodologic and editorial processes. No single portal lists them all, but many can be found through the New York Academy of Medicine (http://www.nyam.org/fellows-members/ebhc/eb_resources.html) or the Cochrane Collaboration (http://www.cochrane.org/about-us/webliography-evidence-based-health-care-resources) websites.

It is beyond the scope of this chapter to discuss the pros and cons of each resource. Instead, we will focus on how to navigate across the pyramid of EBM resources and discuss how these resources can complement each other. We provide examples of resources to illustrate important aspects both from research on evidence retrieval and from our own practice but do not aim to be comprehensive or prescriptive on which resource to use.

Summaries and Guidelines

Start your searches by using resources at the top of the pyramid for summaries and guidelines that address your question. These resources can provide a comprehensive view of the body of evidence at a topic level. Imagine, for example, that you are looking for antithrombotic therapies most appropriate for prevention of stroke in patients with atrial fibrillation. Available options include aspirin; other antiplatelet agents, such as clopidogrel; a combination of aspirin plus other antiaggregants; warfarin; or new anticoagulants, such as direct thrombin inhibitors or factor Xa inhibitors. To fully address your question from lower levels of the pyramid, you would need to retrieve, read, and integrate several systematic reviews or trials that cover all the relevant comparisons and important outcomes. Summaries and guidelines aim to integrate this body of evidence and also often provide actionable recommendations for practice.

Table 5-3 lists examples of 10 widely used online summaries and their corresponding URLs. A recent analytical survey compared them on 3 aspects: the timeliness of updates, coverage of clinical topics, and quality of processing and reporting of the evidence.[19] At the time of this assessment (2011), the mean time since update ranged from 3.5 months (DynaMed) to 29 months (First Consult), and the percentage of clinical topics covered ranged from 25% (Clinical Evidence) to 83% (UpToDate). Quality substantially varied across the resources. For example, despite its limited coverage, the authors rated Clinical

TABLE 5-3

Rank Orderings of 10 Online Summaries Compared on 3 Aspects[19]

Summary Resource	URL	Updates	Coverage, No. (%)	Quality
DynaMed	https://dynamed.ebscohost.com	1	3 (70)	2
UpToDate	http://www.uptodate.com	5	1 (83)	2
Micromedex	http://www.micromedex.com	2	8 (47)	2
Best Practice	http://bestpractice.bmj.com	3	4 (63)	7
Essential Evidence Plus	http://www.essentialevidenceplus.com	7	7 (48)	2
First Consult	http://www.firstconsult.com	9	5 (60)	2
Medscape Reference	http://reference.medscape.com	6	2 (82)	9
Clinical Evidence	http://clinicalevidence.bmj.com	8	10 (25)	1
ACP PIER	http://acpjc.acponline.org	4	9 (33)	7
PEPID	http://www.pepidonline.com	NA	6 (58)	10

Abbreviation: NA, data not available.

Reproduced with permission from the *Journal of Clinical Epidemiology*.[19]

Evidence as the highest-quality resource. Because EBM resources continuously evolve, these numbers may be outdated but illustrate that online summaries can be complementary. Summaries also differ on their methods and commitment to providing actionable recommendations (eg, UpToDate now formulates recommendations using the *GRADE* [*Grading of Recommendations Assessment, Development and Evaluation*] framework, whereas Clinical Evidence focuses more on the summary of evidence, also using GRADE) and their editorial style (eg, structured bullet points in DynaMed and Best Practice vs textbook-like structured chapters in UpToDate).

Unlike summaries, most guidelines are scattered across journals or websites from individual countries or health organizations. One of the most comprehensive portals to search for guidelines is the US National Guideline Clearinghouse (http://www.guideline.gov). It includes the full text of many US guidelines and thousands of international guidelines. Searching is easy, although initial retrievals are often relatively large. Other international guidelines can be found through the UK National Institute for Health and Care Excellence (https://www.evidence.nhs.uk) or the Guideline International Network (http://www.g-i-n.net/library/international-guidelines-library).

Perhaps even more than other types of preappraised evidence, practice guidelines are extremely variable in their trustworthiness.[22,23] When you conduct your search, look for guidelines that are transparent in how they process the evidence and formulate recommendations (see Chapter 26, How to Use a Patient Management Recommendation: Clinical Practice Guidelines and Decision Analyses). The US National Guideline Clearinghouse website also allows side-by-side comparisons of the guideline process and components for guidelines on the same topic.

Finally, the top of the EBM pyramid also includes decision analyses, which process a body of evidence in a similar way to guidelines, map out the options with outcomes and probabilities, and help you judge the benefits and harms of different treatment options for a specific patient (see Chapter 26, How to Use a Patient Management Recommendation: Clinical Practice Guidelines and Decision Analyses). These decision analyses often can be found in stand-alone studies, *economic evaluation* reports, and health technology assessment reports. An efficient way to locate decision analyses is through the Centre for Reviews and Dissemination at the UK University of York (http://www.crd.york.ac.uk/crdweb) by selecting the search filters "HTA" and "NHS EED" (for economic evaluation).

FIGURE 5-2

Example of Preappraised Research: McMaster PLUS

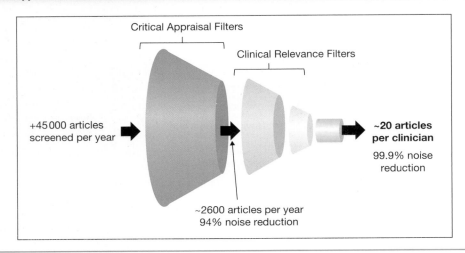

Preappraised Research

If you do not find a satisfactory answer in summaries or guidelines, either because your question is not covered or because you have reasons to doubt what you found, you may need to look for preappraised research. You also might search preappraised research to look for more recent evidence published since the summary or guideline was last updated.[24] You might wonder how often this additional searching would be worth the trouble. A recent study of the quality of online summaries found that, on average, new high-quality evidence providing potentially different conclusions than existing summaries was available for approximately 52% of the topics evaluated in UpToDate, 60% in Best Practice, and 23% in DynaMed.[18] This potential discrepancy between newly published evidence and existing recommendations would occur more frequently, and likely with greater adverse consequences, for most clinical practice guidelines, which are usually updated every 2 to 8 years.[25]

Consider, for example, the question of whether cardiac resynchronization therapy (CRT) reduces mortality in patients with heart failure and a narrow QRS complex. An initial search in mid-September 2013 in DynaMed or UpToDate provided an excellent summary of available evidence on the efficacy of CRT according to the degree of heart failure and the QRS duration but did not yet identify a more recent trial published in the *New England Journal of Medicine*.[26] This trial found that CRT did not reduce the composite rate of death or hospitalization for heart failure and actually may increase mortality. This important new evidence will of course be included in subsequent updates, but this process typically takes a couple of months to up to 29 months, depending on the online summary.[19]

A quick and efficient way to find preappraised research is to search specific databases, which include only studies and reviews that are more likely to be methodologically sound and clinically relevant. Figure 5-2 shows a typical example of this improved selection process from McMaster *PLUS* (Premium LiteratUre Service), a large database created by the McMaster Health Knowledge Refinery (http://hiru.mcmaster.ca/hiru/HIRU_McMaster_PLUS_Projects.aspx). The selection process used is as follows: trained research staff continually critically appraise more than 45 000 articles per year, from more than 125 empirically selected, high-quality clinical journals, and identify studies and systematic reviews that meet prespecified methodologic standards. For example, studies of prevention or therapy must have random allocation, a follow-up rate of at least 80%, and at least 1 patient-important outcome. These selected articles are then rated for relevance and newsworthiness by frontline clinicians from around the globe.[27] McMaster *PLUS* is thus a continuously updated database of more than 32 000 highly selective articles (with approximately 3300 added every year) that also feeds several other EBM resources and journals (eg, *ACP Journal Club*, Clinical Evidence, and DynaMed). A simple way to access McMaster *PLUS* is through the free search engine of BMJ EvidenceUpdates (http://plus. mcmaster.ca/EvidenceUpdates/QuickSearch.aspx) or through the McMaster search engine, ACCESSSS, which we discuss further below (see Searching All Levels of the Pyramid at the Same Time). McMaster *PLUS* also has distinct databases for nursing (http:// plus.mcmaster.ca/np) and rehabilitation studies (http://plus.mcmaster.ca/rehab).

In a further level of preappraisal, the more clinically relevant studies and systematic reviews are selected to become *synopses* (<1% of the initial selection). These synopses are usually a 1-page, structured summary of the research findings, along with a brief commentary from an expert in the field. You can find various types of synopses in specialized evidence-based *secondary evidence-based journals*. Figure 5-3 shows an example of a synopsis of a systematic review from *ACP Journal Club* (http://acpjc.acponline.org) on the impact of eplerenone on mortality compared with other aldosterone antagonists in heart failure. The abstract summarizes salient elements of the methods and results and an expert provides a commentary. This appraisal is not always systematic or as thorough as a full critical appraisal, but it usually provides the gist of the strengths and weaknesses of a study. Similar resources include *Evidence-Based Medicine* (http://ebm.bmj.com), *Evidence-Based Mental Health* (http://ebmh.bmj.com), *Evidence-based Oncology* (www.sciencedirect.com/science/journal/13634054), or POEMs (Patient-Oriented Evidence that Matters) (www.essentialevidenceplus.com/content/poems). The New York Academy of Medicine keeps a current

list of specialized EBM journals in many health care disciplines (www.nyam.org/fellows-members/ebhc/ eb_publications.html).

When searching preappraised research, make synopses of systematic reviews your first priority because they summarize the body of evidence on a question. In addition to evidence-based journals, you can find synopses of systematic reviews in DARE (Database of Abstracts of Reviews of Effects) (http:// www.cochrane.org/editorial-and-publishing-policy- resource/database-abstracts-reviews-effects-dare). If no synopses answer your question, move to a direct search for other systematic reviews. A useful resource is the Cochrane Library (http://www. thecochranelibrary.com).

Regardless of the resources you use, remember that preappraisal and the collection of these synopses can only increase the likelihood of finding sound evidence efficiently. It does not guarantee it. You should also apply your own critical appraisal to the research findings that are summarized, as explained throughout the *Users' Guides to the Medical Literature*.

Alerts to Important New Evidence

In addition to building continuously updated databases of preappraised research, an increasing number of resources offer e-mail *alerting services*. To make the volume of new evidence manageable, these alerts are usually tailored to your information needs when you register (eg, clinical disciplines, quality choices, and frequency of alerts).

For example, the whole process leading to McMaster *PLUS*, including clinicians' ratings for relevance and newsworthiness, results in up to a 99.9% noise (non–clinically relevant) reduction and produces a manageable stream of approximately 20 to 50 key articles per year in a clinical area that may influence your practice (Figure 5-2).[28] You can receive these alerts by subscribing to BMJ EvidenceUpdates or ACCESSSS. Several other free or fee-based alerting systems are available for both a wide scope of disciplines (eg, NEJM Journal Watch, http://www.jwatch.org) and specific subspecialties (eg, OrthoEvidence, http://www. myorthoevidence.com). When using any of these alerting resources, check whether their process of selecting and appraising the evidence is explicit, trustworthy, and meeting your needs.

FIGURE 5-3

Example of Synopsis of a Systematic Review From *ACP Journal Club*

Therapeutics

Review: Eplerenone is not more effective for reducing mortality than other aldosterone antagonists

Chatterjee S, Moeller C, Shah N, et al. Eplerenone is not superior to older and less expensive aldosterone antagonists. Am J Med. 2012; 125:817-25.

Clinical impact ratings: ⓐ ★★★★★☆☆ ⓖ ★★★★★☆☆

Question
In patients with left ventricular (LV) dysfunction, what is the relative efficacy of eplerenone and other aldosterone antagonists (AAs)?

Review scope
Included studies compared eplerenone or other AAs with control (placebo, angiotensin-converting enzyme inhibitor, angiotensin-receptor blocker, or β-blocker) in patients > 18 years of age with symptomatic or asymptomatic LV dysfunction, had ≥ 8 weeks of follow-up, and reported ≥ 1 outcome of interest. Studies comparing AAs with each other were excluded. Outcomes were all-cause mortality, cardiovascular (CV) mortality, gynecomastia {per trial definition in individual studies}*, and hyperkalemia {serum potassium > 5.5 mEq/L}*.

Review methods
MEDLINE, EMBASE/Excerpta Medica, CINAHL, and Cochrane Central Register of Controlled Trials (all to Jul 2011); reference lists; and reviews were searched for randomized controlled trials (RCTs). 16 RCTs (n = 12 505, mean age 55 to 69 y, 54% to 87% men) met selection criteria. 4 RCTs included patients after acute myocardial infarction LV dysfunction, and 12 included patients with heart failure. Study drugs were spironolactone (10 RCTs), canrenone (3 RCTs), and eplerenone (3 RCTs). Risk for bias (Cochrane criteria) was low for 8 RCTs, intermediate for 7, and high for 1.

Main results
Eplerenone and other AAs reduced all-cause mortality and CV mortality compared with no AA (Table). Eplerenone increased risk for hyperkalemia, and other AAs increased risk for gynecomastia, compared with no AA (Table). Based on an indirect comparison, other AAs reduced mortality more than eplerenone (P = 0.009).

Conclusion
Based on an indirect comparison, eplerenone is not more effective for reducing mortality in adults with left ventricular dysfunction than other aldosterone antagonists.

Information provided by author.

Source of funding: No external funding.

For correspondence: Dr. S. Chatterjee, Maimonides Medical Center, Brooklyn, NY, USA. E-mail sauravchatterjeemd@gmail.com. ■

Commentary
In their thorough review of the use of AAs in systolic heart failure, Chatterjee and colleagues conclude that data are insufficient to recommend eplerenone over spironolactone. Only 3 large outcome trials actually address the issue: RALES, assessing spironolactone (1), and EPHESUS (2) and EMPHASIS-HF (3), assessing eplerenone. Although the populations evaluated in each study were quite different, the relative reductions in mortality were similar (25%, 14%, and 19%, respectively). Indirect comparisons of drug efficacy across clinical trials with different patient populations and study protocols are challenging. Without head-to-head trials of AAs, we should not draw conclusions about their relative efficacy.

Chatterjee and colleagues confirm that spironolactone increases risk for gynecomastia. Hyperkalemia is a known adverse effect of any AA, although potassium increases were "not clinically important" in RALES (1). After RALES was published, however, there was a marked increase in the number of spironolactone prescriptions, with an increase in hyperkalemia and associated mortality (4). Gynecomastia can be distressing to male patients, but hyperkalemia may be fatal to either sex.

A strict, evidence-based practitioner would base drug and dosage selection on the clinical trial most closely matching a patient's presentation. While waiting for a definitive head-to-head trial—noting that benefits seem similar in the studied populations—I start with the less expensive spironolactone, switching to eplerenone if troublesome sexual adverse effects develop (while closely monitoring potassium!).

Ellis Lader, MD, FACC
Mid Valley Cardiology, New York University School of Medicine
Kingston, New York, USA

References
1. Pitt B, Zannad F, Remme WJ, et al. The effect of spironolactone on morbidity and mortality in patients with severe heart failure. Randomized Aldactone Evaluation Study Investigators. N Engl J Med. 1999;341:709-17.
2. Pitt B, Remme W, Zannad F, et al; Eplerenone Post-Acute Myocardial Infarction Heart Failure Efficacy and Survival Study Investigators. Eplerenone, a selective aldosterone blocker, in patients with left ventricular dysfunction after myocardial infarction. N Engl J Med. 2003;348:1309-21.
3. Zannad F, McMurray JJ, Krum H, et al; EMPHASIS-HF Study Group. Eplerenone in patients with systolic heart failure and mild symptoms. N Engl J Med. 2011;364:11-21.
4. Juurlink DN, Mamdani MM, Lee DS, et al. Rates of hyperkalemia after publication of the Randomized Aldactone Evaluation Study. N Engl J Med. 2004;351:543-51.

Eplerenone or other AAs vs control in patients with left ventricular dysfunction†

Outcomes	Number of trials (n)	Weighted event rates		At 2 to 24 mo	
		Eplerenone	Control‡	RRR (95% CI)	NNT (CI)
All-cause mortality	2 (9369)	14%	16%	15% (7 to 23)	41 (27 to 88)
CV mortality	2 (9369)	12%	14%	17% (8 to 25)	42 (29 to 88)
Gynecomastia	2 (9361)	0.49%	0.66%	26% (−27 to 57)	NS
				RRI (CI)	NNH (CI)
Hyperkalemia	3 (9489)	6.1%	3.8%	72% (19 to 147)	37 (19 to 140)
		Other AA§	Control‡	RRR (95% CI)	NNT (CI)
All-cause mortality	12 (3569)	19%	25%	26% (17 to 34)	16 (12 to 24)
CV mortality	4 (2553)	26%	34%	25% (16 to 33)	12 (9 to 19)
				RRI (CI)	NNH (CI)
Gynecomastia	6 (2279)	5.4%	0.86%	526% (238 to 1057)	23 (11 to 49)
Hyperkalemia	10 (3342)	8.1%	4.5%	80% (−17 to 291)	NS

†AA = aldosterone antagonist; CV = cardiovascular; NS = not significant; other abbreviations defined in Glossary. Weighted event rates, RRR, RRI, NNT, NNH, and CI calculated from control event rates and risk ratios in article using a random-effects model.
‡Placebo, angiotensin-converting enzyme inhibitor, angiotensin-receptor blocker, or β-blocker.
§Other AAs were spironolactone or canrenone.

FIGURE 5-4

Clinical Queries in PubMed: Accessing From Main Page and Choosing of Filter (Category and Scope)

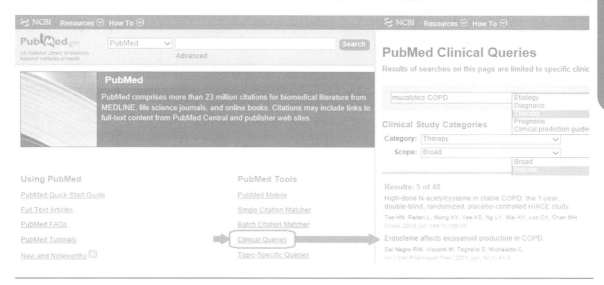

Reproduced with permission of the US National Library of Medicine and PubMed.

Nonpreappraised Research

Only when summaries, guidelines, and preappraised research have failed to provide an answer should you search among the tens of millions of nonpreappraised research articles. They are stored in many different databases (the ones usually searched in systematic reviews), such as PubMed's MEDLINE, EMBASE, CINAHL, or Web of Science. These databases can be accessed directly or through different search engines. Some search engine companies, such as Ovid (http://www.ovid.com), are designed to facilitate complex search strategies, such as those done by medical librarians or authors of systematic reviews. For clinical purposes, PubMed is the most popular search engine, providing free access to the entire MEDLINE database (http://www.ncbi.nlm.nih.gov/pubmed).

Consider, for example, the question of whether statins can prevent dementia. Summaries and preappraised research provide limited or selected evidence to answer that question. Because of its volume, searching PubMed to find relevant evidence requires more advanced searching skills, particularly in the choice and combination of search terms. Simple searches typically yield large outputs with few easily identified relevant studies in the first pages.

To limit irrelevant studies in the outputs, use methodologic filters, such as Clinical Queries. As shown in Figure 5-4, instead of typing your search terms on the main page of PubMed, select Clinical Queries or go directly to http://www.ncbi.nlm.nih.gov/pubmed/clinical. Empirically validated "methods" search terms are added to your search, according to your type of question. For example, Table 5-4 lists the filters used for questions of therapy that facilitate the retrieval of randomized clinical trials.[30] Two filters are available for each search category, 1 broad (sensitive) and 1 narrow (specific), the latter being more adapted to clinical practice. Use of a filter will increase the proportion of relevant studies from approximately 2% to 30% in the first 2 pages of PubMed's output (first 40 citations).[2] Similar filters are available for questions of diagnosis, etiology, prognosis, and *clinical prediction rules*.

Table 5-5 lists similar broad and narrow filters to find systematic reviews from PubMed.[31] In contrast with Clinical Queries, these filters are not implemented in PubMed; the search strategy needs

TABLE 5-4

Clinical Queries "Therapy" Filter: Performance and Strategy Used[a]

	Sensitivity, %	Specificity, %	PubMed Equivalent
Broad filter	99	70	((clinical[Title/Abstract] AND trial[Title/Abstract]) OR clinical trials[MeSH Terms] OR clinical trial[Publication Type] OR random*[Title/Abstract] OR random allocation[MeSH Terms] OR therapeutic use[MeSH Subheading])
Narrow filter	93	97	(randomized controlled trial[Publication Type] OR (randomized[Title/Abstract] AND controlled[Title/Abstract] AND trial[Title/Abstract]))

Abbreviation: MeSH, medical subject headings.
[a]Reproduced with permission of the US National Library of Medicine.

TABLE 5-5

Filters to Retrieve Systematic Reviews From PubMed[a][31]

	Sensitivity, %	Specificity, %	PubMed Equivalent
Broad filter	99.9	52	search*[Title/Abstract] OR meta analysis[Publication Type] OR meta analysis[Title/Abstract] OR meta analysis[MeSH Terms] OR review[Publication Type] OR diagnosis[MeSH Subheading] OR associated[Title/Abstract]
Narrow filter	71	99	MEDLINE[Title/Abstract] OR (systematic[Title/Abstract] AND review[Title/Abstract]) OR meta analysis[Publication Type]

Abbreviation: MeSH, medical subject headings.
[a]These filters are not implemented in PubMed; the search strategy needs to be copy and pasted right after the search to optimally filter systematic reviews. Reproduced with permission from the *BMJ*.

to be copy and pasted right after your search. Going back to our example of the search phrase "statins for the prevention of dementia," an unfiltered search retrieves hundreds of citations that cannot be reliably screened in clinical practice. When adding the narrow filter of Table 5-5 to your search, the output shrinks to 19 citations (in October 2013), and a quick review will identify 6 systematic reviews, including 1 Cochrane Review, updated in 2009, and the most recent review, published in *Mayo Clinic Proceedings* in September 2013, Statins and Cognition: A Systematic Review and Meta-analysis of Short- and Long-term Cognitive Effects. The University of York keeps a comprehensive list of available filters and the publications that describe their development and

validations. For example, in addition to the ones we have already discussed, you will find filters for adverse events, economic evaluation, observational studies, and even qualitative studies (https://sites. google.com/a/york.ac.uk/issg-search-filters-resource/home/search-filters-by-design).

Another useful database for clinical practice is the Cochrane Controlled Trials Registry, the largest electronic compilation of controlled trials, built from MEDLINE, EMBASE, and other sources, including hand searches of most major health care journals. Because it includes only trials, this registry is the fastest, most reliable method of determining whether a controlled trial has been published on any topic. You can search the registry in the Cochrane Library's

TABLE 5-6

Example of a Federated Search: EBM Resources Searched in Parallel in ACCESSSS[a]

Summaries	DynaMed
	UpToDate
	Best Practice
	ACP PIER
Preappraised research	
Synopses of systematic reviews	*ACP Journal Club* DARE
Systematic reviews	McMaster *PLUS* (including Cochrane reviews)
Synopses of studies	McMaster *PLUS*
Nonpreappraised research	
Filtered studies	Clinical Queries in PubMed
Unfiltered studies	PubMed (MEDLINE)

Abbreviations: ACCESSSS, ACCess to Evidence-based Summaries, Synopses, Systematic Reviews and Studies; DARE, Database of Abstracts of Reviews of Effects; EBM, evidence-based medicine.

[a]Reproduced with permission of the Health Information Research Unit, McMaster University.

advanced search function (http://onlinelibrary.wiley.com/cochranelibrary/search; select "Search Limits," then "Trials"). However, to access the full text of articles, you will need a subscription to the Cochrane Library or several Ovid Evidence-Based Medicine Review packages of databases (http://www.ovid.com/site/catalog/DataBase/904.jsp).

Searching All Levels of the Pyramid at the Same Time

At this point, you may wonder if you can search across all levels of the pyramid of resources, instead of having sequential searches in different resources to get the current best evidence. Federated search engines do this easily. One of the most comprehensive and transparent federated resources is ACCESSSS (http://plus.mcmaster.ca/accessss). Typing a single question in ACCESSSS will run parallel searches in major resources from each level of the pyramid, from summaries to all types of preappraised research and all Clinical Queries filters in PubMed. Table 5-6 presents the resources searched by ACCESSSS. Results are given in 1 page organized by level in the pyramid of EBM resources, with the most relevant and useful for clinical practice on the top (see Figure 5-5). Subscribing to ACCESSSS is free, although access to

the full text of some resources will depend on institutional or personal subscriptions. To directly link your own subscriptions to all features of ACCESSSS, you can ask to add your institution to its list.

Other interesting and free federated searches that similarly search multiple resources at more or less each level of the pyramid are available. Instead of looking into summaries at the top, Trip (http://www.tripdatabase.com) has an algorithm to retrieve clinical practice guidelines, classified by country, along with many sources of synopses and other preappraised and nonpreappraised research. Its navigation is easy, and additional interesting features include the ability to structure your search with PICO (patient, intervention, comparison, outcome) and tailor your search to issues in developing countries. SumSearch (http://sumsearch.org) shares similar features, particularly for the retrieval of practice guidelines, but it organizes output according to level of processing (original studies, systematic reviews, and guidelines; Figure 5-1, middle box). SumSearch is linked to alerts from NEJM JournalWatch (http://www.jwatch.org). Finally, Epistemonikos (http://www.epistemonikos.org) is innovative both in simultaneously searching multiple resources and in indexing and interlinking relevant evidence. For example, Epistemonikos connects systematic reviews and

FIGURE 5-5

Output of a Federated Search in ACCESSSS

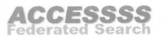

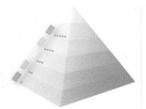

6S model explained
Criteria for articles in **PLUS**

■ Summaries ★★★★★
  UpToDate
  DynaMed
  Best Practice
  Stat!Ref PIER

■ Synopses of Syntheses ★★★★☆
  ACP Journal Club (via PLUS)
  DARE

☐ Syntheses ★★★☆☆
  PLUS Syntheses

■ Synopses of Studies ★★☆☆☆
  ACP Journal Club (via PLUS)

■ Studies ★☆☆☆☆
  PLUS Studies

■ Non-Appraised ★★★★★
  PubMed CQ
  PubMed

McMaster
PLUS

History
dabigatran atrial fibrillation   **Search**
                             Advanced Options
Current PLUS Database: Physician ▾
Resource Portal: ⓘ **McMaster University**
Add your institution   Change

Summaries ★★★★★

■ UpToDate
    Antithrombotic therapy to prevent embolization in atrial fibrillation
    Dabigatran: Drug information
    More Results...

■ DynaMed
    Atrial fibrillation
    Dabigatran
    More Results...

Synopses of Syntheses ★★★★☆

■ ACP Journal Club (selected via PLUS)
    Review: New oral anticoagulants reduced stroke and systemic embolism compared with warfarin in AF
    Review: Dabigatran increases MI and reduces mortality compared with warfarin, enoxaparin, or placebo

Syntheses ★★★☆☆

☐ PLUS Syntheses
    Stroke Prevention in Atrial Fibrillation *(Systematic Review)*
    Combined anticoagulation and antiplatelet therapy for high-risk patients with atrial fibrillation: a systematic review. *(Systematic Review)*

Synopses of Studies ★★☆☆☆

■ ACP Journal Club (selected via PLUS)
    $CHADS_2$ score predicted bleeding and death in atrial fibrillation treated with anticoagulants
    Dabigatran led to less major bleeding than warfarin in younger but not older patients with atrial fibrillation

Studies (pre-appraised by these criteria) ★☆☆☆☆

■ PLUS Studies
    Dabigatran versus warfarin in patients with mechanical heart valves. *(Original Study)*
    Intracranial hemorrhage in atrial fibrillation patients during anticoagulation with warfarin or dabigatran: the RE-LY trial. *(Original Study)*
    More Results...

Below this bar you must do your own critical appraisal. (and can use these criteria if you wish)

■ PubMed Clinical Queries
    These results are yielded from your search term combined with Search Filters which are a modified version of our PubMed Clinical Queries.

    Systematic Reviews
        Meta-Analysis of Randomized Controlled Trials on Risk of Myocardial Infarction from the Use of Oral Direct Thrombin Inhibitors.
        Cost-effectiveness of pharmacogenetic guided warfarin therapy versus alternative anticoagulation in **atrial fibrillation**.
        More Results...

    Therapy
        The new oral anti-coagulants and the phase 3 clinical trials - a systematic review of the literature.
        Safety and Efficacy of **Dabigatran** Compared With Warfarin for Patients Undergoing Radiofrequency Catheter Ablation of **Atrial Fibrillation**: A Meta-analysis.

their included studies and thus allows clustering of systematic reviews based on the primary studies they have in common. Epistemonikos is also unique in offering an appreciable multilingual user interface, multilingual search, and translation of abstracts in more than 9 languages.

When to Use Google

Google (http://www.google.com) has brought a revolution in the way we search the Internet. Its powerful algorithm retrieves answers to any type of question. Many factors seem to influence its output, including the relevance to your query but also the number of times a specific website has been previously accessed or cited, the computer IP and server from which you conduct your search, your nationality, and possibly other financial and nonfinancial interests. Because of its lack of transparency, Google is not a reliable way to filter current best evidence from unsubstantiated or nonscientifically supervised sources. When searching the Web, be aware that you are not searching defined databases but rather surfing the constantly shifting seas of electronic communications. The material you need that is supported by evidence may not float to the surface at any particular time.

On the other hand, "Googling" can be useful for defined purposes. It is often the fastest way to answer general background questions, often through multilingual resources such as Wikipedia (http://www.wikipedia.org), or research new topics, conditions, or treatments that have attracted media attention before being included in any EBM resources (eg, at the time of viral outbreaks around the globe, you may have wondered what Middle East respiratory syndrome coronavirus is). Google also can help you refine the wording of your search terms by rapidly finding 1 relevant citation. For example, you might want to learn whether incretins are associated with pancreatic cancer, but you are unclear about the different types of incretins. By searching Google and Wikipedia, you will rapidly remember how to spell (or copy and paste) dipeptidyl peptidase 4 inhibitor or glucagon-like peptide 1 analogs. Finally, Google can be a surprisingly powerful tool to search for uncommon patterns of symptoms and findings by simply typing them together as a query. These uncommon combinations would usually retrieve little or no information in most medical databases. Google can sometimes find the rare citation that would give you a clue about that syndrome.

A better alternative to Google for answering foreground questions is Google Scholar, which applies Google algorithms to scholarly literature (http://www.google.com/scholar). Although Google Scholar's search algorithms are not transparent, comparisons have found Google Scholar to be comparable to other databases,[32] and an analysis has found increasing evidence that Google Scholar retrieves twice as many relevant articles as PubMed, with almost 3 times greater access to free full-text articles,[33] as well as access to conference abstracts that might be useful for rare topics. Google Scholar has a complex searching system, and the help feature provides useful guidance in refining your searches (http://scholar.google.com/intl/en/scholar/help.html).

TRANSLATING A QUESTION INTO SEARCH TERMS

How to Choose and Combine Search Terms

Table 5-7 illustrates how you can break down a question into its PICO components and corresponding search terms. You next choose and combine search terms into a variety of search strategies, adapted to each resources. One advantage of searching the top EBM resources is that you can keep searches simple because the databases are highly selective and relatively small. One or 2 search terms for the population or problem and for your intervention or exposure will find most relevant topics. For example, if you are interested in the impact of mucolytics on patients with chronic obstructive pulmonary disease (COPD) who are stable, simply searching with the terms "COPD mucolytic" in summaries (eg, UpToDate) and preappraised research (eg, DARE) will usually suffice. Being too specific in your search can cause you to lose important information. In contrast, searching nonpreappraised research (eg, PubMed) usually requires more specific and structured searches.

TABLE 5-7

Combining Search Terms Into Different Search Strategies

PICO Components		Potential Search Terms
P	Patients with stable chronic bronchitis	COPD OR (chronic bronchitis)
I	Any mucolytic agent	Mucolytic
C	Placebo (and current best care)	Placebo
O	Number of exacerbation, mortality	Exacerbation OR mortality
Level of the Pyramid		**Examples of Search Strategies[a]**
Summaries and preappraised research		Chronic bronchitis mucolytic
		COPD mucolytic
Nonpreappraised research		COPD mucolytic exacerbation
		(COPD OR (chronic bronchitis)) AND mucolytic
		(COPD OR (chronic bronchitis)) AND mucolytic AND exacerbation
		(COPD OR (chronic bronchitis)) AND mucolytic AND (exacerbation OR mortality)

Abbreviation: COPD, chronic obstructive pulmonary disease.

[a]OR and AND are Boolean operators in these searches.

To find the evidence you need in large databases, your search terms should closely relate to the components of your PICO question (see Chapter 4, What Is the Question?). For some components, the corresponding search terms are straightforward. For example, if your population is patients with diabetes, you may simply use "diabetes" or "diabetic." Other components of PICO may prove more challenging, such as "antithyroid drug therapy" as an intervention. Indeed, you might choose "antithyroid" as a single term or consider combining several drugs, such as "carbimazole OR propylthiouracil OR methimazole." Notice that the latter example combines search terms with "OR" in capital letters to signify this is a *Boolean operator*: the search will retrieve studies for either of these treatments. In contrast, adding no operator actually corresponds to linking search terms with "AND." For example, typing "neuraminidase inhibitors" is equivalent to typing "neuraminidase AND inhibitors" and will retrieve only studies that include both terms, instead of all studies that include any type of inhibitor.

Efficient wording of search terms is based in part on your familiarity with the topic but is also based on trial and error. The Medical Subject Headings (MeSH) Thesaurus (http://www.nlm.nih.gov/mesh/MBrowser.html) can help you find words generally used by indexers for a given medical concept. A quick Google search often can give you a sense of appropriate wording in a faster way. If you are surprised that a search yields little relevant evidence, ask yourself if you misspelled a term or were too specific (eg, adding too many words that will automatically be linked with "AND"). Definitions also can differ. For example, in MeSH, "ventilation" refers to "supplying a building or house, their rooms and corridors, with fresh air." "Pulmonary ventilation" is the preferred term for clinicians because it indicates "the total volume of gas inspired or expired per unit of time, usually measured in liters per minute."

Broad vs Narrow Searches

Table 5-8 indicates how to refine your search. If you initially found little evidence, you can broaden your search (eg, increase its sensitivity) by adding synonyms for each concept or using truncated terms

TABLE 5-8

Refining the Search Strategy[1,19,31,35]

Ways to Increase Sensitivity	Ways to Increase Specificity
Many search terms for a similar PICO component, linked with "OR"	More PICO concepts linked with "AND": (P) AND (I) AND (C) AND (O)
Truncated terms, wildcards (eg, diabet*, wom?n)	Use of NOT to exclude irrelevant terms
Synonyms (pressure sore, decubitus ulcer)	Use of NOT as Boolean operator
Variant spelling (tumour, tumor)	Limits (date, age group, etc)
Explosion of MeSH terms	Methodological filters (Clinical Queries)
Use of PubMed "Related citations" or bibliography of relevant articles	Content filters (topic or disease specific)

Abbreviation: MeSH, medical subject headings.

(eg, diabet* will retrieve diabetes, diabetic, and many other similar terms with different endings). Conversely, if your initial search retrieved too many citations to be screened, you can narrow your search (eg, increase its specificity) by linking more PICO components with "AND" or by adding limits and methodologic filters (eg, narrow Clinical Queries; http://www.ncbi.nlm.nih.gov/pubmed/clinical). More sophisticated approaches include entering PICO components sequentially according to their importance to obtain a manageable number of articles in large databases, such as PubMed.[34]

Finding Related Articles

When your PubMed search seems laborious, a useful trick is to find at least 1 potentially relevant article to your question and use the "Related citations" feature, as highlighted in Figure 5-6. It will automatically look for other articles that are similar in their titles, abstracts, and index terms. You then can screen the new output and select "Related citations" for each potentially relevant article you find. To keep track of potentially relevant citations, send them to the PubMed clipboard as you screen, and they will be labeled as items in the clipboard (Figure 5-6). This strategy may help you gather relevant articles rapidly in a snowball sampling.

Getting Help

Finally, because of the complexity and interconnections of medical databases, some searches simply require the help of information specialists. In anticipation of such cases in your clinical practice, befriend your medical librarians. They can be a great resource to help answer difficult questions or those that require elaborate search strategies.

CONCLUSION: IMPROVING YOUR SEARCHING SKILLS IN DAILY PRACTICE

Box 5-2 presents a few practical tips to help you improve your searching skills in daily practice. Because of the continuous flow of new research findings of variable quality, finding current best evidence is challenging. However, this process has been greatly facilitated by the development of numerous EBM resources that can provide fast answers at the point of care. No resource is sufficient for all information needs, and you will need to use several in combination to find current best evidence. This chapter provides guidance on how to navigate across the pyramid of resources efficiently, ideally by using federated search engines.

FIGURE 5-6

Features in PubMed: Related Citations and Clipboard

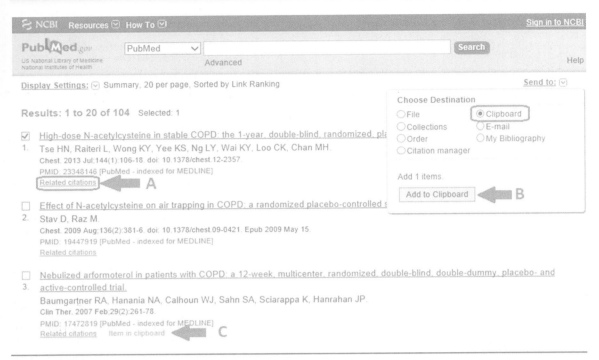

A, Link to "Related citations" from a relevant article. B, Dialogue box allowing user to send relevant articles to the clipboard. C, After having sent an article to the clipboard, it is labeled so in the output.

Reproduced with permission of the US National Library of Medicine.

BOX 5-2

Tips to Help Improve Searching Skills

With the pyramid of EBM resources in mind, map the EBM resources that are accessible to you through your affiliations or personal subscriptions.

Choose which resources you would like to explore next, according to your information needs and the criteria described in this chapter.

Bookmark these resources in the browsers of all your devices—your desktop computer, smartphone, or tablet. Find out if you can get remote access from your institution and implement it so that access is automatic.

Subscribe to an e-mail alerting system for newly published evidence that is transparent and trustworthy.

Train yourself on questions that are familiar to you and compare EBM resources.

Keep track of your questions. It can enhance your learning and help you reflect back on your evidence-based practice.

Finally, always keep the patient perspective. This will help you focus on the appropriate body of evidence that informs all patient important outcomes, instead of being driven by the evidence that is first presented to you.

References

1. Straus SE. *Evidence-Based Medicine: How to Practice and Teach EBM*. 4th ed. New York, NY: Elsevier/Churchill Livingstone; 2011.

2. Agoritsas T, Merglen A, Courvoisier DS, et al. Sensitivity and predictive value of 15 PubMed search strategies to answer clinical questions rated against full systematic reviews. *J Med Internet Res*. 2012;14(3):e85.

3. Green ML, Ciampi MA, Ellis PJ. Residents' medical information needs in clinic: are they being met? *Am J Med*. 2000;109(3):218-223.

4. González-González AI, Dawes M, Sánchez-Mateos J, et al. Information needs and information-seeking behavior of primary care physicians. *Ann Fam Med*. 2007;5(4):345-352.

5. Graber MA, Randles BD, Ely JW, Monnahan J. Answering clinical questions in the ED. *Am J Emerg Med*. 2008;26(2):144-147.

6. Hoogendam A, Stalenhoef AF, Robbé PF, Overbeke AJ. Answers to questions posed during daily patient care are more likely to be answered by UpToDate than PubMed. *J Med Internet Res*. 2008;10(4):e29.

7. Hoogendam A, Stalenhoef AF, Robbé PF, Overbeke AJ. Analysis of queries sent to PubMed at the point of care: observation of search behaviour in a medical teaching hospital. *BMC Med Inform Decis Mak*. 2008;8:42.

8. Thiele RH, Poiro NC, Scalzo DC, Nemergut EC. Speed, accuracy, and confidence in Google, Ovid, PubMed, and UpToDate: results of a randomised trial. *Postgrad Med J*. 2010;86(1018):459-465.

9. McKibbon KA, Fridsma DB. Effectiveness of clinician-selected electronic information resources for answering primary care physicians' information needs. *J Am Med Inform Assoc*. 2006;13(6):653-659.

10. Glasziou P, Burls A, Gilbert R. Evidence based medicine and the medical curriculum. *BMJ*. 2008;337:a1253.

11. Bastian H, Glasziou P, Chalmers I. Seventy-five trials and eleven systematic reviews a day: how will we ever keep up? *PLoS Med*. 2010;7(9):e1000326.

12. Guyatt GH, Akl EA, Crowther M, Schunemann HJ, Gutterman DD, Zelman Lewis S. Introduction to the ninth edition: Antithrombotic Therapy and Prevention of Thrombosis, 9th ed: American College of Chest Physicians Evidence-Based Clinical Practice Guidelines. *Chest*. 2012;141(2 suppl):48S-52S.

13. Haynes RB, Cotoi C, Holland J, et al; McMaster Premium Literature Service (PLUS) Project. Second-order peer review of the medical literature for clinical practitioners. *JAMA*. 2006;295(15):1801-1808.

14. Holland J, Haynes RB; McMaster PLUS Team Health Information Research Unit. McMaster Premium Literature Service (PLUS): an evidence-based medicine information service delivered on the Web. *AMIA Annu Symp Proc*. 2005;2005:340-344.

15. Garg AX, Adhikari NK, McDonald H, et al. Effects of computerized clinical decision support systems on practitioner performance and patient outcomes: a systematic review. *JAMA*. 2005;293(10):1223-1238.

16. Del Fiol G, Curtis C, Cimino JJ, et al. Disseminating context-specific access to online knowledge resources within electronic health record systems. *Stud Health Technol Inform*. 2013;192:672-676.

17. Roshanov PS, Fernandes N, Wilczynski JM, et al. Features of effective computerised clinical decision support systems: meta-regression of 162 randomised trials. *BMJ*. 2013;346:f657.

18. Jeffery R, Navarro T, Lokker C, Haynes RB, Wilczynski NL, Farjou G. How current are leading evidence-based medical textbooks? an analytic survey of four online textbooks. *J Med Internet Res*. 2012;14(6):e175.

19. Prorok JC, Iserman EC, Wilczynski NL, Haynes RB. The quality, breadth, and timeliness of content updating vary substantially for 10 online medical texts: an analytic survey. *J Clin Epidemiol*. 2012;65(12):1289-1295.

20. Vandvik PO, Lincoff AM, Gore JM, et al. Primary and secondary prevention of cardiovascular disease: Antithrombotic Therapy and Prevention of Thrombosis, 9th ed: American College of Chest Physicians Evidence-Based Clinical Practice Guidelines. *Chest*. 2012;141(2 suppl):e637S-e668S.

21. Wentz R. Visibility of research: FUTON bias. *Lancet*. 2002;360(9341):1256.

22. Kung J, Miller RR, Mackowiak PA. Failure of clinical practice guidelines to meet institute of medicine standards: two more decades of little, if any, progress. *Arch Intern Med*. 2012;172(21):1628-1633.

23. Vandvik PO, Brandt L, Alonso-Coello P, et al. Creating clinical practice guidelines we can trust, use, and share: a new era is imminent. *Chest*. 2013;144(2):381-389.

24. Banzi R, Cinquini M, Liberati A, et al. Speed of updating online evidence based point of care summaries: prospective cohort analysis. *BMJ*. 2011;343:d5856.

25. Martínez García L, Arévalo-Rodríguez I, Solà I, Haynes RB, Vandvik PO, Alonso-Coello P; Updating Guidelines Working Group. Strategies for monitoring and updating clinical practice guidelines: a systematic review. *Implement Sci*. 2012;7:109.

26. Ruschitzka F, Abraham WT, Singh JP, et al; EchoCRT Study Group. Cardiac-resynchronization therapy in heart failure with a narrow QRS complex. *N Engl J Med*. 2013;369(15):1395-1405.

27. Haynes RB, Holland J, Cotoi C, et al. McMaster PLUS: a cluster randomized clinical trial of an intervention to accelerate clinical use of evidence-based information from digital libraries. *J Am Med Inform Assoc*. 2006;13(6):593-600.

28. Haynes RB. ACP Journal Club: the best new evidence for patient care. *ACP J Club*. 2008;148(3):2.

29. Lader E. Review: Eplerenone is not more effective for reducing mortality than other aldosterone antagonists. *Ann Intern Med*. 2012;157:JC6-10.

30. Haynes RB, McKibbon KA, Wilczynski NL, Walter SD, Werre SR; Hedges Team. Optimal search strategies for retrieving scientifically strong studies of treatment from Medline: analytical survey. *BMJ*. 2005;330(7501):1179.

31. Montori VM, Wilczynski NL, Morgan D, Haynes RB; Hedges Team. Optimal search strategies for retrieving systematic reviews from Medline: analytical survey. *BMJ*. 2005;330(7482):68.

32. Kulkarni AV, Aziz B, Shams I, Busse JW. Comparisons of citations in Web of Science, Scopus, and Google Scholar for articles published in general medical journals. *JAMA*. 2009;302(10):1092-1096.

33. Shariff SZ, Bejaimal SA, Sontrop JM, et al. Retrieving clinical evidence: a comparison of PubMed and Google Scholar for quick clinical searches. *J Med Internet Res*. 2013;15(8):e164.

34. Dans AL, Dans LF, Silvestre MAA. Literature searches. In: Dans AL, Dans LF, Silvestre MAA, eds. *Painless Evidence-Based Medicine*. Chichester, England: John Wiley & Sons; 2008:115-136.

35. DiCenso A, Bayley L, Haynes RB. ACP Journal Club. Editorial: Accessing preappraised evidence: fine-tuning the 5S model into a 6S model. *Ann Intern Med*. 2009;151(6):JC3-JC2, JC3-JC3.

6

Why Study Results Mislead: Bias and Random Error

Gordon Guyatt, Roman Jaeschke, and Maureen O. Meade

IN THIS CHAPTER

Random Error

Bias

Strategies for Reducing the Risk of Bias

Our clinical questions have correct answers that correspond to an underlying reality or truth. For instance, there is a true underlying magnitude of the impact of β-blockers on mortality in patients with heart failure, the impact of inhaled corticosteroids on exacerbations in patients with asthma, the impact of reamed vs unreamed nailing of tibial fractures, the *prognosis* of patients with hip osteoarthritis, and the diagnostic properties of a pregnancy test. Research studies attempt to estimate that underlying truth. Unfortunately, however, we will never know the exact truth. Studies may be flawed in their design or conduct and introduce *systematic error* (or *bias*). Even if a study could be perfectly designed and executed, the estimated *treatment effect* may miss the mark because of *random error.* The next section explains why.

RANDOM ERROR

Consider a perfectly balanced coin. Every time we flip the coin, the *probability* of it landing with its head up or tail up is equal—50%. Assume, however, that we as investigators do not know that the coin is perfectly balanced—in fact, we have no idea how well balanced it is, and we would like to find out. We can state our question formally: What is the true underlying probability of a resulting head or tail on any

given coin flip? Our first experiment addressing this question is a series of 10 coin flips; the result: 8 heads and 2 tails. What are we to conclude? Taking our result at face value, we infer that the coin is very unbalanced (ie, biased in such a way that it yields heads more often than tails) and that the probability of heads on any given flip is 80%.

Few would be happy with this conclusion. The reason for our discomfort is that we know that the world is not constructed so that a perfectly balanced coin will always yield 5 heads and 5 tails in any given set of 10 coin flips. Rather, the result is subject to the play of chance, otherwise known as random error. Some of the time, 10 flips of a perfectly balanced coin will yield 8 heads. On occasion, 9 of 10 flips will turn up heads. On rare occasions, we will find heads on all 10 flips. Figure 6-1 shows the actual distribution of heads and tails in repeated series of coin flips.

What if the 10 coin flips yield 5 heads and 5 tails? Our awareness of the play of chance leaves us uncertain that the coin is balanced: a series of 10 coin flips of a very biased coin (a true probability of heads of 0.8, for instance) could, by chance, yield 5 heads and 5 tails.

Let us say that a funding agency, intrigued by the results of our first small experiment, provides us with resources to conduct a larger

FIGURE 6-1

Theoretical Distribution of Results of an Infinite Number of Repetitions of 10 Flips of an Unbiased Coin

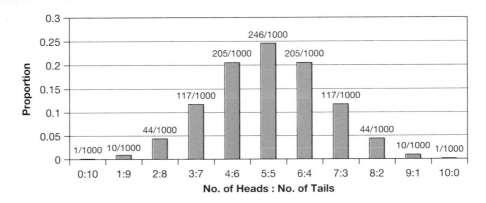

study. This time, we increase the sample size of our experiment markedly, conducting a series of 1000 coin flips. If we end up with 500 heads and 500 tails, are we ready to conclude that we are dealing with a true coin? We are much more confident but still not completely sure. The reason for our remaining uncertainty is that we know that, were the true underlying probability of heads 51%, we would sometimes see 1000 coin flips yield the result we have just observed.

We can apply the above logic to the results of studies that address questions of prognosis, diagnosis, and *harm* and also to *randomized clinical trials* (RCTs) that address treatment issues. For instance, an RCT finds that 10 of 100 treated patients die during treatment, as do 20 of 100 control patients. Does treatment really reduce the death rate by 50%? Maybe, but awareness of chance will leave us with some degree of uncertainty about the magnitude of the treatment effect—and perhaps about whether treatment helps at all.

In a study of congestive heart failure, 228 of 1320 patients (17%) with moderate to severe heart failure allocated to receive *placebo* died, as did 156 of 1327 (12%) allocated to receive bisoprolol.[1] Although the true underlying reduction in the *relative risk* of dying is likely to be in the vicinity of the 32% suggested by the study, we must acknowledge that appreciable uncertainty remains about the true magnitude of the effect (see Chapter 10, Confidence Intervals: Was the Single Study or Meta-analysis Large Enough?).

We have now addressed the question with which we started: "Why is it that no matter how powerful and well designed a study, we will never be sure of the truth?" The answer is that chance is directionless, and it is equally likely, for instance, to overestimate or underestimate treatment effects.

BIAS

Bias is the term we use for the other reason study results may be misleading. In contrast to random error, bias leads to systematic deviations (ie, the error has direction) from the underlying truth. In studies of prognosis, bias leads us to falsely optimistic or pessimistic conclusions about a patient's fate. In studies of diagnosis, bias leads us to an overly optimistic (usually) or pessimistic assessment of a test's value in differentiating between those with and without a target condition. In treatment or *harm studies*, bias leads to either an underestimate or an overestimate of the underlying benefit or harm (Box 6-1).

Bias may intrude as a result of differences, other than the *experimental intervention*, between patients in treatment and *control groups* at the time they enter a study. At the start of a study, each patient, if left untreated, is destined to do well—or poorly. To do poorly means to have an adverse event (eg, a stroke) during the study. We often refer to the adverse event that is the focus of a study as the *target outcome* or *target event*. Bias will result if treated and control patients differ in their prognosis (ie, their likelihood of experiencing the target outcome) at the start of the study. For instance, if patients in the control group have more

---

BOX 6-1
How Can a Study of an Intervention (Treatment) Be Biased?

Intervention and control groups may be different at the start

> Example: patients in control group are sicker or older

Intervention and control groups may, independent of the experimental treatment, become different as the study proceeds

> Example: patients in the intervention group receive effective additional medication

Intervention and control groups may differ, independent of treatment, at the end

> Example: more sick patients lost to follow-up in the intervention group

severe atherosclerosis or are older than their counterparts, their destiny will be to have a greater proportion of adverse events than those in the intervention or treatment group, and the results of the study will be biased in favor of the treatment group; that is, the study will yield a larger treatment effect than would be obtained were the study groups prognostically similar at baseline.

Even if patients in the intervention and control groups begin the study with the same *prognosis*, the result may still be biased. This will occur if, for instance, effective interventions are differentially administered to treatment and control groups. For instance, in a study of a novel agent for the *prevention* of complications of atherosclerosis, the intervention group might receive more intensive statin therapy than the control group.

Finally, patients may begin prognostically similar, and stay prognostically similar, but the study may end with a biased result. This could occur if, for example, the study loses patients to *follow-up* (see Chapter 7, Therapy [Randomized Trials]) or because a study is *stopped early* because of an apparent large treatment effect (see Chapter 11.3, Randomized Trials Stopped Early for Benefit).

STRATEGIES FOR REDUCING THE RISK OF BIAS

This book teaches you how to recognize *risk of bias* not only in studies that address issues of therapy and harm but also in studies of prognosis and diagnosis. In studies of prognosis, investigators can reduce bias by enrolling a representative sample and ensuring they are completely followed up. In studies of diagnosis, investigators can ensure that they have chosen an appropriate *criterion* or *gold standard* for diagnosis and that those interpreting test results are unaware of the gold standard findings. In the remainder of this chapter, however, we focus on issues of therapy and harm.

We have noted that bias arises from differences in *prognostic factors* in treatment and control groups at the start of a study or from differences in prognosis that arise as a study proceeds. What can investigators do to reduce these biases? Table 6-1 summarizes the available strategies to reduce biases in RCTs and *observational studies*.

TABLE 6-1

Ways of Reducing Bias in Studies of Therapy and Harm

Source of Bias	Therapy: Strategy for Reducing Bias	Harm: Strategy for Reducing Bias
Differences Observed at the Start of the Study		
Treatment and control patients differ in prognosis	Randomization	Statistical adjustment for prognostic factors in the analysis of data
	Randomization with stratification	Matching
Differences That Arise as the Study Proceeds		
Placebo effects	Blinding of patients	Choice of outcomes (such as mortality) less subject to placebo effects
Cointervention	Blinding of caregivers	Documentation of treatment differences and statistical adjustment
Bias in assessment of outcome	Blinding of assessors of outcome	Choice of outcomes (such as mortality) less subject to observer bias
Differences at the Completion of the Study		
Loss to follow-up	Ensuring complete follow-up	Ensuring complete follow-up
Stopping study early because of large effect	Completing study as initially planned by sample size calculation	Not applicable
Omitting patients who did not receive assigned treatment	Including all patients for whom data are available in the arm to which they were randomized	Not applicable

When studying new treatments, investigators can implement a large of number of strategies to limit the risk of bias. They can reduce the likelihood of differences in the prognostic features in treated and untreated patients at baseline by *randomly allocating* patients to the 2 groups. They can balance placebo effects by administering identical-appearing but biologically inert treatments—placebos—to patients in the control group. *Blinding* clinicians to whether patients are receiving active or placebo therapy can eliminate the risk of important *cointerventions*, and blinding outcome assessors minimizes bias in the assessment of event rates.

Investigators studying either treatment effects or harm using observational study designs have far less control over the risk of bias. They must be content to compare patients whose *exposure* is determined by their choice or circumstances, and they can address potential differences in patients' fate only by statistical adjustment for known prognostic factors. Blinding is impossible, so their best defense against placebo effects and bias in outcome assessment is to choose *end points*, such as death, that are less subject to these biases. Investigators who address both sets of questions can reduce bias by minimizing loss to follow-up (Table 6-1).

Note that when investigators choose observational study designs to study treatment issues, clinicians must apply the risk of bias criteria developed primarily for questions of harm. Similarly, if the potentially harmful exposure is a drug with beneficial effects, investigators may be able to randomize patients to intervention and control groups. In this case, clinicians can apply the risk of bias criteria designed primarily for therapy questions. Whether for issues of therapy or harm, the strength of inference from RCTs will almost invariably be greater than the strength of inference from observational studies.

Reference

1. CIBIS-II Investigators and Committees. The Cardiac Insufficiency Bisoprolol Study II (CIBIS-II): a randomised trial. *Lancet*. 1999;353(9146):9-13.

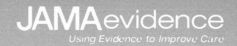

THERAPY

THERAPY

observational study that addresses a potential treatment that has not yet been evaluated in an RCT.

HOW SERIOUS IS THE RISK OF BIAS?

Did Intervention and Control Groups Start With the Same Prognosis?

Were Patients Randomized?

Consider the question of whether hospital care prolongs life. A study finds that more sick people die in the hospital than in the community. We would easily reject the naive conclusion that hospital care kills people because we recognize that hospitalized patients are sicker than patients in the community.

Although the logic of prognostic balance is vividly clear in comparing hospitalized patients with those in the community, it may be less obvious in other contexts. Many people believe that a diet rich in ω3 fatty acids will decrease their risk of a cardiovascular event. This belief arose from many observational studies in which people who ingested larger quantities of ω3 fatty acids had fewer cardiovascular events than those that who ate lesser quantities.[5] However, large randomized trials did not find any benefits with ω3 fatty acid supplementation.[6,7]

Other surprises generated by randomized trials include the demonstration that antioxidant vitamins fail to reduce gastrointestinal cancer[8]—and one such agent, vitamin E, may actually increase all-cause mortality[9]—and that a variety of initially promising drugs increase mortality in patients with heart failure.[10-12] Such surprises occur periodically when investigators conduct randomized trials to test the observations from studies in which patients and physicians determine which treatment a patient receives.

The reason that studies in which patient or physician preference determines whether a patient receives treatment or control (observational studies) often yield misleading results is that morbidity and mortality result from many causes. Treatment studies attempt to determine the impact of an intervention on events such as stroke, myocardial infarction, and death—occurrences that we call the trial's *target outcomes*. A patient's age, the underlying severity of illness, the presence of *comorbidity*, and a host of other factors typically determine the frequency with which a trial's target outcome occurs (*prognostic factors* or

---

BOX 7-1

Users' Guides for an Article About Therapy

How serious was the risk of bias?

Did intervention and control groups start with the same prognosis?

Were patients randomized?

Was randomization concealed?

Were patients in the study groups similar with respect to known prognostic factors?

Was prognostic balance maintained as the study progressed?

To what extent was the study blinded?

Were the groups prognostically balanced at the study's completion?

Was follow-up complete?

Were patients analyzed in the groups to which they were randomized?

Was the trial stopped early?

What are the results?

How large was the treatment effect?

How precise was the estimate of the treatment effect?

How can I apply the results to patient care?

Were the study patients similar to my patient?

Were all patient-important outcomes considered?

Are the likely treatment benefits worth the potential harm and costs?

---

determinants of outcome). If prognostic factors—either those we know about or those we do not know about—prove unbalanced between a trial's treatment and *control groups*, the study's outcome will be biased, either underestimating or overestimating the treatment's effect. Because known prognostic factors often influence clinicians' recommendations and patients' decisions about taking treatment, observational studies often yield biased results that may get the magnitude or even the direction of the effect wrong.

Observational studies can theoretically match patients, either in the selection of patients for study or in the subsequent statistical analysis, for known *prognostic factors* (see Chapter 14, Harm [Observational

Studies], and Chapter 11.1, An Illustration of Bias and Random Error). However, not all prognostic factors are easily measured or characterized, and in many diseases only a few are known. Therefore, even the most careful patient selection and statistical methods are unable to completely address the *bias* in the estimated *treatment effect*. The power of randomization is that treatment and control groups are more likely to have a balanced distribution of known and unknown prognostic factors.

Consider again our example of the ω3 fatty acid studies. What was the cause of bias in the ω3 fatty acids observational studies? People who eat larger amounts of ω3 fatty acids may typically have a higher socioeconomic status than those who eat smaller amounts. In addition, patients who eat larger amounts of ω3 fatty acids may eat fewer unhealthy foods and may be more careful with other important risk factors (eg, smoking and exercise). Their apparent benefit from ω3 fatty acids may reflect their healthier lifestyle. Whatever the explanation, we are now confident that it was their previous *prognosis*, rather than the ω3 fatty acids, that led to lower rates of cardiovascular events.

Although randomization is a powerful technique, it does not always succeed in creating groups with similar prognosis. Investigators may make mistakes that compromise randomization, or randomization may fail because of chance—unlikely events sometimes happen. The next 2 sections address these issues.

When those enrolling patients are unaware and cannot control the arm to which the patient is allocated, we refer to randomization as concealed. In unconcealed trials, those responsible for recruitment may systematically enroll sicker—or less sick—patients to either a treatment or control group. This behavior will compromise the purpose of randomization, and the study will yield a biased result.[13-15] Careful investigators will ensure that randomization is concealed through strategies such as remote randomization, in which the individual recruiting the patient makes a call to a methods center to discover the arm of the study to which the patient is assigned.

Consider, for instance, a trial of β-blockers vs angiotensin-converting enzyme (ACE) inhibitors for hypertension treatment that used

opaque numbered envelopes to conceal randomization.[16] At the time the study was conducted, evidence suggested that β-blockers were better for patients with heart disease. Significantly more patients with heart disease were assigned to receive β-blockers ($P = .037$). In addition, evidence suggested that ACE inhibitors were better for patients with diabetes mellitus. Significantly more patients with diabetes were assigned to receive ACE inhibitors ($P = .048$). It is possible that clinicians were opening envelopes and violating the randomization to ensure patients received what the clinicians believed was the best treatment. Thus, the prognostic balance that randomization could have achieved was prevented.

Were Patients in the Treatment and Control Groups Similar With Respect to Known Prognostic Factors?

The purpose of randomization is to create groups whose prognosis, with respect to the target outcomes, is similar. Sometimes, through bad luck, randomization will fail to achieve this goal. The smaller the sample size, the more likely the trial will have prognostic imbalance.

Picture a trial testing a new treatment for heart failure that is enrolling patients classified as having New York Heart Association functional class III and class IV heart failure. Patients with class IV heart failure have a much worse prognosis than those with class III heart failure. The trial is small, with only 8 patients. One would not be surprised if all 4 patients with class III heart failure were allocated to the treatment group and all 4 patients with class IV heart failure were allocated to the control group. Such a result of the allocation process would seriously bias the study in favor of the treatment. Were the trial to enroll 800 patients, one would be startled if randomization placed all 400 patients with class III heart failure in the treatment arm. The larger the sample size, the more likely randomization will achieve its goal of prognostic balance.

You can check how effectively randomization has balanced known prognostic factors by looking for a display of patient characteristics of the treatment and control groups at the study's commencement—the baseline or entry prognostic features. Although we will never know whether similarity exists for the unknown prognostic factors, we are reassured when the known prognostic factors are well balanced.

All is not lost if the treatment groups are not similar at baseline. Statistical techniques permit adjustment of the study result for baseline differences. When both *adjusted analyses* and unadjusted analyses generate the same conclusion, clinicians gain confidence that the *risk of bias* is not excessive.

Was Prognostic Balance Maintained as the Study Progressed?

To What Extent Was the Study Blinded?

If randomization succeeds, treatment and control groups begin with a similar prognosis. Randomization, however, provides no guarantees that the 2 groups will remain prognostically balanced. *Blinding* is the optimal strategy for maintaining prognostic balance.

Box 7-2 describes 5 groups involved in clinical trials that, ideally, will remain unaware of whether patients are receiving the *experimental therapy* or control therapy. Patients who take a treatment that they believe is effective may feel and perform better than those who do not, even if the treatment has no biologic activity. Although the magnitude and consistency of this *placebo effect* remain uncertain,[17-20] investigators interested in determining the biologic impact of a treatment will ensure patients are blind to treatment allocation. Similarly, rigorous research designs will ensure blinding of those caring for participants, as well as those collecting, evaluating, and analyzing data (Box 7-2). Demonstrations of bias introduced by unblinding, such as the results of a trial in multiple sclerosis in which a treatment benefit judged by unblinded outcome assessors disappeared when adjudicators of outcome were blinded,[21] highlight the importance of blinding. The more subjectivity involved in judging whether a patient has had a target outcome, the more important blinding becomes. For example, blinding of an outcome assessor is unnecessary when the outcome is all-cause mortality.

BOX 7-2

Five Groups That Should, if Possible, Be Blind to Treatment Assignment

Patients	To avoid placebo effects
Clinicians	To prevent differential administration of therapies that affect the outcome of interest (cointervention)
Data collectors	To prevent bias in data collection
Adjudicators of outcome	To prevent bias in decisions about whether or not a patient has had an outcome of interest
Data analysts	To avoid bias in decisions regarding data analysis

---

Finally, differences in patient care other than the intervention under study—*cointerventions*—can, if they affect study outcomes, bias the results. Effective blinding eliminates the possibility of either conscious or unconscious differential administration of effective interventions to treatment and control groups. When effective blinding is not possible, documentation of potential cointerventions becomes important.

Were the Groups Prognostically Balanced at the Study's Completion?

It is possible for investigators to effectively conceal and blind treatment assignment and still fail to achieve an unbiased result.

Was Follow-up Complete?

Ideally, at the conclusion of a trial, investigators will know the status of each patient with respect to the target outcome. The greater the number of patients whose outcome is unknown—patients *lost to follow-up*—the more a study is potentially compromised. The reason is that patients who are lost to follow-up often have different prognoses from those who are retained—they may disappear because they have adverse outcomes or because they are doing well and so did not return for assessment.[22] The magnitude of the bias may be substantial. A systematic review suggested that up to a third of positive trials reported in high-impact journals may lose significance given plausible assumptions regarding differential loss to follow-up in treatment and control groups.[23]

When does loss to follow-up pose a serious risk of bias? Although you may run across thresholds such as 20% for a serious risk of bias, such rules of thumb are misleading. Consider 2 hypothetical randomized trials, each of which enters 1000 patients into both the treatment and control groups, of whom 30 (3%) are lost to follow-up (Table 7-1). In trial A, treated patients die at half the rate of the control group (200 vs 400), a *relative risk* (RR) of 50%. To what extent does the loss to follow-up threaten our inference that treatment reduces the death rate by half? If we assume the worst (ie, that all treated patients lost to follow-up died), the number of deaths in the *experimental group* would be 230 (23%). If there were no deaths among the control patients who were lost to follow-up, our best estimate of the effect of treatment in reducing the RR of death decreases from 200/400, or 50%, to 230/400, or 58%. Thus, even assuming the worst makes little difference to the best estimate of the magnitude of the treatment effect. Our inference is therefore secure.

Contrast this with trial B. Here, the RR of death is also 50%. In this case, however, the total number of deaths is much lower; of the treated patients, 30 die, and the number of deaths in control patients is 60. In trial B, if we make the same worst-case assumption about the fate of the patients lost to follow-up, the results would change markedly. If we assume that all patients initially allocated to treatment—but subsequently lost to follow-up—die, the number of deaths among treated patients increases from 30 to 60, which is equal to the number of control group deaths. If this assumption is accurate, we would have 60 deaths in both the treatment and control groups, and the effect of treatment would decrease to 0. Because of this marked change in the treatment effect (50% RR if we ignore those lost to follow-up; 100% RR if we assume all patients in the treatment group who were lost to follow-up died), the 3% loss to follow-up in trial B threatens our inference about the magnitude of the RR.

Of course, this worst-case scenario is unlikely. When a worst-case scenario, were it true, substantially alters the results, you must judge the plausibility of a markedly different outcome *event rate* in the treatment and control group patients lost to follow-up. Ideally, investigators would conduct *sensitivity analyses* to deal with this issue. Because they seldom do, guidelines are available to help you should you choose to make your own judgment of the trial's vulnerability to loss to follow-up.[23]

TABLE 7-1

When Does Loss to Follow-up Seriously Increase Risk of Bias?

	Trial A		Trial B	
	Treatment	**Control**	**Treatment**	**Control**
No. of patients randomized	1000	1000	1000	1000
No. (%) lost to follow-up	30 (3)	30 (3)	30 (3)	30 (3)
No. (%) of deaths	200 (20)	400 (40)	30 (3)	60 (6)
RR not counting patients lost to follow-up	0.2/0.4 = 0.50		0.03/0.06 = 0.50	
RR for worst-case scenario[a]	0.23/0.4 = 0.58		0.06/0.06 = 1	

Abbreviation: RR, relative risk.

[a]The worst-case scenario assumes that all patients allocated to the treatment group and lost to follow-up died and all patients allocated to the control group and lost to follow-up survived.

Thus, loss to follow-up may substantially increase the risk of bias. If assuming a worst-case scenario does not change the inferences arising from study results, then loss to follow-up is unlikely a problem. If such an assumption would significantly alter the results, the extent to which bias is introduced depends on how likely it is that treatment patients lost to follow-up fared badly, whereas control patients lost to follow-up fared well. That decision is a matter of judgment.

Was the Trial Stopped Too Early?

Stopping trials early (ie, before enrolling the planned sample size) when one sees an apparent large benefit is risky and may compromise randomization (see Chapter 11.3, Randomized Trials Stopped Early for Benefit). These *stopped early trials* run the risk of greatly overestimating the treatment effect.[24]

A trial designed with too short a follow-up also may compromise crucial information that adequate length of follow-up would reveal. For example, consider a trial that randomly assigned patients with an abdominal aortic aneurysm to either an open surgical repair or a less invasive, endovascular repair technique.[25] At the end of the 30-day follow-up, mortality was significantly lower in the endovascular technique group (*relative risk reduction* [RRR], 0.61; 95% CI, 0.13-0.82). The investigators followed up participants for an additional 2 years and found that there was no difference in mortality between groups after the first year. Had the trial ended earlier, the endovascular technique may have been considered substantially better than the open surgical technique.

Were Patients Analyzed in the Groups to Which They Were Randomized?

Investigators will undermine the benefits of randomization if they omit from the analysis patients who do not receive their assigned treatment or, worse yet, count events that occur in *nonadherent* patients who were assigned to treatment against the control group. Such analyses will bias the results if the reasons for nonadherence are related to prognosis. In a number of randomized trials, patients who did not adhere to their assigned drug regimens fared worse than those who took their medication as instructed, even after taking into account all known prognostic factors.[26-31] When adherent patients are destined to have a better

outcome, omitting those who do not receive assigned treatment undermines the unbiased comparison provided by randomization. Investigators prevent this bias when they follow the *intention-to-treat* principle and analyze all patients in the group to which they were randomized irrespective of what treatment they actually received (see Chapter 11.4, The Principle of Intention to Treat and Ambiguous Dropouts).[32] Following the intention-to-treat principle does not, however, reduce bias associated with loss to follow-up.[33]

USING THE GUIDE

Returning to our opening clinical scenario, did the experimental and control groups begin the study with a similar prognosis? The study was randomized and allocation was concealed; 212 patients participated and 95% were followed up.[4] The investigators followed the intention-to-treat principle, including all patients they had followed up in the arm to which they were randomized, and stopped when they reached the planned sample size. There were more patients who had occlusive arterial disease (39.6% vs 22.7%) in the ramipril group. This finding could bias the results in favor of the placebo group, and the investigators do not provide an adjusted analysis for the baseline differences. Clinicians, patients, data collectors, outcomes assessors, and data analysts were all blind to allocation.

The final risk of bias assessment represents a continuum from studies that are at very low risk of bias to others that are at very high risk of yielding a biased estimate of effect. Inevitably, where a study lies in this continuum involves some judgment. In this case, despite uncertainty about baseline differences between the groups, we conclude that the risk of bias is low.

WHAT ARE THE RESULTS?

How Large Was the Treatment Effect?

Most frequently, RCTs monitor *dichotomous* outcomes (eg, "yes" or "no" classifications for cancer recurrence, myocardial infarction, or death). Patients

TABLE 7-2

Results From a Hypothetical Randomized Trial

Exposure	Outcome, No. of Patients		
	Death	Survival	Total
Treatment (experimental)	15	85	100
Control	20	80	100

Control group risk (CGR): 20/100 = 20%

Experimental group risk (EGR): 15/100 = 15%

Absolute risk reduction or risk difference: CGR − EGR, 20% − 15% = 5%

Relative risk: EGR/CGR = (15/100)/(20/100) × 100% = 75%

Relative risk reduction: [1 − (EGR/CGR)] × 100% = 1 − 75% = 25%

Abbreviations: CGR, control group risk; EGR, experimental group risk.

either have such an event or they do not, and the article reports the proportion of patients who develop such events. Consider, for example, a study in which 20% of a control group died but only 15% of those receiving a new treatment died (Table 7-2). How might one express these results?

One possibility is the absolute difference (known as the *absolute risk reduction* [ARR] or *risk difference*) between the proportion who died in the control group (*control group risk* [CGR]) and the proportion who died in the experimental group (*experimental group risk* [EGR]), or CGR − EGR = 0.20 − 0.15 = 0.05. Another way to express the impact of treatment is as the RR: the risk of events among patients receiving the new treatment relative to that risk among patients in the control group, or EGR/CGR = 0.15/0.20 = 0.75.

The most commonly reported measure of dichotomous treatment effects is the complement of the RR, the RRR. It is expressed as a percentage: 1 − (EGR/CGR) = 100% = (1 − 0.75) × 100% = 25%. An RRR of 25% means that of those who would have died had they been in the control group, 25% will not die if they receive treatment; the greater the RRR, the more effective the therapy. Investigators may compute the RR during a specified period, as in a *survival analysis*; the relative measure of effect in such a time-to-event analysis is called the *hazard ratio* (see Chapter 9, Does Treatment Lower Risk? Understanding the Results). When people do not specify whether they

are talking about RRR or ARR—for instance, "Drug X was 30% effective in reducing the risk of death" or "The efficacy of the vaccine was 92%"—they are almost invariably talking about RRR (see Chapter 9, Does Treatment Lower Risk? Understanding the Results).

How Precise Was the Estimate of the Treatment Effect?

We can never be sure of the true risk reduction; the best estimate of the true treatment effect is what we observe in a well-designed randomized trial. This estimate is called a *point estimate* to remind us that, although the true value lies somewhere in its neighborhood, it is unlikely to be precisely correct. Investigators often tell us the neighborhood within which the true effect likely lies by calculating CIs, a range of values within which one can be confident the true effect lies.[34]

We usually use the 95% CI (see Chapter 10, Confidence Intervals: Was the Single Study or Meta-analysis Large Enough?). You can consider the 95% CI as defining the range that—assuming the study has low risk of bias—includes the true RRR 95% of the time. The true RRR will generally lie beyond these extremes only 5% of the time, a property of the CI that relates closely to the conventional level of *statistical significance* of P <.05. We illustrate the use of CIs in the following examples.

Example 1

If a trial randomized 100 patients each to experimental and control groups, and there were 20 deaths in the control group and 15 deaths in the experimental group, the authors would calculate a point estimate for the RRR of 25% [CGR = 20/100 or 0.20, EGR = 15/100 or 0.15, and 1 − EGR/CGR = (1 − 0.75) × 100 = 25%]. You might guess, however, that the true RRR might be much smaller or much greater than 25%, based on a difference of only 5 deaths. In fact, you might surmise that the treatment might provide no benefit (an RRR of 0%) or might even do harm (a negative RRR). And you would be right; in fact, these results are consistent with both an RRR of −38% (that is, patients given the new treatment might be 38% more likely to die than control patients) and an RRR of nearly 59% (that is, patients subsequently receiving the new treatment might have a risk of dying almost 60% less than those who are not treated). In other words, the 95% CI on this RRR is −38% to 59%, and the trial really has not helped us decide whether or not to offer the new treatment (Figure 7-1).

Example 2

What if the trial enrolled 1000 patients per group rather than 100 patients per group, and the same event rates were observed as before, so that there were 200 deaths in the control group (CGR = 200/1000 = 0.20) and 150 deaths in the experimental group (EGR = 150/1000 = 0.15)? Again, the point estimate of the RRR is 25% (1 − EGR/CGR = 1 − [0.15/0.20] × 100 = 25%).

In this larger trial, you might think that our confidence that the true reduction in risk is close to 25% is much greater; again, you would be right. The 95% CI on the RRR for this set of results is all on the positive side of 0 and runs from 9% to 41% (Figure 7-1).

These examples show that the larger the sample size and higher the number of outcome events in a trial, the greater our confidence that the true RRR (or any other measure of effect) is close to what we observed. The point estimate—in this case, 25%—is the one value most likely to represent the true RRR. As one considers values farther and farther from the point estimate, they become less and less likely to represent the truth. By the time one crosses the upper or lower boundaries of the 95% CI, the values are unlikely to represent the true RRR. All of this assumes the study is at low risk of bias.

Not all randomized trials have dichotomous outcomes, nor should they. In a study of respiratory muscle training for patients with chronic airflow limitation, one primary outcome measured how far patients could

FIGURE 7-1

Confidence Intervals in Trials of Various Sample Size

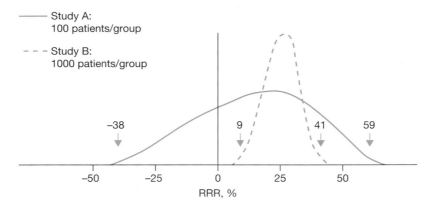

Abbreviation: RRR, relative risk reduction.

Two studies with the same point estimate, a 25% RRR, but different sample sizes and correspondingly different CIs. The x-axis represents the different possible RRR, and the y-axis represents the likelihood of the true RRR having that particular value. The solid line represents the CI around the first example, in which there were 100 patients per group, and the number of events in the active and control groups were 15 and 20, respectively. The dashed line represents the CI around the second example, in which there were 1000 patients per group, and the number of events in the active and control groups were 150 and 200, respectively.

walk in 6 minutes in an enclosed corridor.[35] This 6-minute walk improved from a mean of 406 to 416 m (up 10 m) in the experimental group receiving respiratory muscle training, and 409 to 429 m (up 20 m) in the control group. The point estimate for improvement in the 6-minute walk due to respiratory muscle training therefore was negative, at −10 m (or a 10-m difference in favor of the control group).

Here, too, you should look for the 95% CIs around this difference in changes in exercise capacity and consider their implications. The investigators tell us that the lower boundary of the 95% CI was −26 (ie, the results are consistent with a difference of 26 m in favor of the control treatment) and the upper boundary was 5 m. Even in the best of circumstances, patients are unlikely to perceive adding 5 m to the 400 recorded at the start of the trial as important, and this result effectively excludes an important benefit of respiratory muscle training as applied in this study.

Having determined the magnitude and precision of the treatment effect, clinicians can turn to the final question of how to apply the article's results to their patients.

USING THE GUIDE

Using the numbers provided in the article,[4] patients in the ramipril group walked 75 seconds (95% CI, 60-89 seconds) longer without pain than the placebo group and 255 seconds (95% CI, 215-295 seconds) longer overall. The effect of ramipril is convincing given that the 95% CIs are narrow and the lower boundaries are far from showing no effect (ie, 0 seconds). The clinical importance of walking 75 seconds without pain is likely noticeable given that they could walk a mean of 140 seconds without pain at baseline. This finding is consistent with a substantial improvement in a secondary outcome, a measure of health-related quality of life, for patients in the ramipril group.

HOW CAN I APPLY THE RESULTS TO PATIENT CARE?

Were the Study Patients Similar to the Patient in My Practice?

If the patient before you would have qualified for enrollment in the study, you can apply the results with considerable confidence or consider the results *generalizable*. Often, your patient has different attributes or characteristics from those enrolled in the trial and would not have met a study's eligibility criteria. Patients may be older or younger, may be sicker or less sick, or may have comorbid disease that would have excluded them from participation in the study.

A study result probably applies even if, for example, adult patients are 2 years too old for enrollment in the study, had more severe disease, had previously been treated with a competing therapy, or had a comorbid condition. A better approach than rigidly applying the study *inclusion* and *exclusion criteria* is to ask whether there is some compelling reason why the results do not apply to the patient. You usually will not find a compelling reason, in which case you can generalize the results to your patient with confidence.

A related issue has to do with the extent to which we can generalize findings from a study using a particular drug to another closely (or not so closely) related agent. The issue of drug *class effects* and how conservative one should be in assuming class effects remains controversial (see Chapter 28.4, Understanding Class Effects). Generalizing findings of surgical treatment may be even riskier. Randomized trials of carotid endarterectomy, for instance, demonstrate much lower perioperative rates of stroke and death than one might expect in one's own community, which may reflect on either the patients or surgeons (and their relative expertise) selected to participate in randomized trials.[36] An example of how expertise might be considered is provided below.

Expertise in Procedural Interventions

Unlike pharmacologic interventions in which we expect the intervention to vary minimally between patients, procedural interventions may differ substantially based on the expertise of the physician and the technology available to deliver the intervention.

For example, it is suggested that "off-pump" coronary artery bypass surgery reduces the risk of postoperative complications compared with the traditional "on-pump" technique. When the 2 techniques are compared in a randomized trial, one must be careful interpreting the results because of potential differences in expertise. For example, if surgeons participating in the trial are, on average, less skilled with the off-pump technique, the outcomes of patients in the off-pump group may reflect surgeon inexperience more than the true risks and merits of the technique. Further, surgeons may choose to switch from off-pump to on-pump technique more frequently than they would switch from on-pump to off-pump. This will bias the result toward demonstrating no difference between the techniques. One way of preventing these misleading results is by ensuring only surgeons with sufficient expertise in both on-pump and off-pump techniques are allowed to participate in the trial, as was done in the CABG Off or On Pump Revascularization Study (CORONARY) trial.[37] Another method of preventing this differential expertise bias is to randomize patients to a surgeon with expertise in one technique or to a surgeon with expertise in the alternate technique rather than randomize the patient to a surgeon who will perform either procedure to which the patient is randomized.[38]

A final issue arises when a patient fits the features of a subgroup of patients in the trial report. We encourage you to be skeptical of *subgroup analyses*.[39] The treatment is likely to benefit the subgroup more or less than the other patients only if the difference in the effects of treatment in the subgroups is large and unlikely to occur by chance. Even when these conditions apply, the results may be misleading, particularly when investigators did not specify their hypotheses before the study

began, if they had a large number of hypotheses, or if other studies fail to replicate the finding.[40]

Were All Patient-Important Outcomes Considered?

Treatments are indicated when they provide important benefits. Demonstrating that a bronchodilator produces small increments in forced expiratory volume in patients with chronic airflow limitation, that a vasodilator improves cardiac output in heart failure patients, or that a lipid-lowering agent improves lipid profiles does not provide sufficient justification for administering these drugs (see Chapter 13.4, Surrogate Outcomes). In these instances, investigators have chosen *substitute outcomes* or *surrogate outcomes* rather than those that patients would consider important. What clinicians and patients require is evidence that the treatments improve outcomes that are important to patients, such as reducing shortness of breath during the activities required for daily living, avoiding hospitalization for heart failure, or decreasing the risk of a major stroke.[41]

Trials of the impact of antiarrhythmic drugs after myocardial infarction illustrate the danger of using substitute outcomes or end points. Because abnormal ventricular depolarizations were associated with a high risk of death and antiarrhythmic drugs demonstrated a reduction in abnormal ventricular depolarizations (the substitute end point), it made sense that they should reduce death. A group of investigators performed randomized trials on 3 agents (encainide, flecainide, and moricizine) that were previously found to be effective in suppressing the substitute end point of abnormal ventricular depolarizations. The investigators had to stop the trials when they discovered that mortality was substantially higher in patients receiving antiarrhythmic treatment than in those receiving placebo.[42,43] Clinicians relying on the substitute end point of arrhythmia suppression would have continued to administer the 3 drugs, to the considerable detriment of their patients (for additional examples of misleading surrogates, see Chapter 11.2, Surprising Results of Randomized Trials).

Even when investigators report favorable effects of treatment on a patient-important outcome, you must consider whether there may be deleterious effects on other outcomes. For instance, cancer chemotherapy

TABLE 7-3

Considerations in the Decision to Treat 2 Patients With Myocardial Infarction With Clopidogrel and Aspirin or Aspirin Alone

	Risk of Death or MI 1 Year After MI With Aspirin Alone (CER)	Risk With Clopidogrel Plus Aspirin (EGR) (ARR = CGR − EGR)	NNT (100/ARR When ARR Is Expressed as a Percentage)
40-year-old man with small MI	5.3%	4.2% (1.1% or 0.011)	91
70-year-old man with large MI and heart failure	36%	28.8% (7.2% or 0.072)	14

Abbreviations: ARR, absolute risk reduction; CER, control event rate; CGR, control group risk; EGR, experimental group risk; MI, myocardial infarction; NNT, number needed to treat.

may lengthen life but decrease its quality. Randomized trials often fail to adequately document the toxicity or adverse effects of the experimental intervention.[44]

Composite end points represent a final dangerous trend in presenting outcomes (see Chapter 12.4, Composite End Points). Like surrogate outcomes, composite end points are attractive for reducing sample size and decreasing length of follow-up. Unfortunately, they can mislead. For example, a trial that reduced a composite outcome of death, nonfatal myocardial infarction, and admission for an acute coronary syndrome actually demonstrated a trend toward increased mortality with the experimental therapy and convincing effects only on admission for an acute coronary syndrome.[45] The composite outcome would most strongly reflect the treatment effect of the most common of the components, admission for an acute coronary syndrome, even though there is no convincing evidence the treatment reduces the risk of death or myocardial infarction.

Another long-neglected outcome is the resource implications of alternative management strategies. Health care systems face increasing resource constraints that mandate careful attention to *economic analysis* (see Chapter 28.2, Economic Analysis).

Are the Likely Treatment Benefits Worth the Potential Harm and Costs?

If the results of a study apply to your patient and the outcomes are important to your patient, the next question concerns whether the probable treatment benefits are worth the associated *risks*, *burden*, and resource requirements. A 25% reduction in the RR of death may sound impressive, but its impact on your patient may nevertheless be minimal. This notion is illustrated by using a concept called *number needed to treat* (NNT), the number of patients who must receive an intervention of therapy during a specific period to prevent 1 adverse outcome or produce 1 positive outcome.[46]

The impact of a treatment is related not only to its RRR but also to the risk of the adverse outcome it is designed to prevent. One large trial in myocardial infarction suggests that clopidogrel in addition to aspirin reduces the RR of death from a cardiovascular cause, nonfatal myocardial infarction, or stroke by approximately 20% in comparison to aspirin alone.[47] Table 7-3 considers 2 patients presenting with acute myocardial infarction without elevation of ST segments on their electrocardiograms.

In the first case, a 40-year-old man presents with electrocardiographic findings that suggest an inferior myocardial infarction without ST-segment elevation. You find no signs of heart failure; the patient is in normal sinus rhythm, with a rate of 80/min; and he does not have elevated troponin. This individual's risk of death or recurrent myocardial infarction in the next year is estimated to be 5.3%. Compared with aspirin alone, clopidogrel in addition to aspirin would reduce this risk by 20% to 4.2%, an ARR of 1.1% (0.011). The inverse of this

ARR (ie, 100 divided by the ARR expressed as a percentage) is equal to the number of such patients we would have to treat to prevent 1 event (ie, 1 death, or recurrent myocardial infarction after a mild myocardial infarction in a low-risk patient), the NNT. In this case, we would have to treat approximately 91 such patients to prevent 1 recurrent myocardial infarction or save 1 life (100/1.1 = 91). Given the small decrease in the outcome of death, recurrent myocardial infarction, or stroke (most noticeably recurrent myocardial infarction) with clopidogrel, the small increased risk of major bleeding associated with clopidogrel, and its additional cost, many clinicians might prefer aspirin alone in this patient.

In the second case, a 70-year-old man presents with electrocardiographic signs of anterior myocardial infarction with pulmonary edema and cardiogenic shock. His risk of dying or having a recurrent myocardial infarction in the subsequent year is approximately 36%. A 20% RRR of death in such a high-risk patient generates an ARR of 7.2% (0.072), and we would have to treat only 14 such individuals to avert a recurrent myocardial infarction or death (100/7.2 = 13.8). Many clinicians would consider clopidogrel in addition to aspirin.

A key element of the decision to start therapy, therefore, is to consider the patient's risk of the event if left untreated. For any given RRR, the higher the probability that a patient will experience an adverse outcome if we do not treat, the more likely the patient will benefit from treatment and the fewer such patients we need to treat to prevent 1 adverse outcome (see Chapter 9, Does Treatment Lower Risk? Understanding the Results). Knowing the NNT assists clinicians in helping patients weigh the benefits and downsides associated with their management options.

Trading off benefits and risks also requires an accurate assessment of the adverse effects of treatment. Randomized trials with relatively small sample sizes are unsuitable for detecting rare but catastrophic adverse effects of therapy. Clinicians often must look to other sources of information—often characterized by higher risk of bias—to obtain an estimate of the adverse effects of therapy (see Chapter 14, Harm [Observational Studies]).

When determining the optimal treatment choice based on the relative benefits and harms of a therapy, the *values and preferences* of each individual patient must be considered. How best to communicate information to patients and how to incorporate their values into clinical decision making remain areas of active investigation in *evidence-based medicine* (see Chapter 27, Decision Making and the Patient).

CLINICAL SCENARIO RESOLUTION

The study that we identified found an increase in pain-free and total walking time of patients with peripheral arterial disease treated with ramipril compared with placebo.[4] The authors did not describe any harmful effects of ramipril other than more withdrawals due to cough than placebo-treated patients. This finding may leave some uncertainty as to the net benefits to patients. In particular, there is no mention of kidney failure or hyperkalemia-induced cardiac arrest, the most serious adverse effects associated with ramipril. However, there is a large body of literature on patients with other types of vascular disease that suggests that ramipril, at the dose used in this study, is well tolerated and safe, particularly if clinicians monitor patients periodically for the precursors to these adverse effects (ie, changes in kidney function or serum potassium).

Your patient is significantly limited by his intermittent claudication. He is similar to patients included in this study. Given the treatment effect on walking time and the observed effect on health-related quality of life, as well as an apparently minimal side effect profile, the study suggests patient-important benefits to taking ramipril.

The patient finds his limited walking ability and the pain he experiences debilitating. He believes that being able to walk for 1 additional minute would be worthwhile. He is, however, under financial stress and is concerned that ramipril costs $1.20 per pill, or approximately $450 in the next year. You explain that the investigators' choice of medication leaves some doubt about the best drug to use. The investigators could have chosen lisinopril, an ACE inhibitor with marginal differences from ramipril, which the patient can purchase for approximately one-third the price. Ultimately, implicitly accepting a class effect, the patient chooses the lisinopril.

References

1. Momsen AH, Jensen MB, Norager CB, Madsen MR, Vestersgaard-Andersen T, Lindholt JS. Drug therapy for improving walking distance in intermittent claudication: a systematic review and meta-analysis of robust randomised controlled studies. *Eur J Vasc Endovasc Surg*. 2009;38(4):463-474.

2. Wong PF, Chong L-Y, Stansby G. Antiplatelet therapy to prevent cardiovascular events and mortality in patients with intermittent claudication. *JAMA*. 2013;309(9):926-927.

3. Jaar BG. ACP Journal Club. Ramipril improved walking times and QOL in peripheral artery disease and intermittent claudication. *Ann Intern Med*. 2013;158(12):JC7.

4. Ahimastos AA, Walker PJ, Askew C, et al. Effect of ramipril on walking times and quality of life among patients with peripheral artery disease and intermittent claudication: a randomized controlled trial. *JAMA*. 2013;309(5):453-460.

5. Hu FB, Bronner L, Willett WC, et al. Fish and omega-3 fatty acid intake and risk of coronary heart disease in women. *JAMA*. 2002;287(14):1815-1821.

6. Kotwal S, Jun M, Sullivan D, Perkovic V, Neal B. Omega 3 fatty acids and cardiovascular outcomes: systematic review and meta-analysis. *Circ Cardiovasc Qual Outcomes*. 2012;5(6):808-818.

7. Bosch J, Gerstein HC, Dagenais GR, et al; ORIGIN Trial Investigators. n-3 fatty acids and cardiovascular outcomes in patients with dysglycemia. *N Engl J Med*. 2012;367(4):309-318.

8. Bjelakovic G, Nikolova D, Simonetti RG, Gluud C. Antioxidant supplements for prevention of gastrointestinal cancers: a systematic review and meta-analysis. *Lancet*. 2004;364(9441):1219-1228.

9. Miller ER III, Pastor-Barriuso R, Dalal D, Riemersma RA, Appel LJ, Guallar E. Meta-analysis: high-dosage vitamin E supplementation may increase all-cause mortality. *Ann Intern Med*. 2005;142(1):37-46.

10. Ikram H, Crozier IG. Xamoterol in severe heart failure. *Lancet*. 1990;336(8713):517-518.

11. Califf RM, Adams KF, McKenna WJ, et al. A randomized controlled trial of epoprostenol therapy for severe congestive heart failure: The Flolan International Randomized Survival Trial (FIRST). *Am Heart J*. 1997;134(1):44-54.

12. Hampton JR, van Veldhuisen DJ, Kleber FX, et al; Second Prospective Randomised Study of Ibopamine on Mortality and Efficacy (PRIME II) Investigators. Randomised study of effect of ibopamine on survival in patients with advanced severe heart failure. *Lancet*. 1997;349(9057):971-977.

13. Schulz KF, Chalmers I, Hayes RJ, Altman DG. Empirical evidence of bias: dimensions of methodological quality associated with estimates of treatment effects in controlled trials. *JAMA*. 1995;273(5):408-412.

14. Moher D, Pham B, Jones A, et al. Does quality of reports of randomised trials affect estimates of intervention efficacy reported in meta-analyses? *Lancet*. 1998;352(9128):609-613.

15. Balk EM, Bonis PA, Moskowitz H, et al. Correlation of quality measures with estimates of treatment effect in meta-analyses of randomized controlled trials. *JAMA*. 2002;287(22):2973-2982.

16. Hansson L, Lindholm LH, Niskanen L, et al. Effect of angiotensin-converting-enzyme inhibition compared with conventional therapy on cardiovascular morbidity and mortality in hypertension: the Captopril Prevention Project (CAPPP) randomised trial. *Lancet*. 1999;353(9153):611-616.

17. Kaptchuk TJ. Powerful placebo: the dark side of the randomised controlled trial. *Lancet*. 1998;351(9117):1722-1725.

18. Hróbjartsson A, Gøtzsche PC. Is the placebo powerless? An analysis of clinical trials comparing placebo with no treatment. *N Engl J Med*. 2001;344(21):1594-1602.

19. McRae C, Cherin E, Yamazaki TG, et al. Effects of perceived treatment on quality of life and medical outcomes in a double-blind placebo surgery trial. *Arch Gen Psychiatry*. 2004;61(4):412-420.

20. Rana JS, Mannam A, Donnell-Fink L, Gervino EV, Sellke FW, Laham RJ. Longevity of the placebo effect in the therapeutic angiogenesis and laser myocardial revascularization trials in patients with coronary heart disease. *Am J Cardiol*. 2005;95(12):1456-1459.

21. Noseworthy JH, Ebers GC, Vandervoort MK, Farquhar RE, Yetisir E, Roberts R. The impact of blinding on the results of a randomized, placebo-controlled multiple sclerosis clinical trial. *Neurology*. 1994;44(1):16-20.

22. Ioannidis JP, Bassett R, Hughes MD, Volberding PA, Sacks HS, Lau J. Predictors and impact of patients lost to follow-up in a long-term randomized trial of immediate versus deferred antiretroviral treatment. *J Acquir Immune Defic Syndr Hum Retrovirol*. 1997;16(1):22-30.

23. Akl EA, Briel M, You JJ, et al. Potential impact on estimated treatment effects of information lost to follow-up in randomised controlled trials (LOST-IT): systematic review. *BMJ*. 2012;344:e2809.

24. Montori VM, Devereaux PJ, Adhikari NK, et al. Randomized trials stopped early for benefit: a systematic review. *JAMA*. 2005;294(17):2203-2209.

25. Greenhalgh RM, Brown LC, Powell JT, Thompson SG, Epstein D, Sculpher MJ; United Kingdom EVAR Trial Investigators. Endovascular versus open repair of abdominal aortic aneurysm. *N Engl J Med*. 2010;362(20):1863-1871.

26. The Coronary Drug Project Research Group. Influence of adherence to treatment and response of cholesterol on mortality in the coronary drug project. *N Engl J Med*. 1980;303(18):1038-1041.

27. Asher WL, Harper HW. Effect of human chorionic gonadotrophin on weight loss, hunger, and feeling of well-being. *Am J Clin Nutr*. 1973;26(2):211-218.

28. Hogarty GE, Goldberg SC. Drug and sociotherapy in the aftercare of schizophrenic patients: one-year relapse rates. *Arch Gen Psychiatry*. 1973;28(1):54-64.

29. Fuller R, Roth H, Long S. Compliance with disulfiram treatment of alcoholism. *J Chronic Dis*. 1983;36(2):161-170.

30. Pizzo PA, Robichaud KJ, Edwards BK, Schumaker C, Kramer BS, Johnson A. Oral antibiotic prophylaxis in patients with cancer: a double-blind randomized placebo-controlled trial. *J Pediatr*. 1983;102(1):125-133.

31. Horwitz RI, Viscoli CM, Berkman L, et al. Treatment adherence and risk of death after a myocardial infarction. *Lancet*. 1990;336(8714):542-545.

32. Montori VM, Guyatt GH. Intention-to-treat principle. *CMAJ*. 2001;165(10):1339-1341.

33. Alshurafa M, Briel M, Akl EA, et al. Inconsistent definitions for intention-to-treat in relation to missing outcome data: systematic review of the methods literature. *PLoS One*. 2012;7(11):e49163.

34. Altman DG, Gore SM, Gardner MJ, Pocock SJ. Statistical guidelines for contributors to medical journals. *Br Med J (Clin Res Ed)*. 1983;286(6376):1489-1493.

35. Guyatt G, Keller J, Singer J, Halcrow S, Newhouse M. Controlled trial of respiratory muscle training in chronic airflow limitation. *Thorax*. 1992;47(8):598-602.

36. Walker MD, Marler JR, Goldstein M, et al; Executive Committee for the Asymptomatic Carotid Atherosclerosis Study. Endarterectomy for asymptomatic carotid artery stenosis. *JAMA*. 1995;273(18):1421-1428.

37. Lamy A, Devereaux PJ, Prabhakaran D, et al; CORONARY Investigators. Off-pump or on-pump coronary-artery bypass grafting at 30 days. *N Engl J Med*. 2012;366(16):1489-1497.

38. Devereaux PJ, Bhandari M, Clarke M, et al. Need for expertise based randomised controlled trials. *BMJ*. 2005;330(7482):88.

39. Oxman AD, Guyatt GH. A consumer's guide to subgroup analyses. *Ann Intern Med*. 1992;116(1):78-84.

40. Sun X, Briel M, Walter SD, Guyatt GH. Is a subgroup effect believable? updating criteria to evaluate the credibility of subgroup analyses. *BMJ*. 2010;340:c117.

41. Guyatt G, Montori V, Devereaux PJ, Schünemann H, Bhandari M. Patients at the center: in our practice, and in our use of language. *ACP J Club*. 2004;140(1):A11-A12.

42. Echt DS, Liebson PR, Mitchell LB, et al. Mortality and morbidity in patients receiving encainide, flecainide, or placebo: The Cardiac Arrhythmia Suppression Trial. *N Engl J Med*. 1991;324(12):781-788.

43. Rogers W, Epstein A, Arciniegas J, et al; The Cardiac Arrhythmia Suppression Trial II Investigators. Effect of the antiarrhythmic agent moricizine on survival after myocardial infarction. *N Engl J Med*. 1992;327(4):227-233.

44. Ioannidis JP, Lau J. Completeness of safety reporting in randomized trials: an evaluation of 7 medical areas. *JAMA*. 2001;285(4):437-443.

45. Pfisterer M, Buser P, Osswald S, et al; Trial of Invasive versus Medical therapy in Elderly patients (TIME) Investigators. Outcome of elderly patients with chronic symptomatic coronary artery disease with an invasive vs optimized medical treatment strategy: one-year results of the randomized TIME trial. *JAMA*. 2003;289(9):1117-1123.

46. Laupacis A, Sackett DL, Roberts RS. An assessment of clinically useful measures of the consequences of treatment. *N Engl J Med*. 1988;318(26):1728-1733.

47. Yusuf S, Zhao F, Mehta SR, Chrolavicius S, Tognoni G, Fox KK; Clopidogrel in Unstable Angina to Prevent Recurrent Events Trial Investigators. Effects of clopidogrel in addition to aspirin in patients with acute coronary syndromes without ST-segment elevation. *N Engl J Med*. 2001;345(7):494-502.

THERAPY

8

How to Use a Noninferiority Trial

Sohail M. Mulla, Ian A. Scott, Cynthia A. Jackevicius,
John J. You, and Gordon Guyatt

THERAPY

IN THIS CHAPTER

You are an internist seeing a 51-year-old woman with severe osteoarthritis and limited mobility who presents with progressive dyspnea for a 3-day period. She is subjectively in distress, with a pulse of 105/min, a respiratory rate of 28/min, and an arterial oxygen saturation of 85% while breathing room air. Aside from her arthritis, the physical examination findings are unremarkable, and a lower-extremity examination reveals no sign of deep venous thrombosis. A computed tomographic (CT) pulmonary angiogram reveals unequivocal clot in 2 lobar arteries.

Recently, you have been treating patients with deep venous thrombosis without hospital admission using low-molecular-weight heparin (LMWH) administration in the outpatient setting. You are less comfortable not admitting a patient in the more dangerous setting of pulmonary embolism. You recall receiving, from the updating service to which you subscribe (see Chapter 5, Finding Current Best Evidence), a recent *randomized trial* that addressed this issue. Before discussing the issue of inpatient vs outpatient treatment with your patient, you quickly review the article.[1] In doing so, you find that the trial tested for *noninferiority* and you wonder, as you begin to read the methods and results, if there are special issues you should consider when using this article to guide your clinical care.

INTRODUCTION

Traditionally, randomized clinical trials (RCTs) have sought to ascertain whether an experimental treatment is superior to standard treatment or *placebo* in improving quality of life or preventing morbid or mortal events—what we will refer to as effectiveness outcomes. In these superiority trials, the primary objective is to determine the magnitude of increased benefit of the experimental intervention over standard therapy on effectiveness outcomes.

Recently, another paradigm has emerged that offers novel experimental treatments not on the basis of superiority in effectiveness outcomes but instead

because they reduce harms or other treatment burdens relative to standard treatment. In modern medicine, clinicians are fortunate to have many effective treatments; unfortunately, these treatments are often associated with *harms*, inconvenience, or excessive cost. For these interventions, reducing treatment *burden*, including limitations and inconvenience, becomes a legitimate goal of innovative therapy.

In such instances, a question arises: can clinicians be confident that the experimental treatment's impact on effectiveness outcomes—the prime reason for wanting to prescribe it—is sufficiently close to that of standard treatment that they are comfortable substituting it for the existing standard? In technical terms, is the novel treatment noninferior to the standard treatment?

Noninferiority trials provide an alternative to *equivalence trials*, which endeavor to establish that an experimental treatment is neither better nor worse (beyond a specified margin) than the standard. In contrast, the noninferiority trialist is unconcerned if the experimental treatment is better as long as it is "not much worse." Perhaps illustrating the limitations of the term, a noninferior treatment may thus be inferior, just not so inferior that it would cause concern. How much worse (ie, how much less effective) clinicians should consider acceptable will depend on the importance of the effectiveness outcome and the magnitude of the reduction in harms or burden achieved by the new treatment.

Consider how the concept of "not much worse" plays out for the patient in the previously presented scenario. She may dislike spending time in the hospital and may strongly prefer treatment at home, but there may be risks she incurs in choosing home management. Perhaps the care she would receive in the hospital would result in a lower risk of recurrent venous thromboembolism (VTE) and a lower risk of serious bleeding, which can complicate antithrombotic therapy. Would our patient be willing to incur the additional risk of VTE or serious bleeding that may be associated with home management? If so, what level of increased risk would she be willing to tolerate?

The example illustrates the following point: given that patients will choose the new experimental treatment only if the risks are not much worse than the standard treatment, the critical issue in interpreting noninferiority trials is the choice of an acceptable threshold of "not much worse." This noninferiority threshold (the dashed line labeled Δ in Figure 8-1) is the maximum allowable excess of outcome events that arises from the experimental treatment compared with the standard treatment.

When designing noninferiority trials, investigators set their own thresholds, typically using statistically based criteria. However, there is no universally accepted method for defining an appropriate threshold. It depends on the eye of the beholder. Experts have recommended using sound statistical reasoning and clinical judgment in determining noninferiority thresholds.[2,3] What is sound reasoning for one observer, however, may strike another as misguided.

The US Food and Drug Administration (FDA) has produced draft guidance regarding noninferiority thresholds that has proved highly influential.[4] The logic of the FDA's approach begins by considering the smallest plausible benefit achieved by the existing standard treatment with which the experimental—and it is hoped noninferior—treatment is compared. One establishes the smallest plausible benefit of the existing standard treatment by examining the results of a trial of that treatment against the previous best

care or placebo. To establish the smallest plausible benefit, one focuses on the *confidence interval* (CI) around the observed estimate of effect (in technical terms, the CI around the point estimate) and, in particular, the boundary of the CI nearest to no effect.

For instance, the point estimate may suggest that the existing standard treatment decreases the absolute incidence of stroke, relative to placebo, by an absolute difference of 3%, with a 95% CI of 2% to 4% (Figure 8-2, top graph). The smallest plausible benefit of the standard drug is then 2%, or 2 fewer strokes for every 100 patients treated.

If the 95% CIs around the difference in strokes in a subsequent trial testing an experimental drug for noninferiority include an increase in strokes of 2% (for instance, a point estimate of no difference, with a CI of a 2% decrease to a 2% increase), the results are consistent with the new drug being no better than placebo (Figure 8-2, scenario A). This is because the absolute benefit of the existing standard may be a reduction in strokes of as little as 2%, and those receiving the experimental treatment may have a stroke rate of 2% more than the standard treatment—exactly equivalent to the rate on placebo.

The logic then goes that we should insist on some preservation of the treatment effect. Commonly, drug regulatory authorities stipulate that at least 50% of that minimal treatment effect be preserved. The threshold would, in this example, be 1%; if the experimental

FIGURE 8-1

Possible Outcome Scenarios in Noninferiority Trials

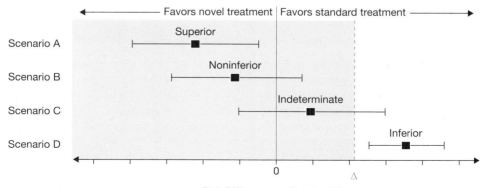

The dashed line labeled Δ represents the noninferiority threshold or the maximum allowable excess of outcome events arising from the experimental treatment compared with the standard treatment. The tinted area represents the noninferiority zone.

FIGURE 8-2

Setting an Acceptable Noninferiority Threshold

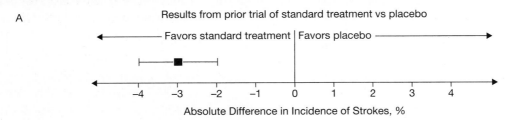

A   Results from prior trial of standard treatment vs placebo

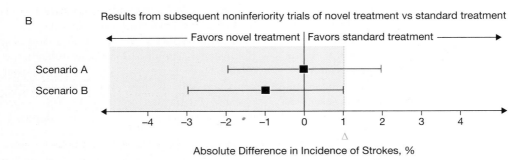

B   Results from subsequent noninferiority trials of novel treatment vs standard treatment

A, Standard treatment decreases the absolute incidence of stroke, relative to placebo, by 3%, with a 95% CI of 2% to 4%. B, The blue dashed line represents the noninferiority zone. In scenario A, the 95% CIs around the difference in strokes between the experimental treatment and the standard treatment include an increase in incidence of strokes by as much as 2% with the experimental treatment, thereby failing to retain 50% of the minimal treatment effect of the standard treatment. In scenario B, the same 95% CIs suggest that the experimental treatment increases the incidence of strokes by no more than 1%, thus successfully preserving at least 50% of the 2% absolute reduction in stroke with the standard treatment.

treatment increases strokes by no more than 1% relative to the existing standard, at least 50% of the 2% absolute reduction in stroke has been preserved[5,6] (Figure 8-2, scenario B). Depending on the seriousness of the outcome, some may argue for retaining a greater proportion of benefit, resulting in a more challenging noninferiority margin. We have focused herein on expression of the noninferiority margin in absolute terms; sometimes, the choice of threshold is based on a relative rather than an absolute effect.

USING THE GUIDE

Sometimes, the standard approaches to setting noninferiority thresholds are not applicable, as was the case in the trial of inpatient vs outpatient treatment for pulmonary embolism. Because there are no randomized trials that compare anticoagulation to no anticoagulation in pulmonary embolism, the authors could not use the procedure for setting the noninferiority margin described in the previously presented scenario. As an alternative, they first considered the likelihood of recurrent VTE at 90 days in low-risk inpatients with pulmonary embolism, which they estimated at 0.9%. They then specified a noninferiority margin of 4% (implying that patients would find it acceptable if the rate of recurrent VTE for outpatients would be <4.9%). They justified their choice by saying that it was similar to the noninferiority margins—3% to 5%—set in other trials of different anticoagulant regimens in acute VTE and outpatient vs inpatient treatment for deep venous thrombosis. The authors implicitly chose the same noninferiority margin (4%) for bleeding, although they provide no justification for this choice.

When subsequently reviewing their results, if investigators find that the CI around the estimate for the difference in primary outcome events lies entirely below their chosen noninferiority threshold, they will claim noninferiority (Figure 8-1, scenario B) or even, in some instances, superiority of the experimental treatment (Figure 8-1, scenario A). If, on the other hand, the CI crosses the threshold, the trial has failed to establish noninferiority (Figure 8-1, scenario C). If the CI lies wholly above the noninferiority threshold, then the experimental treatment is inferior to standard treatment (Figure 8-1, scenario D).

If noninferiority trials choose insufficiently stringent thresholds, they run the risk of concluding noninferiority when, actually, many patients would be unwilling to accept the experimental treatment if they were informed of the largest possible increased risk (ie, decreased effectiveness) associated with its use. If these choices of thresholds go uncontested, wide uptake of experimental treatments could prove detrimental to patients. In interpreting noninferiority thresholds, we will encourage you to use your own judgment rather than accepting that of the investigators, relieving you of the need to decipher what many may experience as obscure statistical reasoning used to define the thresholds.

Although others have explained the rationale and provided criteria for interpreting noninferiority trials,[2,3,5-9] this chapter strives to present a simple and practical approach based on *Users' Guides* principles. We will use contemporary examples to illustrate concepts that can guide optimal clinical practice. In doing so, we follow the 3-step approach of other *Users' Guides* chapters, focusing on issues of validity, interpretation of results, and applicability of results specific to noninferiority trials (Box 8-1).

ARE THE RESULTS VALID?

Limitations of study design of noninferiority trials include issues beyond risk of bias. Thus, in this chapter, we continue to use the term "validity" to address both risk of bias and these additional issues.

The question "Are the results valid?" asks to what extent the results are likely to represent an

---

BOX 8-1

Users' Guides Approach to Evaluating a Noninferiority Trial

Are the results valid?[a]

Did experimental and standard treatment groups start with the same prognosis?

Was prognostic balance maintained as the trial progressed?

Were the groups prognostically balanced at the completion of the trial?

Did the investigators guard against an unwarranted conclusion of noninferiority?[b]

Was the effect of the standard treatment preserved?

Did the investigators analyze patients according to the treatment they received and to the groups to which they were assigned?

What are the results?

How can I apply the results to patient care?

Were the study patients similar to my patient?

Were all patient-important outcomes considered?

Are the likely advantages of the experimental treatment worth the potential harm and costs?[b]

---

[a]Limitations of study design of noninferiority trials include issues beyond risk of bias. Thus, in this chapter, we continue to use the term "validity" to address both risk of bias and these additional issues.

[b]Includes issues specific to noninferiority trials.

---

unbiased estimate of effect vs systematic overestimates or underestimates. As with other studies that address disease management questions, noninferiority trials will reduce the risk of bias if they ensure concealed randomization; demonstrate balance of known *prognostic factors*; *blind* patients, clinicians, and outcome assessors; and ensure complete *follow-up* (see Chapter 7, Therapy [Randomized Trials]). Noninferiority trials are, however, vulnerable to misleading conclusions in ways that superiority trials are not. Although not strictly related to the risk of bias, we have classified the relevant concerns, italicized in Box 8-1, as issues of validity.

Did the Investigators Guard Against an Unwarranted Conclusion of Noninferiority?

Was the Effect of the Standard Treatment Preserved?

One way to achieve apparent noninferiority is to suboptimally administer the standard treatment. Suboptimal treatment can include enrolling patients less likely to be adherent or responsive to standard treatment; enrolling a population at low risk of the effectiveness outcome, particularly if the noninferiority threshold is expressed in absolute terms; reducing treatment intensity or administering treatment by a suboptimal route (eg, orally rather than intravenously); or terminating follow-up before treatment effects are fully manifest. One strategy to assess whether the treatment effect was likely to have been preserved would be to evaluate the extent to which the design and conduct of the study attempted to overcome each of these threats to the standard treatment effect.

Another way to determine whether the effect of standard treatment has been preserved is to compare the event rate in the noninferiority trial with those seen in historical trials that involve the standard treatment. A higher *control event rate* in the standard treatment group in the noninferiority trial compared with the typical rate seen in historical trials would raise the suspicion of suboptimal administration of the standard treatment. Unfortunately, the competing explanation—prognostic differences between the populations enrolled in noninferiority vs historical trials—is also likely. Comparing patient characteristics among the trials could help decide which of the competing explanations is more likely, but the possibility remains that unmeasured prognostic features are responsible for the observed difference in event rates.

Take, for instance, the trial Rivaroxaban Once Daily Oral Direct Factor Xa Compared With Vitamin K Antagonism for Prevention of Stroke and Embolism in Atrial Fibrillation (ROCKET AF), in which investigators declared rivaroxaban to be noninferior to warfarin in managing patients with atrial fibrillation.[10] Concerns exist about the extent to which the patients treated with warfarin remained within the therapeutic range of anticoagulation throughout this study in comparison with previous RCTs comparing warfarin with placebo. Investigators documented a mean time in therapeutic range (TTR) of 55% in the warfarin group in ROCKET AF—considerably less than rates of approximately 75% (range, 42%-83%) seen in prior studies[11,12] and in contemporary noninferiority trials.[12] Hence, we cannot be confident that the warfarin treatment effect was preserved in ROCKET AF. The apparent noninferiority of rivaroxaban to warfarin may be because the latter was suboptimally administered.[13]

Using the second criterion to determine whether the effect of standard treatment has been preserved, the rate of stroke or systemic embolism in the warfarin group was lower in the ROCKET AF trial than has been seen historically,[14] despite the fact that patients in the ROCKET AF trial were older and had a higher prevalence of hypertension and type 2 diabetes mellitus than those in the previous trials.[11] Thus, control event rates fail to support the suspicion of suboptimal warfarin administration in the control group. The low TTR, nevertheless, remains concerning.

Did the Investigators Analyze Patients According to the Treatment They Received and to the Groups to Which They Were Assigned?

Another issue has to do with how investigators dealt with patients who were randomized and followed up to the end of the study but who did not take their medication as intended or did not use it at all. The purpose of randomization is to ensure that prognostic factors for the outcome of interest are balanced between treatment groups. It is likely that those who do not adhere to the allocated treatment as set out in the study protocol are prognostically different from those who do.[15]

Investigators may be tempted to include only those individuals who were adherent to study protocol and omit those who were not (often called a *per-protocol analysis*). This is likely, however, to compromise the prognostic balance that randomization created in the first place. Because, more often than not, *nonadherent* patients are prognostically worse than adherent patients, the omission of those who failed to adhere to the experimental treatment is likely to bias results toward an overestimation of treatment benefit in a superiority trial. In contrast, an analyze-as-randomized approach (intention-to-treat analysis) analyzes patients in the groups to which they were assigned irrespective of the level of patient adherence (see Chapter 11.4, The Principle of Intention to Treat and Ambiguous Dropouts). As a result, it yields an unbiased—and typically more conservative—estimate of treatment effectiveness in a superiority trial.[16]

Unfortunately, the analyze-as-randomized approach has serious limitations in the context of noninferiority trials. Picture a noninferiority trial in which the experimental treatment is actually substantially inferior to the current standard. Let us further suppose that, in this trial, many patients in the standard treatment group do not, for whatever reason, adhere to treatment. In the analyze-as-randomized approach, inclusion of these nonadherent patients may result in a substantial underestimate of the benefit of standard treatment and thus cause a misleading inference of noninferiority in comparison with the experimental treatment.

The per-protocol analysis, which focuses only on those who use the treatment more or less as directed, likely introduces prognostic imbalance but can nevertheless provide some reassurance regarding noninferiority. If the results of such an analysis are consistent with those from the analyze-as-randomized approach and if both lie below the noninferiority threshold, our inference regarding noninferiority is strengthened. If, however, there are important differences between the results of the 2 analyses, the inference of noninferiority is weakened.

For example, the Cardiac Insufficiency Bisoprolol Study (CIBIS) III trial addressed the initial use of a ß-blocker rather than an angiotensin-converting enzyme (ACE) inhibitor for preventing deaths or hospitalization in patients with heart failure.[17] The investigators set a noninferiority threshold of a 5% absolute increase in the primary *end point* of death or hospitalization with ß-blocker use. The as-randomized analysis met their noninferiority threshold: the upper limit of the CI suggested that an increase in death or hospitalization greater than 4.4% with ß-blockers was unlikely. In the per-protocol analysis, however, the upper limit of the CI was 5.1%, just above the investigators' chosen threshold. Were one to accept the authors' threshold, the inference of noninferiority is weakened by the results of the per-protocol analysis. Whether one should accept the authors' threshold at all is a point to which we will return.

USING THE GUIDE

In the pulmonary embolism treatment trial,[1] the investigators randomized 344 patients with acute symptomatic pulmonary embolus at low risk of death to outpatient treatment for 5 or more days of inpatient treatment. *Allocation concealment* was ensured via a central computer randomization system. Neither patients nor their caregivers were blinded to the allocated treatment, but adjudicators of outcome were. Patients in the treatment and *control* groups were similar with respect to known prognostic factors, including location of the embolus, comorbidity, and clinical findings. Complete follow-up was achieved in all but 5 patients. Although the lack of blinding raises concern, blinding of the outcome assessors provides a safeguard against *risk of bias*.

The crucial issues in optimal administration of the standard intervention in this study are the duration patients in the hospitalized group received LMWH and the TTR during subsequent warfarin treatment. Patients spent a mean of 8.9 days receiving LMWH, as long or longer than the standard in many settings (and thus satisfactory). The TTR was only 52%, which is suboptimal and raises concern. However, the TTR in the outpatient group was also 52%, substantially ameliorating the concern.

The investigators conducted both an analysis-as-randomized and a per-protocol analysis, which excluded patients in the hospitalized group discharged within 24 hours and those in the outpatient group discharged more than 24 hours after randomization. As you will see in the results that we present below, the per-protocol results do not substantially differ from the as-randomized results.

In conclusion, although the trial has some limitations in risk of bias, we would conclude moderate to high credibility of its findings.

WHAT ARE THE RESULTS?

The relevant results of a noninferiority trial focus on the following: (1) the difference between experimental and standard treatment in the effectiveness outcome that is the primary target of treatment, (2) the harm and burden outcomes that should favor the experimental over the standard treatment, and (3) whether the results provide reassurance that the standard treatment was optimally administered.

USING THE GUIDE

For pulmonary embolism, the primary effectiveness outcome is reducing recurrent VTE, and the treatment burden (staying in the hospital rather than being treated at home) is easily measured. Another important issue is the incidence of major bleeding, which could be conceptualized as an additional outcome warranting a noninferiority inquiry. Even if outpatient care was noninferior to inpatient care with respect to the primary effectiveness outcome, patients may choose to remain in the hospital if the risks of serious bleeding are substantially higher at home.

For each outcome, we are interested in the *point estimate* (the best estimate) of the difference in event rates between experimental and standard treatments and its associated CI. The boundaries of the CI represent the range of

plausible truth—less likely than the point estimate but still plausible (see Chapter 10, Confidence Intervals: Was the Single Study or Meta-analysis Large Enough?). Herein, we focus on the absolute differences between groups at 90 days. In the as-randomized analysis, recurrent VTE occurred in 1 individual in the outpatient group and none in the inpatient group, a difference of 0.6% or 6 in 1000, with an upper boundary of the 95% CI of 2.7% (27 more VTEs in 1000 outpatients).[1] This result suggests that it is unlikely that the recurrent VTE rate among outpatients is more than 4% (40 in 1000) greater than among inpatients ($P = .01$), the authors' noninferiority threshold.

For serious bleeding, the investigators observed 3 events in the outpatient group and none in the inpatient group (1.8%, or 18 in 1000 more bleeds in outpatients). The upper boundary of the 95% CI is 4.5%, which exceeds the authors' 4% threshold and therefore fails the statistical test of noninferiority ($P = .09$).

The authors also present a per-protocol analysis, the results of which are consistent with the as-randomized results. The major bleeding outcome is actually more favorable to outpatient management (a difference of 1.2% favoring inpatient management, with an upper boundary of the 95% CI of 3.8%; the P against the 4% threshold is .04).

HOW CAN I APPLY THE RESULTS TO PATIENT CARE?

In applying findings from the medical literature to individual patient care, we suggest asking 3 questions (Box 8-1), of which one—assessing trade-offs between an experimental treatment's likely advantages and potential harm and costs—includes issues specific to noninferiority trials.

Are the Likely Advantages of the Experimental Treatment Worth the Potential Harm and Costs?

Is a particular noninferiority trial simply a failed superiority trial, portrayed to put a happy face on a sad result? When investigators plan their trials, they specify the analysis, and this specification has implications for how results are interpreted. It is the job of the editors to ensure that only trials planned as noninferiority are in fact reported in published articles as noninferiority trials. Unfortunately, editors are not always thorough in performing due diligence in this aspect (and others) of reporting.[18]

The risk that a trial reported as noninferiority may not have been planned as noninferiority again highlights the importance of an independent judgment of the noninferiority threshold. You may be tempted to turn to the authors of a study for guidance on assessing the key inferences from a noninferiority trial: are the advantages of the experimental treatment worth the risks of loss of effectiveness? In doing so, you are implicitly accepting the authors' noninferiority threshold. For various reasons, investigators may have an incentive to be as lenient as possible with the choice of noninferiority threshold. Thus, accepting that threshold may not serve your patients' best interests.

Consider first the CIBIS-III trial, which investigates the substitution of ß-blockers for ACE inhibitors in the initial treatment of heart failure that we used to illustrate the desirability of a per-protocol analysis.[17] The as-randomized and per-protocol results straddled the authors' noninferiority margin of 5%. But is that margin appropriate? The harms or convenience advantages of ß-blockers over ACE inhibitors are few, if any. Thus, patients are unlikely to accept starting with ß-blockers if it really meant an absolute increase of up to 5% in the end point of death or hospitalization.

Consider next the Post-Operative Radiation Therapy for Endometrial Carcinoma 2 (PORTEC-2) trial, which investigated the effect of vaginal brachytherapy (VBT) vs pelvic external beam radiotherapy (EBRT) on the primary outcome of vaginal recurrence of endometrial carcinoma.[19] The investigators set a noninferiority threshold of a risk difference of 6%—an increase in the primary outcome

of 6 events in 100 patients—between the 2 groups at 5 years. After analyzing the data, they declared the VBT regimen to be noninferior to EBRT on the basis that the upper boundary of the CI—an absolute difference of 5%—fell below their threshold. Although patients undergoing VBT report better health-related quality of life than those receiving EBRT,[19] for an outcome as serious as cancer recurrence, we suspect that few patients would be willing to choose the VBT approach if the actual increase was as great as 5%.

The noninferiority threshold implies a trade-off between the advantages of the experimental treatment and the potential loss in effectiveness. Making this trade-off may be a challenging judgment, but it is not fundamentally different from other patient management decisions: they all involve trading off the desirable and undesirable consequences of the alternatives. They therefore involve *value and preference* judgments, and it is the preferences of the individual patient that must drive the decision. When the trade-off between desirable and undesirable consequences is a close one, the best—some would argue the only—way to ensure the chosen course of action is right for the individual is through shared decision making (see Chapter 27, Decision Making and the Patient).

In preparing for shared decision making with your patients, and being cognizant of the limited time you and they may have to spend on this activity, it may be worthwhile to reflect on the values and preferences of your typical patient and the implications for the noninferiority threshold. To gain a better understanding of how your typical patient perceives benefits and risks, you may want to refer to published studies that provide insight into patients' values and preferences.[20]

If, given the benefits and harms of an experimental intervention, you perceive all or virtually all patients would make the same decision, you and your patient may be able to quickly come to a fully satisfactory decision (see Chapter 26, How to Use a Patient Management Recommendation: Clinical Practice Guidelines and Decision Analyses).

If, however, the desirable and undesirable consequences are more closely balanced, you will need to have a detailed discussion with your patients.

Considering the most appropriate noninferiority margin will help distinguish between these 2 situations. First, look at the upper boundary of the CI for the primary outcome; then, note the extent to which it exceeds the maximum increase in risk of the primary outcome that your patients would, on average, be willing to accept in exchange for the experimental treatment's reduction in harms or burden.

If the upper boundary is substantially greater than your threshold and very few, if any, of your patients would choose the intervention, decision making may be expeditious. If, however, the upper boundary of the CI is near your threshold—that is, the balance between desirable and undesirable consequences is a close one—ensuring the right decision will involve full exploration of your patients' views of the trade-off at hand.

CLINICAL RESOLUTION

Your patient's clinical profile suggests a relatively low risk of death from pulmonary embolism. She would thus have been eligible for the trial,[1] and its results are directly applicable to her care. Point estimates suggest similar and low risks of recurrent VTE (6 in 1000); the difference in important bleeding is somewhat greater (18 more bleeds per 1000 in the outpatient group). The CIs raise more concern and include an increase in embolism of 2.7% (27 in 1000) and an increase in bleeding of 4.5% (45 in 1000), both within 90 days, in the outpatient care group.

Because their noninferiority margin for VTE has been met, the authors of the pulmonary embolism trial conclude that "[i]n selected low-risk patients with pulmonary embolism, outpatient care can safely and effectively be used in place of inpatient care."[1] Individuals who, all else being equal, would much prefer home treatment and are ready to focus on the point estimates that suggest that rates of adverse events (at least VTE) are likely similar with outpatient management might agree. On the other hand, risk-averse individuals who perceive the possibility of increased risk of VTE and bleeding with outpatient management as not being worth the benefit of receiving treatment at home would not agree with this conclusion. We believe that there are likely to be a substantial number of such risk-averse individuals. Reliance on the authors' noninferiority would not serve such patients well.

CONCLUSIONS

Critical appraisal of noninferiority studies closely follows the principles and criteria for assessing any study of experimental management strategies. With respect to validity, assessment of a noninferiority study requires special attention to the optimal use of the standard treatment and to the results of the as-randomized and per-protocol analyses. With respect to the trade-offs between desirable and undesirable consequences in noninferiority trials, close attention to best estimates and CIs around the difference in effectiveness outcomes between experimental and standard treatments is needed. In particular, clinicians should consider whether patients would be willing to accept loss in the effectiveness outcome suggested by the upper boundary of the 95% CI, irrespective of whether this interval lies below or above the investigators' choice of noninferiority threshold.

References

1. Aujesky D, Roy PM, Verschuren F, et al. Outpatient versus inpatient treatment for patients with acute pulmonary embolism: an international, open-label, randomised, non-inferiority trial. *Lancet.* 2011;378(9785):41-48.
2. Fleming TR. Current issues in non-inferiority trials. *Stat Med.* 2008;27(3):317-332.
3. Kaul S, Diamond GA. Good enough: a primer on the analysis and interpretation of noninferiority trials. *Ann Intern Med.* 2006;145(1):62-69.
4. Temple R, O'Neill R. *Guidance for Industry Non-Inferiority Clinical Trials.* Rockville, MD: Food and Drug Administration, Dept of Health and Human Services; 2010.

5. Le Henanff A, Giraudeau B, Baron G, Ravaud P. Quality of reporting of noninferiority and equivalence randomized trials. *JAMA*. 2006;295(10):1147-1151.

6. Piaggio G, Elbourne DR, Pocock SJ, Evans SJW, Altman DG; CONSORT Group. Reporting of noninferiority and equivalence randomized trials: extension of the CONSORT 2010 statement. *JAMA*. 2012;308(24):2594-2604.

7. Scott IA. Non-inferiority trials: determining whether alternative treatments are good enough. *Med J Aust*. 2009;190(6):326-330.

8. Gøtzsche PC. Lessons from and cautions about noninferiority and equivalence randomized trials. *JAMA*. 2006; 295(10):1172-1174.

9. Schumi J, Wittes JT. Through the looking glass: understanding non-inferiority. *Trials*. 2011;12:106.

10. Patel MR, Mahaffey KW, Garg J, et al; ROCKET AF Investigators. Rivaroxaban versus warfarin in nonvalvular atrial fibrillation. *N Engl J Med*. 2011;365(10):883-891.

11. Jackson K, Gersh BJ, Stockbridge N, et al; Duke Clinical Research Institute/American Heart Journal Expert Meeting on Antithrombotic Drug Development for Atrial Fibrillation. Antithrombotic drug development for atrial fibrillation: proceedings, Washington, DC, July 25-27, 2005. *Am Heart J*. 2008;155(5):829-840.

12. Granger CB, Alexander JH, McMurray JJ, et al; ARISTOTLE Committees and Investigators. Apixaban versus warfarin in patients with atrial fibrillation. *N Engl J Med*. 2011;365(11): 981-992.

13. Fleming TR, Emerson SS. Evaluating rivaroxaban for nonvalvular atrial fibrillation—regulatory considerations. *N Engl J Med*. 2011;365(17):1557-1559.

14. Hart RG, Benavente O, McBride R, Pearce LA. Antithrombotic therapy to prevent stroke in patients with atrial fibrillation: a meta-analysis. *Ann Intern Med*. 1999;131(7):492-501.

15. Kunz R, Guyatt G. Which patients to include in the analysis? *Transfusion*. 2006;46(6):881-884.

16. Montori VM, Guyatt GH. Intention-to-treat principle. *CMAJ*. 2001;165(10):1339-1341.

17. Willenheimer R, van Veldhuisen DJ, Silke B, et al; CIBIS III Investigators. Effect on survival and hospitalization of initiating treatment for chronic heart failure with bisoprolol followed by enalapril, as compared with the opposite sequence: results of the randomized Cardiac Insufficiency Bisoprolol Study (CIBIS) III. *Circulation*. 2005;112(16):2426-2435.

18. Yank V, Rennie D, Bero LA. Financial ties and concordance between results and conclusions in meta-analyses: retrospective cohort study. *BMJ*. 2007;335(7631):1202-1205.

19. Nout RA, Smit VT, Putter H, et al; PORTEC Study Group. Vaginal brachytherapy versus pelvic external beam radiotherapy for patients with endometrial cancer of high-intermediate risk (PORTEC-2): an open-label, non-inferiority, randomised trial. *Lancet*. 2010;375(9717):816-823.

20. MacLean S, Mulla S, Akl EA, et al; American College of Chest Physicians. Patient values and preferences in decision making for antithrombotic therapy: a systematic review: Antithrombotic Therapy and Prevention of Thrombosis, 9th ed: American College of Chest Physicians Evidence-Based Clinical Practice Guidelines. *Chest*. 2012;141(2)(suppl):e1S-e23S.

THERAPY

9

Does Treatment Lower Risk? Understanding the Results

Waleed Alhazzani, Stephen D. Walter, Roman Jaeschke, Deborah J. Cook, and Gordon Guyatt

THERAPY

IN THIS CHAPTER

When clinicians consider the results of clinical trials, they are interested in the association between a treatment and an outcome. This chapter will help you understand and interpret study results related to outcomes that are either present or absent (*dichotomous* or binary) for each patient. Such binary outcomes include death, stroke, myocardial infarction, hospitalization, or disease exacerbations. A guide for teaching the *concepts* in this chapter is also available.[1]

THE 2 × 2 TABLE

Table 9-1 is a 2 × 2 table that captures the information for a dichotomous outcome of a clinical trial.

For instance, during a *randomized trial* that compares mortality rates in patients with bleeding esophageal varices that were controlled by endoscopic ligation or endoscopic sclerotherapy,[2] 18 of 64 participants assigned to ligation died, as did 29 of 65 patients assigned to sclerotherapy (Table 9-2).

THE RISK

The simplest measure of occurrence to understand is the *risk* (or *absolute risk*). We often refer to the risk of the adverse outcome in the *control group* as the *baseline risk,* the *control group risk,* or, occasionally, the *control event rate.*

The risk of dying in the ligation group is 28% (18/64 or $[a/(a + b)]$), and the risk of dying in the sclerotherapy group is 45% (29/65 or $[c/(c + d)]$).

THE RISK DIFFERENCE (ABSOLUTE RISK REDUCTION)

One way of comparing 2 risks is by calculating the absolute difference between them. We refer to this difference as the *absolute risk reduction* (ARR) or the *risk difference* (RD). Algebraically, the formula for the RD (the control group risk minus the treatment group risk) is $[c/(c + d)] - [a/(a + b)]$ (Table 9-1). This measure of effect uses absolute rather than relative terms in looking at the proportion of patients who are spared the adverse outcome.

In our example, the RD is 0.446 − 0.281 or 0.165 (ie, an RD of 16.5%).

THE RELATIVE RISK

Another way to compare the risks in the 2 groups is to take their ratio; this is called the *relative risk* or *risk ratio* (RR). The RR tells us the proportion of the original risk (in this case, the risk of death in patients who received sclerotherapy) that is still present when patients receive the *experimental treatment* (in this case, ligation). From our 2 × 2 table, the formula for this calculation is $[a/(a + b)]/[c/(c + d)]$ (Table 9-1).

TABLE 9-1

The 2 × 2 Table

Exposure	Outcome	
	Yes	**No**
Yes	a	b
No	c	d

Risk with exposure = $a/(a + b)$
Risk without exposure = $c/(c + d)$

Odds with exposure = a/b
Odds without exposure = c/d

Relative risk = $\dfrac{a/(a + b)}{c/(c + d)}$

Relative risk reduction = $\dfrac{c/(c + d) - a/(a + b)}{c/(c + d)}$

Relative difference[a] = $\dfrac{c}{c + d} = \dfrac{a}{a + b}$

Number needed to treat = 100 / (risk difference expressed as %)

Odds ratio = $\dfrac{a/b}{c/d} = \dfrac{ad}{cb}$

[a] Also known as the absolute risk reduction.

In our example, the RR of dying after receiving initial ligation vs sclerotherapy is 18/64 (the risk in the ligation group) divided by 29/65 (the risk in the sclerotherapy group) or 0.63. In everyday English, we would say that the risk of death with ligation is approximately two-thirds of that with sclerotherapy.

THE RELATIVE RISK REDUCTION

An alternative relative measure of treatment effectiveness is the *relative risk reduction* (RRR), an estimate of the proportion of baseline risk that is removed by the therapy. It may be calculated as 1 − RR. One also can calculate the RRR by dividing the RD (amount of risk removed) by the absolute risk in the control group (Table 9-1).

In our bleeding varices example, where the RR was 0.63, the RRR is thus 1 − 0.63 (or 16.5% divided by 44.6%, the risk in the sclerotherapy group); either way, it comes to 0.37. In other words, ligation decreases the risk of death by just more than one-third compared with sclerotherapy.

THE ODDS RATIO

Instead of looking at the risk of an event, we could estimate the odds of having vs not having an event. When considering the effects of therapy, you usually will not go far wrong if you interpret the *odds ratio* (OR) as equivalent to the RR. The exception is when the risk of having an event is very high—for instance, when more than 40% of control patients experience myocardial infarction or death (see Chapter 12.2, Understanding the Results: More About Odds Ratios).

RELATIVE RISK VS RISK DIFFERENCE: WHY THE FUSS?

Failing to distinguish between the OR and the RR when interpreting randomized trial results will

TABLE 9-2

Results From a Randomized Trial of Endoscopic Sclerotherapy Compared With Endoscopic Ligation for Bleeding Esophageal Varices[a]

Exposure	Outcome		Total
	Death	**Survival**	
Ligation	18	46	64
Sclerotherapy	29	36	65
Relative risk = (18/64) / (29/65) = 0.63 or 63%			
Relative risk reduction = 1 − 0.63 = 0.37 or 37%			
Risk difference = 0.446 − 0.281 = 0.165 or 16.5%			
Number needed to treat = 100 / 16.5 = 6			
Odds ratio = (18/46) / (29/36) = 0.39 / 0.80 = 0.49 or 49%			

[a]Data from Stiegmann et al.[2]

seldom mislead you; you must, however, distinguish between the RR and the RD. The reason is that the RR is generally far larger than the RD, and presentations of results in the form of RR (or RRR) can convey a misleading message. Furthermore, it is the risk difference in which the patient is ultimately interested. Reducing a patient's risk by 50% sounds impressive. That may, however, represent a reduction in risk from 2% to 1%. The corresponding 1% RD sounds considerably less impressive and in fact conveys the crucial information.

As depicted in Figure 9-1, consider a treatment that is administered to 3 different subpopulations of patients and that, in each case, decreases the risk by one-third (RRR, 0.33; RR, 0.67). When administered to a subpopulation with a 30% risk of dying, treatment reduces the risk to 20%. When administered to a population with a 10% risk of dying, treatment reduces the risk to 6.7%. In the third population, treatment reduces the risk of dying from 1% to 0.67%.

Although treatment reduces the risk of dying by one-third in each population, this piece of information is not adequate to fully capture the impact of treatment. What if the treatment under consideration is a toxic cancer chemotherapeutic drug associated with severe adverse effects in 50% of those to whom it is administered? Under these circumstances, most patients in the lowest risk group in Figure 9-1, whose RD is only 0.3%, would likely decline treatment.

THERAPY

FIGURE 9-1

Constant Relative Risk With Varying Risk Differences

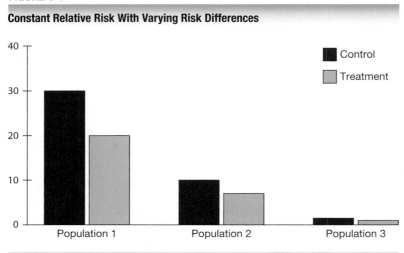

In the intermediate population, those with an absolute reduction in risk of death of approximately 3%, some might accept the treatment, but many would likely decline. Many in the highest-risk population with an absolute benefit of 10% would likely accept the treatment, but some may not.

We suggest that you consider the RRR in light of your patient's baseline risk. For instance, you might expect an RRR of approximately 25% in vascular events in patients with possible cardiovascular disease with administration of statins. You would view this RRR differently in a 40-year-old woman without hypertension, diabetes mellitus, or a history of smoking with a mildly elevated low-density lipoprotein level (5-year risk of a cardiovascular event of approximately 2%, ARR of approximately 0.5%) and a 70-year-old woman with hypertension and diabetes who smokes (5-year risk of 30%, ARR of 7.5%). All of this assumes a constant RRR across risk groups; fortunately, a more or less constant RRR is usually the case, and we suggest you make that assumption unless there is evidence that suggests it is incorrect.[3-5]

THE NUMBER NEEDED TO TREAT

The impact of treatment also can be expressed by the number of patients you would need to treat to prevent an adverse event, the *number needed to treat* (NNT).[6]

Table 9-2 indicates that the risk of dying is 28.1% in the ligation group and 44.6% in the sclerotherapy group, an RD of 16.5%. If treating 100 patients results in avoiding 16.5 events, how many patients do we need to treat to avoid 1 event? The answer: 100 divided by 16.5, or approximately 6, is the NNT.

The NNT calculation always implies a given time of *follow-up* (ie, do we need to treat 50 patients for 1 year or 5 years to prevent an event?). When trials with long follow-ups are analyzed by survival methods, there are a variety of ways of calculating the NNT (see the following subsection, Survival Data). These different methods will, however, rarely lead to results with different clinical implications.[7]

Assuming a constant RRR, the NNT is inversely related to the proportion of patients in the control group who have an adverse event. For instance, if the control group risk doubles, the NNT will decrease by a factor of 2 (ie, be half of what it was). If the risk of an adverse event doubles (eg, if we deal with patients at a higher risk of death than those included in the clinical trial), we need to treat only half as many patients to prevent an adverse event. On the other hand, if the risk decreases by a factor of 4 (patients are younger and have less *comorbidity* than those in the study), we will have to treat 4 times as many people.

The NNT also is inversely related to the RRR. With the same baseline risk, a more effective treatment with twice the RRR will reduce the NNT by half.

TABLE 9-3

Association Among the Baseline Risk, Relative Risk Reduction, and Number Needed to Treat[a]

Control Group Risk	Experimental Group Risk	Relative Risk, %	Relative Risk Reduction, %	Risk Difference, %	Number Needed to Treat
0.02 or 2%	0.01 or 1%	50	50	1	100
0.4 or 40%	0.2 or 20%	50	50	20	5
0.04 or 4%	0.02 or 2%	50	50	2	50
0.04 or 4%	0.03 or 3%	75	25	1	100
0.4 or 40%	0.3 or 30%	75	25	10	10
0.01 or 1%	0.005 or 0.5%	50	50	0.5	200

[a]Relative risk = experimental group risk/control group risk; relative risk reduction = 1 − relative risk; risk difference = control group risk − experimental group risk; number needed to treat = 100/risk difference in %.

If the RRR with one treatment is only a quarter of that achieved by an alternative strategy, the NNT will be 4 times greater.

Table 9-3 presents hypothetical data that illustrate these relationships.

THE NUMBER NEEDED TO HARM

Clinicians can calculate the *number needed to harm* (NNH) in a similar way. If you expect 5 of 100 patients to become fatigued when taking a β-blocker for a year, of 20 patients you treat, 1 will become tired; therefore, the NNH is 20.

CONFIDENCE INTERVALS

We have presented all of the measures of association of the treatment with ligation vs sclerotherapy as if they represented the true effect. The results of any experiment, however, represent only an estimate of the truth. The true effect of treatment may be somewhat greater—or less—than what we observed. The *confidence interval* (CI) tells us, within the bounds of plausibility (and assuming a low *risk of bias*), how much greater or smaller the true effect is likely to be (see Chapter 10, Confidence Intervals: Was the Single Study or Meta-analysis Large Enough?).

SURVIVAL DATA

Analysis of a 2 × 2 table implies an examination of the data at a specific point in time. This analysis is satisfactory if we are looking for events that occur within relatively short periods and if all patients have the same duration of follow-up. In longer-term studies, however, we are interested not only in the total number of events but also in their timing. For instance, we may focus on whether therapy for patients with a uniformly fatal condition (unresectable lung cancer, for example) delays death.

When the timing of events is important, investigators could present the results in the form of several 2 × 2 tables constructed at different points of time after the study began. For example, Table 9-2 represents the situation after the study was finished. Similar tables could be constructed describing the fate of all patients available for analysis after their enrollment in the trial for 1 week, 1 month, 3 months, or whatever time we chose to examine. The analysis of accumulated data that takes into account the timing of events is called *survival analysis*. Do not infer from the name, however, that the analysis is restricted to deaths; in fact, any dichotomous outcome occurring over time will qualify.

The *survival curve* of a group of patients describes their status at different times after a defined

FIGURE 9-2

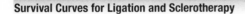

Survival Curves for Ligation and Sclerotherapy

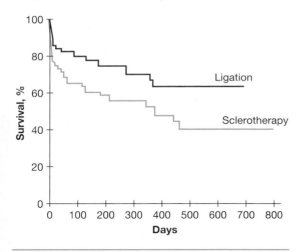

starting point.[8] In Figure 9-2, we show the survival curve from the bleeding varices trial. Because the investigators followed up some patients for a longer time, the survival curve extends beyond the mean follow-up of approximately 10 months. At some point, prediction becomes imprecise because there are few patients remaining to estimate the *probability of survival*. The CIs around the survival curves capture the precision of the estimate.

Even if the true RR, or RRR, is constant throughout the duration of follow-up, the play of chance will ensure that the *point estimates* differ. Ideally then, we would estimate the overall RR by applying an average, weighted for the number of patients available, for the entire survival experience. Statistical methods allow just such an estimate. The probability of events occurring at any point in each group is referred to as the hazard for that group, and the weighted RR during the entire study duration is known as the *hazard ratio*.

A major advantage of using survival analysis is the ability to account for differential length of follow-up. In many trials of a fixed duration, some patients are enrolled early and thus have long follow-up and some later with consequently shorter follow-up. Survival analysis takes into account both those with shorter (by a process called *censoring*) and those with longer follow-up, and all contribute to estimates of

hazard and the hazard ratio. Patients are censored at the point at which they are no longer being followed up. Appropriate accounting for those with differential length of follow-up is not possible in 2×2 tables that deal only with the number of events.

"Competing risks" is an issue that arises when one event influences the likelihood of another event. The most extreme example is death: if the outcome is stroke, people who die can no longer have a stroke. Competing risks also can arise when there are 2 or more outcome events among living patients (for instance, if a patient has a stroke, the likelihood of a subsequent transient ischemic attack may decrease). Investigators can deal with the problem of competing risks by censoring patients at the time of the "competing" events (death and stroke in the previous examples). The censoring approach, however, has its limitations.[9]

Specifically, the usual assumption is that the censored events are independent of the main outcome of interest, but in practice this assumption may not be correct. In our example, it is probable that patients who experience myocardial infarction have a higher death rate than those without myocardial infarction, and this would violate the assumption of independence. Investigators also sometimes use censoring for those *lost to follow-up*. This is much more problematic because the censoring assumes that those with shorter follow-up are similar to those with longer follow-up—the only difference, indeed, being length of follow-up. Because loss to follow-up may be associated with a higher or lower likelihood of events (and thus, those lost differ from those who are followed up), the censoring approach does not deal with the risk of bias associated with loss to follow-up.[9]

WHICH MEASURE OF ASSOCIATION IS BEST?

As *evidence-based practitioners*, we must decide which measure of association deserves our focus. Does it matter? The answer is yes. The same results, when presented in different ways, may lead to different treatment decisions.[9-13] For example, Forrow et al[10] found that clinicians were less inclined to treat patients after presentation of trial results as the absolute change in the outcome compared with the relative change in the outcome. In a similar study, Naylor et al[11] found that clinicians rated the effectiveness of an intervention lower when events were presented in absolute terms rather than using RRR. Moreover, clinicians offered lower effectiveness ratings when they viewed results expressed in terms of NNT than when they saw the same data as RRRs or ARRs. The awareness of this phenomenon in the pharmaceutical industry may be the reason for their propensity to present physicians with treatment-associated RRRs.

Patients are as susceptible as clinicians to how results are communicated. In one study, when researchers presented patients with a hypothetical scenario of life-threatening illness, the patients were more likely to choose a treatment described in terms of RRR than in terms of the corresponding ARR.[14] Other investigators found similar results.[15,16]

Considering how our interpretations differ with data presentations, we are best advised to consider all of the data (as either a 2 × 2 table or a survival analysis) and then reflect on both the relative and the absolute figures. As you examine the results, you will find that if you can estimate your patient's baseline risk, knowing how well the treatment works—expressed as an RR or RRR—allows you to estimate the patient's risk with treatment. Considering the RD—the difference between the risk with and without treatment—and its reciprocal, the NNT, in an individual patient will be most useful in guiding the treatment decision.

THERAPY

References

1. Barratt A, Wyer PC, Hatala R, et al. Tips for learners of evidence-based medicine, 1: relative risk reduction, absolute risk reduction and number needed to treat. *CMAJ.* 2004;171(4:online-1 to online-8):353-358. http://www.cmaj.ca/cgi/data/171/4/353/DC1/1. Accessed August 25, 2014.

2. Stiegmann GV, Goff JS, Michaletz-Onody PA, et al. Endoscopic sclerotherapy as compared with endoscopic ligation for bleeding esophageal varices. *N Engl J Med.* 1992;326(23):1527-1532.

3. Deeks JJ. Issues in the selection of a summary statistic for meta-analysis of clinical trials with binary outcomes. *Stat Med.* 2002;21(11):1575-1600.

4. Schmid CH, Lau J, McIntosh MW, Cappelleri JC. An empirical study of the effect of the control rate as a predictor of treatment efficacy in meta-analysis of clinical trials. *Stat Med.* 1998;17(17):1923-1942.

5. Furukawa TA, Guyatt GH, Griffith LE. Can we individualize the 'number needed to treat'? an empirical study of summary effect measures in meta-analyses. *Int J Epidemiol.* 2002;31(1):72-76.

6. Laupacis A, Sackett DL, Roberts RS. An assessment of clinically useful measures of the consequences of treatment. *N Engl J Med.* 1988;318(26):1728-1733.

7. Barratt AL, Wyer PC, Guyatt G, et al. NNT for studies with long-term follow-up. *CMAJ.* 2005;172(5):613-615.

8. Coldman AJ, Elwood JM. Examining survival data. *Can Med Assoc J.* 1979;121(8):1065-1068, 1071.

9. Kleinbaum DG, Klein M. *Survival Analysis: A Self-Learning Text.* New York, NY: Springer; 2012.

10. Forrow L, Taylor WC, Arnold RM. Absolutely relative: how research results are summarized can affect treatment decisions. *Am J Med.* 1992;92(2):121-124.

11. Naylor CD, Chen E, Strauss B. Measured enthusiasm: does the method of reporting trial results alter perceptions of therapeutic effectiveness? *Ann Intern Med.* 1992;117(11):916-921.

12. Hux JE, Levinton CM, Naylor CD. Prescribing propensity: influence of life-expectancy gains and drug costs. *J Gen Intern Med.* 1994;9(4):195-201.

13. Redelmeier DA, Tversky A. Discrepancy between medical decisions for individual patients and for groups. *N Engl J Med.* 1990;322(16):1162-1164.

14. Bobbio M, Demichelis B, Giustetto G. Completeness of reporting trial results: effect on physicians' willingness to prescribe. *Lancet.* 1994;343(8907):1209-1211.

15. Malenka DJ, Baron JA, Johansen S, Wahrenberger JW, Ross JM. The framing effect of relative and absolute risk. *J Gen Intern Med.* 1993;8(10):543-548.

16. McNeil BJ, Pauker SG, Sox HC Jr, Tversky A. On the elicitation of preferences for alternative therapies. *N Engl J Med.* 1982;306(21):1259-1262.

10

Confidence Intervals: Was the Single Study or Meta-analysis Large Enough?

Gordon Guyatt, Stephen D. Walter, Deborah J. Cook, and Roman Jaeschke

IN THIS CHAPTER

In discussions of whether trials were large enough, you may have heard people refer to the power of the trial as the authors presented in their sample size calculations. Such discussions are complex and confusing. As we illustrate in this chapter, whether a trial or *meta-analysis* is large enough depends only on the *confidence interval* (CI).

Hypothesis testing, on which sample size calculations are typically based, involves estimating the probability that observed results would have occurred by chance if a *null hypothesis*, which states that there is no difference between a treatment condition and a control condition, were true. Health researchers and medical educators have increasingly recognized the limitations of hypothesis testing[1-5]; consequently, an alternative approach, estimation, is becoming more popular.

HOW SHOULD WE TREAT PATIENTS WITH HEART FAILURE? A PROBLEM IN INTERPRETING STUDY RESULTS

In a *blinded randomized clinical trial* of 804 men with heart failure, investigators compared treatment with enalapril (an angiotensin-converting enzyme [ACE] inhibitor) to treatment with a combination of hydralazine and nitrates.[6] In the *follow-up* period, which ranged from 6 months to 5.7 years, 132 of 403 patients (33%) assigned to receive enalapril died, as did 153 of 401 patients (38%) assigned to receive hydralazine and nitrates. The *P* value associated with the difference in mortality is .11.

Looking at this study as an exercise in hypothesis testing and adopting the usual 5% risk of obtaining a *false-positive* result, we would conclude that chance remains a plausible explanation for the apparent differences between groups. We would classify this as a *negative study* (ie, we would conclude that no important difference existed between the treatment and *control groups*).

The investigators also conducted an additional analysis that compared the time pattern of the deaths occurring in both groups. This *survival analysis*, which generally is more sensitive than the test of the difference in proportions

(see Chapter 9, Does Treatment Lower Risk? Understanding the Results), had a nonsignificant *P* value of .08, a result that leads to the same conclusion as the simpler analysis that focused on relative proportions at the end of the study. The authors also tell us that the *P* value associated with differences in mortality at 2 years (a point predetermined to be a major *end point* of the trial) was significant at .016.

At this point, one might excuse clinicians who feel a little confused. Ask yourself, is this a *positive trial,* dictating use of an ACE inhibitor instead of the combination of hydralazine and nitrates, or is it a negative study, showing no difference between the 2 regimens and leaving the choice of drugs open?

SOLVING THE PROBLEM: WHAT ARE CONFIDENCE INTERVALS?

How can clinicians deal with the limitations of hypothesis testing and resolve the confusion? The solution involves posing 2 questions: (1) "What is the single value most likely to represent the true difference between experimental and control treatments?" and (2) "Given the observed difference between experimental and control groups, what is the plausible range of differences within which the true difference might actually lie?" Confidence intervals provide an answer to this second question: they offer a range of values within which it is probable that the true value of a parameter (eg, a mean or a *relative risk*) lies. Before applying CIs to resolve the issue of enalapril vs hydralazine and nitrates in patients with heart failure, we illustrate the use of CIs with a thought experiment.

Imagine a series of 5 trials (of equal duration but different sample sizes) wherein investigators have experimented with treating patients with elevated low-density lipoprotein cholesterol and a previous myocardial infarction (MI) to determine whether a drug (a novel cholesterol-lowering agent) would work better than *placebo*

TABLE 10-1

Confidence Intervals Around the Relative Risk Reduction for the Hypothetical Results of 5 Successively Larger Trials[a]

Control Group Risk	Experimental Group Risk	RR, %	RRR, %	Calculated 95% CI Around the RRR, %
2/4	1/4	50	50	−174 to 92
10/20	5/20	50	50	−14 to 79.5
20/40	10/40	50	50	9.5-73.4
50/100	25/100	50	50	26.8-66.4
500/1000	250/1000	50	50	43.5-55.9

Abbreviations: RR, relative risk; RRR, relative risk reduction.

Reproduced from Montori et al,[7] by permission of the publisher. © 2004 Canadian Medical Association.

in complementing a statin to *prevent* recurrent MI (Table 10-1). The smallest trial enrolled only 8 patients, and the largest enrolled 2000 patients.

Now imagine that all of the trials showed a *relative risk reduction* (RRR) for the treatment group of 50% (meaning that patients in the drug treatment group were 50% as likely as those in the placebo group to have a stroke). In each trial, how confident can we be about the true value of the RRR? If you were looking at the studies individually, which ones would lead you to recommend the treatment to your patients?

Most clinicians know intuitively that we can be more confident in the results of a larger vs a smaller trial. Why is this? In the absence of *bias* or *systematic error*, one can interpret the trial as providing an estimate of the true effect that would occur if all possible eligible patients had participated. When only a few patients participate, chance may lead to a best estimate of the *treatment effect*—the *point estimate*—which is far removed from the true value. Confidence intervals provide the range within which such variation is likely to occur. The 95% CIs that we often see in biomedical publications represent the range in which it is very likely that the true effect lies. More precision (narrower CIs) results from larger sample sizes and, consequently, a larger number of events. Statisticians (and clinician-friendly statistical software) can calculate 95% CIs around any estimate of treatment effect.

To gain a better appreciation of CIs, go back to Table 10-1. Consider the first trial, in which 2 of 4 patients receiving the control intervention and 1 of 4 patients receiving the experimental intervention have a stroke. The risk in the experimental group was thus half of that in the control group, giving a relative risk (RR) of 50% and an RRR of 50%.

Would you be ready to recommend this treatment to a patient in view of the substantial RRR? Before you answer this, consider whether it is plausible that, with so few patients in the study, we could have just been lucky in our sample and the true treatment effect could really be a 50% increase in RR. In other words, is it plausible that the true *event rate* in the group that received treatment was 3 of 4 instead of 1 of 4?

Most clinicians answer yes to this question, and they are correct. Indeed, calculation of the CIs tells us that the results of the first trial are consistent with close to a tripling of the death rate in the intervention group.

The second trial, enrolling 40 patients, has results that are still consistent with treatment increasing the rate of deaths by, in relative terms, 17%. The third trial results tell us it is very likely that the treatment is beneficial, but the effect may be small (an RRR of less than 10%). Finally, a trial of 2000 patients with the same rate of events in the treatment and control groups provides confidence that the true effect is close to the 50% RRR we observed.

USING CONFIDENCE INTERVALS TO INTERPRET THE RESULTS OF CLINICAL TRIALS

How do CIs help us understand the results of the trial of vasodilators in patients with heart failure?[6] By the end of the study, the mortality was 33% in the ACE inhibitor arm and 38% in the hydralazine plus nitrate group, an *absolute difference* of 5% and an RR of 0.86. The 5% absolute difference and the 14% RRR represent our best single estimate of the mortality benefit from using an ACE inhibitor. The 95% CI around the RRR is −3.5% to 29%. Note that when the CI crosses an RR of 1.0, the negative RRR represents a benefit for the comparator—in this case, an RRR of 3.5% for hydralazine.

How can we now interpret the study results? We can conclude that patients offered ACE inhibitors will quite possibly (but far from certainly) die later than patients offered hydralazine and nitrates. The magnitude of the true difference may be either trivial or large, and there remains the possibility of a marginally lower mortality with the hydralazine-nitrate regimen.

Use of the CI avoids the yes/no dichotomy of hypothesis testing. It also obviates the need to argue whether the study result should be considered positive or negative. One can conclude that, all else being equal, an ACE inhibitor is the appropriate choice for patients with heart failure, but our confidence in the estimate of effect on mortality is, at best, moderate. Thus, toxicity, expense, and *evidence* from other studies would all bear on the final treatment decision (see Chapter 26, How to Use a Patient Management Recommendation: Clinical Practice Guidelines and Decision Analyses). Because a number of large randomized trials have now shown a mortality benefit from ACE inhibitors in patients with heart failure,[8] one can confidently recommend this class of agents as the treatment of choice. Another study has suggested that for black patients, the hydralazine-nitrate combination offers additional mortality reduction beyond ACE inhibitors.[9]

NEGATIVE TRIALS OFTEN FAIL TO EXCLUDE AN IMPORTANT BENEFIT

Another example of the use of CIs in interpreting study results comes from a randomized trial of low vs high positive end-expiratory pressure (PEEP) in patients with adult respiratory distress syndrome.[10] Of 273 patients in the low-PEEP group, 24.9% died; of 276 in the high-PEEP group, 27.5% died. The point estimate from these results is a 2.6% *absolute risk increase* in deaths in the high-PEEP group.

This trial of more than 500 patients might appear to exclude any possible benefit from high PEEP. The 95% CI on the absolute difference of 2.6% in favor of low PEEP, however, is 10.0% in favor of low PEEP to 4.7% in favor of high PEEP. Were it true that high PEEP reduces the risk of dying by almost 5%, all patients would want to receive the high-PEEP strategy. This would mean one would need to treat approximately 20 patients to prevent a premature death. One can thus conclude that the trial has not excluded a patient-important benefit and, in that sense, was not large enough. As in this example, negative studies seldom indicate that a treatment is not effective; rather, they fail to demonstrate a benefit.

WAS THE INDIVIDUAL TRIAL OR META-ANALYSIS LARGE ENOUGH? JUST CHECK THE CONFIDENCE INTERVALS

The examples thus far demonstrate the limitations of individual trials that seldom enroll sufficient patients to generate satisfactorily narrow CIs. This illustrates why we recommend that, whenever possible, clinicians turn to *systematic reviews* and meta-analyses that pool data from multiple studies and thus achieve narrower CIs than are possible for any single study (see Chapter 5, Finding Current Best Evidence).

As implied in our discussion to this point, CIs provide a way of answering the question, "Was the meta-analysis or individual trial large enough?" In the subsequent discussion, we will focus on meta-analyses. If you are relying on an individual study, however, the principles are identical.

We illustrate the approach in Figure 10-1. In this figure, we present the *pooled estimates* of 4 meta-analyses. The width of CIs from meta-analyses are driven by the number of patients (and for *binary outcomes*, even more by the number of events; see Chapter 12.3, What Determines the Width of the Confidence Interval?) rather than the number of studies. Thus, the narrower CIs (A and C) come from meta-analyses with larger numbers of events and patients, though not necessarily larger numbers of studies.

Although most *forest plots* (visual plots of trial results) focus on RRs or *odds ratios*, Figure 10-1 presents the results in absolute terms. Thus, the solid vertical line in the center of the figure represents a *risk difference* (RD) (or *absolute risk reduction*) of 0: the experimental and control groups have the same mortality. Values to the left of the vertical line represent results in which treated groups had a lower mortality than the control groups. Values to

the right of the vertical line represent results in which the treated group fared worse and had a higher mortality rate than the control group.

Assume that the treatment carries sufficient toxicity or risk such that, in each case, patients would choose treatment only if the RD were 1% or greater. That is, if the reduction in death rates were greater than 1%, patients would consider it worth enduring the toxic effects and risk of treatment, but if the reduction in event rates were less than 1%, they would not. The dashed line in Figure 10-1 represents this threshold reduction in death rates of 1%.

Now consider the pooled estimate from meta-analysis A: Would you recommend this therapy to your patients if the point estimate represented the truth? What if the upper boundary of the CI (representing the largest plausible effect) represented the truth? What about the lower boundary (representing the smallest plausible effect)?

For all 3 of these questions, the answer is yes, given that 1% is the smallest patient-important difference, and all suggest a benefit of greater than 1%. Thus, the meta-analysis is definitive and provides a strong inference about the treatment decision.

In the case of meta-analysis B, would your patients choose to take the treatment if either the pooled estimate or the upper boundary of the CI represented the true effect? The answer is yes, the patients would because the reduction in death rate would be greater than the 1% threshold. What about the lower boundary? The answer here is no because the effect is less than the smallest difference that patients would consider large enough to undergo treatment. Although meta-analysis B reveals a positive result (ie, the CI excludes an effect of 0), the sample size was inadequate and yielded a result that remains compatible with risk reductions below the minimal patient-important difference.

For negative studies, those that fail to exclude a true treatment effect of 0, you should focus on the other end of the CI, that which represents the largest plausible treatment effect

FIGURE 10-1

When Is a Meta-analysis Sample Size Sufficiently Large? Four Hypothetical Meta-analysis Results

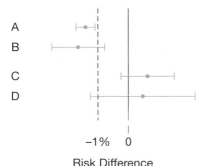

Risk Difference

consistent with the data. You should consider whether that upper boundary of the CI falls below the smallest difference that patients might consider important. If so, the sample size is adequate, and the meta-analysis is definitive: the treatment benefit is not worth the undesirable consequences (Figure 10-1, meta-analysis C). If the boundary representing the largest plausible effect exceeds the smallest patient-important difference, then the meta-analysis is not definitive and more trials with larger sample sizes are needed (Figure 10-1, meta-analysis D).[7]

Application of the logic we have described can sometimes yield surprising inferences. In a blinded trial in patients with vascular disease, 19 185 patients were randomized to clopidogrel or aspirin (Figure 10-2).[11] Patients receiving clopidogrel experienced a 5.32% annual risk of ischemic stroke, MI, or vascular death vs 5.83% with aspirin, an RRR of 8.7% in favor of clopidogrel (95% CI, 0.3%-16.5%; $P = .04$). Clopidogrel is much more expensive than aspirin. Consider patients with a risk of major vascular events of 10% in the next year (1000 per 10 000). Using the trial's point estimate of the RRR of 8.7%, such patients could expect an absolute reduction in events of 0.87% (8.7% of 10%) or 87 fewer events in 10 000

treated patients. Those averse to vascular events may well choose clopidogrel, and were the upper boundary of the CI the true effect (16.5% RRR or, assuming again *baseline risk* of 1000 in 10 000, 165 fewer events in 10 000), they most likely would. If the lower boundary represented the truth, an absolute reduction of only 3 events in 10 000 patients, few, if any, would choose the more expensive drug. Given the different choices at different ends of the CI, we can conclude that the sample size—almost 20 000 patients—was insufficient to provide a definitive answer.

Our logic depends on specifying a threshold benefit below which, given the toxicity, cost, and burden of treatment, patients are unlikely to choose to use the intervention. Investigators seldom engage in the discussion of the threshold; however, if you are to avoid subjecting patients to treatments with marginal benefits and substantial downsides while incorporating their *values and preferences*, you and your patients should do so.

The advent of studies designed to help determine whether we should substitute a treatment that is less expensive, easier to administer, or less toxic for an existing treatment has forced investigators to be explicit about thresholds. In such *noninferiority trials*, we will be ready to make the substitution only if we are sure that the experimental treatment is not substantially less effective than the standard treatment. We deal in detail with the logic of the noninferiority trial in Chapter 8, How to Use a Noninferiority Trial.

CONCLUSION

To decide on your confidence in results, in a positive trial or meta-analysis establishing that the effect of treatment is greater than 0, look to the lower boundary of the CI to determine whether the sample size has been adequate. If this lower boundary—the smallest plausible treatment effect compatible with the data—is greater than the smallest difference that you consider important, the sample size is adequate

FIGURE 10-2

Clopidogrel or Acetylsalicylic Acid for Threatened Vascular Events

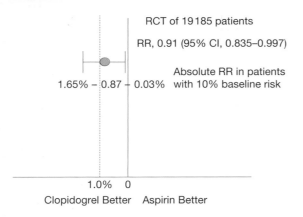

RCT of 19 185 patients

RR, 0.91 (95% CI, 0.835–0.997)

Absolute RR in patients with 10% baseline risk

1.65% – 0.87 – 0.03%

1.0% 0

Clopidogrel Better   Aspirin Better

and the trial or meta-analysis is definitive. If the lower boundary is less than this smallest important difference, the results are nondefinitive and further trials are required.

In a negative trial or meta-analysis, look to the upper boundary of the CI to determine whether the sample size has been adequate. If this upper boundary, the largest treatment effect plausibly compatible with the data, is less than the smallest difference that you consider important, the sample size is adequate and the results are definitively negative. If the upper boundary exceeds the smallest important difference, there may still be an important positive treatment effect, the trial is nondefinitive, and further trials are required.

Acknowledgment

Portions of this material were previously published in Montori et al.[7]

References

1. Simon R. Confidence intervals for reporting results of clinical trials. *Ann Intern Med*. 1986;105(3):429-435.

2. Gardner M. *Statistics With Confidence: Confidence Intervals and Statistical Guidelines*. London, England: BMJ Publishing Group; 1989.

3. Bulpitt CJ. Confidence intervals. *Lancet*. 1987;1(8531):494-497.

4. Pocock SJ, Hughes MD. Estimation issues in clinical trials and overviews. *Stat Med*. 1990;9(6):657-671.

5. Braitman LE. Confidence intervals assess both clinical significance and statistical significance. *Ann Intern Med*. 1991;114(6):515-517.

6. Cohn JN, Johnson G, Ziesche S, et al. A comparison of enalapril with hydralazine-isosorbide dinitrate in the treatment of chronic congestive heart failure. *N Engl J Med*. 1991;325(5):303-310.

7. Montori VM, Kleinbart J, Newman TB, et al; Evidence-Based Medicine Teaching Tips Working Group. Tips for learners of evidence-based medicine, 2: measures of precision (confidence intervals). *CMAJ*. 2004;171(6):611-615.

8. Garg R, Yusuf S; Collaborative Group on ACE Inhibitor Trials. Overview of randomized trials of angiotensin-converting enzyme inhibitors on mortality and morbidity in patients with heart failure. *JAMA*. 1995;273(18):1450-1456.

9. Taylor AL, Ziesche S, Yancy C, et al; African-American Heart Failure Trial Investigators. Combination of isosorbide dinitrate and hydralazine in blacks with heart failure. *N Engl J Med*. 2004;351(20):2049-2057.

10. Brower RG, Lanken PN, MacIntyre N, et al; National Heart, Lung, and Blood Institute ARDS Clinical Trials Network. Higher versus lower positive end-expiratory pressures in patients with the acute respiratory distress syndrome. *N Engl J Med*. 2004;351(4):327-336.

11. CAPRIE Steering Committee. A randomised, blinded, trial of clopidogrel versus aspirin in patients at risk of ischaemic events (CAPRIE). *Lancet*. 1996;348(9038):1329-1339.

THERAPY

11.1

ADVANCED TOPICS IN THE RISK OF BIAS OF THERAPY TRIALS

An Illustration of Bias and Random Error

Toshi A. Furukawa and Gordon Guyatt

THERAPY

As is true of any area of intellectual endeavor, students of *evidence-based medicine* face challenges both in understanding *concepts* and in becoming familiar with technical language. When asked to say what makes a study valid or reduces its *risk of bias*, students often respond, "large sample size." Small sample size does not produce *bias*, but it can increase the likelihood of a misleading result through *random error.*

An error refers to any deviation from the truth. It can be random, occurring by chance, or systematic, tending in a certain direction. The way we use technical language, "bias" is a synonym for *systematic error*. You may find the following exercise helpful in clarifying these notions.

Consider a set of studies with identical design and sample size. Each study recruits from the same patient pool. Will these studies, with exactly the same type of patients and exactly the same study design, yield identical results? No, they will not. Just as an experiment of 10 coin flips will not always yield 5 heads and 5 tails, the play of chance will ensure that, despite their identical design, each study will have a different result.

Consider 4 sets of such studies. Within each set, the design and sample size of each trial are identical. Two of the 4 sets of studies have a small sample size and 2 have a large sample size.

Two sets of studies include only *randomized clinical trials* (RCTs) in which patients, caregivers, and those assessing outcome are all *blinded*. Design features, such as blinding and *complete follow-up*, reduce bias. The remaining sets of studies use an *observational study design* (eg, patients are in

treatment or *control groups* according to their choice or their clinician's choice), which is far more vulnerable to bias. In this exercise, we are in the unique position of knowing the true *treatment effect*. In Figure 11.1-1, each of the bull's-eyes in the center of the 4 components of the figure represents the truth. Each smaller dot represents not a single patient but the results of 1 repetition of the study. The farther a smaller dot lies from the central bull's-eye, the larger the difference between the study result and the underlying true treatment effect.

Each set of studies represents the results of RCTs or observational studies and of studies of large or small sample size. Before reading further, examine Figure 11.1-1 and draw your own conclusions about the study designs and number of patients in each of the 4 (A through D) components.

Figure 11.1-1A represents the results of a series of randomized trials with large sample sizes. The results are valid and thus uniformly distributed around the true effect, represented by the central bull's-eye, resulting from the strong study design. The results also do not fall exactly on target because of chance or random error. Nevertheless, the large sample size, which minimizes random error, ensures that the result of any study is relatively close to the truth.

Contrast this set of results with the trials depicted in Figure 11.1-1B. Again, the strong study design results in the individual study results being distributed uniformly around the truth. Because the sample size is small and random error is large, however, the results of individual studies may be far from the truth.

FIGURE 11.1-1

Four Sets of Identically Conducted Studies Showing Various Degrees of Bias and Random Error

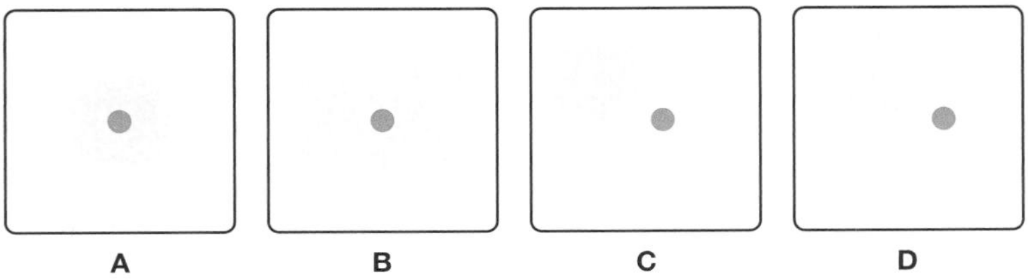

A   B   C   D

A and B represent randomized trials. C and D represent observational studies. In each part, the studies are of identical sample size and identical design.

Thinking back to the coin flip experiments from Chapter 6 (Why Study Results Mislead: Bias and Random Error) clarifies the difference between the studies in Figure 11.1-1A and 11.1-1B. In a series of experiments in which each study involves 10 flips of a true coin, individual results may fall far from the truth. Findings of 7 to 3 (70%) or even 8 to 2 (80%) heads (or tails) will not be unusual. This situation is analogous to Figure 11.1-1B. If our experiments involve 1000 coin flips, analogous to Figure 11.1-1A, we will seldom see distributions more extreme than, say, 540 to 460, or a 54% probability of heads or tails. With the smaller sample size, individual results are far from the truth; with the larger sample size, they are all close to the truth.

In Figure 11.1-1C, the center of the set of dots is far from the truth because studies with observational designs, even large ones, are vulnerable to bias. Because the studies share an identical design, each will be subject to the same magnitude and direction of bias. The results are precise, with minimal random error; however, they are wrong.

One example of this phenomenon is the apparent benefit of vitamin E on reducing mortality from coronary artery disease, suggested by the results of a number of large observational studies. By contrast, a subsequent, large, well-conducted RCT[1] and a meta-analysis[2] of all available randomized trials failed to demonstrate any beneficial effect of vitamin E on coronary deaths or all-cause mortality. There are many additional examples of this phenomenon (see Chapter 11.2, Surprising Results of Randomized Trials).

The situation depicted in Figure 11.1-1C is a particularly dangerous one because the large size of the studies instills confidence in clinicians that their results are accurate. Chapter 11.2, Surprising Results of Randomized Trials, provides many examples of misleading results of observational studies, some of which had a major, if temporary, influence on clinical practice. Had the subsequent RCTs not been conducted, the misleading results would have continued to hold sway.

Like Figure 11.1-1C, Figure 11.1-1D depicts a series of observational studies leading to biased results that are far from the truth. However, because the sample sizes are all small, the results vary widely from study to study. One might be tempted to conduct a meta-analysis of these data. This is dangerous because we risk converting imprecise estimates with large random error to precise estimates with small random error; both, however, are biased and will therefore yield misleading estimates of the true effect.

Finally, note that, even in a situation such as depicted in Figure 11.1-1A, let alone Figure 11.1-1B, any study may be as far away from the underlying truth as the studies in Figure 11.1-1C or 11.1-1D. To put it another way: in any study, random error can lead to differences from the truth as great as systematic error. This is one important reason why you should always seek, and attend to, systematic summaries of all available studies.

THERAPY

References

1. Yusuf S, Dagenais G, Pogue J, Bosch J, Sleight P; The Heart Outcomes Prevention Evaluation Study Investigators. Vitamin E supplementation and cardiovascular events in high-risk patients. *N Engl J Med*. 2000;342(3):154-160.

2. Miller ER III, Pastor-Barriuso R, Dalal D, Riemersma RA, Appel LJ, Guallar E. Meta-analysis: high-dosage vitamin E supplementation may increase all-cause mortality. *Ann Intern Med*. 2005;142(1):37-46.

11.2

ADVANCED TOPICS IN THE RISK OF BIAS OF THERAPY TRIALS

Surprising Results of Randomized Trials

Romina Brignardello-Petersen, John P. A. Ioannidis, George Tomlinson, and Gordon Guyatt

THERAPY

IN THIS CHAPTER

MOST MAJOR BASIC SCIENCE AND PRECLINICAL PROMISES FOR EFFECTIVE INTERVENTIONS DISAPPOINT IN CLINICAL TRIALS

Ideally, *evidence* for the effectiveness of diagnostic, preventive, or therapeutic interventions will come from rigorous *randomized clinical trials* (RCTs) measuring effects on *patient-important outcomes*, such as stroke, myocardial infarction, and death. Whenever an intervention is tested to see whether it is effective for patient-important outcomes, typically some other evidence of variable quantity and quality already exists. This evidence includes combinations of basic science findings, preclinical results, *observational studies*, and *phase 1 or 2 clinical trials.*

Sometimes, clinicians adopt interventions even though randomized trials have never been performed to test their effect on patient-important outcomes. This is very common for acute surgical interventions, common for elective surgical interventions and mental health interventions, and somewhat less common for medical interventions.[1] Nevertheless, even for medical interventions, randomized trials are usually unavailable for interventions that need to be applied for specialized decisions after some major first decision has been made. For example, in the hematology-oncology field there is little evidence from randomized trials for the treatment of recurrent diseases.[2] For interventions such as these, their adoption and continued use in clinical practice have been based on various combinations of basic science, preclinical, and observational evidence.

Moreover, there is a strong undercurrent in many scientific circles that supports the use of *surrogate end points* for adopting interventions for common diseases. Trials using surrogate end points require smaller sample sizes and shorter *follow-up* periods than trials of patient-important end points. Thus, drugs and other interventions can be rapidly tested and approved for clinical use.[3]

Given this patchy and uneven availability of evidence, surprises often occur when interventions that seem promising—or that have even been established according to relatively high-quality evidence—prove disappointing in large randomized trials. Typically, fewer and fewer promising interventions retain their postulated claims to effectiveness as we move from basic science experimentation to RCTs with patient-important outcomes. An empirical evaluation[4] examined 101 major findings published in the top basic science journals between 1979 and 1983 in which the investigators confidently declared that their work would be translated to a major therapeutic or preventive intervention. Of those, only 27 eventually had a randomized trial, and by 2002 only 19 had positive results in at least 1 randomized trial with any kind of end point. At that time, only 5 interventions were approved for clinical use, with only 1 of them having a major effect in therapeutics and the other 4 having uncommon or questionable clinical indications. The credibility of basic science and preclinical claims or observational discoveries, fascinating as they may be, is often low.[5]

TYPES OF LOW-QUALITY EVIDENCE

There are a number of reasons evidence may warrant low confidence[6]; here, we will highlight 3 categories. First, although the methods of a study may be pristine, the participants may be very different from those of interest. For instance, demonstrating that a type of therapy hastens the resolution of experimentally induced renal failure in rats is provocative, but it provides very limited evidence for administration of that therapy to humans.

Second, the outcomes may be interesting but not important to patients. For example, demonstrating the effect of an intervention on cardiac output or pulmonary capillary wedge pressure may herald the introduction of a beneficial drug for patients with heart failure, but trials examining daily function, the frequency of hospitalization, or mortality are essential before clinicians can confidently offer the medication to patients (see Chapter 13.4, Surrogate Outcomes).

Third, investigators examining the effect of a drug, device, procedure, or program on patient-important outcomes, such as stroke, myocardial infarction, or death, may choose the right population and outcome but use a weak study design (eg, an observational study) that leads to a biased estimate of the *treatment effect.*

Evidence may have combinations of these limitations. For example, investigators may use observational study designs to test the effects of interventions using surrogate outcomes on other species.

Our message is not to dismiss evidence warranting low confidence. Studies at higher *risk of bias* may occasionally provide such compelling results that they strongly support clinical use of an intervention. They may even dissuade patients, clinicians, and researchers from performing large clinical trials with patient-important outcomes because of perceived ethical constraints. Evidence-based decision making demands reliance on the best available evidence, even if that evidence is low quality. Moreover, sometimes RCTs with patient-important outcomes still may be highly biased, whereas observational studies of the same question may be more rigorous and their results closer to the truth.

Allowing for these caveats, we suggest that when clinicians rely on low-quality evidence, they acknowledge the risk of administering useless or even harmful interventions.[7] Our concern is empirically strengthened by examples of conclusions clinicians have drawn based on a nonhuman, surrogate end point, or observational studies subsequently refuted by RCTs. In most cases, the lower-quality evidence

suggested that a therapy should be used, but this was later found to be misleading. In a few cases, the opposite was seen: an intervention deemed useless or harmful according to low-quality evidence was eventually, on the basis of higher-quality evidence, found to be effective.

In the following sections, we present examples of instances in which RCT results addressing patient-important end points contradicted the results of previous, lower-quality studies. We categorize the examples according to the type of low-quality previous evidence. All of these examples suggest the same message: clinician, beware!

WHEN RANDOMIZED CLINICAL TRIAL RESULTS HAVE CONTRADICTED NONHUMAN STUDIES

Table 11.2-1 provides examples in which findings from studies using animals or tissues led to

TABLE 11.2-1

Evidence From Studies of Animals or Tissues Subsequently Refuted by RCTs[a]

Question	Evidence From Animal or Tissue Studies	RCT Evidence in Humans
What effect does atrial natriuretic peptide (anaritide) have on renal function?	An experiment evaluated α-human atrial natriuretic peptide in experimental ischemic renal failure induced by renal artery occlusion in renally intact rats. After ischemia, a 4-hour intrarenal infusion restored 14C-inulin clearances ($P < .001$). There was progressive decrease in medullary hyperemia and prevention of intratubular cell shedding and granulocyte margination; at 24-48 hours, tissue histologic findings were essentially normal.[8]	A multicenter RCT studied administration of anaritide in 504 critically ill patients with acute tubular necrosis. Among 120 patients with oliguria, dialysis-free survival was 8% in the placebo group and 27% in the anaritide group ($P = .008$). However, among the 378 patients without oliguria, dialysis-free survival was 59% in the placebo group and 48% in the anaritide group ($P = .03$).[9]
Does acetylcysteine prevent doxorubicin-induced acute myocardial morphologic damage?	An experiment investigated the effect of acetylcysteine administration on the toxicity of doxorubicin in mice. Results suggested that pretreatment with acetylcysteine 1 hour before doxorubicin significantly decreased lethality, long-term	Twenty patients with normal cardiovascular function were randomized to 2 groups. Group 1 received placebo and group 2 received NAC, both 1 hour before doxorubicin. Endomyocardial biopsies were performed and specimens viewed by electron microscopy and stereoscopic

(Continued)

TABLE 11.2-1

Evidence From Studies of Animals or Tissues Subsequently Refuted by RCTs[a] *(Continued)*

Question	Evidence From Animal or Tissue Studies	RCT Evidence in Humans
	mortality, and loss in total body weight and heart weight. Acetylcysteine pretreatment also ablated electron microscopic evidence of doxorubicin cardiomyopathy.[10]	techniques. The change of the tubular area and mitochondrial swelling were similar in the 2 groups and were proportionate throughout the cell. This study found that the acute doxorubicin-induced damage was diffuse and not prevented by NAC.[11]
Does treatment with naloxone (opiate antagonist) improve neurologic outcomes in patients with spinal cord injury?	The opiate antagonist naloxone has been used to treat cats subjected to cervical spinal trauma. In contrast to saline-treated controls, naloxone treatment significantly improved the hypotension observed after cervical spinal injury. More critically, naloxone therapy significantly improved neurologic recovery.[12]	A multicenter, randomized, blinded trial evaluated the efficacy and safety of naloxone (and other drugs) in patients with acute spinal cord injury. Naloxone was given to 154 patients and placebo to 171 patients. Motor and sensory functions were assessed by systematic neurologic examination. Results revealed that patients treated with naloxone did not differ in their neurologic outcomes from those given placebo. Mortality and major morbidity were also similar between groups. Investigators concluded that treatment with naloxone in the dose used in this study does not improve neurologic recovery after acute spinal cord injury.[13]
What is the efficacy of rhRlx as a cervical ripening agent?	Relaxin, a peptide hormone synthesized in the corpora lutea of ovaries during pregnancy, is released into the bloodstream before parturition. Synthetic relaxin exhibited relaxin-like bioactivity assessed by the standard uterine contraction bioassay. Results suggested "synthetic human relaxin … may lead to the development of clinical treatments to alleviate some of the problems encountered at childbirth."[14]	A multicenter, blinded, placebo-controlled trial evaluated the efficacy and safety of rhRlx as a cervical ripening agent in women with an unfavorable cervix before induction of labor. Ninety-six women at 37-42 weeks of gestation were treated with 0, 1, 2, or 4 mg of rhRlx. Results revealed no significant differences in the change in modified Bishop score among the 4 treatment groups, and the lengths of the first and second stages of labor were similar in all 4 groups. Investigators concluded that 1-4 mg of rhRlx has no effect as a cervical ripening agent before induction of labor at term.[15]
What is the therapeutic effect of vitamin D_3 metabolite in patients with leukemia?	HL-60 cells from patients with promyelocytic leukemia responded to near physiologic levels of vitamin D_3 by rapidly acquiring a number of monocyte-like features. These phenotypic changes were preceded by a marked decrement in the expression of the c-*myc* oncogene (a gene related to the process of development of cancer).	An RCT evaluated 63 patients with myelodysplastic syndromes and 15 with acute myelogenous leukemia. Patients were randomized between low-dose cytosine ara-C and low-dose ara-C in combination with 13-CRA and vitamin D_3. Results suggested that the addition of 13-CRA and vitamin D_3 had no positive influence on survival of the patients, remission rates, or duration of remissions.[17]

(Continued)

TABLE 11.2-1

Evidence From Studies of Animals or Tissues Subsequently Refuted by RCTs[a] *(Continued)*

Question	Evidence From Animal or Tissue Studies	RCT Evidence in Humans
	In addition, removal of vitamin D_3, after the onset of maturational change, resulted in the reappearance of elevated *myc* mRNA levels. Authors concluded that "this is the first demonstration of a sequential relationship between the application of an exogenous inducing agent, a reduction in *myc* mRNA levels and the development of characteristics associated with normal cell maturation."[16]	
What is the efficacy of treatment with CA in patients with herpes zoster?	Several investigations of the in vitro antiviral action of CA revealed that CA had antiviral activity in cell cultures against DNA viruses, including herpes. Results also suggested that the presence of CA in the medium feeding actively growing cells inhibited some cellular function necessary for replication.[18]	A randomized, blinded study investigating the treatment of disseminated herpes zoster with CA found that the duration of the dissemination was greater in the treated than placebo group ($P = .03$). Authors concluded that CA at a dose of 100 mg/m²/24 h has no beneficial effects on the disease.[19]
What is the effect of the TNF Fc-fusion protein receptor in patients with septic shock?	Animal models of gram-positive and gram-negative bacterial sepsis have revealed that the fusion protein receptor has an inhibitory effect against TNF-α, protecting animals from death.[20-23]	A multicenter, randomized, blinded, placebo-controlled trial assessing the effects of 3 different doses of TNF Fc receptor found no reduction in mortality when administering the receptor and suggested that higher doses may increase mortality (30% mortality in placebo group vs 30%, 48%, and 53% mortality in the low-dose, medium-dose, and high-dose groups, respectively).[24]

Abbreviations: 1-α-D3, 1 α-hydroxy-vitamin D3; ara-C, cytarabine; CA, cytosine arabinoside; 13-CRA, 13-*cis*-retinoic acid; mRNA, messenger RNA; NAC, *N*-acetylcysteine; RCT, randomized clinical trial; rhRlx, recombinant human relaxin; TNF, tumor necrosis factor.

[a]Data are expressed as reported in the original literature.

misleading inferences. In the typical scenario, an attractive promise in nonhuman research remains unfulfilled when tested in humans, as has been found in recent empirical studies.[25-28] It is uncommon to see negative results in nonhuman experiments being followed by proof of effectiveness on human studies, probably because interventions that do not have promise at the basic science and animal experimentation level are unlikely to move to human experimentation.

WHEN RANDOMIZED CLINICAL TRIAL RESULTS HAVE CONTRADICTED HUMAN STUDIES OF SURROGATE END POINTS

Table 11.2-2 gives examples in which RCTs of patient-important outcomes refuted results of studies using physiologic or surrogate end points. Surrogate

THERAPY

end point studies were either observational or randomized. Whereas in most cases the studies with surrogate end points were overly optimistic, in others surrogates did not suggest any benefit (or even suggested *harm*), but patient-important outcomes indicated benefit.

TABLE 11.2-2

Refuted Evidence From Studies of Physiologic or Surrogate End Points

Question	Evidence From Surrogate End Points	RCT Evidence of Patient-Important End Points
In patients with chronic heart failure, what impact does β-adrenergic blockade have on mortality?	In a before-after study, intravenous propranolol produced decreases in ejection fraction (range, 0.05-0.22) and increases in end-diastolic volume (range, 30-135 mL) in 4 patients with advanced coronary disease and previous myocardial infarction. Abnormalities of wall motion after propranolol developed in 2 patients. Investigators suggested that "results are consistent with the thesis that β-adrenergic blocking drugs may inhibit compensatory sympathetic mechanisms."[29]	A meta-analysis of 18 RCTs of β-blockers in patients with heart failure found a 32% reduction in the RR of death (95% CI, 12%-47%; *P* = .003) and a 41% reduction in the RR of hospitalization for heart failure (95% CI, 26%-52%; *P* < .001) with β-blockers. Significant improvements were also seen in New York Heart Association status.[30]
What effect does clofibrate have on mortality in men without clinically evident ischemic heart disease?	A before-after study of the effects of clofibrate on total and β-cholesterol found, after a 4-week treatment regimen with 750-1500 mg of clofibrate, a significant reduction in total cholesterol level in 86% of patients (30/35) and a significant decrease in β-cholesterol in 91% of patients (21/23). Furthermore, in every case, the tolerance to clofibrate was excellent, and no adverse effects were observed.[31]	An RCT of men without clinical ischemic heart disease randomized participants in the upper third of the cholesterol distribution to clofibrate therapy or placebo. After a mean observation of 9.6 years, there were 20% fewer incidents of ischemic heart disease (*P* < .05) but 25% more deaths (*P* < .01) in the clofibrate group compared with those in the high-cholesterol control group (*P* < .05).[32]
What effect do the antiarrhythmic drugs encainide and flecainide have on mortality from ventricular arrhythmias in patients after myocardial infarction?	A before-after study of patients with symptomatic, recurrent, previously drug-refractory ventricular tachycardia found that encainide completely eliminated recurrence of ventricular tachycardia in 54% of patients after 6 months of therapy and in 29% of patients after 18-30 months of therapy. Investigators concluded that "encainide is a safe, well-tolerated antiarrhythmic agent."[33]	An RCT evaluating the effect of encainide and flecainide in survivors of acute myocardial infarction with ventricular ectopy found an RR of 2.64 (95% CI, 1.60-4.36) for cardiac deaths and cardiac arrests among patients receiving active drug vs those receiving placebo.[34]
In patients with chronic heart failure, does	A before-after study in 12 patients with congestive heart failure found	In an RCT of 1088 patients with severe chronic heart failure and

(Continued)

TABLE 11.2-2

Refuted Evidence From Studies of Physiologic or Surrogate End Points *(Continued)*

Question	Evidence From Surrogate End Points	RCT Evidence of Patient-Important End Points
treatment with milrinone alter mortality?	that milrinone treatment produced an improvement in left ventricular function during exercise, with significant changes in cardiac index, stroke volume index, and pulmonary capillary wedge pressure ($P < .001$). Systemic oxygen consumption increased ($P < .05$), as did maximum exercise capacity ($P < .001$). Beneficial effects on exercise hemodynamics and tolerance were sustained throughout the 4-week treatment period. No drug-related adverse effects occurred.[35]	advanced left ventricular dysfunction, milrinone (compared with placebo) was associated with a 28% relative increase in overall mortality (95% CI, 1%-61%; $P = .04$) and a 34% increase in cardiovascular mortality (95% CI, 6%-69%; $P = .02$). The effect of milrinone was adverse in all predefined subgroups, defined by left ventricular fraction, cause of heart failure, functional class, serum sodium and creatinine levels, age, sex, angina, cardiothoracic ratio, and ventricular tachycardia.[36]
In patients with heart failure, what is the effect of treatment with vesnarinone on morbidity and mortality?	A before-after study of 11 patients with moderate congestive heart failure receiving OPC-8212 found, after 8 hours, that cardiac and stroke work indexes increased by 11% ($P < .01$) and 20% ($P < .005$), respectively, with concomitant decreases in diastolic pulmonary-artery (25%; $P < .005$) and right atrial pressures (33%; $P < .01$). Inotropic effects were confirmed by a shifting function curve. Researchers claimed that "OPC-8212 clearly improves rest hemodynamics … and may be particularly useful for the treatment of mild to moderate cardiac failure."[37]	An RCT evaluated the effects of daily doses of 60 mg or 30 mg of vesnarinone compared with placebo on mortality and morbidity. Results revealed 18.9%, 21.0%, and 22.9% death rates in the placebo, 30-mg vesnarinone, and 60-mg vesnarinone groups, respectively. The HR for sudden death was 1.35 (95% CI, 1.08-1.69) in the 60-mg group and 1.15 (95% CI, 0.91-1.17) in the 30-mg group compared with the placebo group. The increase in mortality with vesnarinone was attributed to an increase in sudden death, presumably from arrhythmia.[38]
In cardiac arrest patients, what is the effect of ACD CPR vs standard CPR on mortality?	Patients in cardiac arrest were randomized to receive 2 minutes of either standard CPR or ACD CPR followed by 2 minutes of the alternate technique. The mean (SD) end-tidal carbon dioxide was 4.3 (3.8) mm Hg vs 9.0 (0.9) mm Hg, respectively ($P < .001$). Systolic arterial pressure was 52.5 (14.0) mm Hg vs 88.9 (24.7) mm Hg, respectively ($P < .003$). The velocity time integral increased from 7.3 (2.6) cm to 17.5 (5.6) cm ($P < .001$), and diastolic filling times increased from 0.23 (0.09) seconds	An RCT allocated 1784 adults in cardiac arrest to receive either standard CPR or ACD CPR throughout resuscitation and found, in patients who arrested in the hospital, no significant difference between the standard and ACD CPR groups in survival for 1 hour (35.1% vs 34.6%; $P = .89$) or until hospital discharge (11.4% vs 10.4%; $P = .64$). For patients who collapsed outside the hospital, there were no significant differences in survival between the standard and ACD CPR groups for 1 hours (16.5% vs 18.2%; $P = .48$)

THERAPY

(Continued)

TABLE 11.2-2

Refuted Evidence From Studies of Physiologic or Surrogate End Points *(Continued)*

Question	Evidence From Surrogate End Points	RCT Evidence of Patient-Important End Points
	to 0.37 (0.12) seconds, respectively ($P < .004$).[39]	or until hospital discharge (3.7% vs 4.6%; $P = .49$).[40]
In patients with myocarditis, what is the effect of immunosuppressive therapy on mortality?	Authors of a before-after study of 16 patients with myocarditis receiving azathioprine and prednisolone in addition to standard measures found a significant decrease in cardiothoracic ratio (62.3% [4.7%] to 50.6% [1.5%]; $P < .001$), mean pulmonary-artery pressure (34.3 [13.05] to 20.0 [2.75] mm; $P < .01$), and mean pulmonary wedge pressure (26.0 [9.1] to 13.2 [4.6] mm; $P < .001$) after 6 months of therapy. Left ventricular ejection fraction improved from 24.3% (8.4%) to 49.8% (18.2%) ($P < .001$).[41]	An RCT assigned 111 patients with myocarditis to receive conventional therapy alone or combined with a 24-week regimen of immunosuppressive therapy (prednisolone plus cyclosporine or azathioprine). A change in the left ventricular ejection fraction at 28 weeks did not differ significantly between the compared groups. There was no significant difference in survival between the 2 groups (RR, 0.98; 95% CI, 0.52-1.87; $P = .96$).[42]
In ventilated preterm neonates, is morphine safe and effective?	Twenty-six preterm infants with hyaline membrane disease requiring ventilatory assistance were randomized to morphine or placebo. Results revealed that morphine-treated infants spent a significantly greater percentage of total ventilated time breathing in synchrony with their ventilators (median [IQR], 72% [58%-87%] vs 31% [17%-51%]; $P = .001$). Heart rate and respiratory rate were reduced in morphine-treated infants. Duration of oxygen therapy was reduced (median [IQR], 4.5 [3-7] days vs 8 [4.75-12.5] days; $P = .046$).[43]	Preterm neonates receiving ventilatory support were randomly assigned masked placebo (n = 449) or morphine (n = 449). Open-label morphine could be given on clinical judgment. The placebo and morphine groups had similar rates of neonatal death (11% vs 13%), severe intraventricular hemorrhage (11% vs 13%), and periventricular leukomalacia (9% vs 7%).[44]
In patients with advanced colorectal cancer, what is the effect of 5-FU plus LV on survival?	A total of 343 patients with previously untreated metastatic measurable colorectal carcinoma were studied to evaluate the effect on toxicity, response, and survival of LV-modulated 5-FU. A maximally tolerated intravenous bolus loading-course regimen of 5-FU alone was compared with a high-dose LV regimen and with a similar low-dose LV regimen. Significant improvements in response rates were observed, with a response rate of 30.3% on the high-dose LV regimen ($P < .01$ vs control), 12.1% on the 5-FU control, and	A meta-analysis was performed on 9 RCTs that compared 5-FU with 5-FU plus intravenous LV for the treatment of advanced colorectal cancer. The end points of interest were tumor response and overall survival. Results revealed that therapy with 5-FU plus LV had a highly significant benefit over single-agent 5-FU in terms of tumor response rate (23% vs 11%; response OR, 0.45; $P < .001$). This increase in response did not result in a discernable improvement of overall survival (survival OR, 0.97; $P = .57$). Authors concluded that "...in

(Continued)

TABLE 11.2-2

Refuted Evidence From Studies of Physiologic or Surrogate End Points *(Continued)*

Question	Evidence From Surrogate End Points	RCT Evidence of Patient-Important End Points
	18.8% on the low-dose LV regimen. Authors concluded that "leucovorin was shown to significantly enhance the therapeutic effect of 5-FU in metastatic colorectal carcinoma."[45]	planning future trials, tumor response should not be considered a valid surrogate endpoint for survival in patients with advanced colorectal cancer."[46]
In patients with breast cancer, what is the effect of neoadjuvant therapy on mortality?	An RCT in 196 premenopausal and postmenopausal patients with operable breast cancer compared neoadjuvant and adjuvant regimens of chemotherapy with radiotherapy with or without surgery. Results revealed that tumor response, evaluated after 2 cycles of neoadjuvant chemotherapy, was significantly associated with dose ($P = .003$).[47]	Clinical end points of patients with breast cancer treated preoperatively with systemic therapy (neoadjuvant therapy) and of those treated post-operatively with the same regimen (adjuvant therapy) were compared in a meta-analysis of RCTs. Nine randomized studies compared neoadjuvant therapy with adjuvant. No statistically or clinically significant difference was found between neoadjuvant therapy and adjuvant therapy arms associated with death (RR, 1.00; 95% CI, 0.90-1.12), disease progression (RR, 0.99; 95% CI, 0.91-1.07), or distant disease recurrence (RR, 0.94; 95% CI, 0.83-1.06). However, neoadjuvant therapy was statistically significantly associated with an increased risk of locoregional disease recurrences (RR, 1.22; 95% CI, 1.04-1.43) compared with adjuvant therapy, especially in trials in which more patients in the neoadjuvant than the adjuvant arm received radiation therapy without surgery (RR, 1.53; 95% CI, 1.11-2.10).[48]
In patients with chronic granulomatous disease, what is the effect of interferon-γ treatment on infection?	A blinded study randomized 128 patients with chronic granulomatous disease to receive interferon-γ or placebo subcutaneously 3 times a week for up to a year. As a secondary measure, phagocyte function was monitored. Results revealed no significant changes in the measures of superoxide production by phagocytes.[49]	The same randomized, double-blind, placebo-controlled study in 128 patients with chronic granulomatous disease considered time to the first serious infection, defined as an event that required hospitalization and parenteral antibiotics as a primary outcome. Results revealed a clear benefit from interferon-γ compared with placebo in time to the first serious infection ($P = .001$). Of the 63 patients assigned to interferon-γ, 14 had serious infections compared with 30 of the 65 patients assigned to placebo ($P = .002$). There was also a

THERAPY

TABLE 11.2-2

Refuted Evidence From Studies of Physiologic or Surrogate End Points *(Continued)*

Question	Evidence From Surrogate End Points	RCT Evidence of Patient-Important End Points
		reduction in the total number of serious infections—20 with interferon-γ compared with 56 with placebo (P < .001).[49]
In adults with cardiac arrest, what is the effect of treatment with high-dose epinephrine on mortality?	The effect of standard and high doses of epinephrine on coronary perfusion pressure was studied in 32 patients. Patients remaining in cardiac arrest after multiple 1-mg doses of epinephrine received a high dose of 0.2 mg/kg. The increase in the coronary perfusion pressures after a standard dose was not statistically significant. The increase after a high dose was statistically different from before administration and larger than after a standard dose. High-dose epinephrine was more likely to raise the coronary perfusion pressure above the previously found critical value of 15 mm Hg. Authors concluded that because coronary perfusion pressure is a good predictor of outcome in cardiac arrest, the increase after high-dose epinephrine may improve rates of return of spontaneous circulation.[50]	An RCT randomly assigned 650 cardiac arrest patients to receive up to 5 doses of high-dose (7 mg) or standard-dose (1 mg) epinephrine at 5-minute intervals according to standard protocols for advanced cardiac life support. Results revealed no significant difference between the high-dose group and the standard-dose group in the proportions of patients who survived for 1 hour (18% vs 23%) or who survived until hospital discharge (3% vs 5%). Among the survivors, there was no significant difference in the proportions that remained in the best category of cerebral performance (90% vs 94%) and no significant difference in the median Mini-Mental State Examination score (36 vs 37). The exploration of subgroups, including those with out-of-hospital and in-hospital arrest, failed to identify any patients who appeared to benefit from high-dose epinephrine and suggested that some patients may have worse outcomes after high-dose epinephrine.[51]
In patients with acute lung injury or acute respiratory distress syndrome, what is the effect of inhaled NO on mortality?	Nine of 10 consecutive patients with severe adult respiratory distress syndrome were made to inhale NO in 2 concentrations for 40 minutes each to investigate whether inhaling NO gas would cause selective vasodilation of ventilated lung regions, thereby reducing pulmonary hypertension and improving gas exchange. Results revealed that inhalation of NO in a concentration of 18 ppm reduced the mean pulmonary-artery pressure (P = .008) and decreased intrapulmonary shunting (P = .03). The ratio of	To evaluate the clinical efficacy of low-dose inhaled NO in patients with acute lung injury, a multicenter, randomized, placebo-controlled study was conducted in the intensive care units of 46 hospitals in the United States. Patients (n = 385) were randomly assigned to placebo (nitrogen gas) or inhaled NO at 5 ppm until 28 days, discontinuation of assisted breathing, or death. An intention-to-treat analysis revealed that inhaled NO at 5 ppm did not increase the number of days patients were alive

(Continued)

TABLE 11.2-2

Refuted Evidence From Studies of Physiologic or Surrogate End Points (Continued)

Question	Evidence From Surrogate End Points	RCT Evidence of Patient-Important End Points
	the partial pressure of arterial oxygen to the fraction of inspired oxygen increased during NO administration ($P = .03$). Authors concluded that inhalation of NO by patients with severe adult respiratory distress syndrome reduces the pulmonary-artery pressure and increases arterial oxygenation by improving the matching of ventilation with perfusion, without producing systemic vasodilation.[52]	and not receiving assisted breathing ($P = .97$). Mortality was similar between groups (20% placebo vs 23% NO; $P = .54$). Days patients were alive after a successful 2-hour unassisted ventilation trial were a mean (SD) of 11.9 (9.9) for placebo and 11.4 (9.8) for NO patients ($P = .54$).[53]
What are the efficacy and safety of moxonidine in patients with heart failure?	An RCT designed to evaluate the effects of central sympathetic inhibition on clinical and neurohumoral status in patients with congestive heart failure evaluated 25 patients with symptomatic heart failure, stabilized while receiving standard therapy. Patients were titrated in a blinded fashion to 11 weeks of oral therapy with placebo (n = 9) or SR moxonidine (n = 16). PNE was substantially reduced after 6 weeks at the maximum dose by 50% vs placebo ($P < .001$). A reduction in 24-hour mean heart rate ($P < .01$) was correlated to the reduction in PNE ($r = 0.70$; $P < .05$). Abrupt cessation of long-term therapy resulted in substantial increases in PNE, blood pressure, and heart rate.[54]	An RCT of SR moxonidine or matching placebo found an early increase in death rate and adverse events in the moxonidine SR group. This led to the premature termination of the trial because of safety concerns after 1934 patients were entered. Final analysis revealed 54 deaths (5.5%) in the moxonidine SR group and 32 deaths (3.4%) in the placebo group during the active treatment phase. Survival curves revealed a significantly worse outcome ($P = .012$) in the moxonidine SR group. Hospitalization for heart failure, acute myocardial infarction, and adverse events was also more frequent in the moxonidine SR group.[55]
In patients with hypoxemic ARF, what is the effect of prone positioning on mortality?	A clinical follow-up study in an intensive care setting examined 13 patients with severe acute lung insufficiency caused by trauma, septicemia, aspiration, and burn injury. Patients were treated in the prone position, without changing of other ventilatory settings other than fraction of inspired oxygen when saturation increased. Results revealed that 12 of the 13 patients responded to treatment in the prone position. No patient needed extracorporeal membrane oxygenation. In the prone position, the oxygenation index increased	A multicenter RCT of 791 ARF patients investigated whether prone positioning improves mortality in ARF patients. Patients were randomly assigned to prone position placement (n = 413), applied as early as possible for at least 8 hours per day on standard beds, or to supine position placement (n = 378). The 28-day mortality rate was 31.5% in the supine group and 32.4% in the prone group (RR, 0.97; 95% CI, 0.79-1.19; $P = .77$). Ninety-day mortality for the supine group was 42.2% vs 43.3% for the prone group (RR, 0.98;

THERAPY

TABLE 11.2-2

Refuted Evidence From Studies of Physiologic or Surrogate End Points *(Continued)*

Question	Evidence From Surrogate End Points	RCT Evidence of Patient-Important End Points
	$(P < .001)$ and the alveolar-arterial oxygen gradient decreased significantly $(P < .001)$. Authors concluded that the prone position significantly improves impaired gas exchange caused by severe acute lung insufficiency and suggested that this treatment be used before more complex modalities.[56]	95% CI, 0.84-1.13; $P = .74$). Authors concluded that this trial revealed no beneficial outcomes and some safety concerns associated with prone positioning.[57]
In patients with severe emphysema, what is the effect of LVRS on mortality?	Eighty-nine consecutive patients with severe emphysema who underwent bilateral LVRS were prospectively followed up for up to 3 years. Patients underwent preoperative pulmonary function testing, 6-minute walk, and chest computed tomography and answered a baseline dyspnea questionnaire. CTs in 65 patients were analyzed for emphysema extent and distribution using the percentage of emphysema in the lung, percentage of normal lower lung, and the CT emphysema ratio. Results revealed that, compared with baseline, FEV_1 was significantly increased up to 36 months after surgery $(P \leq .008)$. The 6-minute walk distance increased from 871 ft (baseline) to 1326 ft (12 months), 1342 ft (18 months), 1371 ft (24 months), and 1390 ft (36 months) after surgery. Despite a decline in FEV_1 over time, 6-minute walk distance was preserved. Dyspnea improved at 3, 6, 12, 18, 24, and 36 months after surgery. Authors concluded that LVRS improves pulmonary function, decreases dyspnea, and enhances exercise capacity in many patients with severe emphysema.[58]	A multicenter RCT randomly assigned 1033 patients to undergo LVRS or receive medical treatment. Results revealed that for 69 patients who had an FEV_1 that was no more than 20% of their predicted value and either a homogeneous distribution of emphysema on CT or a carbon monoxide–diffusing capacity that was no more than 20% of their predicted value, the 30-day mortality rate after surgery was 16% (95% CI, 8.2%-26.7%) compared with a rate of 0% among 70 medically treated patients $(P < .001)$. Among these high-risk patients, the overall mortality rate was higher in surgical patients than medical patients (0.43 deaths per person-year vs 0.11 deaths per person-year; RR, 3.9; 95% CI, 1.9-9.0). Authors cautioned that the use of LVRS in patients with emphysema who have a low FEV_1 and either homogeneous emphysema or a very low carbon monoxide–diffusing capacity comes with a high risk for death after surgery and that such patients are unlikely to benefit from the surgery.[59]
What is the efficacy of indomethacin therapy in low-birth-weight infants?	Thirty-seven infants with symptomatic PDA were in the historical comparison group, and 39 infants were given low-dose indomethacin continuously from 6 to 12 postnatal hours until the recognition of closing PDA.	An RCT randomly assigned 1202 infants with birth weights of 500-999 g to receive either indomethacin or placebo once daily for 3 days. Results revealed that, of the 574 infants with data on the primary outcome who

TABLE 11.2-2

Refuted Evidence From Studies of Physiologic or Surrogate End Points *(Continued)*

Question	Evidence From Surrogate End Points	RCT Evidence of Patient-Important End Points
	Low-dose continuous indomethacin significantly decreased the incidence of symptomatic PDA at 5 days of age (*P* < .01) compared with the historical comparison group. There was no episode of decreasing urinary output and necrotizing enterocolitis in the indomethacin group. Authors concluded that the low-dose continuous indomethacin therapy results in a decrease in the incidence of symptomatic PDA, without significant adverse reactions.[60]	were assigned to indomethacin, 271 (47%) died or survived with impairments compared with 261 of the 569 infants (46%) assigned to placebo (OR, 1.1; 95% CI, 0.8-1.4; *P* = .61). Indomethacin reduced the incidence of PDA (24% vs 50% in the placebo group; OR, 0.3; *P* < .001) and of severe periventricular and intraventricular hemorrhage (9% vs 13% in the placebo group; OR, 0.6; *P* = .02). Authors concluded that in extremely low-birth-weight infants, prophylaxis with indomethacin does not improve the rate of survival without neurosensory impairment at 18 months, despite a reduction in the frequency of PDA and severe periventricular and intraventricular hemorrhage.[61]
What is the effect of salbutamol in patients with acute respiratory distress syndrome?	An RCT in which 40 mechanically ventilated patients were assigned to treatment with either intravenous salbutamol (15 µg kg⁻¹ h⁻¹) or placebo for 7 days measured as the primary end point the extravascular lung water by thermodilution. Patients in the salbutamol group had lower lung water (mean difference, 4 mL kg⁻¹; 95% CI, 0.2-8.3 mL kg⁻¹). Plateau airway pressure was also lower in the salbutamol group.[62]	A multicenter RCT assigned 326 intubated, mechanically ventilated patients to receive either intravenous salbutamol (15 µg kg⁻¹ h⁻¹) or placebo for 7 days. There was a higher mortality in the salbutamol group (35% vs 23% in the placebo group; RR, 1.47; 95% CI, 1.03-2.08). Treatment with salbutamol also was poorly tolerated in the early stages of acute respiratory distress syndrome because of tachycardia, arrhythmias, and lactic acidosis. The trial was stopped early because of safety concerns.[63]
What is the effect of aliskiren in patients hospitalized with heart failure?	An RCT assigned 302 patients with class II-IV heart failure and history of hypertension to treatment with aliskiren, 150 mg/d, or placebo. Patients in the aliskiren group had a decrease in their mean (SD) brain natriuretic peptide plasma levels (244 [2025] pg/mL), whereas patients in the placebo group increased their levels (762 [6123] pg/mL). Aldosterone also was reduced in the treatment group.[64]	An RCT allocated 1639 hemodynamically stable hospitalized heart failure patients to aliskiren, 150 mg/d, or placebo. There were no differences in the primary outcomes of post-discharge mortality or subsequent hospitalization at 6 months (HR, 0.92; 95% CI, 0.76-1.12; *P* = .41) and at 12 months (HR, 0.93; 95% CI, 0.79-1.09; *P* = .36). Authors concluded that aliskiren has no effect on cardiovascular deaths and additional heart failure hospitalizations.[65]

(Continued)

THERAPY

TABLE 11.2-2

Refuted Evidence From Studies of Physiologic or Surrogate End Points *(Continued)*

Question	Evidence From Surrogate End Points	RCT Evidence of Patient-Important End Points
What is the effect of NOS inhibition in patients with septic shock?	Small, clinical, uncontrolled studies assessed the effect of NOS inhibition in patients with septic shock. A study with 11 enrolled patients reported an increase in the mean arterial pressure (from 65 [3] to 93 [4] mm Hg), vascular resistance (from 426 [54] to 700 [75] dyne second/cm⁵), pulmonary arterial pressure (from 31 [2] to 36 [2] mm Hg), and pulmonary vascular resistance (from 146 [13] to 210 [23] dyne second/cm⁵).[66] Another study that enrolled 36 patients reported an increase in the vascular tone and in the cardiac index.[67]	A multicenter, blinded, placebo-controlled RCT assigned 797 patients with septic shock to receive either the NOS inhibitor 546C88 or placebo in addition to standard therapy. Mortality at 28 days was 59% in the NOS inhibitor group and 49% in the placebo group ($P < .001$). Cardiovascular deaths had a higher incidence in the intervention group (14% vs 6% in the placebo group).[68]
What is the effect of ultrafiltration in patients with decompensated heart failure with cardiorenal syndrome?	A trial randomized 24 patients with moderate congestive heart failure to either ultrafiltration or control. Ultrafiltration reduced the radiologic score of extravascular lung water, ventricular filling pressures, and increased oxygen consumption.[69] These findings were similar to those of uncontrolled clinical studies.[70,71] Another study found beneficial effects in the right atrial and pulmonary artery and in pulmonary capillary wedge pressure.[72]	An RCT assigned 188 patients with acute decompensated heart failure to undergo ultrafiltration or receive pharmacologic treatment. There was no difference in weight loss between the groups (12.1 [11.3] lb in the pharmacologic therapy group vs 12.6 [8.5] lb in the ultrafiltration group; $P = .58$). There was a higher incidence of adverse events, such as kidney failure, bleeding complications, and intravenous catheter-related complications, in the ultrafiltration group (72% vs 57% in the pharmacologic treatment group; $P = .03$).[73]

Abbreviations: ACD, active compression-decompression; ARF, acute respiratory failure; CA, cytosine arabinoside; CI, confidence interval; CPR, cardiopulmonary resuscitation; CT, computed tomography; 5-FU, fluorouracil; FEV₁, forced expiratory volume in 1 second; HR, hazard ratio; IQR, interquartile range; LV, leucovorin; LVRS, lung volume reduction surgery; NO, nitric oxide; NOS, nitric oxide synthase; OR, odds ratio; PDA, patent ductus arteriosus; PNE, plasma norepinephrine; RCT, randomized clinical trial; RR, relative risk; SR, sustained release.

Surrogate end points can generate misleading inferences for the efficacy and harms of an intervention. Surrogates that capture adequately the eventual clinical benefits and the clinical harms of an intervention are difficult to develop let alone validate.[3,7,74] In some of the examples herein, both study design and reliance on a surrogate were problematic (the RCT failed to identify the apparent effect on the surrogate in a study with a higher risk of bias and also failed to reveal an effect on the related patient-important outcome). An empirical evaluation has found that effect sizes tend to be much larger on average for surrogate end points than for patient-important end points in trials published in high-impact journals.[75]

WHEN RANDOMIZED CLINICAL TRIAL RESULTS HAVE CONTRADICTED OBSERVATIONAL STUDIES OF PATIENT-IMPORTANT END POINTS

Table 11.2-3 indicates that the results of observational studies are often an inadequate guide for therapeutic decisions, even if they pertain to patient-important outcomes. Some investigators have suggested that evidence from randomized trials and observational studies usually agree.[124-126] An empirical evaluation, however, examined 45 topics for which both RCTs and observational studies were available on the same clinical question and used the same outcome. Observational studies found, on average, larger benefits, and in 7 of these questions, the 2 designs gave results that were different beyond chance.[127] Overall, estimates from observational studies may be more variable than estimates from randomized trials of a similar sample size, reflecting the noise introduced by uncontrolled aspects of study design.[128] Some observational studies may use very large sample sizes (much larger than what randomized trials can achieve), and therefore they produce spuriously tight *confidence intervals* (CIs). Young and Karr[129] have described 52 claims for significant effects made by observational studies, none of which were validated in the subsequent RCTs.

TABLE 11.2-3

Refuted Evidence From Observational Studies[a]

Question	Evidence From Same End Points	RCT Evidence
In patients with cerebral malaria, what is the effect of dexamethasone on morbidity and mortality?	A case report of a 40-year-old man with cerebral malaria in a coma for 24 hours suggested dexamethasone had a strong lifesaving effect and thus "dexamethasone should be given routinely, together with antimalarial therapy, to patients with cerebral malaria."[76]	A blinded, placebo-controlled trial of 100 comatose patients found no significant difference in total deaths between the dexamethasone and placebo groups, but dexamethasone prolonged coma among survivors ($P = .02$). Complications, including pneumonia and gastrointestinal bleeding, occurred in 52% of patients given dexamethasone vs 22% given placebo ($P = .004$).[77]
In patients in need of a pacemaker to correct symptomatic bradycardia, what effect does physiologic (AAI) and ventricular (VVI) pacing have on risks of cardiovascular morbidity and death?	A cohort study of the effect of AAI vs VVI pacing with respect to cardiovascular morbidity and mortality found, after a mean follow-up of 4 years in 168 patients, significantly higher incidence of permanent physiologic fibrillation in patients treated with VVI pacing (47%) compared with AAI pacing (6.7%) (RR, 7.0; $P < .001$). Congestive heart failure occurred significantly more often in the VVI group than in the AAI group (37% vs 15%; RR, 2.5; $P < .005$). Analysis of survival data revealed a higher overall mortality rate in the VVI group (23%) than in the AAI group (8%) (RR, 2.9; $P < .05$).[78]	Investigators randomized 2568 patients to an AAI or VVI pacemaker and found that the type of pacemaker had virtually no effect on the annual rate of death (6.3% in the AAI group vs 6.6% in the VVI group; RRR, 4%; 95% CI, −29% to 29%). There was no significant difference in the incidence of hospitalization for congestive heart failure between the 2 groups (3.1% vs 3.5%; RRR, 12%; 95% CI, −35% to 42%). The annual stroke rate was 1.0% vs 1.1%. There were significantly more perioperative complications with AAI pacing than with VVI pacing (9.0% vs 3.8%; $P < .001$).[79]

THERAPY

(Continued)

TABLE 11.2-3

Refuted Evidence From Observational Studies[a] *(Continued)*

Question	Evidence From Same End Points	RCT Evidence
What effect does plasma exchange have in patents with dermato-myositis and polymyositis?	Authors of a before-after study of 38 patients who had undergone plasma exchanges between 1980 and 1986 found that, according to changes in muscle force, 24 patients (63%) improved (10 appreciably and 14 moderately) and 14 remained unchanged. Plasma exchange was well tolerated in 23 patients.[80]	An RCT of 39 patients with definite polymyositis or dermatomyositis assigned to receive plasma exchange, leukapheresis, or sham apheresis found no significant differences among the 3 treatment groups in final muscle strength or functional capacity; investigators concluded that leukapheresis and plasma exchange are no more effective than sham apheresis.[81]
What is the effect of sodium fluoride on vertebral fractures?	In a before-after study using quantitative computed tomography to measure TVBD in the lumbar spine of 18 female patients with osteoporosis, TVBD was significantly greater in the experimental group than mean TVBD for an age-matched group of untreated female patients with osteoporosis ($P < .001$). Only 1 of the 18 fluoride-treated patients had spinal fractures during therapy. Incidence (4 fractures per 87.2 patient-years of observation) was significantly lower than the published incidence of 76 fractures per 91 patient-years for untreated patients ($P < .001$).[82]	An RCT studied patients receiving either sodium fluoride or placebo, in addition to daily supplements of calcium. Compared with the placebo group, the treatment group had increases in median bone mineral density of 35% ($P < .001$) in the lumbar spine, 12% ($P < .001$) in the femoral neck, and 10% ($P < .001$) in the femoral trochanter. However, the number of new vertebral fractures was similar in the 2 groups (163 and 136, respectively; $P = .32$), whereas the fluoride-treated patients had nonvertebral fractures 3.2 times more often than patients given placebo (95% CI, 1.8-5.6; $P < .01$).[83]
Does ERT alter the risk of stroke in postmenopausal women?	A national sample of 1910 (of 2371 eligible) white postmenopausal women who were 55–74 years old and who did not report a history of stroke at that time were examined. Results revealed that there were 250 incident cases of stroke identified, including 64 deaths with stroke listed as the underlying cause. The age-adjusted incidence rate of stroke among postmenopausal hormone ever-users was 82 per 10 000 woman-years of follow-up compared with 124 per 10 000 among never-users. Postmenopausal hormone use remained a protective factor against stroke incidence (RR, 0.69; 95% CI, 0.47-1.00) and stroke mortality (RR, 0.37; 95% CI, 0.14-0.92) after adjustment for the baseline risk factors.[84]	A multicenter, blinded, placebo-controlled RCT involving 16 608 women aged 50 through 79 years assigned patients to receive conjugated equine estrogen plus medroxyprogesterone acetate (n = 8506) or placebo (n = 8102). Results revealed that 1.8% of patients in the estrogen plus progestin and 1.3% in the placebo groups had strokes. For combined ischemic and hemorrhagic strokes, the intention-to-treat HR for estrogen plus progestin vs placebo was 1.31 (95% CI, 1.02-1.68). The HRs were 1.44 (95% CI, 1.09-1.90) for ischemic stroke and 0.82 (95% CI, 0.43-1.56) for hemorrhagic stroke.[85]

(Continued)

TABLE 11.2-3

Refuted Evidence From Observational Studies[a] (Continued)

Question	Evidence From Same End Points	RCT Evidence
Does ERT alter the risk of dementia in postmenopausal women?	A prospective, longitudinal study of 472 postmenopausal or perimeno-pausal women, followed for up to 16 years, found that approximately 45% of the women in the cohort had used ERT and diagnosed 34 incident cases of AD (National Institute of Neurological and Communicative Disorders and Stroke and the Alzheimer's Disease and Related Disorders Association criteria) during follow-up, including 9 estrogen users. After adjusting for education, the RR for AD in ERT users compared with nonusers was 0.46 (95% CI, 0.21-1.00), suggesting a reduced risk of AD for women who had reported the use of estrogen.[84]	A randomized, blinded, placebo-controlled clinical trial enrolled 4532 eligible postmenopausal women 65 years or older and free of prob-able dementia at baseline. Participants received conjugated equine estrogen with medroxyprogesterone acetate (n = 2145) or matching placebo (n = 2236). More women in the estrogen plus progestin group had a substan-tial and clinically important decrease ($\geq$2 SDs) in Modified Mini-Mental State Examination total score (6.7%) com-pared with the placebo group (4.8%) (P = .008).[85]
In patients with diabetes who have ISH, what is the effect of diuretic-based antihyper-tensive treatment on mortality?	In a cohort analytic study of 759 par-ticipants aged 35 to 69 years with normal serum creatinine levels, cardiovascular mortality in individu-als with diabetes, after adjusting for differences in risk factors, was 3.8 times higher in patients treated with diuretics alone than in patients with untreated hypertension (P < .001). Investigators concluded that "there is an urgent need to reconsider its con-tinued usage in this population."[86]	Authors of an RCT of diuretic treatment vs placebo in 4736 patients aged $\geq$60 years with ISH found an RRR in 5-year major cardiovascular death rate of 34% for active treatment compared with pla-cebo for patients with diabetes (95% CI, 6%-54%) and for those without diabe-tes (95% CI, 21%-45%). Absolute risk reduction with active treatment com-pared with placebo was twice as great for patients with vs without diabetes (101/1000 vs 51/1000 at 5 years).[87]
In critically ill patients, what is the effect of treat-ment with growth hormone on mortality?	A before-after study of 53 patients in whom standard ventilator weaning protocols had failed and who were subsequently treated with HGH found that 81% of the previously unwean-able patients were eventually weaned from mechanical ventilation, with overall survival of 76%. Predicted mortality of the study group was significantly greater than the actual mortality rate (P < .05). Researchers concluded that "this study presents clinical evidence supporting the safety and efficacy of HGH in pro-moting respiratory independence in a selected group of surgical ICU patients."[88]	Two multicenter RCTs were performed in patients in ICUs. The patients received either HGH or placebo until discharge from intensive care or for a maximum of 21 days. The in-hospital mortality rate was higher in the HGH arms (P < .001 for both studies). The RR of death was 1.9 (95% CI, 1.3-2.9) in the Finnish study and 2.4 (95% CI, 1.6-3.5) in the multinational study. Among sur-vivors, the length of stay in the ICU and in the hospital and the duration of mechanical ventilation were prolonged in the HGH group.[89]

(Continued)

THERAPY

TABLE 11.2-3

Refuted Evidence From Observational Studies[a] *(Continued)*

Question	Evidence From Same End Points	RCT Evidence
In patients with DVT, what is the effect of vena cava filters (vs no filter) on pulmonary embolism and recurrent DVT?	A before-after study followed up the insertion of 61 vena cava filters (47 permanent and 14 temporary) in patients with DVT and recorded no deaths or clinically evident pulmonary embolism in any patient in whom a vena cava filter was inserted. Researchers concluded that "vena cava filters represent an effective prevention of pulmonary embolism together with medical and surgical treatment."[90]	Investigators randomized 400 patients with proximal DVT who were at risk for pulmonary embolism to receive a vena caval filter or no filter. Results revealed an OR of 0.22 (95% CI, 0.05-0.90) for pulmonary embolism at 12 days. However, this benefit was counterbalanced by an excess of recurrent DVT (OR, 1.87; 95% CI, 1.10-3.20) at 2 years, without any significant differences in mortality.[91]
Do educational and community interventions modify the risk of adolescent pregnancy?	A meta-analysis of observational studies found a statistically significant delay in initiation of sexual intercourse (OR, 0.64; 95% CI, 0.44-0.93) and a reduction in pregnancy (OR, 0.74; 95% CI, 0.56-0.98) with educational and community interventions.[92]	A meta-analysis of randomized trials provided no support for the effect of educational or community interventions on initiation of sexual intercourse (OR, 1.09; 95% CI, 0.90-1.32) or pregnancy (OR, 1.08; 95% CI, 0.91-1.27).[92]
What is the efficacy of arthroscopic surgery of the knee in relieving pain and improving function?	A retrospective review of medical records and operative videotapes, along with follow-up evaluation, was undertaken for 43 knees in 40 patients with degenerative joint disease. Mean follow-up was 24 months; 72.1% of patients had good results at follow-up, 16.3% had fair results, and 11.6% had treatment failures. Preoperative clinical status, severity of degenerative changes, and number of pathologic entities encountered at surgery correlated with the results of treatment. Authors concluded that arthroscopic debridement is an effective means of treatment for mild to moderate degenerative joint disease after failure of conservative measures.[93]	A randomized, blinded, placebo-controlled trial of 180 patients with osteoarthritis of the knee randomly assigned patients to receive arthroscopic debridement, arthroscopic lavage, or placebo surgery. Patients in the placebo group received skin incisions and underwent a simulated debridement without insertion of the arthroscope. Results revealed that at no point did either of the intervention groups report less pain or better function than the placebo group. The 95% CIs for the differences between the placebo group and intervention groups exclude any patient-important differences.[94]
What effect do statins have on cancer incidence and mortality?	A nested case-control study was performed with administrative health databases on a cohort of 6721 beneficiaries of the health care plan of Quebec who were free of cancer for at least 1 year at cohort entry, 65 years and older, and treated with lipid-modifying agents. Of the cohort,	A meta-analysis of 26 RCTs investigated the effect of statin therapy on cancer incidence and cancer death. Analyses that included 6662 incident cancers and 2407 cancer deaths revealed that statins did not reduce the incidence of cancer (OR, 1.02; 95% CI, 0.97-1.07) or cancer deaths (OR, 1.01; 95% CI, 0.93-1.09).

(Continued)

TABLE 11.2-3

Refuted Evidence From Observational Studies[a] *(Continued)*

Question	Evidence From Same End Points	RCT Evidence
	542 cases of first malignant neoplasm were identified, and 5420 controls were randomly selected. Users of HMG-CoA reductase inhibitors were compared with users of bile acid–binding resins as to their risk of cancer. Specific cancer sites were also considered. Users of HMG-CoA reductase inhibitors were found to be 28% less likely than users of bile acid–binding resins to be diagnosed as having any cancer (RR, 0.72; 95% CI, 0.57-0.92). All specific cancer sites under study were not or were inversely associated with the use of HMG-CoA reductase inhibitors.[95]	No reductions were noted for any individual cancer type. Authors concluded that statins have a neutral effect on cancer and cancer death risk in RCTs. They found that no type of cancer was affected by statin use and no subtype of statin affected the risk of cancer.[96]
What effect does gastric freezing have on duodenal ulcers?	Clinical observations in 24 patients with duodenal ulcers revealed that short periods of gastric freezing, with inflowing coolant temperatures of −17°C to −20°C, were well tolerated. Patients had subjective relief of symptoms, disappearance of duodenal ulcer craters, and significant decreases in gastric secretory responses.[97]	A blinded, randomized trial of gastric freezing in the treatment of duodenal ulcer allocated patients to either a true freeze with coolant at −10°C or a sham procedure with coolant at 37°C. The results revealed no significant difference in the relief of pain, secretory suppression, the number and severity of recurrences, development of perforation, hospitalization, obstruction, hemorrhage, surgery, repeated hypothermia, or radiograph therapy to the stomach in the 2 groups.[98]
Do occlusive hydrocolloid wound dressings heal venous leg ulcers quicker than simple NA dressings?	Eighteen patients with a total of 24 dermal ulcers of varying causes and unresponsive to other conservative treatments were treated with a new hydrocolloid dressing. The case report revealed that all lesions healed in less time than with other modalities. Authors concluded that the hydrocolloid dressing is more effective than others currently available for the treatment of noninfected dermal ulcers.[99]	An RCT of 56 patients with chronic venous ulcers, present for a mean of 2.4 years, randomized the patients to a new occlusive hydrocolloid dressing or a porous NA dressing. In all patients, dressings were applied beneath a standard graduated compression bandage. There was no difference between the 2 groups, with complete healing in 21 of 28 occlusive dressing patients (75%) and 22 of 28 NA dressing patients (78%) by 12 weeks. Careful graduated compression bandaging achieves healing even in most of the so-called resistant chronic venous ulcers; there was no additional benefit of applying occlusive dressings, which tend to be expensive.[100]

(Continued)

TABLE 11.2-3

Refuted Evidence From Observational Studies[a] *(Continued)*

Question	Evidence From Same End Points	RCT Evidence
What are the effects of folic acid and vitamin B in women at high risk for cardiovascular disease?	A systematic review of 30 observational studies assessed the association between homocysteine levels and cardiovascular disease. After adjusting for potential confounders, authors found that a 25% lower homocysteine level was associated with an 11% lower risk of ischemic heart disease and a 19% lower stroke risk. The effects were stronger in women (OR for ischemic heart disease in women, 0.68; 95% CI, 0.55-0.85; vs OR for ischemic heart disease in men, 0.85; 95% CI, 0.79-0.92). Authors discussed the potential implications of reducing homocysteine levels for public health.[101]	An RCT assessed the effects of lowering homocysteine levels by administering either a combination of folic acid (2.5 mg) and vitamins B_6 (50 mg) and B_{12} (1 mg) or placebo in women at high risk for cardiovascular disease. After 7 years of follow-up, similar rates of the composite outcome of stroke, myocardial infarction, coronary revascularization, or mortality were observed in both groups (RR, 1.03; 95% CI, 0.90-1.19). There also were no differences between the groups in each of the outcomes, despite the higher reduction in plasma homocysteine levels observed in patients in the intervention group.[102]
What are the effects of lowering homocysteine levels in patients with cardiovascular disease?	A systematic review included 20 prospective observational studies that assessed the association between homocysteine and ischemic heart disease, DVT, pulmonary embolism, and stroke. Authors found statistically significant associations; for a 5-μmol/L homocysteine increase, the OR for ischemic heart disease was 1.32 (95% CI, 1.19-1.45) and the OR for stroke was 1.59 (95% CI, 1.29-1.76).[103]	A systematic review included 12 RCTs that assessed the effects of lowering homocysteine levels in people with or without cardiovascular disease. Information from 47 429 participants identified no differences between the intervention and placebo groups for the outcomes myocardial infarction (RR, 1.02; 95% CI, 0.95-1.10), stroke (RR, 0.91; 95% CI, 0.82-1.00), and death by any cause (RR, 1.01; 95% CI, 0.96-1.07). Authors concluded that interventions for lowering homocysteine levels are not effective for preventing cardiovascular events.[104]
What is the effect of an intra-aortic balloon support in patients with myocardial infarction with cardiogenic shock?	A systematic review of 9 cohort studies reported that the risk of mortality at 30 days was lower in patients who had intra-aortic balloon support (RD, 0.11; 95% CI, 0.09-0.13) than in those who did not have it. Authors concluded that this evidence supported the use of intra-aortic balloon support adjunctive to thrombolysis.[105]	The same systematic review[105] performed a meta-analysis of 7 RCTs (n = 1009 patients) and reported no difference in 30-day mortality between patients with and without intra-aortic balloon support (RD, 0.01; 95% CI, −0.03 to 0.04). An open-label, multicenter RCT was performed after this systematic review was published (n = 600 patients), and the researchers did not find differences in 30-day mortality (RR, 0.96; 95% CI, 0.79-1.17).[106]

(Continued)

TABLE 11.2-3

Refuted Evidence From Observational Studies[a] (Continued)

Question	Evidence From Same End Points	RCT Evidence
What is the effect of vitamin B therapy on disease progression in patients with diabetic nephropathy?	A prospective cohort study followed up 396 patients with type 2 diabetes to determine whether there was an association between homocysteine levels and microvascular complications, such as nephropathy and retinopathy. After adjusting for sex, age, and duration of diabetes, the incidence rate ratio was 1.42 for each 5 μmol/L of homocysteine difference (95% CI, 1.09-1.84). Authors concluded that higher homocysteine concentrations are related to the incidence of nephropathy.[107]	A multicenter, blinded RCT assessed the effects of vitamin B to reduce homocysteine levels on nephropathy in 238 patients with type 1 and type 2 diabetes. Authors assessed the progression of nephropathy by measuring the change in renal function. A greater decrease in the glomerular filtration rate was observed among patients who received B vitamin compared with those who received placebo (-5.8 mL/min/1.73 m^2; 95% CI, -10.6 to -1.1). Authors concluded that they demonstrated a harmful effect and that the use of vitamin B to lower homocysteine levels should be discouraged.[108]
Do antioxidant supplements have any effect on primary and secondary prevention of mortality due to chronic diseases?	Antioxidants, such as vitamins C and E, carotenoids, and other nutrients, are thought to prevent and protect against the chronic diseases that account for an important proportion of deaths.[109,110] Data from epidemiologic studies reveal that people who consume a diet rich in these antioxidants have a smaller risk of developing cancer and cardiovascular diseases.[109]	A systematic review included 78 RCTs that assessed the effect of antioxidant supplements on mortality. The information from 296 707 patients revealed no association between the consumption of any antioxidant supplement and mortality (RR, 1.02; 95% CI, 0.98-1.05).[111]
What is the effect of vitamins E and C in the prevention of cardiovascular disease in men?	A meta-analysis of 9 cohort studies that followed up 293 172 patients for 10 years found a trend of lowest incidence of CHD with higher consumption of vitamin E ($P = .01$). It also was reported that those taking >700 mg/d of supplemental vitamin C had a lower risk of CHD than those who did not (RR, 0.75; 95% CI, 0.60-0.93).[112]	An RCT assessed whether men with long-term consumption of vitamins E and C had a lower risk of cardiovascular events. The factorial trial enrolled 14 641 male physicians and followed them up for 10 years. There were no differences when comparing vitamin E vs placebo (HR, 1.01; 95% CI, 0.90-1.13) or vitamin C vs placebo (HR, 0.99; 95% CI, 0.89-1.11). Authors concluded that there is no support for using vitamins E and C for preventing cardiovascular disease in men.[113]
What is the effect of PTAS in patients who had a recent ischemic attack or stroke?	Case series of 8,[114] 61,[115] and 100 patients[116] suggested that PTAS was useful for preventing recurrent stroke and that patients had a low rate of adverse events and a high rate of good outcomes.	An RCT enrolled 451 patients with a recent ischemic attack or stroke due to stenosis of an intracranial artery to receive PTAS adjunct to aggressive medical management or aggressive medical management alone. The 30-day rate of stroke was higher in the PTAS group (14.7% vs 5.8% in the non-PTAS group), and the trial was stopped early because of harm.[117]

(Continued)

TABLE 11.2-3

Refuted Evidence From Observational Studies[a] (Continued)

Question	Evidence From Same End Points	RCT Evidence
What is the effect of revascularization in patients with atherosclerotic renovascular disease undergoing treatment?	A retrospective study assessed the clinical outcomes of transluminal renal artery angioplasty. Authors reported statistically significant reductions in mean arterial pressure and need for antihypertensive medications. Of the patients with atherosclerotic renovascular disease, 70% benefited from the angioplasty.[118]	An open-label RCT enrolled 806 patients with atherosclerotic renovascular disease and assigned them to receive medical therapy alone or medical therapy plus revascularization. When comparing the groups, researchers found no differences in systolic blood pressure ($P = .63$). There also were no differences in the risk of renal events (HR, 0.97; 95% CI, 0.67-1.40), major cardiovascular events (HR, 0.94; 95% CI, 0.75-1.19), and mortality (HR, 0.90; 95% CI, 0.69-1.18). In addition, severe complications associated with revascularization were observed in the trial. Authors concluded that the benefits did not justify the substantial risks of treatment.[119]
What are the effects of vitamin E and selenium on the risk of prostate cancer?	Evidence from observational studies suggested that higher selenium plasma levels were associated with lower risk of prostate cancer. A nested case-control study reported an OR of 0.39 (95% CI, 0.16-0.97) when comparing patients of the highest vs the lowest quintiles of selenium plasma levels.[120] No associations were found between vitamin E and the risk of prostate cancer.[121,122]	A multicenter trial assessed the long-term effects of vitamin E and selenium on the risk of prostate cancer. After following up 35 533 men and observing 2279 cases of prostate cancer, it was found that patients in the vitamin E group had a higher risk of developing prostate cancer (HR, 1.17; 99% CI, 1.004-1.36) than patients in the placebo group. No differences were observed when comparing patients in the selenium group vs patients in the placebo group (HR, 1.09; 99% CI, 0.93-1.27).[123]

Abbreviations: AD, Alzheimer disease; CABG, coronary artery bypass grafting; CHD, coronary heart disease; CR, coronary artery revascularization; DVT, deep venous thrombosis; ERT, estrogen replacement therapy; HGH, human growth hormone; HMG-CoA, 3-hydroxy-3-methylglutaryl coenzyme A; HR, hazard ratio; ICU, intensive care unit; ISH, isolated systolic hypertension; NA, nonadherent; OR, odds ratio; PTAS, percutaneous transluminal angioplasty and stenting; PTCA, percutaneous transluminal coronary angioplasty; PTS, preoperative thallium scanning; RCT, randomized clinical trial; RD, risk difference; RR, relative risk; RRR, relative risk reduction; TVBD, trabecular vertebral body density.

[a]Data are expressed as reported in the original literature.

RANDOMIZED CLINICAL TRIAL RESULTS ALSO MAY CONTRADICT PREVIOUS RANDOMIZED CLINICAL TRIAL RESULTS

Although well-designed RCTs with patient-important outcomes (and *meta-analyses* of these trials) represent the *reference standard* for therapeutic decisions, even this reference standard is not always perfect. Accumulating examples highlight how RCTs may be refuted by subsequent trials that are larger, more carefully protected from *bias*, or more *generalizable*.[5] Even large, confirmatory randomized trials with little or no obvious bias and statistically significant results ($P < .05$) may ultimately prove misleading. For small, underpowered randomized trials at high risk of bias, a statistically significant result is likely to be misleading more often than not.[5,130] The interplay of small sample sizes, small or negligible true effects, risk of bias, and scouring data for significant results can generate spurious literature even for trials with patient-important outcomes. For instance, a number of small trials in early human immunodeficiency virus research that were conducted before the advent of effective treatments revealed major differences in survival that seemed unexplained, implausible, and probably false[131] based on subsequent evidence.

Although small and poorly designed trials are likely to be refuted, even the most prominent, highly cited randomized trials sometimes prove misleading. Among the 39 randomized trials published between 1990 and 2003 that received more than 1000 citations each, 9 had been entirely contradicted or found to have had potentially exaggerated results by 2004, according to subsequent better and larger studies.[132] A typical example of an initially widely cited RCT, the results of which ultimately proved misleading, is an RCT of monoclonal antibody to endotoxin for the treatment of gram-negative sepsis. A trial of 200 patients found that mortality could be halved with this intervention.[133] However, a 10-fold larger trial[134] found that this antibody has no effect in mortality in these patients.

Large randomized trials[135] eventually refuted observational studies and even a randomized trial[136] that suggested that vitamin E decreases cardiovascular mortality. A subsequent summary of trials in a meta-analysis and *meta-regression*[137] suggests that vitamin E does not reduce mortality but also may increase mortality when given in high doses.

EVOLUTION OF EVIDENCE

Clinicians should view evidence on any therapeutic question as a continuum that evolves across time and research designs. The composite evidence may change little or a lot over time as more results become available. Surprises, such as those described herein, comprise the end of the spectrum in these continuous fluctuations. Ideally, one would like to know that once a certain amount of evidence of a certain quality has been reached, then results are not going to change in any important manner even if more studies are conducted. Unfortunately, this point is not reached in practice for many important medical questions.[138,139]

One should be particularly skeptical of very large treatment effects that arise from very small studies, even randomized ones. An evaluation of more than 85 000 meta-analyses of RCTs revealed that it is common to see *odds ratios* that exceed 5 in small trials, but when additional trials are performed on the same question, the effects almost always become much smaller and may even disappear.[140] Small trials with results that suggest large effects that are published in journals with high impact factors may be particularly susceptible to such regression to the mean (see Chapter 11.3, Randomized Trials Stopped Early for Benefit, and Chapter 13.3, Dealing With Misleading Presentations of Clinical Trial Results).[141] The *GRADE (Grading of Recommendations Assessment, Development and Evaluation)* approach to looking at evidence provides guidance for trustworthiness of results,[6] including guidance regarding when sufficient evidence has accumulated to warrant high confidence[142] (see Chapter 23, Understanding and Applying the Results of a Systematic Review and Meta-analysis).

CONCLUSION

Physiologic and pathophysiologic rationale—or an observational study—may accurately predict the results of RCTs. However, this is not always the case. Unfortunately, one never knows in advance whether specific preliminary data will predict the results of RCTs or whether they are misleading. Therefore, confident clinical action must generally await the results of RCTs. Even then, evidence may not be final. Clinicians should consider evidence as an evolving continuum in which even the best classics of old may not stand the test of time.

THERAPY

References

1. Gray JAM. *Evidence-Based Healthcare*. London, England: Churchill Livingstone; 1997.

2. Djulbegovic B, Loughran TP Jr, Hornung CA, et al. The quality of medical evidence in hematology-oncology. *Am J Med*. 1999;106(2):198-205.

3. Fleming TR. Surrogate endpoints and FDA's accelerated approval process. *Health Aff (Millwood)*. 2005;24(1):67-78.

4. Contopoulos-Ioannidis DG, Ntzani E, Ioannidis JP. Translation of highly promising basic science research into clinical applications. *Am J Med*. 2003;114(6):477-484.

5. Ioannidis JP. Why most published research findings are false. *PLoS Med*. 2005;2(8):e124.

6. Guyatt GH, Oxman AD, Kunz R, Vist GE, Falck-Ytter Y, Schünemann HJ; GRADE Working Group. What is "quality of evidence" and why is it important to clinicians? *BMJ*. 2008;336(7651):995-998.

7. Fleming TR, DeMets DL. Surrogate end points in clinical trials: are we being misled? *Ann Intern Med*. 1996;125(7):605-613.

8. Shaw SG, Weidmann P, Hodler J, Zimmermann A, Paternostro A. Atrial natriuretic peptide protects against acute ischemic renal failure in the rat. *J Clin Invest*. 1987;80(5):1232-1237.

9. Allgren RL, Marbury TC, Rahman SN, et al; Auriculin Anaritide Acute Renal Failure Study Group. Anaritide in acute tubular necrosis. *N Engl J Med*. 1997;336(12):828-834.

10. Doroshow JH, Locker GY, Ifrim I, Myers CE. Prevention of doxorubicin cardiac toxicity in the mouse by N-acetylcysteine. *J Clin Invest*. 1981;68(4):1053-1064.

11. Unverferth DV, Jagadeesh JM, Unverferth BJ, Magorien RD, Leier CV, Balcerzak SP. Attempt to prevent doxorubicin-induced acute human myocardial morphologic damage with acetylcysteine. *J Natl Cancer Inst*. 1983;71(5):917-920.

12. Faden AI, Jacobs TP, Holaday JW. Opiate antagonist improves neurologic recovery after spinal injury. *Science*. 1981;211(4481):493-494.

13. Bracken MB, Shepard MJ, Collins WF, et al. A randomized, controlled trial of methylprednisolone or naloxone in the treatment of acute spinal-cord injury: results of the Second National Acute Spinal Cord Injury Study. *N Engl J Med*. 1990;322(20):1405-1411.

14. Hudson P, Haley J, John M, et al. Structure of a genomic clone encoding biologically active human relaxin. *Nature*. 1983;301(5901):628-631.

15. Brennand JE, Calder AA, Leitch CR, Greer IA, Chou MM, MacKenzie IZ. Recombinant human relaxin as a cervical ripening agent. *Br J Obstet Gynaecol*. 1997;104(7):775-780.

16. Reitsma PH, Rothberg PG, Astrin SM, et al. Regulation of myc gene expression in HL-60 leukaemia cells by a vitamin D metabolite. *Nature*. 1983;306(5942):492-494.

17. Hellström E, Robèrt KH, Samuelsson J, et al; The Scandinavian Myelodysplasia Group (SMG). Treatment of myelodysplastic syndromes with retinoic acid and 1 alpha-hydroxy-vitamin D3 in combination with low-dose ara-C is not superior to ara-C alone: results from a randomized study. *Eur J Haematol*. 1990;45(5):255-261.

18. Buthala DA. Cell culture studies on antiviral agents, I: action of cytosine arabinoside and some comparisons with 5-iodo-2-deoxyuridine. *Proc Soc Exp Biol Med*. 1964;115:69-77.

19. Stevens DA, Jordan GW, Waddell TF, Merigan TC. Adverse effect of cytosine arabinoside on disseminated zoster in a controlled trial. *N Engl J Med*. 1973;289(17):873-878.

20. Mohler KM, Torrance DS, Smith CA, et al. Soluble tumor necrosis factor (TNF) receptors are effective therapeutic agents in lethal endotoxemia and function simultaneously as both TNF carriers and TNF antagonists. *J Immunol*. 1993;151(3):1548-1561.

21. Opal SM, Palardy JE, Romulo RLC, Cross AS, Rousfeau A-M, Widmer M. Tumor necrosis factor receptor-Fc fusion protein (sTNFR:Fc) in the treatment of experimental *Pseudomonas* sepsis. Paper presented at: 33rd Interscience Conference on Antimicrobial Agents and Chemotherapy; October 17–20, 1993; New Orleans, Louisiana.

22. Evans T, Carpenter A, Martin R, Coehn J. Protective effect of soluble tumor necrosis factor receptor in experimental gram-negative sepsis. Paper presented at: 33rd Interscience Conference on Antimicrobial Agents and Chemotherapy; October 17-20, 1993; New Orleans, Louisiana.

23. MacVittie T, Kittell C, Kirschner K, Agosti J, Williams D, Widmer M. Effect of soluble rhu IL-1 and TNF receptors on hemodynamics, metabolism, hematology and circulating levels of inflammatory cytokines in a nonhuman primate model of endotoxin shock. Paper presented at: Second Conference of the International Endotoxin Society; August 17-20, 1992; Vienna, Austria.

24. Fisher CJ Jr, Agosti JM, Opal SM, et al; The Soluble TNF Receptor Sepsis Study Group. Treatment of septic shock with the tumor necrosis factor receptor:Fc fusion protein. *N Engl J Med*. 1996;334(26):1697-1702.

25. Tsilidis KK, Panagiotou OA, Sena ES, et al. Evaluation of excess significance bias in animal studies of neurological diseases. *PLoS Biol*. 2013;11(7):e1001609.

26. Landis SC, Amara SG, Asadullah K, et al. A call for transparent reporting to optimize the predictive value of preclinical research. *Nature*. 2012;490(7419):187-191.

27. O'Collins VE, Macleod MR, Donnan GA, Horky LL, van der Worp BH, Howells DW. 1,026 experimental treatments in acute stroke. *Ann Neurol*. 2006;59(3):467-477.

28. Begley CG, Ellis LM. Drug development: raise standards for preclinical cancer research. *Nature*. 2012;483(7391):531-533.

29. Coltart J, Alderman EL, Robison SC, Harrison DC. Effect of propranolol on left ventricular function, segmental wall motion, and diastolic pressure-volume relation in man. *Br Heart J*. 1975;37(4):357-364.

30. Lechat P, Packer M, Chalon S, Cucherat M, Arab T, Boissel JP. Clinical effects of beta-adrenergic blockade in chronic heart failure: a meta-analysis of double-blind, placebo-controlled, randomized trials. *Circulation*. 1998;98(12):1184-1191.

31. Delcourt R, Vastesaeger M. Action of Atromid on total and beta-cholesterol. *J Atheroscler Res*. 1963;3:533-537.

32. Report from the Committee of Principal Investigators. A co-operative trial in the primary prevention of ischaemic heart disease using clofibrate. *Br Heart J*. 1978;40(10):1069-1118.

33. Mason JW, Peters FA. Antiarrhythmic efficacy of encainide in patients with refractory recurrent ventricular tachycardia. *Circulation*. 1981;63(3):670-675.

34. Echt DS, Liebson PR, Mitchell LB, et al. Mortality and morbidity in patients receiving encainide, flecainide, or placebo: The Cardiac Arrhythmia Suppression Trial. *N Engl J Med*. 1991; 324(12):781-788.

35. Timmis AD, Smyth P, Jewitt DE. Milrinone in heart failure. Effects on exercise haemodynamics during short term treatment. *Br Heart J*. 1985;54(1):42-47.

36. Packer M, Carver JR, Rodeheffer RJ, et al; The PROMISE Study Research Group. Effect of oral milrinone on mortality in severe chronic heart failure. *N Engl J Med*. 1991;325(21): 1468-1475.

37. Asanoi H, Sasayama S, Iuchi K, Kameyama T. Acute hemodynamic effects of a new inotropic agent (OPC-8212) in patients with congestive heart failure. *J Am Coll Cardiol*. 1987;9(4):865-871.

38. Cohn JN, Goldstein SO, Greenberg BH, et al; Vesnarinone Trial Investigators. A dose-dependent increase in mortality with vesnarinone among patients with severe heart failure. *N Engl J Med*. 1998;339(25):1810-1816.

39. Cohen TJ, Tucker KJ, Lurie KG, et al; Cardiopulmonary Resuscitation Working Group. Active compression-decompression: a new method of cardiopulmonary resuscitation. *JAMA*. 1992;267(21):2916-2923.

40. Stiell IG, Hébert PC, Wells GA, et al. The Ontario trial of active compression-decompression cardiopulmonary resuscitation for in-hospital and prehospital cardiac arrest. *JAMA*. 1996;275(18):1417-1423.

41. Talwar KK, Goswami KC, Chopra P, Dev V, Shrivastava S, Malhotra A. Immunosuppressive therapy in inflammatory myocarditis: long-term follow-up. *Int J Cardiol*. 1992;34(2):157-166.

42. Mason JW, O'Connell JB, Herskowitz A, et al; The Myocarditis Treatment Trial Investigators. A clinical trial of immunosuppressive therapy for myocarditis. *N Engl J Med*. 1995;333(5):269-275.

43. Dyke MP, Kohan R, Evans S. Morphine increases synchronous ventilation in preterm infants. *J Paediatr Child Health*. 1995;31(3):176-179.

44. Anand KJ, Hall RW, Desai N, et al; NEOPAIN Trial Investigators Group. Effects of morphine analgesia in ventilated preterm neonates: primary outcomes from the NEOPAIN randomised trial. *Lancet*. 2004;363(9422):1673-1682.

45. Petrelli N, Douglass HO Jr, Herrera L, et al; Gastrointestinal Tumor Study Group. The modulation of fluorouracil with leucovorin in metastatic colorectal carcinoma: a prospective randomized phase III trial. *J Clin Oncol*. 1989;7(10):1419-1426.

46. Advanced Colorectal Cancer Meta-Analysis Project. Modulation of fluorouracil by leucovorin in patients with advanced colorectal cancer: evidence in terms of response rate. *J Clin Oncol*. 1992;10(6):896-903.

47. Scholl SM, Asselain B, Palangie T, et al. Neoadjuvant chemotherapy in operable breast cancer. *Eur J Cancer*. 1991;27(12):1668-1671.

48. Mauri D, Pavlidis N, Ioannidis JP. Neoadjuvant versus adjuvant systemic treatment in breast cancer: a meta-analysis. *J Natl Cancer Inst*. 2005;97(3):188-194.

49. The International Chronic Granulomatous Disease Cooperative Study Group. A controlled trial of interferon gamma to prevent infection in chronic granulomatous disease. *N Engl J Med*. 1991;324(8):509-516.

50. Paradis NA, Martin GB, Rosenberg J, et al. The effect of standard- and high-dose epinephrine on coronary perfusion pressure during prolonged cardiopulmonary resuscitation. *JAMA*. 1991; 265(9):1139-1144.

51. Stiell IG, Hebert PC, Weitzman BN, et al. High-dose epinephrine in adult cardiac arrest. *N Engl J Med*. 1992;327(15): 1045-1050.

52. Rossaint R, Falke KJ, López F, Slama K, Pison U, Zapol WM. Inhaled nitric oxide for the adult respiratory distress syndrome. *N Engl J Med*. 1993;328(6):399-405.

53. Taylor RW, Zimmerman JL, Dellinger RP, et al; Inhaled Nitric Oxide in ARDS Study Group. Low-dose inhaled nitric oxide in patients with acute lung injury: a randomized controlled trial. *JAMA*. 2004;291(13):1603-1609.

54. Dickstein K, Manhenke C, Aarsland T, McNay J, Wiltse C, Wright T. The effects of chronic, sustained-release moxonidine therapy on clinical and neurohumoral status in patients with heart failure. *Int J Cardiol*. 2000;75(2-3):167-177.

55. Cohn JN, Pfeffer MA, Rouleau J, et al; MOXCON Investigators. Adverse mortality effect of central sympathetic inhibition with sustained-release moxonidine in patients with heart failure (MOXCON). *Eur J Heart Fail*. 2003;5(5):659-667.

56. Mure M, Martling CR, Lindahl SG. Dramatic effect on oxygenation in patients with severe acute lung insufficiency treated in the prone position. *Crit Care Med*. 1997;25(9):1539-1544.

57. Guerin C, Gaillard S, Lemasson S, et al. Effects of systematic prone positioning in hypoxemic acute respiratory failure: a randomized controlled trial. *JAMA*. 2004;292(19):2379-2387.

58. Flaherty KR, Kazerooni EA, Curtis JL, et al. Short-term and long-term outcomes after bilateral lung volume reduction surgery: prediction by quantitative CT. *Chest*. 2001;119(5):1337-1346.

59. National Emphysema Treatment Trial Research Group. Patients at high risk of death after lung-volume-reduction surgery. *N Engl J Med*. 2001;345(15):1075-1083.

60. Nakamura T, Tamura M, Kadowaki S, Sasano T. Low-dose continuous indomethacin in early days of age reduce the incidence of symptomatic patent ductus arteriosus without adverse effects. *Am J Perinatol*. 2000;17(5):271-275.

61. Schmidt B, Davis P, Moddemann D, et al; Trial of Indomethacin Prophylaxis in Preterms Investigators. Long-term effects of indomethacin prophylaxis in extremely-low-birth-weight infants. *N Engl J Med*. 2001;344(26):1966-1972.

62. Perkins GD, McAuley DF, Thickett DR, Gao F. The beta-agonist lung injury trial (BALTI): a randomized placebo-controlled clinical trial. *Am J Respir Crit Care Med*. 2006;173(3):281-287.

63. Gao Smith F, Perkins GD, Gates S, et al; BALTI-2 study investigators. Effect of intravenous β-2 agonist treatment on clinical outcomes in acute respiratory distress syndrome (BALTI-2): a multicentre, randomised controlled trial. *Lancet*. 2012;379(9812):229-235.

64. McMurray JJ, Pitt B, Latini R, et al; Aliskiren Observation of Heart Failure Treatment (ALOFT) Investigators. Effects of the oral direct renin inhibitor aliskiren in patients with symptomatic heart failure. *Circ Heart Fail*. 2008;1(1):17-24.

65. Gheorghiade M, Böhm M, Greene SJ, et al; ASTRONAUT Investigators and Coordinators. Effect of aliskiren on postdischarge mortality and heart failure readmissions among patients hospitalized for heart failure: the ASTRONAUT randomized trial. *JAMA*. 2013;309(11):1125-1135.

THERAPY

66. Avontuur JA, Tutein Nolthenius RP, van Bodegom JW, Bruining HA. Prolonged inhibition of nitric oxide synthesis in severe septic shock: a clinical study. *Crit Care Med*. 1998;26(4):660-667.

67. Grover R, Zaccardelli D, Colice G, Guntupalli K, Watson D, Vincent JL; Glaxo Wellcome International Septic Shock Study Group. An open-label dose escalation study of the nitric oxide synthase inhibitor, N(G)-methyl-L-arginine hydrochloride (546C88), in patients with septic shock. *Crit Care Med*. 1999;27(5):913-922.

68. López A, Lorente JA, Steingrub J, et al. Multiple-center, randomized, placebo-controlled, double-blind study of the nitric oxide synthase inhibitor 546C88: effect on survival in patients with septic shock. *Crit Care Med*. 2004;32(1):21-30.

69. Pepi M, Marenzi GC, Agostoni PG, et al. Sustained cardiac diastolic changes elicited by ultrafiltration in patients with moderate congestive heart failure: pathophysiological correlates. *Br Heart J*. 1993;70(2):135-140.

70. Rimondini A, Cipolla CM, Della Bella P, et al. Hemofiltration as short-term treatment for refractory congestive heart failure. *Am J Med*. 1987;83(1):43-48.

71. Agostoni PG, Marenzi GC, Pepi M, et al. Isolated ultrafiltration in moderate congestive heart failure. *J Am Coll Cardiol*. 1993;21(2):424-431.

72. Marenzi G, Lauri G, Grazi M, Assanelli E, Campodonico J, Agostoni P. Circulatory response to fluid overload removal by extracorporeal ultrafiltration in refractory congestive heart failure. *J Am Coll Cardiol*. 2001;38(4):963-968.

73. Bart BA, Goldsmith SR, Lee KL, et al; Heart Failure Clinical Research Network. Ultrafiltration in decompensated heart failure with cardiorenal syndrome. *N Engl J Med*. 2012; 367(24):2296-2304.

74. Albert JM, Ioannidis JP, Reichelderfer P, et al. Statistical issues for HIV surrogate endpoints: point/counterpoint: an NIAID workshop. *Stat Med*. 1998;17(21):2435-2462.

75. Ciani O, Buyse M, Garside R, et al. Comparison of treatment effect sizes associated with surrogate and final patient relevant outcomes in randomised controlled trials: meta-epidemiological study. *BMJ*. 2013;346:f457.

76. Woodruff AW, Dickinson CJ. Use of dexamethasone in cerebral malaria. *Br Med J*. 1968;3(5609):31-32.

77. Warrell DA, Looareesuwan S, Warrell MJ, et al. Dexamethasone proves deleterious in cerebral malaria: a double-blind trial in 100 comatose patients. *N Engl J Med*. 1982;306(6):313-319.

78. Rosenqvist M, Brandt J, Schüller H. Long-term pacing in sinus node disease: effects of stimulation mode on cardiovascular morbidity and mortality. *Am Heart J*. 1988;116(1, pt 1):16-22.

79. Connolly SJ, Kerr CR, Gent M, et al; Canadian Trial of Physiologic Pacing Investigators. Effects of physiologic pacing versus ventricular pacing on the risk of stroke and death due to cardiovascular causes. *N Engl J Med*. 2000;342(19):1385-1391.

80. Herson S, Lok C, Roujeau JC, et al. Echanges plasmatiques au cours des dermatomyosites et polymyosites: etude rétrospective de 38 séries d'échanges [Plasma exchange in dermatomyositis and polymyositis: retrospective study of 38 cases of plasma exchange]. *Ann Med Interne (Paris)*. 1989;140(6):453-455.

81. Miller FW, Leitman SF, Cronin ME, et al. Controlled trial of plasma exchange and leukapheresis in polymyositis and dermatomyositis. *N Engl J Med*. 1992;326(21):1380-1384.

82. Farley SM, Libanati CR, Odvina CV, et al. Efficacy of long-term fluoride and calcium therapy in correcting the deficit of spinal bone density in osteoporosis. *J Clin Epidemiol*. 1989;42(11):1067-1074.

83. Riggs BL, Hodgson SF, O'Fallon WM, et al. Effect of fluoride treatment on the fracture rate in postmenopausal women with osteoporosis. *N Engl J Med*. 1990;322(12):802-809.

84. Finucane FF, Madans JH, Bush TL, Wolf PH, Kleinman JC. Decreased risk of stroke among postmenopausal hormone users: results from a national cohort. *Arch Intern Med*. 1993;153(1):73-79.

85. Wassertheil-Smoller S, Hendrix SL, Limacher M, et al; WHI Investigators. Effect of estrogen plus progestin on stroke in postmenopausal women: the Women's Health Initiative: a randomized trial. *JAMA*. 2003;289(20):2673-2684.

86. Warram JH, Laffel LM, Valsania P, Christlieb AR, Krolewski AS. Excess mortality associated with diuretic therapy in diabetes mellitus. *Arch Intern Med*. 1991;151(7):1350-1356.

87. Curb JD, Pressel SL, Cutler JA, et al; Systolic Hypertension in the Elderly Program Cooperative Research Group. Effect of diuretic-based antihypertensive treatment on cardiovascular disease risk in older diabetic patients with isolated systolic hypertension. *JAMA*. 1996;276(23):1886-1892.

88. Knox JB, Wilmore DW, Demling RH, Sarraf P, Santos AA. Use of growth hormone for postoperative respiratory failure. *Am J Surg*. 1996;171(6):576-580.

89. Takala J, Ruokonen E, Webster NR, et al. Increased mortality associated with growth hormone treatment in critically ill adults. *N Engl J Med*. 1999;341(11):785-792.

90. Cotroneo AR, Di Stasi C, Cina A, Di Gregorio F. Venous interruption as prophylaxis of pulmonary embolism: vena cava filters. *Rays*. 1996;21(3):461-480.

91. Decousus H, Leizorovicz A, Parent F, et al; Prévention du Risque d'Embolie Pulmonaire par Interruption Cave Study Group. A clinical trial of vena caval filters in the prevention of pulmonary embolism in patients with proximal deep-vein thrombosis. *N Engl J Med*. 1998;338(7):409-415.

92. Guyatt GH, DiCenso A, Farewell V, Willan A, Griffith L. Randomized trials versus observational studies in adolescent pregnancy prevention. *J Clin Epidemiol*. 2000;53(2):167-174.

93. Gross DE, Brenner SL, Esformes I, Gross ML. Arthroscopic treatment of degenerative joint disease of the knee. *Orthopedics*. 1991;14(12):1317-1321.

94. Moseley JB, O'Malley K, Petersen NJ, et al. A controlled trial of arthroscopic surgery for osteoarthritis of the knee. *N Engl J Med*. 2002;347(2):81-88.

95. Blais L, Desgagné A, LeLorier J. 3-Hydroxy-3-methylglutaryl coenzyme A reductase inhibitors and the risk of cancer: a nested case-control study. *Arch Intern Med*. 2000;160(15): 2363-2368.

96. Dale KM, Coleman CI, Henyan NN, Kluger J, White CM. Statins and cancer risk: a meta-analysis. *JAMA*. 2006;295(1):74-80.

97. Wangensteen OH, Peter ET, Nicoloff DM, Walder AI, Sosin H, Bernstein EF. Achieving "physiological gastrectomy" by gastric freezing. A preliminary report of an experimental and clinical study. *JAMA*. 1962;180:439-444.

98. Ruffin JM, Grizzle JE, Hightower NC, McHardy G, Shull H, Kirsner JB. A co-operative double-blind evaluation of gastric "freezing" in the treatment of duodenal ulcer. *N Engl J Med*. 1969;281(1):16-19.

99. Mulder GD, Albert SF, Grimwood RE. Clinical evaluation of a new occlusive hydrocolloid dressing. *Cutis*. 1985;35(4):396-397, 400.

100. Backhouse CM, Blair SD, Savage AP, Walton J, McCollum CN. Controlled trial of occlusive dressings in healing chronic venous ulcers. *Br J Surg*. 1987;74(7):626-627.

101. Homocysteine Studies Collaboration. Homocysteine and risk of ischemic heart disease and stroke: a meta-analysis. *JAMA*. 2002;288(16):2015-2022.

102. Albert CM, Cook NR, Gaziano JM, et al. Effect of folic acid and B vitamins on risk of cardiovascular events and total mortality among women at high risk for cardiovascular disease: a randomized trial. *JAMA*. 2008;299(17):2027-2036.

103. Wald DS, Law M, Morris JK. Homocysteine and cardiovascular disease: evidence on causality from a meta-analysis. *BMJ*. 2002;325(7374):1202.

104. Martí-Carvajal AJ, Solà I, Lathyris D, Karakitsiou DE, Simancas-Racines D. Homocysteine-lowering interventions for preventing cardiovascular events. *Cochrane Database Syst Rev*. 2013;1:CD006612.

105. Sjauw KD, Engström AE, Vis MM, et al. A systematic review and meta-analysis of intra-aortic balloon pump therapy in ST-elevation myocardial infarction: should we change the guidelines? *Eur Heart J*. 2009;30(4):459-468.

106. Thiele H, Zeymer U, Neumann FJ, et al; IABP-SHOCK II Trial Investigators. Intraaortic balloon support for myocardial infarction with cardiogenic shock. *N Engl J Med*. 2012;367(14):1287-1296.

107. Looker HC, Fagot-Campagna A, Gunter EW, et al. Homocysteine as a risk factor for nephropathy and retinopathy in Type 2 diabetes. *Diabetologia*. 2003;46(6):766-772.

108. House AA, Eliasziw M, Cattran DC, et al. Effect of B-vitamin therapy on progression of diabetic nephropathy: a randomized controlled trial. *JAMA*. 2010;303(16):1603-1609.

109. Stanner SA, Hughes J, Kelly CN, Buttriss J. A review of the epidemiological evidence for the 'antioxidant hypothesis'. *Public Health Nutr*. 2004;7(3):407-422.

110. Willcox JK, Ash SL, Catignani GL. Antioxidants and prevention of chronic disease. *Crit Rev Food Sci Nutr*. 2004;44(4):275-295.

111. Bjelakovic G, Nikolova D, Gluud LL, Simonetti RG, Gluud C. Antioxidant supplements for prevention of mortality in healthy participants and patients with various diseases. *Cochrane Database Syst Rev*. 2012;3:CD007176.

112. Knekt P, Ritz J, Pereira MA, et al. Antioxidant vitamins and coronary heart disease risk: a pooled analysis of 9 cohorts. *Am J Clin Nutr*. 2004;80(6):1508-1520.

113. Sesso HD, Buring JE, Christen WG, et al. Vitamins E and C in the prevention of cardiovascular disease in men: the Physicians' Health Study II randomized controlled trial. *JAMA*. 2008;300(18):2123-2133.

114. Rasmussen PA, Perl J II, Barr JD, et al. Stent-assisted angioplasty of intracranial vertebrobasilar atherosclerosis: an initial experience. *J Neurosurg*. 2000;92(5):771-778.

115. SSYLVIA Study Investigators. Stenting of Symptomatic Atherosclerotic Lesions in the Vertebral or Intracranial Arteries (SSYLVIA): study results. *Stroke*. 2004;35(6):1388-1392.

116. Suh DC, Kim JK, Choi JW, et al. Intracranial stenting of severe symptomatic intracranial stenosis: results of 100 consecutive patients. *AJNR Am J Neuroradiol*. 2008;29(4):781-785.

117. Chimowitz MI, Lynn MJ, Derdeyn CP, et al; SAMMPRIS Trial Investigators. Stenting versus aggressive medical therapy for intracranial arterial stenosis. *N Engl J Med*. 2011;365(11):993-1003.

118. Bonelli FS, McKusick MA, Textor SC, et al. Renal artery angioplasty: technical results and clinical outcome in 320 patients. *Mayo Clin Proc*. 1995;70(11):1041-1052.

119. Wheatley K, Ives N, Gray R, et al; ASTRAL Investigators. Revascularization versus medical therapy for renal-artery stenosis. *N Engl J Med*. 2009;361(20):1953-1962.

120. Li H, Stampfer MJ, Giovannucci EL, et al. A prospective study of plasma selenium levels and prostate cancer risk. *J Natl Cancer Inst*. 2004;96(9):696-703.

121. Gilbert R, Metcalfe C, Fraser WD, et al. Associations of circulating retinol, vitamin E, and 1,25-dihydroxyvitamin D with prostate cancer diagnosis, stage, and grade. *Cancer Causes Control*. 2012;23(11):1865-1873.

122. Gill JK, Franke AA, Steven Morris J, et al. Association of selenium, tocopherols, carotenoids, retinol, and 15-isoprostane F(2t) in serum or urine with prostate cancer risk: the multiethnic cohort. *Cancer Causes Control*. 2009;20(7):1161-1171.

123. Klein EA, Thompson IM Jr, Tangen CM, et al. Vitamin E and the risk of prostate cancer: the Selenium and Vitamin E Cancer Prevention Trial (SELECT). *JAMA*. 2011;306(14):1549-1556.

124. Benson K, Hartz AJ. A comparison of observational studies and randomized, controlled trials. *N Engl J Med*. 2000;342(25):1878-1886.

125. Concato J, Shah N, Horwitz RI. Randomized, controlled trials, observational studies, and the hierarchy of research designs. *N Engl J Med*. 2000;342(25):1887-1892.

126. Ioannidis JP, Haidich AB, Lau J. Any casualties in the clash of randomised and observational evidence? *BMJ*. 2001;322(7291):879-880.

127. Ioannidis JP, Haidich AB, Pappa M, et al. Comparison of evidence of treatment effects in randomized and nonrandomized studies. *JAMA*. 2001;286(7):821-830.

128. Deeks JJ, Dinnes J, D'Amico R, et al; International Stroke Trial Collaborative Group; European Carotid Surgery Trial Collaborative Group. Evaluating non-randomised intervention studies. *Health Technol Assess*. 2003;7(27):iii-x, 1-173.

129. Young S, Karr A. Deming, data and observational studies. *Significance*. 2011;8(3):116-120.

130. Ioannidis JP, Cappelleri JC, Sacks HS, Lau J. The relationship between study design, results, and reporting of randomized clinical trials of HIV infection. *Control Clin Trials*. 1997;18(5):431-444.

131. Ioannidis JP, Lau J. The impact of high-risk patients on the results of clinical trials. *J Clin Epidemiol*. 1997;50(10):1089-1098.

132. Ioannidis JP. Contradicted and initially stronger effects in highly cited clinical research. *JAMA*. 2005;294(2):218-228.

133. Ziegler EJ, Fisher CJ Jr, Sprung CL, et al. Treatment of gram-negative bacteremia and septic shock with HA-1A human monoclonal antibody against endotoxin. A randomized, double-blind, placebo-controlled trial. The HA-1A Sepsis Study Group. *N Engl J Med*. 1991;324(7):429-436.

134. McCloskey RV, Straube RC, Sanders C, Smith SM, Smith CR; CHESS Trial Study Group. Treatment of septic shock with human monoclonal antibody HA-1A. A randomized, double-blind, placebo-controlled trial. *Ann Intern Med*. 1994;121(1):1-5.

135. Yusuf S, Dagenais G, Pogue J, Bosch J, Sleight P; The Heart Outcomes Prevention Evaluation Study Investigators. Vitamin E supplementation and cardiovascular events in high-risk patients. *N Engl J Med.* 2000;342(3):154-160.

136. Stephens NG, Parsons A, Schofield PM, Kelly F, Cheeseman K, Mitchinson MJ. Randomised controlled trial of vitamin E in patients with coronary disease: Cambridge Heart Antioxidant Study (CHAOS). *Lancet.* 1996;347(9004):781-786.

137. Miller ER III, Pastor-Barriuso R, Dalal D, Riemersma RA, Appel LJ, Guallar E. Meta-analysis: high-dosage vitamin E supplementation may increase all-cause mortality. *Ann Intern Med.* 2005;142(1):37-46.

138. Ioannidis J, Lau J. Evolution of treatment effects over time: empirical insight from recursive cumulative metaanalyses. *Proc Natl Acad Sci U S A.* 2001;98(3):831-836.

139. Trikalinos TA, Churchill R, Ferri M, et al; EU-PSI project. Effect sizes in cumulative meta-analyses of mental health randomized trials evolved over time. *J Clin Epidemiol.* 2004;57(11):1124-1130.

140. Pereira TV, Horwitz RI, Ioannidis JP. Empirical evaluation of very large treatment effects of medical interventions. *JAMA.* 2012;308(16):1676-1684.

141. Siontis KC, Evangelou E, Ioannidis JP. Magnitude of effects in clinical trials published in high-impact general medical journals. *Int J Epidemiol.* 2011;40(5):1280-1291.

142. Guyatt GH, Oxman AD, Kunz R, et al. GRADE guidelines 6: rating the quality of evidence—imprecision. *J Clin Epidemiol.* 2011;64(12):1283-1293.

ADVANCED TOPICS IN THE RISK OF BIAS OF THERAPY TRIALS

Randomized Trials Stopped Early for Benefit

Dirk Bassler, Victor M. Montori, PJ Devereaux, Holger J. Schünemann, Maureen O. Meade, Deborah J. Cook, and Gordon Guyatt

THERAPY

IN THIS CHAPTER

Randomized Clinical Trials Stopped Early for Benefit Play a Prominent Role in the Medical Literature

Truncated Randomized Clinical Trials Are at Risk of Overestimating Treatment Effects

Estimates From Truncated Randomized Clinical Trials Are Frequently Too Good to Be True

Truncated Randomized Clinical Trials May Prevent a Comprehensive Assessment of Treatment Effect

Ethical Considerations

Was There a Planned Stopping Rule?

Did the Planned Stopping Rule Involve Few Interim Looks, and Did the Trial Enroll a Large Proportion of the Planned Sample Size?

Were There a Large Number of Events?

What Are the Results of Other Studies That Ask the Same Question?

Conclusion: Guidance for the Clinician

RANDOMIZED CLINICAL TRIALS STOPPED EARLY FOR BENEFIT PLAY A PROMINENT ROLE IN THE MEDICAL LITERATURE

Investigators may stop *randomized clinical trials* (RCTs) earlier than planned because of perceived harm of the *experimental intervention*, because they lose hope in achieving a positive result, or because the sponsor wishes to save money.[1] The reason for early stopping that may have the most effect on clinical practice, however, is that investigators note *treatment effects* that appear to be unlikely by chance—and that are usually large—that persuade them that the experimental intervention is beneficial. Trials stopped early for apparent benefit—which we will refer to as *truncated RCTs* (tRCTs)—often receive considerable attention. They appear in the most prominent journals and in the popular press[2,3] markedly increasing the likelihood of widespread dissemination and subsequent citation. These trials may, with remarkable rapidity, form the basis of *practice guidelines* and criteria for quality of medical care—and such recommendations may persist after subsequent studies have debunked the results of the tRCTs. For example, such has been the fate of

stopped-early RCTs documenting the effect of tight glucose control with insulin in patients in the intensive care unit, β-blockers in patients undergoing vascular surgery, and activated protein C in sepsis.[4]

Truncated Randomized Clinical Trials Are at Risk of Overestimating Treatment Effects

Truncated RCTs will, on average, overestimate treatment effects, and this overestimation may be large, particularly when tRCTs have a small number of outcome events. To understand this overestimation, imagine a number of similar RCTs that address a particular research question in which the truth is a small treatment effect. If trials are at low *risk of bias*, their results will vary only because of chance. Some trials will start and continue near the truth. However, because of imprecision when the sample size is still small, some will reveal apparent *harm* early on, and some will reveal large overestimates: the latter 2 categories of trials will approach the truth as the data accumulate (Figure 11.3-1).

Truncated RCTs will belong to the group of trials that overestimate because they are at the high end of the random distribution of results. Correspondingly, the non-tRCTs will tend to slightly underestimate. Thus, the overestimation from tRCTs is largely the result of random error. If such studies were to

FIGURE 11.3-1

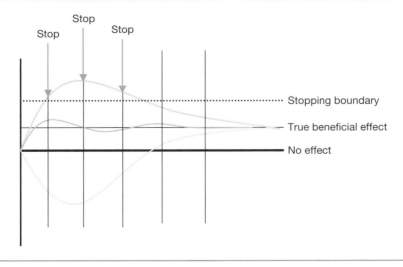

Theoretical Distribution of Randomized Clinical Trial Results as Data Accumulate

continue to their planned sample sizes, then because of what Pocock and White[5] have described as "regression to the truth," they would still produce overestimates of effect, but those overestimates would be smaller than those seen with early stopping.

As Figure 11.3-1 suggests, large random differences from the true effect are more likely to happen early in a trial when sample sizes are small.[5,6] Thus, trials stopped early with extreme stopping boundaries will often produce effect estimates much larger than the truth. The smaller the sample size at the time of an interim look at the data, and in particular the smaller the number of outcome events (see Chapter 12.3, What Determines the Width of the Confidence Interval?), the larger an effect estimate needs to be to qualify for standard *stopping rules*, and thus the larger the overestimate of effect is likely to be.

Although statistical simulation can readily reveal how tRCTs will overestimate treatment effects,[5] trials in which investigators have looked at the data as they accumulated but refrained from stopping early also provide compelling evidence. For example, investigators conducted a trial that compared 5 vs 4 courses of chemotherapy for acute myeloid leukemia.[7] They observed an extremely large treatment effect early in their RCT (Figure 11.3-2). Their results crossed their prespecified stopping boundary. Nevertheless, because they correctly concluded that the effect was too good to be true, they continued recruiting and following up patients. Ultimately, the apparent beneficial effect disappeared, and the final result revealed a weak trend toward harm.

THERAPY

FIGURE 11.3-2

A Near Miss in a Trial of Chemotherapy for Leukemia

Time Point	Deaths/Patients		Statistics		HR and 95% CI		Odds Reduction
	5 Courses	4 Courses	(O–E)	Var.	5 Courses :	4 Courses	(SD)
1997	7/102	15/100	–4.6	5.5			57% (29); 2P = 0.05
1998 (1)	23/171	42/169	–12.0	15.9			53% (18); 2P = 0.003
1998 (2)	41/240	66/240	–16.0	26.7			45% (15); 2P = 0.002
1999	51/312	69/309	–11.9	30.0			33% (15); 2P = 0.03
2000	79/349	91/345	–9.5	42.4			20% (14); 2P = 0.1
2001	106/431	113/432	–6.2	53.7			11% (13); 2P = 0.4
2002	157/537	140/541	6.7	74.0			–9% (12); 2P = 0.4

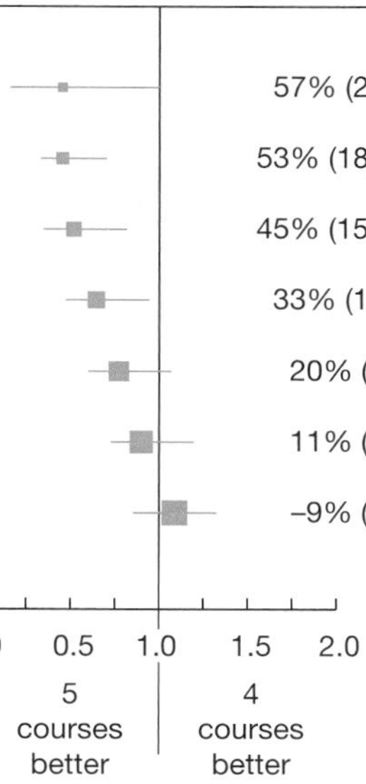

0.0   0.5   1.0   1.5   2.0

5 courses better | 4 courses better

Abbreviations: CI, confidence interval; HR, hazard ratio; P, patients.

Reproduced from Wheatley and Clayton.[7] Copyright © 2003, with permission from Elsevier.

Had the investigators adhered to their initial plan to stop early if they saw a sufficiently large effect and published this erroneous result, subsequent leukemia patients would have undergone additional toxic chemotherapy without benefit.

Estimates From Truncated Randomized Clinical Trials Are Frequently Too Good to Be True

A *systematic review* and *meta-analysis* that compared the treatment effect from tRCTs with that from meta-analyses of RCTs addressing the same research question but not stopped early found the pooled ratio of *relative risks* (RRs) in tRCTs vs matching nontruncated RCTs was 0.71 (95% *confidence interval* [CI], 0.65-0.77).[3] This implies that, for instance, if the RR from non-tRCTs was 0.8 (a 20% *relative risk reduction* [RRR]), the RR from the tRCTs would be, on average, approximately 0.57 (a 43% RRR—more than double the apparent benefit). Non-tRCTs with no evidence of benefit (ie, with an RR of 1.0) would, on average, be associated with a 29% RRR in tRCTs that addressed the same research question.

This overestimation could not be explained by differences in methodologic quality (*allocation concealment* and *blinding*) or by the presence of a statistical stopping rule, but it was associated with the total number of outcome events.[3] As we describe subsequently, the results of the meta-analysis provide guidance regarding numbers of events that provide protection against large overestimates.

Truncated Randomized Clinical Trials May Prevent a Comprehensive Assessment of Treatment Effect

In 32 of 143 tRCTs included in another systematic review, the decision to stop was based on a *composite end point* (an aggregate of end points of various importance).[2] Use of a composite end point compounds the *risk* of misleading results: the least *patient-important outcome* that makes up the composite end point (eg, angina in a composite of death, myocardial infarction, and angina) (see Chapter 12.4, Composite End Points) may drive the decision to stop early. Consequently, few events that are most important to patients may accrue.

Even when investigators do not use composite end points, few events are likely to accrue in the end points not driving the decision to stop early for benefit. These end points may include patient-important beneficial events (eg, overall survival rather than progression-free survival[8]) or adverse events. Lack of adequate safety data as a result of stopping the trial early may in turn affect the perceived and actual risk-benefit ratios (ie, overestimating the benefit and underestimating the risk) of implementing the intervention in clinical practice.[9]

ETHICAL CONSIDERATIONS

Readers may, at this point, experience a dilemma. Even if investigators are aware of the dangers of stopping early—overestimating treatment effects and failing to provide precise estimates of effect on all patient-important benefits and risks[10]—how can they continue to ethically enroll patients who have a 50% chance of receiving *placebo* when results indicate an apparent large benefit of treatment? The answer to the question lies in ethical responsibilities toward the many patients who are at risk of basing their subsequent treatment decisions on false information.[11] For instance, the prospect of patients with leukemia undergoing toxic chemotherapy without benefit, as in our previous example, is not ethically attractive. Patients deserve robust, accurate, and precise estimates of the effects of treatments they are considering.

WAS THERE A PLANNED STOPPING RULE?

If investigators check their data periodically and stop as soon as they observe an apparent large treatment effect, the risk of overestimation of the treatment effect is substantial (Figure 11.3-1). A previous plan to look at the data only periodically (eg, at 250, 500, and 750 completed patients of a trial planning to enroll 1000 patients) and stop only if the results meet certain criteria (eg, $P < .001$) reduces considerably the chances of stopping early.

There are, however, 3 serious limitations of formal stopping rules. First, investigators sometimes choose unsatisfactory criteria for termination. In one trial, after finding an apparent trend in favor of treatment after 28 patients, investigators decided to review the data after every subsequent 5 patients and to stop as soon as their P value reached .001 (which it did after another 25 patients, for a total of 53 enrolled, of whom 28 had died).[12]

Second, trials that stop early without formal stopping rules often fail to inform you that their trial was indeed stopped early. This is one reason to be skeptical of small trials with very large effects—they may represent instances of stopping in response to a large treatment effect discovered because of repeated looks at the data (see Chapter 13.3, Dealing With Misleading Presentations of Clinical Trial Results).

Third, trials that hit preplanned stopping boundaries early, after relatively few events, are still likely to overestimate the treatment effect. Even those with more events will, on average, overestimate treatment effects; however, as we have pointed out, in those with very large sample sizes, the overestimates will be modest. Without a prior rule, the risk of substantial overestimates of effect is very high.

Did the Planned Stopping Rule Involve Few Interim Looks, and Did the Trial Enroll a Large Proportion of the Planned Sample Size?

Trials with stopping rules that involve multiple looks at short intervals, such as the every-5-patients criterion described above, provide little protection against the play of chance and the risk of an inflated estimate of treatment effect. Somewhat more rigorous criteria with excessively lenient P values (for instance, .02) are also problematic.[13,14] More rigorous criteria that demand a $P \le .001$ provide increasing protection.

Stringent P values, however, still leave a major danger: although they will decrease the likelihood of stopping early, the more stringent the P value, the greater the likelihood that, in instances in which the boundary is crossed, the overestimate of the treatment effect will be large. In other words, the stringent P value decreases the likelihood of stopping early but does nothing to protect against the overestimate of effect

when the boundary is crossed. Added protection comes from looking infrequently and late in the trial (when most of the anticipated events have occurred) and from the continuation of enrollment in combination with having another look after the stopping criteria are met. That is particularly true when, as the next criterion suggests, the trial included large numbers of patients, a large proportion of whom experienced the outcome of interest.

WERE THERE A LARGE NUMBER OF EVENTS?

As events accumulate, the likelihood of chance producing a substantially inflated effect decreases (Figure 11.3-1). The systematic review and meta-analysis that compared treatment effects from tRCTs with those from meta-analyses of RCTs that addressed the same research question but were not stopped early found a substantial overestimation of effect in the tRCTs.[3] Very large overestimates were common when the total number of events was less than 100, with large overestimates up to 200 events; smaller but important overestimates occurred with 200 to 500 events; and trials with more than 500 events showed small overestimates. Thus, when true underlying treatment effects are modest—as is usually the case—small trials that are stopped early with few outcome events (<200 events) will result in large overestimates. Larger trials still will, on average, overestimate effects, and these overestimates also may lead to important spurious inferences. Thus, skepticism is warranted for any stopped-early trial, but high levels of skepticism are mandatory when numbers of events are small.

WHAT ARE THE RESULTS OF OTHER STUDIES THAT ASK THE SAME QUESTION?

The first principle of evidence-based medicine is that patient management should be based on systematic summaries of all the best evidence (see Chapter 2, What Is Evidence-Based Medicine?). This principle is

THERAPY

nowhere more necessary than in a tRCT. Simulations reveal that, on average, meta-analyses that include a substantial number of RCTs of which one or more are tRCTS with appropriate stopping rules and that include a large number of events will lead to only trivial overestimation of treatment effects. Thus, meta-analyses that meet these specifications should solve the problem of potential overestimation caused by early stopping.[15]

However, under certain circumstances tRCTs will disproportionally contribute to meta-analytic estimates, again running the risk of substantial overestimation of effects. This will be true when tRCTs occur early in the sequence of trials with few subsequent studies, when publication of nontruncated RCTs is delayed, or when there is *publication bias*. Much more serious, the tRCTs may impede the conduct of future trials.[15] The danger of overestimation will be particularly high when the following 3 conditions exist: (1) tRCTs have a relatively small number of outcome events (eg, <200), (2) there is a substantial difference (eg, RR <0.7) in the RRs between the tRCTs and the non-tRCTs, and (3) the tRCTs have a substantial (>20%) weight in the meta-analysis. When these 3 conditions do not exist and RCTs have instituted safeguards against *bias* and yield precise estimates that are consistent across trials,[16,17] readers of systematic reviews and meta-analyses can, regardless of the presence of tRCTs, have a high level of confidence in the results.

CONCLUSION: GUIDANCE FOR THE CLINICIAN

How should a clinician respond to a trial stopped early? If the conventional risk of bias criteria are met (see Chapter 7, Therapy [Randomized Trials]) and the tRCT has a very large number of events (>500 events), the trial may well represent an accurate estimate of the true patient benefit, and the clinician can proceed with confidence. If not, the clinician faces a situation not dissimilar to acting on the basis of trials with high risk of bias: the results are likely to represent an overestimate of the effect and, particularly if the number of events is relatively small (<200 events), the degree of the overestimate may be large.

As with any individual trial, clinicians should seek systematic reviews of all trials that address the question or, short of that, information sources that will summarize the existing evidence (although not in the form of a systematic review). If the body of evidence is dominated by a tRCT, patients' underlying *values and preferences* (how they feel about receiving treatment with uncertain benefit and some inconvenience, risk, and possibly cost) become particularly salient in decision making (see Chapter 27, Decision Making and the Patient).

References

1. Psaty BM, Rennie D. Stopping medical research to save money: a broken pact with researchers and patients. *JAMA*. 2003;289(16):2128-2131.

2. Montori VM, Devereaux PJ, Adhikari NK, et al. Randomized trials stopped early for benefit: a systematic review. *JAMA*. 2005;294(17):2203-2209.

3. Bassler D, Briel M, Montori VM, et al; STOPIT-2 Study Group. Stopping randomized trials early for benefit and estimation of treatment effects: systematic review and meta-regression analysis. *JAMA*. 2010;303(12):1180-1187.

4. Guyatt GH, Briel M, Glasziou P, Bassler D, Montori VM. Problems of stopping trials early. *BMJ*. 2012;344:e3863. doi:10.1136/bmj.e3863.

5. Pocock S, White I. Trials stopped early: too good to be true? *Lancet*. 1999;353(9157):943-944.

6. Schulz KF, Grimes DA. Multiplicity in randomised trials II: subgroup and interim analyses. *Lancet*. 2005;365(9471):1657-1661.

7. Wheatley K, Clayton D. Be skeptical about unexpected large apparent treatment effects: the case of an MRC AML12 randomization. *Control Clin Trials*. 2003;24(1):66-70.

8. Cannistra SA. The ethics of early stopping rules: who is protecting whom? *J Clin Oncol*. 2004;22(9):1542-1545.

9. Juurlink DN, Mamdani MM, Lee DS, et al. Rates of hyperkalemia after publication of the Randomized Aldactone Evaluation Study. *N Engl J Med*. 2004;351(6):543-551.

10. Guyatt G, Montori V, Devereaux PJ, Schünemann H, Bhandari M. Patients at the center: in our practice, and in our use of language. *ACP J Club*. 2004;140(1):A11-A12.

11. Bernard GR, Vincent JL, Laterre PF, et al; Recombinant human protein C Worldwide Evaluation in Severe Sepsis (PROWESS) study group. Efficacy and safety of recombinant human activated protein C for severe sepsis. *N Engl J Med*. 2001;344(10):699-709.

12. Amato MB, Barbas CS, Medeiros DM, et al. Effect of a protective-ventilation strategy on mortality in the acute respiratory distress syndrome. *N Engl J Med*. 1998;338(6):347-354.

13. Pocock SJ. When (not) to stop a clinical trial for benefit. *JAMA*. 2005;294(17):2228-2230.

14. DAMOCLES Study Group, NHS Health Technology Assessment Programme. A proposed charter for clinical trial data monitoring committees: helping them to do their job well. *Lancet*. 2005;365(9460):711-722.

15. Bassler D, Montori VM, Briel M, et al. Reflections on meta-analyses involving trials stopped early for benefit: is there a problem and if so, what is it? *Stat Methods Med Res*. 2013;22(2):159-168.

16. Guyatt GH, Oxman AD, Vist G, et al; GRADE Working Group. GRADE: an emerging consensus on rating quality of evidence and strength of recommendations. *BMJ*. 2008;336(7650): 924-926.

17. Guyatt GH, Oxman AD, Kunz R, Vist GE, Falck-Ytter Y, Schünemann HJ; GRADE Working Group. What is "quality of evidence" and why is it important to clinicians? *BMJ*. 2008; 336(7651):995-998.

THERAPY

FIGURE 11.4-1

Results of a Hypothetical Trial of Surgical Therapy in Patients With Cerebrovascular Disease

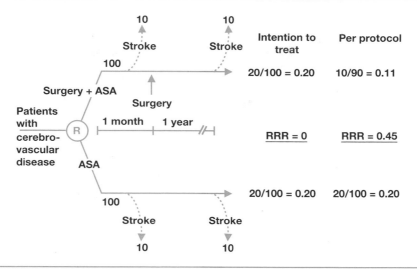

after randomization and another 10 will have a stroke in the subsequent year.

The principle that dictates that we count events in all randomized patients, regardless of whether they received the intended intervention, is the *intention-to-treat principle.* When we apply the intention-to-treat principle in our study of cerebrovascular surgery for stroke, we find 20 events in each group and, therefore, no evidence of a positive *treatment effect.* However, if we use the logic that we should not count events in patients in the surgical group who did not receive surgery, the event rate in the experimental groups would be 10 of 90 (or 11%) compared with the 20% event rate in the control group—a reduction in *relative risk* of 45% instead of the true *relative risk reduction* (RRR) of 0. These data reveal how analyses restricted to patients who adhered to assigned treatment (sometimes referred to as *per-protocol analyses, efficacy analyses,* or *explanatory analyses*) can provide a misleading estimate of surgical therapy's effect.

A REAL-WORLD EXAMPLE OF A RANDOMIZED TRIAL OF DRUG THERAPY

Many years ago, a *placebo*-controlled trial tested the effect of clofibrate, a lipid-lowering agent, to reduce mortality in men between the ages of 30 and 64 years who had experienced a myocardial infarction.[2] After 5 years of *follow-up,* slightly fewer (20% of 1103) patients randomized to clofibrate had died than those randomized to placebo (20.9% of 2789), but this result showed no *statistically significant* difference ($P = .55$). However, the mortality rate in 357 patients treated with clofibrate was 24.6% among those who took less than 80% of their prescribed treatment, whereas it was 15.0% among those who had taken more than 80% of the medication ($P < .001$). The study found parallel results among placebo-treated patients: the mortality rate was 28.2% in low-adherence patients and 15.1% in high-adherence patients ($P < .001$). Patients with high adherence in the experimental group and the control group clearly represent a prognostically better group. The fact that good adherence to drug therapy is associated with positive *health outcomes* supports the existence of a "healthy adherer" effect, whereby adherence to drug therapy is a surrogate marker for overall healthy behavior.[3] In the case of differential adherence to the intervention and control groups, any inferences about treatment effects based on a per-protocol analysis would be extremely misleading.

The intention-to-treat principle applies regardless of the intervention (surgery, medication, or behavioral therapy) and regardless of the outcome (mortality, morbidity, or behavioral outcome, such as smoking cessation). Removing patients after randomization always introduces a *risk of bias* by creating noncomparable groups.

ADHERING TO THE INTENTION-TO-TREAT PRINCIPLE DOES NOT MEAN THAT ALL PATIENTS RANDOMIZED MUST BE INCLUDED IN THE ANALYSIS

The goal of the intention-to-treat principle is to prevent *bias* introduced by prognostic differences between patients in the treatment and control groups included in the analysis. There are circumstances in which one can achieve efficiencies by excluding randomized patients and still avoid imbalance of *prognostic factors*.[4] This requires meeting 2 conditions: (1) allocation to treatment or control could not possibly influence whether a particular randomized patient met criteria for postrandomization exclusion, and (2) the decision about postrandomization exclusion is made without possible bias (usually achieved by a review that is *blinded* to allocation).

For instance, in an RCT of different ways of nailing tibial fractures, because the nailing approach is unlikely to be an important determinant of outcome among patients with previous osteomyelitis in the affected limb, the investigators planned to exclude such individuals.[5] However, when study personnel failed to identify this exclusion criterion, they would occasionally enroll such a patient in error. For these patients, study investigators planned for postrandomization exclusion. A team of reviewers masked to allocation routinely reviewed information available at randomization and, if there was evidence of osteomyelitis in the affected limb, made the decision to exclude patients from the analysis.

LIMITATIONS OF THE INTENTION-TO-TREAT PRINCIPLE

Even after understanding the logic of the intention-to-treat principle, clinicians may find it unpalatable to count adverse *target events* in large numbers of patients who did not receive an experimental treatment against the treatment group. After all, a specific patient will be interested in the effect a specific medication would have if he or she were to take it. The best estimate of this effect would come from a group of patients who all received the *experimental intervention* rather than from a group in which some did and some did not receive that intervention. Regrettably, following the intention-to-treat principle does not produce this best estimate, and the higher the level of nonadherence, the farther an analysis that adheres to the intention-to-treat principle will be from that best estimate. Unfortunately, as we have pointed out, possible solutions (eg, per-protocol analyses) are vulnerable to bias.

Differential nonadherence can produce potentially misleading results, even when investigators analyze the patients in the groups to which they were randomized irrespective of adherence. High rates of nonadherence in trials of effective treatment against placebo or standard care controls will lead to underestimates of treatment effect.

The situation is even more problematic in trials of 2 active treatments in which one (say treatment A) is superior to the other (treatment B). If, in such a trial, nonadherence is greater with treatment A than with treatment B, the apparent benefit from treatment A may be lost. If the differential adherence is large enough, the superior treatment may even appear inferior.

Unfortunately, a per-protocol analysis cannot solve the problem because we cannot distinguish between treatment adherence effects and a bias introduced by baseline differences in *prognosis*. When substantial nonadherence exists, our choice is between a biased estimate of the treatment effect from a per-protocol analysis and an unbiased estimate of the effect of the treatment as administered (rather than as intended) from the analysis that attributes events in all patients to the arm to which they were allocated. Statistical methods to "correct" for nonadherent methods are available but are either limited in their applicability or complex and not widely used.[6]

The safest action for the clinician when faced with a trial of active treatment against placebo or standard care that reveals an apparent effect of treatment, but in which nonadherence was substantial, is to treat the apparent treatment effect as a likely underestimate of the true treatment effect. For instance, in the Heart Protection Study, the overall adherence with simvastatin therapy was approximately 85%, and the overall use of statins in the control group was approximately 17%.[7] Thus, one can consider the apparent 17% RRR in vascular deaths with simvastatin a likely underestimate of the benefit a fully adherent patient might expect from taking the drug vs not taking it. We will deal with the situation of differential nonadherence with 2 active treatments in the next section.

INTENTION TO TREAT, TOXICITY, NONINFERIORITY TRIALS, AND DIFFERENTIAL NONADHERENCE

Investigators sometimes adhere to the intention-to-treat principle in terms of assessing *end points* that reflect potential treatment benefit but not for toxicity outcomes, for which they conduct a per-protocol analysis. Considering only those exposed to an intervention is appropriate if the adverse outcomes occur exclusively in this population (eg, wound dehiscence can only occur in those who have undergone a surgical procedure).

In other instances, unbiased assessment of intervention toxicity requires, as much as assessment of benefit, analyzing patients in the arms to which they

were randomized. The reason is that nonadherent individuals in the experimental and control groups may have a different risk of adverse effects or toxic effects than adherent individuals in the same way that they may have a differential risk of the adverse outcomes that treatment is designed to prevent.

We have noted that an intention-to-treat analysis, in the face of substantial nonadherence, can lead to underestimates of benefit. The same is true of toxicity. We may, however, be more uncomfortable with the prospect of underestimates of toxicity than of benefit. If so, one could argue for a parallel per-protocol analysis of toxicity to reassure us regarding the effect estimate from the intention-to-treat analysis. The same is true for trials of 2 active treatments in which there is differential nonadherence and when the goal of the study is to demonstrate that a new treatment with toxicity or burden advantages has only a modest loss in effectiveness (see Chapter 8, How to Use a Noninferiority Trial).

LOSS TO FOLLOW-UP AND THE MISLEADING USE OF "INTENTION TO TREAT"

Unfortunately, there is considerable ambiguity in the term "intention-to-treat analysis" created by the issue of how to deal with patients lost to follow-up in the analysis of RCTs. In this section, we highlight the reason for the ambiguity and clarify the issue of dealing with patients lost to follow-up.

Patients lost to follow-up can cause the same sort of bias as failure to adhere to the intention-to-treat principle in nonadherent patients whom the investigators have successfully followed up. For instance, picture a hypothetical trial in which 20% of treated patients and 20% of control patients stop taking medication and investigators elect to terminate their follow-up at that point. At the end of the trial, the investigators count events in all patients with available status in the groups to which they are allocated. Technically, they could say they had conducted an intention-to-treat analysis in that they counted all events of which they were aware against the group to which the patient was allocated. Of course, the intention-to-treat analysis has in no way avoided the possible bias introduced by omission of outcome events in patients who discontinued treatment. The investigators could have avoided this problem had they chosen to follow up all patients, irrespective of adherence to treatment.

Clinicians evaluating an RCT need to know whether the researchers followed the intention-to-treat principle. A quick approach is to scan the methods section of the RCT, looking for the phrase "intention-to-treat analysis." Although most RCTs mention this phrase (surely the effect of a campaign about the importance of the intention-to-treat principle), they often misuse it or apply it incorrectly.[8-11] Thus, readers must look not just for this phrase but also for what the trial investigators actually did. In its updated 2010 statement, CONSORT recommends replacing "...intention-to-treat analysis, a widely misused term, by a more explicit request for information about retaining participants in their original assigned groups."[12]

DEALING WITH LOSS TO FOLLOW-UP

Loss to follow-up leading to missing outcome data in RCTs that report an "intention-to-treat analysis" is common.[8,11] Large loss to follow-up may introduce the same sort of bias as a per-protocol analysis. This is particularly so because patients lost to follow-up tend to have poorer outcomes than patients whom investigators successfully follow up.[13]

Clinicians will find it helpful to separate the issues of intention to treat and loss to follow-up.[14] As we have noted in the previous section, making assumptions about patients lost to follow-up (eg, all had the event of interest or none had the event of interest) and then describing the resulting analysis as an "intention-to-treat analysis" in no way minimizes the bias that will occur if the prognosis in those lost to follow-up differs in intervention or control groups or if the magnitude of loss to follow-up differs in the 2 groups.

For instance, Silverstein et al[15] reported the results of an RCT of 8843 patients taking nonsteroidal anti-inflammatory agents for rheumatoid arthritis randomized to receive misoprostol (4404 patients) or placebo (4439 patients) to prevent gastroduodenal complications as judged by outcome assessors masked to treatment allocation. The authors described their analysis as intention to treat. However, they included patients lost to follow-up in the denominator of event rates used for this analysis. Inclusion of these patients in the denominator without inclusion of their outcomes in the numerator assumed that no patient lost to follow-up had gastroduodenal ulcerations. The size of the groups lost (1851 patients in the misoprostol arm and 1617 in the placebo arm) eclipsed the number of patients who experienced the primary end point in each group (25 in the misoprostol group and 42 in the placebo group), leaving the reader uncertain about the true magnitude of the treatment effect. The investigators could have avoided the problem by rigorously following up all patients or, at least, made it controllable by conducting sensitivity analyses with different assumptions for patients lost to follow-up.[16,17]

Investigators should transparently describe how they dealt with loss to follow-up in the analysis section of their reports. Probably the best way of dealing with the situation is to begin by analyzing only those patients for whom one has complete data (called a complete case analysis). Investigators should then conduct one or more *sensitivity analyses* using different assumptions for the missing outcomes to assess the robustness of their results. This is true for individual trials and *systematic reviews* and *meta-analyses* of RCTs.[16,17] In the absence of an explicit approach, clinicians should be wary of studies reporting so-called intention-to-treat analyses in the face of substantial loss to follow-up.

CONCLUSIONS

For RCTs to provide unbiased assessments of treatment efficacy, investigators should adhere to the intention-to-treat principle and present analyses in which all patients are included in the groups to which they were randomized. Scanning the methods section for the phrase "intention-to-treat analysis" is insufficient when critically appraising an RCT report. Readers need to check what was actually done in the analysis, with respect to 2 crucial threats to validity: patients who did not follow the protocol and patients lost to follow-up. In unusual situations (toxicity, differential adherence in trials of 2 active treatments, and *noninferiority trials*), an additional per-protocol analysis may provide reassuring (or not so reassuring) information.

References

1. Montori VM, Guyatt GH. Intention-to-treat principle. *CMAJ*. 2001;165(10):1339-1341.

2. The Coronary Drug Project Research Group. Influence of adherence to treatment and response of cholesterol on mortality in the coronary drug project. *N Engl J Med*. 1980;303(18): 1038-1041.

3. Simpson SH, Eurich DT, Majumdar SR, et al. A meta-analysis of the association between adherence to drug therapy and mortality. *BMJ*. 2006;333(7557):15.

4. Fergusson D, Aaron SD, Guyatt G, Hébert P. Post-randomisation exclusions: the intention to treat principle and excluding patients from analysis. *BMJ*. 2002;325(7365):652-654.

5. Bhandari M, Guyatt G, Tornetta P III, et al; Study to Prospectively Evaluate Reamed Intramedullary Nails in Patients with Tibial Fractures Investigators. Randomized trial of reamed and unreamed intramedullary nailing of tibial shaft fractures. *J Bone Joint Surg Am*. 2008;90(12):2567-2578.

6. Dunn G, Maracy M, Tomenson B. Estimating treatment effects from randomized clinical trials with noncompliance and loss to follow-up: the role of instrumental variable methods. *Stat Methods Med Res*. 2005;14(4):369-395.

7. Heart Protection Study Collaborative Group. MRC/BHF Heart Protection Study of cholesterol lowering with simvastatin in 20,536 high-risk individuals: a randomised placebo-controlled trial. *Lancet*. 2002;360(9326):7-22.

8. Hollis S, Campbell F. What is meant by intention to treat analysis? survey of published randomised controlled trials. *BMJ*. 1999;319(7211):670-674.

9. Ruiz-Canela M, Martínez-González MA, de Irala-Estévez J. Intention to treat analysis is related to methodological quality. *BMJ*. 2000;320(7240):1007-1008.

10. Kruse RL, Alper BS, Reust C, Stevermer JJ, Shannon S, Williams RH. Intention-to-treat analysis: who is in? who is out? *J Fam Pract*. 2002;51(11):969-971.

11. Gravel J, Opatrny L, Shapiro S. The intention-to-treat approach in randomized controlled trials: are authors saying what they do and doing what they say? *Clin Trials*. 2007;4(4):350-356.

12. Schulz KF, Altman DG, Moher D; CONSORT Group. CONSORT 2010 statement: updated guidelines for reporting parallel group randomised trials. *BMJ*. 2010;340:c332.

13. Ioannidis JP, Bassett R, Hughes MD, Volberding PA, Sacks HS, Lau J. Predictors and impact of patients lost to follow-up in a long-term randomized trial of immediate versus deferred antiretroviral treatment. *J Acquir Immune Defic Syndr Hum Retrovirol*. 1997;16(1):22-30.

14. Alshurafa M, Briel M, Akl EA, et al. Inconsistent definitions for intention-to-treat in relation to missing outcome data: systematic review of the methods literature. *PLoS One*. 2012; 7(11):e49163.

15. Silverstein FE, Graham DY, Senior JR, et al. Misoprostol reduces serious gastrointestinal complications in patients with rheumatoid arthritis receiving nonsteroidal anti-inflammatory drugs: a randomized, double-blind, placebo-controlled trial. *Ann Intern Med*. 1995;123(4):241-249.

16. Akl EA, Johnston BC, Alonso-Coello P, et al. Addressing dichotomous data for participants excluded from trial analysis: a guide for systematic reviewers. *PLoS One*. 2013;8(2):e57132.

17. Akl EA, Briel M, You JJ, et al. Potential impact on estimated treatment effects of information lost to follow-up in randomised controlled trials (LOST-IT): systematic review. *BMJ*. 2012;344:e2809.

THERAPY

11.5

ADVANCED TOPICS IN THE RISK OF BIAS OF THERAPY TRIALS

N-of-1 Randomized Clinical Trials

Gordon Guyatt, Yuqing Zhang, Roman Jaeschke, and Thomas McGinn

THERAPY

IN THIS CHAPTER

INTRODUCTION

Clinicians should use the results of *randomized clinical trials* (RCTs) of groups of patients to guide their clinical practice. When deciding which management approach will be best for an individual patient, however, clinicians cannot always rely on the results of RCTs. An RCT that addresses the particular issue may not be available; for example, some conditions are so rare that randomized trials are not feasible. Furthermore, even when a relevant RCT generates a clear answer, its result may not apply to an individual patient. First, if the patient is very different from trial participants, the trial results may not be applicable to that patient (see Chapter 13.1, Applying Results to Individual Patients). Second, regardless of the overall trial results, some similar patients may benefit from a given therapy, whereas others receive no benefit. Clinicians may have particularly strong reservations about applying RCT results to individuals when results have revealed small *treatment effects* of questionable importance.

These considerations lead clinicians to conduct *trials of therapy*, in which the patient begins treatment and the subsequent clinical course determines whether treatment is continued. Many factors may, however, mislead physicians who are conducting conventional trials of therapy. The patient may have improved anyway, even without medication. Physicians' and patients' optimism may result in misinterpretation of the therapeutic trial results. Finally, people often feel better when they are taking a new medication even when it does not have any specific activity against their illness (the *placebo effect*); this may also result in misleading inferences regarding the value of the new treatment.

To avoid these pitfalls, clinicians must conduct trials of therapy with safeguards that minimize these *biases*. Potential safeguards include repeatedly administering and withdrawing the target treatment, performing quantitative measurements of the *target outcomes*, and keeping both patients and clinicians *blind* to the treatment being administered. Investigators routinely use such safeguards in RCTs that involve large numbers of patients.

To determine the best care for an individual patient, clinicians can conduct RCTs in individual patients (*n-of-1 RCTs*). In contrast to most of this book, which provides a guide to using the medical literature, this chapter provides an approach to applying the principles of *evidence-based medicine* to conduct an n-of-1 RCT in your own practice.

N-OF-1 RANDOMIZED CLINICAL TRIALS: STUDY DESIGN

Although there are many ways to conduct n-of-1 RCTs, the following is the method we have found to be most widely applicable:

1. A clinician and patient agree to test a therapy (the *experimental therapy*) for its ability to improve or control the *symptoms, signs*, or other manifestations (the *treatment targets*) of the patient's ailment.

2. The patient then undergoes pairs of treatment periods organized so that one period of each pair applies the experimental therapy and the other period applies either an alternative treatment or placebo (Figure 11.5-1). The order of these 2 periods within each pair is *randomized* by a coin toss or any other method that ensures that the patient is equally likely to receive the experimental or control therapy during any treatment period.

3. Whenever possible, a pharmacist independently prepares medication to ensure that the clinician and the patient are blind to when the patient is receiving the treatment and alternative therapies (see the "Is There a Pharmacist Who Can Help?" section).

4. The clinician monitors the treatment targets, often through a patient diary, to document the effect of the treatment currently being applied.

5. Pairs of treatment periods are replicated until the clinician and patient are convinced that the experimental therapy is effective, causes *harm*, or has no effect on the treatment targets. This usually requires a minimum of 3 pairs of treatment periods.

We now describe an n-of-1 RCT in detail. To facilitate its illustration, each step will address a question that must be answered before proceeding to the next step, as summarized in Box 11.5-1.[1]

FIGURE 11.5-1

Basic Design for N-of-1 Randomized Clinical Trial

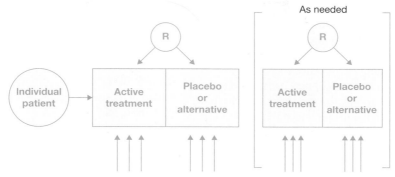

Circled R indicates that the order of placebo and active periods in each pair is determined by random allocation. Bracketed pair with "As needed" indicates that, beyond the first pair of treatment periods, as many additional pairs of treatment periods as necessary are conducted until patient and physician are convinced of the efficacy—or lack of efficacy—of the trial medication.

Reproduced from Carruthers et al.[1] Copyright © 2000, with permission from the McGraw-Hill Companies.

Is an N-of-1 Randomized Clinical Trial Indicated for This Patient?

Because n-of-1 RCTs are unnecessary for some ailments (such as self-limited illnesses) and unsuited for some treatments (such as acute or rapidly evolving illness, surgical procedures, or the *prevention* of distant adverse outcomes, such as death, stroke, or myocardial infarction), at the outset it is important to determine whether an n-of-1 RCT really is indicated for the patient and treatment in question. If an n-of-1 RCT is appropriate, the answer to each of the following questions should be yes (Box 11.5-1).

Is the Effect of the Treatment Really in Doubt?

One or several RCTs may have indicated that the treatment in question is highly effective. If, however, 50% or more of patients in such trials have proved unresponsive, an n-of-1 RCT may still be appropriate. Calculations of *numbers needed to treat* suggest that this will almost always be the case, regardless of whether the treatments are designed to prevent major adverse events or to improve health-related quality of life.[2]

For example, in a randomized trial of selective serotonin reuptake inhibitors (SSRIs) to reduce the frequency of hot flashes in women experiencing

---

BOX 11.5-1

Guidelines for N-of-1 Randomized Clinical Trials

Is an n-of-1 RCT indicated for this patient?

Is the impact of the treatment really in doubt (see Box 11.5-2)?

If effective, will the treatment be continued long term?

Is an n-of-1 RCT feasible in this patient?

Is the patient eager to collaborate in designing and carrying out an n-of-1 RCT?

Does the treatment have rapid onset and termination of action?

Is an optimal duration of treatment feasible?

Are there patient-important targets of treatment amenable to measurement?

Can you identify criteria to end the n-of-1 RCT?

Is there a pharmacist who can help?

Are strategies in place for the interpretation of the data?

Abbreviation: RCT, randomized clinical trial.

Reproduced from Carruthers et al.[1] Copyright © 2000, with permission from the McGraw-Hill Companies.

postmenopausal symptoms, more than 60% of the women in the study experienced a 50% reduction in symptoms.[3] Although these results are impressive, the treatment still leaves a large percentage of women to experience significant symptoms despite effective therapy. In a woman with an equivocal response to SSRIs, an n-of-1 trial may be appropriate to definitively sort out treatment effectiveness.

On the other hand, a patient may have exhibited such a marked response to the treatment that both the clinician and patient are convinced that it works. N-of-1 RCTs are best reserved for the situations presented in Box 11.5-2.

If Effective, Will the Treatment Be Continued on a Long-term Basis?

If the underlying condition is self-limited and treatment will be continued only during the short term,

---

BOX 11.5-2

When to Conduct an N-of-1 Randomized Clinical Trial

1. The clinician is uncertain whether a treatment that has not yet been started will work in a particular patient.

2. The patient has started taking a medication, but neither patient nor clinician is confident that a treatment is really providing benefit.

3. Neither the clinician nor the patient is confident of the optimal dose of a medication the patient is receiving or should receive.

4. A patient has symptoms that both the clinician and the patient suspect—but are not certain—are caused by the adverse effects of the medications.

5. The patient has so far insisted on taking a treatment that the clinician believes is useless or harmful, and although logically constructed arguments have not persuaded a patient, a negative result of an n-of-1 RCT might.

Abbreviation: RCT, randomized clinical trial.

Reproduced from Carruthers et al.[1] Copyright © 2000, with permission from the McGraw-Hill Companies.

---

an n-of-1 RCT is unlikely to be worthwhile. N-of-1 RCTs are most useful when conditions are chronic and maintenance therapy is likely to be prolonged.

Is an N-of-1 Randomized Clinical Trial Feasible in This Patient?

The clinician may wish to determine the efficacy of treatment in an individual patient, but the patient, the ailment, or the treatment may not lend itself to the n-of-1 approach.

Is the Patient Eager to Collaborate in Designing and Performing an N-of-1 Randomized Clinical Trial?

N-of-1 RCTs are indicated only when patients can fully understand the nature of the experiment and are enthusiastic about participating. The n-of-1 RCT is a cooperative venture between clinician and patient.

Does the Treatment Have Rapid Onset and Termination of Action?

N-of-1 RCTs are much easier to perform when positive treatment effects, if they are indeed present, manifest themselves within a few days. Although it may be possible to conduct n-of-1 RCTs with drugs that have a longer latency for the development of signs of efficacy (such as disease-remitting therapy in patients with rheumatoid arthritis or use of antidepressants in patients with depression), the requirement for very long treatment periods before the effect can be evaluated may prove prohibitive.

Similarly, treatments whose effects cease abruptly when they are withdrawn are most suitable for n-of-1 RCTs. If the treatment continues to act long after it is stopped, a prolonged *washout period* may be necessary. If this washout period lasts longer than a few days, the feasibility of the trial is compromised. Similarly, treatments that have the potential to cure the underlying condition—or lead to a permanent change in the treatment target—are not suitable for n-of-1 RCTs.

Is an Optimal Duration of Treatment Feasible?

Although short periods of treatment increase the feasibility of n-of-1 RCTs, the trials may need to be long to be useful. For example, if active therapy takes a few days to reach full effect and a few days to cease acting once it is stopped, avoiding distortion from these delayed peak effects and washout periods requires relatively long treatment periods. Thus, our n-of-1 RCTs of theophylline[4,5] in patients with chronic airflow limitation and asthma used treatment periods of at least 10 days: 3 days to allow the drug to reach steady state or washout and 7 days thereafter to monitor the patient's response to treatment.

In addition, because many n-of-1 RCTs test a treatment's ability to prevent or mitigate attacks or exacerbations (such as migraines or seizures), each treatment period must be long enough to include an attack or exacerbation. A rough rule of thumb, called the *inverse rule of 3s*, tells us the following: If an event occurs, on average, once every x days, we need to observe $3x$ days to be 95% confident of observing at least 1 event. For example, applying this rule in a patient with familial Mediterranean fever with attacks that occur, on average, once every 2 weeks, we chose treatment periods of at least 6 weeks.

Are There Patient-Important Targets of Treatment Amenable to Measurement?

N-of-1 RCTs require assessment of the patient's symptoms and feelings of well-being (or lack of well-being). Clinicians can, in a simple fashion, apply principles of measurement of quality of life to n-of-1 RCTs (see Chapter 12.5, Measuring Patients' Experience). To begin with, ask the patient to identify the most troubling symptoms or problems he/she is experiencing and then decide which of them is likely to respond to the experimental treatment. This responsive subset of symptoms or problems forms the basis of a self-administered patient diary or questionnaire.

For example, a patient with chronic airflow limitation identified the problem as shortness of breath while walking up stairs, bending, or vacuuming.[4] A patient with fibromyalgia identified fatigue, aches and pains, morning stiffness, and sleep disturbance as problems that became the treatment targets for the illness.[6]

You can use a number of formats for the questionnaire to record the patient's symptoms. Figure 11.5-2 shows a data sheet from an n-of-1 RCT that examined the effectiveness of ketanserin in Raynaud phenomenon. For some patients, a daily symptom rating may work best; for others, a weekly summary may be better. The best way of presenting response options to patients

is as graded descriptions of symptoms that range from none to severe. One example of such graded descriptions might be "no shortness of breath," "a little shortness of breath," "moderate shortness of breath," and "extreme shortness of breath." Constructing simple symptom questionnaires allows the patient and the clinician to collaborate in quantifying the patient's symptoms, on which the analysis of the n-of-1 RCT relies.

You can use a patient diary or questionnaire to measure nausea, gastrointestinal disturbances, dizziness, or other common adverse effects, along with symptoms of the primary condition. In n-of-1 RCTs designed to determine whether medication adverse effects are responsible for a patient's symptoms (for example, whether a patient's fatigue is caused by an antihypertensive agent), adverse effects become the primary treatment targets.

Can You Identify Criteria to End the N-of-1 Randomized Clinical Trial?

If the clinician and patient decide not to specify the number of pairs of treatment periods in advance, they can stop anytime they are convinced that the experimental treatment ought to be stopped or continued indefinitely. Thus, if they find a marked improvement in the treatment target between the 2 periods of the first pair, both clinician and patient may want to stop the trial immediately and unblind the sequence of medications. On the other hand, if patient and clinician perceive no or only a minimal difference between the 2 periods of each pair, both the clinician and the patient may need 3, 4, or even 5 pairs before confidently concluding that the treatment is or is not effective.

If, however, one wishes to conduct a formal statistical analysis of data from the n-of-1 RCT, specifying in advance the number of pairs will strengthen the analysis. Regardless of whether they specify the number of treatment periods in advance, we recommend that clinicians resist the temptation and refrain from breaking the code until they are certain they are ready to terminate the study.

Is There a Pharmacist Who Can Help?

In most instances, conducting an n-of-1 RCT that incorporates all of the aforementioned safeguards against bias and misinterpretation requires collaboration

THERAPY

FIGURE 11.5-2

N-of-1 Randomized Clinical Trial—Sample Data Sheet

Physician: _____

Patient: _____

Sex: Male _____ Female _____ Date of birth _____ _____ _____

Diagnosis: _____

Occupation: _____

Present medications: _____

Trial medication: Ketanserin   Dose: _____

Duration of study periods: 2 weeks

Outcomes: Symptom ratings

Informed consent obtained (please sign): _____

Answers to symptom questions, pair 1, period 1:

1. How many episodes of Raynaud phenomenon did you have in the last week?
    First week (to be completed on_____ _____) _____
    Second week (to be completed on _____ _____) _____

2. On average, in comparison with your usual episodes, how long were the
    attacks?
    1. Very long; as long as or longer than they have ever been
    2. Very long; almost as long as they have ever been
    3. Longer than usual
    4. As long as usual
    5. Not as long as usual
    6. Not nearly as long as usual
    7. Very short; as brief as or briefer than they have ever been

    Write in the number that best describes your experience for each week.
    First week (to be completed on _____ _____) _____
    Second week (to be completed on_____ _____) _____

3. On average, in comparison with your usual episodes, how severe were the
    attacks?
    1. Very bad; as severe as or more severe than they have ever been
    2. Very bad; almost as severe as they have ever been
    3. More severe than usual
    4. About as severe as usual
    5. Not as severe as usual
    6. Not nearly as severe as usual
    7. Very mild; as mild as or milder than they have ever been

    Write in the number that best describes your experience for each week.
    First week (to be completed on_____ _____) _____
    Second week (to be completed on_____ _____) _____

between the clinician and a pharmacist who can prepare placebos identical to the active medication in appearance, taste, and texture. Occasionally, pharmaceutical firms can supply such placebos. More often, however, you will want your local pharmacist to repackage the active medication. If it comes in tablet form, the pharmacist can crush and repackage it in capsule form—unless the medication is a modified-release preparation whose absorption characteristics will be altered. Thus, a clinician who is interested in the effect of a modified-release preparation may have to forgo blinding if the duration of action of the medication is a crucial issue.

If you need a placebo, the pharmacist can fill identical-appearing placebo capsules with lactose. Although it is time consuming, preparation of placebos is not technically difficult. Our mean cost for preparing medication for n-of-1 studies in which placebos have not been available from a pharmaceutical company has been $200 (Canadian dollars). In considering the cost, the large savings that follow from abandoning a useless or harmful treatment that might otherwise be continued indefinitely, along with the reassurance of knowing that long-term treatment really works, emphasize the relatively trivial medication cost of the n-of-1 RCT.

The pharmacist is also charged with preparing the randomization schedule (which requires nothing more than a coin toss for each pair of treatment periods). This allows the clinician, along with the patient, to remain blind to allocation. The pharmacist also may be helpful in planning the design of the trial by providing information regarding the anticipated time to onset of action and the washout period, thus helping with decisions about the duration of study periods.

Are Strategies for the Interpretation of the Trial Data in Place?

Once you carefully gather data on the treatment targets in your n-of-1 trial, how will you interpret them? One approach is to simply plot the data and visually inspect the results. Evaluation of results by visual inspection has a long and distinguished record in the psychology literature concerning single-subject designs.[7,8] Visual inspection is simple and easy. Its major disadvantage is that it is vulnerable to viewer or *observer bias*.

An alternative approach to analysis of data from n-of-1 RCTs is to use a test of *statistical significance*. The simplest test would be based on the likelihood of a patient's preferring active treatment in each pair of treatment periods. This situation is analogous to the likelihood of heads coming up repeatedly on a series of coin tosses. For example, the likelihood of a patient's preferring active treatment to placebo during 3 consecutive pairs if the treatment were ineffective would be $(1/2) \times (1/2) \times (1/2) = 1/8$, or 0.125. The disadvantage of this approach (which is called the *sign test*) is that it lacks *power*; 5 pairs must be conducted before there is any chance of reaching conventional levels of statistical significance.

A second statistical strategy is to use the *t* test. The *t* test offers increased power because not only the direction but also the strength of the treatment effect in each pair is taken into account.

To avoid misleading results based on random highs or lows, if you plan a statistical test, you should ideally specify the number of treatment periods before the study begins.

To conduct a paired *t* test, derive a single score for each pair by subtracting the mean score of the placebo period from the mean score of the active period. These differences in scores constitute the data for the paired *t*; the number of *degrees of freedom* is simply the number of pairs minus 1. Statistical software programs that will facilitate quick calculation of the *P* value are available.

Table 11.5-1 presents the results of an n-of-1 RCT. In this trial, we tested the effectiveness of amitriptyline in a dose of 10 mg at bedtime for a patient with fibromyalgia.[8] Each week, the patient separately rated the severity of a number of symptoms, including fatigue, aches and pains, and sleep disturbance, on a 7-point scale in which a higher score represented better function. The treatment periods were 4 weeks long, and 3 pairs were undertaken. Table 11.5-1 presents the mean scores for each of the 24 weeks of the study.

The first step in analyzing the results of the study is to calculate the mean score for each period (presented in the far right-hand column of Table 11.5-1). In each pair, the score favored the active treatment. The sign test tells us that the *probability* of this result occurring by chance if the treatment was ineffective is $(1/2) \times (1/2) \times 1/2 = 1/8$ (or 0.125).

TABLE 11.5-1

Results of an N-of-1 Randomized Clinical Trial in a Patient With Fibrositis[a]

Treatment	Severity Score				
	Week 1	Week 2	Week 3	Week 4	Mean Score
Pair 1					
Active	4.43	4.86	4.71	4.71	4.68
Placebo	4.43	4.00	4.14	4.29	4.22
Pair 2					
Active	4.57	4.89	5.29	5.29	5.01
Placebo	3.86	4.00	4.29	4.14	4.07
Pair 3					
Active	4.29	5.00	5.43	5.43	5.04
Placebo	3.71	4.14	4.43	4.43	4.18

[a]The active drug was amitriptyline hydrochloride. Higher scores represent better function.
Reproduced from Carruthers et al.[1] Copyright © 2000, with permission from the McGraw-Hill Companies.

This analysis, however, ignores the magnitude and consistency of the difference between the active and placebo treatments. A paired *t* test in which data from the same patient during different periods are paired takes these factors into account. We did our *t* test by entering the data from the pairs of results into a simple statistical program: 4.68 and 4.22, 5.01 and 4.07, as well as 5.04 and 4.18. The program tells us that the *t* value is 5.07 and there are 2 *df*; the associated *P* = .04. This analysis makes us considerably more confident that the consistent difference in favor of the active drug is unlikely to have occurred by chance. Clinicians can use simple statistical programs readily available on the Web to conduct this analysis.

The other choice of analysis is *Bayesian* hierarchical models, which are especially suitable when there is available treatment-effect evidence or when both patient-specific and aggregated findings are desired.[9,10] This method can take into account sensible parameter estimates and intervals, embodying prior information and adding covariates and subgroup structure among patients into the model. Furthermore, this method has the advantage of providing probabilistic results for both the individual patient and the group of patients as a whole. Use of this approach, however, requires collaboration with a statistician familiar with its particular methods.[11,12]

The use of n-of-1 RCTs to improve patient care does not depend on statistical analysis of the results. Even if statistical analysis is not used in the interpretation of the trial, the strategies of randomization, blinding, replication, and quantifying outcomes, when accompanied by careful visual inspection of the data, still allow a much more rigorous assessment of effectiveness of treatment than is possible in conventional clinical practice.

ETHICS OF N-OF-1 RANDOMIZED CLINICAL TRIALS

Is conducting an n-of-1 RCT a clinical task or a research undertaking? If the former, is it the sort of clinical procedure, analogous to an invasive diagnostic test, that requires written informed consent? We would argue that the n-of-1 RCT can be—and should be—a part of routine clinical practice.

Nevertheless, there are a number of important ethical issues to consider. Patients should be fully aware of the nature of the study in which they are participating, and there should be no element of deception in the use of placebos as part of the study. Clinicians should obtain written informed consent; see Figure 11.5-3 for an example of a consent form.

FIGURE 11.5-3

Consent Form for N-of-1 Randomized Trial

We think that it would help you to take part in one of these therapeutic trials of [NAME OF DRUG]. We will conduct a number of pairs of periods. Each period will be [DURATION OF PERIOD]. During one period of each pair, you will be taking the active treatment, and during the other you will be using the placebo. The placebo is a pill that looks exactly like the medication but does not contain the active ingredients. If at any time during the study you are feeling worse, we can consider that treatment period at an end and can go on to the next treatment. Therefore, if you begin to feel worse, just call my office at [INSERT NUMBER], and I will get in touch with you.

If you don't think this new way of conducting a therapeutic trial is a good idea for you, we will try the new drug in the usual way. Your decision will not interfere with your treatment in any way. You can decide to stop the trial at any time and this will not interfere with your treatment. All information we collect during the trial will remain confidential.

PATIENT SIGNATURE_____

WITNESS SIGNATURE _____

PHYSICIAN SIGNATURE_____

DATE _____

THERAPY

Patients should be aware that they can terminate the trial at any time without jeopardizing their care or their relationship with their physician. Finally, follow-up should be soon enough to prevent any important deleterious consequences of institution or withdrawal of therapy. Discussing the rationale for, and value of, n-of-1 RCTs with an institutional review board representative can help clarify local policies.

THE EFFECT OF N-OF-1 RANDOMIZED CLINICAL TRIALS ON CLINICAL PRACTICE

We have reported a series of more than 50 n-of-1 RCTs, each designed to improve the care being provided to an individual patient.[5] Patients had a wide variety of conditions, including chronic airflow limitation, asthma, fibrositis, arthritis, syncope, anxiety, insomnia, and angina pectoris. In general, these trials were successful in sorting out whether the treatment was effective. In approximately one-third of the trials, the ultimate treatment differed from that which would have been given had the trial not been conducted. In most of the trials in which treatment differed from treatment that would have been given had the trial not been conducted, the use of medication that otherwise would have been given in the long term was discontinued. Other clinical groups have reported their experience with n-of-1 RCTs, generally confirming the feasibility and usefulness of the approach.[13-15] A systematic review identified 108 n-of-1 trial protocols, including 2154 participants, from 1986 to 2010. Among these trials, the most common conditions (27%) examined were neuropsychiatric (36% of neuropsychiatric were attention-deficit/hyperactivity disorder), pulmonary (13%), and musculoskeletal (12%; 21% of these were osteoarthritis).[16]

TABLE 11.5-2

Examples of N-of-1 Randomized Clinical Trials

Type of Condition	Possible Outcome Measures	Example of Intervention
Chronic headache	Duration, severity, and frequency of headache	Tricyclic antidepressant or β-blockers
Low back pain	Pain or function	Cyclobenzaprine or acupuncture[a]
Recurrent syncope	Syncopal episodes	β-Blockers
Chronic airway obstruction	Dyspnea, peak flow rates	Aerosolized β-agonists, ipratropium, steroids
Fibromyalgia	Aches and pains, fatigue, sleep disruption	Low-dose tricyclic antidepressant
Fatigue	Fatigue	Ginseng tablets[a]
Insomnia	Sleep disruption, satisfaction	Low-dose tricyclic antidepressant
Anxiety	Anxiety, formal anxiety questionnaire such as Beck	Black cohosh[a]
Hot flashes of menopause	Frequency and severity of hot flashes	Clonidine or soy milk[a]

[a]Alternative therapies with limited evidence to support efficacy but frequently used by patients, sometimes with substantial costs.

Reproduced from Carruthers et al.[1] Copyright © 2000, with permission from the McGraw-Hill Companies.

Table 11.5-2 presents a set of conditions and therapeutic options that are excellent candidates for n-of-1 RCTs.

These reports do not definitively answer the question about whether patients who undergo n-of-1 RCTs are better off than those whose treatment regimen is determined by conventional methods. The most rigorous test of the usefulness of n-of-1 RCTs would be a randomized trial. Three such trials, in which investigators randomized patients to conventional care or to n-of-1 RCTs, have addressed the effect of n-of-1 RCTs.

The same group of investigators conducted 2 of these studies[17,18]; both examined the use of theophylline in patients with chronic airflow limitation. The investigators found that, although using n-of-1 RCTs did not affect quality of life or functional status of patients initially receiving theophylline, fewer patients in the n-of-1 RCT groups ended up receiving the drug in the long term. Thus, n-of-1 RCTs saved patients the expense, inconvenience, and potential toxicity of long-term theophylline therapy of no use to them.

The third trial randomized 27 patients with osteoarthritis who were uncertain as to whether adding nonsteroidal anti-inflammatory drugs to conventional management reduced their pain and another 24 similar patients to an n-of-1 randomized trial that compared diclofenac and misoprostol (the latter agent to avoid gastrointestinal adverse effects) to placebo.[19] The results revealed few differences between groups (similar proportion of patients ended up taking diclofenac and had similar quality of life), although all quality-of-life measures revealed trends in favor of the n-of-1 arm. Costs were higher in the n-of-1 arm. These results suggest that n-of-1 RCTs are unlikely to be uniformly superior to conventional trials. Understanding when n-of-1 RCTs will benefit patients will require further study.

CONCLUSIONS

In summary, the n-of-1 approach has the potential to improve the quality of medical care and the judicious use of medication in patients with chronic disease. Using the guidelines offered here, clinicians will find conducting n-of-1 RCTs feasible, highly informative, and stimulating.

References

1. Carruthers SG, Hoffman BB, Melmon KL, Nierenberg DF, eds. *Melmon and Morelli's Clinical Pharmacology: Basic Principles in Therapeutics*. 4th ed. New York, NY: McGraw-Hill; 2000.

2. Guyatt GH, Juniper EF, Walter SD, Griffith LE, Goldstein RS. Interpreting treatment effects in randomised trials. *BMJ*. 1998;316(7132):690-693.

3. Stearns V, Beebe KL, Iyengar M, Dube E. Paroxetine controlled release in the treatment of menopausal hot flashes: a randomized controlled trial. *JAMA*. 2003;289(21):2827-2834.

4. Patel A, Jaeschke R, Guyatt GH, Keller JL, Newhouse MT. Clinical usefulness of n-of-1 randomized controlled trials in patients with nonreversible chronic airflow limitation. *Am Rev Respir Dis*. 1991;144(4):962-964.

5. Guyatt GH, Keller JL, Jaeschke R, Rosenbloom D, Adachi JD, Newhouse MT. The n-of-1 randomized controlled trial: clinical usefulness: our three-year experience. *Ann Intern Med*. 1990;112(4):293-299.

6. Jaeschke R, Adachi J, Guyatt G, Keller J, Wong B. Clinical usefulness of amitriptyline in fibromyalgia: the results of 23 N-of-1 randomized controlled trials. *J Rheumatol*. 1991;18(3):447-451.

7. Kratchowill T. *Single Subject Research: Strategies for Evaluating Change*. New York, NY: Academic Press; 1978.

8. Kazdin A. *Single-case Research Designs: Methods for Clinical and Applied Settings*. New York, NY: Oxford University Press; 1982.

9. Zucker DR, Schmid CH, McIntosh MW, D'Agostino RB, Selker HP, Lau J. Combining single patient (N-of-1) trials to estimate population treatment effects and to evaluate individual patient responses to treatment. *J Clin Epidemiol*. 1997;50(4):401-410.

10. Schluter PJ, Ware RS. Single patient (n-of-1) trials with binary treatment preference. *Stat Med*. 2005;24(17):2625-2636.

11. Berger JO. *Statistical Decision Theory and Bayesian Analysis*. 2nd ed. New York, NY: Springer; 1985.

12. Oleson JJ. Bayesian credible intervals for binomial proportions in a single patient trial. *Stat Methods Med Res*. 2010;19(6):559-574.

13. Ménard J, Serrurier D, Bautier P, Plouin PF, Corvol P. Crossover design to test antihypertensive drugs with self-recorded blood pressure. *Hypertension*. 1988;11(2):153-159.

14. Johannessen T. Controlled trials in single subjects, 1: value in clinical medicine. *BMJ*. 1991;303(6795):173-174.

15. Larson EB, Ellsworth AJ, Oas J. Randomized clinical trials in single patients during a 2-year period. *JAMA*. 1993;270(22):2708-2712.

16. Gabler NB, Duan N, Vohra S, Kravitz RL. N-of-1 trials in the medical literature: a systematic review. *Med Care*. 2011;49(8):761-768.

17. Mahon J, Laupacis A, Donner A, Wood T. Randomised study of n of 1 trials versus standard practice. *BMJ*. 1996;312(7038):1069-1074.

18. Mahon JL, Laupacis A, Hodder RV, et al. Theophylline for irreversible chronic airflow limitation: a randomized study comparing n of 1 trials to standard practice. *Chest*. 1999;115(1):38-48.

19. Pope JE, Prashker M, Anderson J. The efficacy and cost effectiveness of N of 1 studies with diclofenac compared to standard treatment with nonsteroidal antiinflammatory drugs in osteoarthritis. *J Rheumatol*. 2004;31(1):140-149.

THERAPY

11.6

ADVANCED TOPICS IN THE RISK OF BIAS OF THERAPY TRIALS

Clinical Decision Support Systems

Anne M. Holbrook, Adrienne G. Randolph, Linn Brandt, Amit X. Garg, R. Brian Haynes, Deborah J. Cook, and Gordon Guyatt

THERAPY

IN THIS CHAPTER

CLINICAL SCENARIO

On the ambulatory care clinic rotation rounds in which you are the senior attending physician, a senior resident comments that nearly half of the patients seen today have diabetes and many of these patients have complications of diabetes, including previous myocardial infarction, stroke, neuropathy, and nephropathy. Some of the patients are only in their third or fourth decade of life. This leads to a discussion of chronic disease and its effect on disability, quality of life, and mortality, as well as evidence for treatments that improve these outcomes. One of the medical students, who previously worked as a software developer, is convinced that computerized decision support for physicians and patients has to be the way to improve diabetes care. A junior resident from a psychology background points out that a complex chronic disease such as diabetes requires not only awareness of interventions that can decrease mortality and morbidity but also considerable patient investment of learning, time, and expense to address all of the components. You remind the group that diabetes management, with its multiple guideline recommendations, could benefit from *clinical decision support systems* but that one should ask whether the systems improve patient outcomes. The senior resident, intrigued by the discussion, commits to presenting a well-done *randomized clinical trial* (RCT) that addresses the effect of computerized decision support systems on diabetes management at the upcoming morning report for all house staff and attending physicians. You tell her that there have been so many studies in this area that it might be more efficient to look for a well-done *systematic review*.

FINDING THE EVIDENCE

After the final afternoon rounds, you take a few minutes to search the literature. You believe that, given the progress in technology over the years, it is likely that only recent studies will be applicable to current clinical care. Computers on the ward allow you access to PubMed, so you quickly enter "computerized decision support AND diabetes" in the Clinical Queries search field (http://www.ncbi.nlm.nih.gov/pubmed/clinical; see also Chapter 5, Finding Current Best Evidence). The search retrieves 16 publications, including 4 systematic reviews that address your question. After screening the abstracts, the second, a systematic review and *meta-analysis*, stands out as directly relevant[1] (see Chapter 22, The Process of a Systematic Review and Meta-analysis).

In this systematic review, the authors searched for all randomized trials based in ambulatory care that involve patients with diabetes and compare a computerized clinical decision support system with usual care with or without additional educational materials. Outcomes of the trials included measures of process of care or *patient-important outcomes*.

WHAT ARE CLINICAL DECISION SUPPORT SYSTEMS?

Clinicians depend on computers and digital technology. Diagnostic imaging, laboratory data, medication records, and clinical orders and notes are routinely stored, accessed, and presented via computers. Technologies such as barcoding medications, patient-identification bands, diagnostic testing, mechanical ventilators, infusion pumps, and dialysis machines are among the many types of computerized systems that have become integral to hospital and outpatient settings.

Many clinicians and patients are using applications on their mobile devices to use *clinical prediction rules*, check drug interactions, or record an image to send for an electronic consultation via telehealth. These devices and systems capture, transform, display, or analyze data for use in clinical decision making. Clinical decision support systems (CDSSs) are defined as "computer-based information systems

BOX 11.6-1

Functions of a Clinical Decision Support System

Function	Example
Alerts	Highlighting out-of-range (either too high or too low) laboratory values
Reminders	Reminding the clinician to schedule a mammogram
Regulators	"Guardrails" rejecting an inappropriately high dose of a drug requested of the intravenous pump
Interpreting	Analyzing an electrocardiogram
Calculators	Calculating risk of mortality from a severity-of-illness score
Diagnosis aids	Listing a differential diagnosis for a patient with chest pain
Suggestions	Generating suggestions for adjusting a mechanical ventilator
Guidance	Order set for admission and early treatment of sepsis

used to integrate clinical and patient information and provide support for decision-making in patient care."[2]

In CDSSs, individual patient data entered or (preferably) already available via an electronic medical record (EMR) are processed through a series of algorithms to generate patient-specific assessments or recommendations for clinicians.[3] Box 11.6-1 describes the types of CDSSs according to their function.

The reason to invest in computer support is to improve patient outcomes. Merely providing indexed, legible storage of patient records, massive bibliographies of research studies, or even patient-specific advice based on the research synthesis is a poor use of limited resources if they do not improve *health outcomes*. A CDSS should be subject to the same rules of testing as any other health care intervention.

BOX 11.6-2

Using Articles Describing Clinical Decision Support Systems (CDSSs)

How serious is the risk of bias?

Were study participants randomized?

If not, did the investigators find similarity in all known determinants of prognosis or adjust for differences in the analysis?

If the intervention primarily targeted clinicians, was the clinician or clinician group the unit of analysis?

Were participants analyzed in the groups to which they were randomized?

Was the control group unaffected by the CDSS?

Aside from the experimental intervention(s), were the groups treated equally?

Were outcomes assessed uniformly between the experimental and control groups?

What are the results?

What is the effect of the CDSS?

How precise is the estimate of the effect?

How can I apply the results to patient care?

What elements of the CDSS are required?

Is the CDSS exportable to a new site?

Are clinicians in your setting likely to accept the CDSS?

Do the benefits of the CDSS justify the harms and costs?

THERAPY

In this chapter, we describe how to use articles that evaluate the influence of a CDSS, using an approach consistent with other chapters in this book. We consider 3 primary questions related to the *risk of bias* of research methods, the results, and the clinical application of the results (Box 11.6-2). We periodically refer to the systematic review identified in our scenario that addressed the effect of CDSSs on diabetes outcomes.[1]

HOW SERIOUS IS THE RISK OF BIAS?

When clinicians examine the effect of a CDSS on patient management or outcome, they should use the criteria for assessing an intervention. Thus, Box 11.6-2, which summarizes our approach to evaluating an article on the effect of a CDSS, includes some of the criteria from our guide to therapy (see Chapter 7, Therapy [Randomized Trials]) and some criteria from our guide to articles that concern *harm* (see Chapter 14, Harm [Observational Studies]). Although randomized trials have studied CDSSs, most studies that evaluate harms of CDSSs are nonrandomized studies. Our discussion includes only issues of particular importance in the evaluation of a CDSS.[4] Many of these issues overlap with those relevant to studies of quality of care (see Chapter 11.7, How to Use an Article About Quality Improvement), so you may want to consult that chapter for a complementary discussion.

You will note also that although our example article for this chapter is a systematic review and meta-analysis,[1] the criteria for evaluating a CDSS (Box 11.6-2) focus on evaluating individual studies, and we do not include criteria for evaluating the systematic review and meta-analysis (see Chapter 22, The Process of a Systematic Review and Meta-analysis, and Chapter 23, Understanding and Applying the Results of a Systematic Review and Meta-analysis). As it turns out, the example systematic review[1] presented explicit, appropriate eligibility criteria; conducted a comprehensive searching; included a meta-analysis; and undertook duplicate, independent data assessment of *bias*; thus, it meets criteria for a trustworthy process with credible results (see Chapter 22, The Process of a Systematic Review and Meta-analysis).

WERE STUDY PARTICIPANTS RANDOMIZED?

If Not, Did the Investigators Demonstrate Similarity in All Known Determinants of Prognosis or Adjust for Differences in the Analysis?

The risk of bias in observational studies often used to evaluate a CDSS is problematic. One observational design, the before-after design, compares outcomes before a technology is implemented with those after the system is implemented. The validity of this approach is threatened by the possibility that changes over time (called *secular trends* or temporal trends) in patient mix or in other aspects of health care provision are responsible for changes that investigators may attribute to the CDSS.

Consider the CDSS for management of therapy with antibiotics implemented in the late 1980s in the United States that was associated with apparent improvements in the cost-effectiveness of antibiotic ordering throughout the subsequent 5 years.[5] Although this before-after study might appear compelling, changes in the health care system, including the advent of managed care, were occurring simultaneously during the study period. To control for secular trends, study investigators compared antibiotic-prescribing practices to those of other US acute care hospitals for the duration of the study. These other hospitals differed in many ways aside from the CDSS, limiting the validity of the comparison. Nevertheless, the addition of a concurrent *control group* strengthened the study design.

Investigators also may strengthen the before-after design by turning the intervention on and off multiple times, a type of *interrupted time series design*. For example, investigators used this approach to evaluate whether a CDSS that provided recommendations for venous thromboembolism prevention for surgical patients improved thromboprophylaxis use.[6] There were three 10-week intervention periods that alternated with four 10-week control periods, with a 4-week washout between each period. During each intervention period, adherence to practice guidelines improved significantly and then reverted to baseline during each control period.

Although alternating intervention and control periods strengthen a before-after design, *random allocation* of participants to a concurrent control group remains the strongest study design for evaluating therapeutic or preventive interventions. As part of randomization, allocation of groups should be concealed from those involved in the study. Fortunately, randomization has been recognized as an important way to evaluate CDSS.[7]

If the Intervention Primarily Targeted Clinicians, Was the Clinician or Clinician Group (Cluster) the Unit of Analysis?

The *unit of analysis* is a special issue for CDSS evaluation. For most RCTs, the unit of allocation is the patient. Most CDSS evaluations target clinician behavior. Hence, investigators may randomize individual clinicians or clinician clusters, such as health care teams, hospital wards, or outpatient practices.[8] Unfortunately, investigators using such designs often analyze their data as if they had randomized patients.[9,10] This mistake, the *unit of analysis error,* occurs frequently and can generate spuriously low (ie, significant) *P* values.[11] A unit of analysis error should be suspected if a study about a CDSS does not describe the number and characteristics of clinicians (eg, level of clinical experience or specialization, sex, and duration of EMR use) in each arm of a trial.[9-11]

To deepen your understanding of the problem, consider a hypothetical example. Imagine a study in which an investigator randomizes 2 teams of clinicians to a CDSS and another 2 teams to standard practice. During the study, each team sees 5000 patients. If the investigator analyzes the data as if patients were individually randomized, the sample size appears very large. However, if there are underlying differences between the teams in the patient characteristics, or in how the patients are managed, such differences—rather than the intervention—might well explain differences in the outcomes. Were this

the case, we would need to randomize many teams before the patient characteristics or management styles would balance out between groups. At the one extreme, each of the 4 teams is very different; under these circumstances, it is as if we are randomizing only 4 individuals, and the sample size is effectively 4. At the other extreme, the teams are identical in all characteristics other than the intervention, in which case the situation is as if we randomized 20 000 individuals, 10 000 to each group.

A statistic called the *intraclass correlation coefficient* tells us about the correlation of observations (in this case, observations of patients) within clusters. For instance, if one team had a very high proportion of old patients with strokes and uniformly poor outcomes and another team had a high proportion of younger patients with pneumonia and uniformly good outcomes, the intraclass correlation would be high (close to 1.0), and we would be reluctant to attribute differences in outcome to the intervention. On the other hand, if both teams had a similar broad range of patients with widely varying outcomes, the intraclass correlation would be low (close to 0), and we would be more comfortable attributing differences to the intervention. Thus, if the intraclass correlation is high, then the inferences we could make would differ little from those that would be possible if we had randomized only 4 individuals (2 per group), which raises questions about our ability to ensure prognostic similarity in the 2 groups at baseline. If the intraclass correlation is low, the likelihood of prognostic balance at baseline is much greater, and the inferences we can make are similar to those that would be possible if we randomized 10 000 patients to each group.

Obtaining a sufficient sample size and a balance of important *prognostic factors* between groups can therefore be difficult when randomizing physicians and health care teams. If only a few health care teams are available, investigators can pair them according to their similarities on numerous factors, then randomly allocate the intervention within each matched pair.[12-15] A systematic review of 88 RCTs evaluating the effect of CDSSs found that 43 of 88 were *cluster randomized trials* and that 53 of 88 failed to either use cluster as the unit of analysis or adjust for clustering in the analysis (cluster analysis).[7]

Were Participants Analyzed in the Groups to Which They Were Randomized?

Clinicians should particularly attend to an issue regarding randomization. Computer competency varies, and it is common for some clinicians to not use a CDSS or to have technical difficulties accessing a CDSS, even when they are assigned to do so and have help available. Consider the following: If some clinicians assigned to CDSSs fail or refuse to receive the intervention, should these clinicians be included in the analysis? The answer, counterintuitive to some, is yes (see Chapter 11.4, The Principle of Intention to Treat and Ambiguous Dropouts).

Randomization can best accomplish the goal of balancing groups with respect to both known and unknown determinants of outcome if patients (or clinicians) are analyzed according to the groups to which they are randomized. This is the intention-to-treat principle. Deleting or moving patients after randomization compromises or destroys the balance that randomization is designed to achieve (see Chapter 11.4, The Principle of Intention to Treat and Ambiguous Dropouts).

Was the Control Group Unaffected by the Clinical Decision Support System?

The extent to which clinicians or patients in the control group have access to all or part of the CDSS intervention creates a problem of potential contamination. When the control group is influenced by the intervention, the effect of the CDSS may be diluted. Contamination may decrease or even eliminate a true intervention effect.

For example, investigators of a clinical trial randomly allocated patients to have changes in their level of mechanical ventilator support directed by a computer protocol or according to clinical judgment.[16] Because the same physicians and respiratory therapists using the computer protocol were also managing the care of patients not assigned to the protocol, experience with the protocol may have influenced clinicians' management of the control group, thus reducing the effect of the intervention that investigators might have observed had different groups of clinicians been managing each group of patients.

Cluster randomized trials (ie, randomizing groups of physicians) lessen the chance of contamination of the intervention across to the control group,

as long as the clusters do not interact. Ensuring lack of interaction may be challenging. For example, trials that involve medical trainees are difficult to manage even with entire hospitals as a cluster because trainees in many systems have rotations in several hospitals.

Recent randomized trials have attempted to use CDSS interventions that encourage shared decision making by ensuring that decision support is available to both clinicians and patients. One such trial that was included in the systematic review[1] described in our opening clinical scenario randomized patients rather than clinicians or groups of clinicians.[17] The rationale for so doing was that the shared intervention was meant to encourage patients with diabetes to manage their own progress and receive personalized advice on 13 *risk factors* between visits to their family physician.[17] In this case, contamination still may have occurred and would have reduced the differences between the groups.

Imaginative study designs may help deal with contamination. For instance, in a cluster randomized trial, a group of physicians received computerized guidelines for the management of asthma and another group received guidelines for the management of angina.[18] Both groups are part of an intervention but for different diseases, so they may be less likely to pay attention to the other management area for which they serve as a control.

Aside From the Experimental Intervention, Were the Groups Treated Equally?

All CDSS interventions are complex interventions.[4] A CDSS may have a positive influence for unintended reasons. For example, some may be based on the use of structured data collection forms (*checklist effect*) or performance evaluations (*audit and feedback* effect).[19,20] Moreover, a CDSS has multiple components that investigators should describe. For example, ad hoc, unique, locally developed systems are particularly difficult to evaluate without a description of the intervention components. Some have suggested that reports of analyses of CDSS should include figures that show CDSS screenshots, descriptions of CDSS features and functions, and CDSS algorithms and source code.[21] This may be useful for reproducibility and *generalizability* and for addressing the possibility of *cointervention* (ie, interventions associated with but separate from the CDSS). For example, consider a hypothetical report of a venous thrombosis CDSS that does not inform the reader that positive ultrasonography reports always triggered a telephone consultation with a thrombosis specialist. This important cointervention information would have been helpful in understanding the effect of the CDSS itself rather than other associated aspects of the intervention.

The results of studies that evaluated interventions aimed at therapy or prevention are more believable if patients, their caregivers, and the study personnel are *blind* to the treatment (see Chapter 7, Therapy [Randomized Trials]). Blinding also diminishes the *placebo effect*, which in the case of CDSSs may include the tendency of clinicians and patients to ascribe undeserved positive or negative attributes to the use of a computer workstation. Although blinding the clinicians and patients may not be possible, study personnel collecting outcome information usually can—and those analyzing the results always can—be blinded to group allocation. Blinding of the outcome assessment is important to prevent subjective interpretations of data collected that may unduly favor one group over another.[20] Lack of blinding can result in bias if interventions other than the one under scrutiny are differentially applied to the treatment and control groups, particularly if clinicians are permitted to use, at their discretion, effective treatments not included in the study. Investigators can ameliorate concerns regarding lack of blinding if they report details of the intervention and cointerventions.

Cluster randomized trials that involve unblinded clinicians and patients risk differential *loss to follow-up*. Once clinicians and patients learn that they are part of the control group, even if the control group is arranged as delayed access to the intervention, a loss of interest and subsequent unwillingness to participate may occur and bias the results of any study.[22]

Were Outcomes Assessed Uniformly in the Experimental and Control Groups?

In some studies, the computer system may be used as a data collection tool to evaluate the outcome in the CDSS group. Using the information system to log episodes in the treatment group and using a manual system in the non-CDSS group can create a data completeness bias.[19] If the computer logs more episodes than the manual system, it may appear that the CDSS group had more events, which could bias the outcome for or against the CDSS group. To prevent this bias, investigators should collect and measure outcomes similarly in both groups.

USING THE GUIDE

As outlined above, the systematic review and meta-analysis addressing whether a CDSS can improve outcomes in patients with diabetes was judged to be credible[1] (see Chapter 22, The Process of a Systematic Review and Meta-analysis, and Chapter 23, Understanding and Applying the Results of a Systematic Review and Meta-analysis). It included 15 trials that involved 35 557 patients with all types and severity levels of diabetes. Most of the trials assessed compared a CDSS to usual care, 10 of the trials used a cluster randomization, and most concealed allocation, but blinding and follow-up varied. Four of the trials occurred before the year 2000, so they may not be generalizable to current information-technology standards. In terms of clinical outcomes, 2 studies examined hospitalization rates and 3 measured quality of life. Process outcomes (checking hemoglobin A_{1C} [HbA_{1C}], blood pressure, or cholesterol) could not be pooled because of *heterogeneity*. The systematic review authors note an overall lack of high-quality trials in this area in that only 1 trial was judged to be at low risk of bias.[1]

One of the most recent trials in the systematic review was a cluster randomized trial that compared 4 groups.[23] One of the intervention groups in this trial involved patient coaching using mobile CDSS software, Web portal, and telephone access to diabetes educators for patients and primary care clinician decision support that linked the patient-provided data to guidelines.[23] The primary outcome was change in HbA_{1C} at 12 months compared with the usual care group. The report provided no documentation about blinding of final outcome collection or assessment. The investigators used mixed-effects modeling to account for within-practice clustering in the analysis. The authors also discuss additional *sensitivity analyses* to examine the effect of missing data. The intervention package is described in some detail in the text, but screenshots are available only in supplementary files, and algorithms or codes are not provided. In addition, although deploying complex interventions that involve information and communication technology often has significant unforeseen challenges, the authors do not discuss this important issue.

Of 71 physician practices identified, 26 enrolled. Within these 26 practices, 2602 patients were eligible, of whom only 213 enrolled, and 163 were included in the analysis: 62 patients in the intervention group and 56 patients in the control group, as discussed above. The investigators mention imputation techniques to deal with the considerable amount of missing data but do not discuss what influence they had on the results. Similarly, despite reminders to have HbA_{1C} measured at the 12-month end point, it is likely that patients in the intervention group, which was more closely monitored, were more likely to have usable HbA_{1C} test results than the usual care group.

WHAT ARE THE RESULTS?

What Is the Effect of the Clinical Decision Support System?

Chapter 7, Therapy (Randomized Trials), and Chapter 9, Does Treatment Lower Risk? Understanding the Results, provide discussion of *relative risk* (RR), *relative risk reduction* (RRR), *risk difference* (RD), and *absolute risk reduction* (ARR), which inform the magnitude of a treatment effect. As we have discussed, for

patients to benefit, a CDSS must change the behavior of the target (eg, clinician, patient, or both), and that behavior change should positively affect health outcomes. It is now common in health research that addresses electronic systems integrated into clinical care to find that the interventions changed behavior, as evidenced by changes in processes of care, but did not influence clinical outcomes.[7,24,25] Without improvements in patient-important outcomes, the changes required in workflow, documentation practices, knowledge updates, and training are not worthwhile.[26]

Furthermore, CDSS studies rarely report the harms that occur related to the intervention, a problem with potential for serious consequences.[24,27,28] For example, a recent review of medication-related adverse events in the Netherlands found that 16.2% of the 4161 events reported in 12 months were the fault of the information systems themselves, either mistakes made by the software or poor human-computer interfaces that led to error; 9.3% of those originating in hospital caused death or serious temporary harm.[27]

How Precise Is the Estimate of the Effect?

Given a study with low risk of bias, the *confidence interval* (CI) reflects the range in which the true effect of a CDSS might actually lie (see Chapter 7, Therapy [Randomized Trials], and Chapter 10, Confidence Intervals: Was the Single Study or Meta-analysis Large Enough?).

USING THE GUIDE

Results of changes in HbA_{1C} based on the pooled results of 9 studies in the systematic review[1] revealed no significant difference. Similarly, the 2 studies that reported hospitalizations and the 3 studies that reported quality of life did not find a significant benefit from their respective CDSS interventions. Patient-important outcomes, such as mortality or cardiovascular events, were not reported.

In the trial we appraised, HbA_{1C} was decreased by a greater amount (1.2%) at 12 months in the intervention vs usual care group (95% CI, 0.5%-1.9%; $P = .001$).[23] Secondary outcomes, including a depression and diabetes symptom inventory, hospitalizations, and emergency department visits, were not improved.

While recognizing that the summary results of the systematic review may not be accurate given the high risk of bias in most of the trials, it is interesting that there is consistently a lack of evidence that CDSSs for diabetes management improve patient outcomes. Some aspects of clinician performance were said to be improved but could not be combined in meta-analysis. Harm related to the interventions, including increased episodes of severe hypoglycemia due to overly intensive treatment of the diabetes, was not discussed, yet may well have occurred.

HOW CAN I APPLY THE RESULTS TO PATIENT CARE?

Many of the issues specific to a CDSS arise in its application. Implementing a CDSS within your own environment may be challenging.

What Elements of the Clinical Decision Support System Are Required?

There are 2 major elements that compose a CDSS: the logic that has been incorporated and the interface used to present the logic. Unless an RCT specifically compares different logic or presentation components, there is no reliable way to determine which are critical to success or which generally lead to failure. Because CDSS development and deployment tend to be costly in terms of time and resources, determining the factors that lead to success has been an important research endeavor that has, thus far, not yielded reliable results.[25,29]

If the CDSS intervention is poorly described, clinicians may not realize that the intervention requires its own dedicated technical support, clinical care coordinator, or constant "helpline" attention or will not interface with local EMRs. Similarly, it may not be clear that the intervention was developed over many years in a particular institution where the affinity for EMRs and CDSSs might be quite different than in your own setting.

Is the Clinical Decision Support System Exportable to a New Site?

For a CDSS to be exported to a new site, it must have the ability to be integrated with existing information systems and software. In addition, users at the new site must be able to maintain the system, and they must accept the system and ensure that it is kept up-to-date. Systems that require double record keeping generally fail because they increase staff time devoted to documentation, frustrate users, and divert time that could be devoted to patient care. Successful systems are easily integrated into the workflow, address a high-priority area of clinical need, and are timesaving or time neutral for the clinician. Therefore, it is important to assess how the information necessary to run the decision support gets into the system—ideally, through automatic electronic interfaces to existing data-producing systems. Unfortunately, building interfaces to diverse computer systems is often challenging and sometimes impossible.

Applications for CDSSs built on top of proprietary EMR systems are often not portable to other settings. Increasingly, knowledge algorithms are built separately from interface engines to allow for portability of the CDSS, although complexity of the CDSS development may be increased. In addition to technical integration, generalizability of the CDSS to the local clinical environment in terms of relevance, quality, and usability is important to consider. Ideally, each of these items would be thoroughly tested in the local setting to improve the success of CDSS deployment, but the rapid pace of decision making in health care makes this difficult to organize. Simulation laboratories, pilot sites, or staged implementation can be helpful to identify problems before full-scale implementation.

Are Clinicians in Your Setting Likely to Accept the Clinical Decision Support System?

Clinicians who differ in important ways from those in the study may not accept the CDSS. If a study recruited mainly physicians or patients who enjoy using new technology (early adapters), then transfer to regular clinical practice could be disappointing.

Acceptance by clinicians, based on meta-regression and anecdotal evidence, depends on reliability of the system (little downtime and regular upgrades), fast response time, accurate data, and useful information clearly presented.[29] The user interface is an important component of the effectiveness of a CDSS. The CDSS interface should be developed according to potential users' capabilities and limitations, the users' tasks, and the environment in which those tasks are performed.[30]

One of the main difficulties with *alerting systems* is transmitting the information that there is a potential problem (such as an abnormal laboratory value) with the appropriate speed to the individual with the decision-making capability. For example, a group of investigators tried a number of different alerting methods, from a highlighted icon on the computer screen to a flashing yellow light placed on the top of the computer.[31] These investigators later gave the nurses pagers to alert them about abnormal laboratory values.[32] However, this solution might not work well until alerting speed and methods are filtered by the clinical importance of the alert content.

In addition, because a CDSS aims for expert knowledge content, accurate and clear presentation, excellent generalizability, and easy incorporation into daily practice or life, a breakdown in any of these steps may lead to failure.

Patient-oriented CDSSs are also problematic in terms of generalizability because trials tend to recruit a very select group of computer-savvy, usually younger and healthier individuals who are less concerned than others about health information privacy.[33] Typically, older individuals and those who are socially disadvantaged are underrepresented, yet they comprise a high-risk group for many diseases.

Do the Benefits of the Clinical Decision Support System Justify the Harms and Costs?

The costs of CDSSs can be high when including hardware, software, interface, and training.[34] Additional, less obvious costs include the staff required to maintain and upgrade the system. Although cost-effectiveness rather than cost alone should be the determining factor, sometimes the budget effect of a CDSS is so high that it is prohibitive. This is particularly true for community-based physicians who are themselves funding their EMR system and its maintenance, upgrades, and applications.

Systematic reviews have documented that, despite several decades of CDSS development, the quality of research and positive effect on patient outcomes have been disappointing.[35,36] An update of a series of systematic reviews of RCTs that examined the effectiveness and safety of CDSSs for prescribing, ordering diagnostic tests, primary care prevention practices, chronic disease management, and acute care found no significant effect on patient outcomes, such as morbidity, mortality, or quality of life; reported inconsistent effects on processes of care; and documented a lack of attention to potential harms of the CDSS.[37-42] Without reasonable evidence of effectiveness and safety, the concept of cost-effectiveness is moot (see Chapter 28.2, Economic Analysis). However, *economic analyses* attached to randomized trials of diabetes care have been conducted, sometimes based on improvements in surrogate markers, such as HbA_{1C} and cholesterol. Economic analyses based on patient-important outcomes will be a high priority in future research.[34]

CLINICAL SCENARIO RESOLUTION

Your senior resident summarizes the systematic review and meta-analysis[1] of CDSSs for diabetes management at the next morning report. She reports that there is little evidence that CDSSs improve patient outcomes in diabetes. After reviewing concerns about the risk of bias, most of which would tend to overestimate the potential effect of a CDSS, you agree with her assessment. A discussion ensues that ranges from eliminating all computer-based disruptions of care (eg, the unnecessary

pop-up about a clinically irrelevant drug–laboratory test interaction) to developing a computer system that could replace the potential errors of the sleep-deprived resident writing orders in the middle of the night. Everyone recognizes the complexity of the intervention and its components, but the specific facets that might lead to success are uncertain.

In the end, you conclude that although a diabetes tracker system has considerable clinical appeal in terms of organizing patient data, you would have to work with your hospital's information technology department to determine whether an inexpensive "diabetes dashboard" could be purchased or developed for the clinic. You agree that an audit to examine the clinic's performance on diabetes quality benchmarks, as well as a study of the barriers that keep clinicians and patients from meeting those benchmarks, should be completed first.

References

1. Jeffery R, Iserman E, Haynes RB; CDSS Systematic Review Team. Can computerized clinical decision support systems improve diabetes management? a systematic review and meta-analysis. *Diabet Med*. 2013;30(6):739-745.

2. *Medical Subject Headings (MeSH) Database*. Bethesda, MD: National Center for Biotechnology Information; 1998, http://www.ncbi.nlm.nih.gov/mesh/68020000. Accessed February 26, 2014.

3. Johnston ME, Langton KB, Haynes RB, Mathieu A. Effects of computer-based clinical decision support systems on clinician performance and patient outcome: a critical appraisal of research. *Ann Intern Med*. 1994;120(2):135-142.

4. Shcherbatykh I, Holbrook A, Thabane L, Dolovich L; COMPETE III investigators. Methodologic issues in health informatics trials: the complexities of complex interventions. *J Am Med Inform Assoc*. 2008;15(5):575-580.

5. Evans RS, Pestotnik SL, Classen DC, et al. A computer-assisted management program for antibiotics and other antiinfective agents. *N Engl J Med*. 1998;338(4):232-238.

6. Durieux P, Nizard R, Ravaud P, Mounier N, Lepage E. A clinical decision support system for prevention of venous thromboembolism: effect on physician behavior. *JAMA*. 2000;283(21):2816-2821.

7. Garg AX, Adhikari NK, McDonald H, et al. Effects of computerized clinical decision support systems on practitioner performance and patient outcomes: a systematic review. *JAMA*. 2005;293(10):1223-1238.

8. Cornfield J. Randomization by group: a formal analysis. *Am J Epidemiol*. 1978;108(2):100-102.

9. Whiting-O'Keefe QE, Henke C, Simborg DW. Choosing the correct unit of analysis in Medical Care experiments. *Med Care*. 1984;22(12):1101-1114.

10. Divine GW, Brown JT, Frazier LM. The unit of analysis error in studies about physicians' patient care behavior. *J Gen Intern Med*. 1992;7(6):623-629.

11. Calhoun AW, Guyatt GH, Cabana MD, et al. Addressing the unit of analysis in medical care studies: a systematic review. *Med Care*. 2008;46(6):635-643.

12. Klar N, Donner A. The merits of matching in community intervention trials: a cautionary tale. *Stat Med*. 1997;16(15):1753-1764.

13. Thompson SG, Pyke SD, Hardy RJ. The design and analysis of paired cluster randomised trials: an application of meta-analysis techniques. *Stat Med*. 1997;16(18):2063-2079.

14. Campbell MK, Mollison J, Steen N, Grimshaw JM, Eccles M. Analysis of cluster randomised trials in primary care: a practical approach. *Fam Pract*. 2000;17(2):192-196.

15. Mollison J, Simpson J, Campbell M, Grimshaw J. Comparison of analytical methods for cluster randomised trials: an example from a primary care setting. *J Epidemiol Biostat*. 2000;5(6):339-348.

16. Strickland JH Jr, Hasson JH. A computer-controlled ventilator weaning system: a clinical trial. *Chest*. 1993;103(4):1220-1226.

17. Holbrook A, Thabane L, Keshavjee K, et al; COMPETE II Investigators. Individualized electronic decision support and reminders to improve diabetes care in the community: COMPETE II randomized trial. *CMAJ*. 2009;181(1-2):37-44.

18. Eccles M, McColl E, Steen N, et al. Effect of computerised evidence based guidelines on management of asthma and angina in adults in primary care: cluster randomised controlled trial. *BMJ*. 2002;325(7370):941.

19. Friedman C, Wyatt J. The design of demonstration studies. In: Friedman C, Wyatt J, eds. *Evaluation Methods in Biomedical Informatics*. New York, NY: Springer Science and Business Media; 2006:188-223.

20. Guyatt GH, Pugsley SO, Sullivan MJ, et al. Effect of encouragement on walking test performance. *Thorax*. 1984;39(11):818-822.

21. Eysenbach G. CONSORT-EHEALTH: implementation of a checklist for authors and editors to improve reporting of web-based and mobile randomized controlled trials. *Stud Health Technol Inform*. 2013;192:657-661.

22. Hahn S, Puffer S, Torgerson DJ, Watson J. Methodological bias in cluster randomised trials. *BMC Med Res Methodol*. 2005;5(1):10.

23. Quinn CC, Shardell MD, Terrin ML, Barr EA, Ballew SH, Gruber-Baldini AL. Cluster-randomized trial of a mobile phone personalized behavioral intervention for blood glucose control. *Diabetes Care*. 2011;34(9):1934-1942.

24. McKibbon KA, Lokker C, Handler SM, et al. The effectiveness of integrated health information technologies across the phases of medication management: a systematic review of randomized controlled trials. *J Am Med Inform Assoc*. 2012;19(1):22-30.

25. Mollon B, Chong J Jr, Holbrook AM, Sung M, Thabane L, Foster G. Features predicting the success of computerized decision support for prescribing: a systematic review of randomized controlled trials. *BMC Med Inform Decis Mak*. 2009;9(1):11.

26. O'Reilly D, Tarride JE, Goeree R, Lokker C, McKibbon KA. The economics of health information technology in medication management: a systematic review of economic evaluations. *J Am Med Inform Assoc*. 2012;19(3):423-438.

27. Cheung KC, van der Veen W, Bouvy ML, Wensing M, van den Bemt PM, de Smet PA. Classification of medication incidents

associated with information technology. *J Am Med Inform Assoc*. 2014;21(e1):e63-e70.

28. Top 10 health technology hazards for 2013. *Health Devices*. 2012;41(11):342-365.

29. Roshanov PS, Fernandes N, Wilczynski JM, et al. Features of effective computerised clinical decision support systems: meta-regression of 162 randomised trials. *BMJ*. 2013;346:f657.

30. Adams ID, Chan M, Clifford PC, et al. Computer aided diagnosis of acute abdominal pain: a multicentre study. *Br Med J (Clin Res Ed)*. 1986;293(6550):800-804.

31. Bradshaw KE, Gardner RM, Pryor TA. Development of a computerized laboratory alerting system. *Comput Biomed Res*. 1989;22(6):575-587.

32. Tate KE, Gardner RM, Scherting K. Nurses, pagers, and patient-specific criteria: three keys to improved critical value reporting. *Proc Annu Symp Comput Appl Med Care*. 1995;164-168.

33. Brann M, Mattson M. Toward a typology of confidentiality breaches in health care communication: an ethic of care analysis of provider practices and patient perceptions. *Health Commun*. 2004;16(2):231-251.

34. O'Reilly D, Holbrook A, Blackhouse G, Troyan S, Goeree R. Cost-effectiveness of a shared computerized decision support system for diabetes linked to electronic medical records. *J Am Med Inform Assoc*. 2012;19(3):341-345.

35. Black AD, Car J, Pagliari C, et al. The impact of eHealth on the quality and safety of health care: a systematic overview. *PLoS Med*. 2011;8(1):e1000387.

36. Bright TJ, Wong A, Dhurjati R, et al. Effect of clinical decision-support systems: a systematic review. *Ann Intern Med*. 2012;157(1):29-43.

37. Roshanov PS, Misra S, Gerstein HC, et al; CCDSS Systematic Review Team. Computerized clinical decision support systems for chronic disease management: a decision-maker-researcher partnership systematic review. *Implement Sci*. 2011;6(1):92.

38. Sahota N, Lloyd R, Ramakrishna A, et al; CCDSS Systematic Review Team. Computerized clinical decision support systems for acute care management: a decision-maker-researcher partnership systematic review of effects on process of care and patient outcomes. *Implement Sci*. 2011;6:91.

39. Hemens BJ, Holbrook A, Tonkin M, et al; CCDSS Systematic Review Team. Computerized clinical decision support systems for drug prescribing and management: a decision-maker-researcher partnership systematic review. *Implement Sci*. 2011;6:89.

40. Roshanov PS, You JJ, Dhaliwal J, et al; CCDSS Systematic Review Team. Can computerized clinical decision support systems improve practitioners' diagnostic test ordering behavior? a decision-maker-researcher partnership systematic review. *Implement Sci*. 2011;6:88.

41. Souza NM, Sebaldt RJ, Mackay JA, et al; CCDSS Systematic Review Team. Computerized clinical decision support systems for primary preventive care: a decision-maker-researcher partnership systematic review of effects on process of care and patient outcomes. *Implement Sci*. 2011;6(1):87.

42. Nieuwlaat R, Connolly SJ, Mackay JA, et al; CCDSS Systematic Review Team. Computerized clinical decision support systems for therapeutic drug monitoring and dosing: a decision-maker-researcher partnership systematic review. *Implement Sci*. 2011;6(1):90.

11.7

ADVANCED TOPICS IN THE RISK OF BIAS OF THERAPY TRIALS

How to Use an Article About Quality Improvement

Eddy Fan, Andreas Laupacis, Peter J. Pronovost,
Gordon Guyatt, and Dale M. Needham

THERAPY

IN THIS CHAPTER

(continued on following page)

CLINICAL SCENARIO

You, the medical director of an intensive care unit (ICU), discover that mortality has increased for patients with sepsis. You are considering a *quality improvement* (QI) initiative to improve the care and outcomes of your patients. However, you are concerned that many QI studies have weak designs, poor data quality, and often overestimate potential benefits. Before beginning, you decide to identify and evaluate existing QI interventions.

THE SEARCH

You perform a literature search using PubMed and identify a *before-after study* that evaluated an educational QI program for sepsis in 59 medical-surgical ICUs in Spain.[1] This program trained clinicians to recognize and treat severe sepsis based on evidence-based guidelines from the Surviving Sepsis Campaign.[2] The program implemented 2 guideline-based treatment bundles: a resuscitation bundle (ie, a group of interventions that constitute optimal care that need to be implemented together—in this case, 6 tasks started at sepsis recognition and completed within 6 hours) and a management bundle (4 tasks completed within 24 hours). The program looks very promising in the setting of the study, and you wonder about the value of taking this approach in your institution. Your next step is to critically appraise the report.

QUALITY IMPROVEMENT—AN OVERVIEW

Opportunities for QI are common.[3,4] Patients frequently do not receive evidence-based treatments,[5] and more than 9% of hospitalized patients are harmed by adverse events.[6] Quality improvement interventions attempt to change clinician behavior and, through those changes, lead to more consistent, appropriate, and efficient application of established clinical interventions, resulting in improved care and patient outcomes.[7] The target of the intervention in QI research is not ascertaining the efficacy of the intervention but rather determining the effect of the intervention on behavior change, typically manifest as *adherence* to an optimal process of care.

Traditional evaluative clinical research (eg, estimating the efficacy of therapies) typically evaluates interventions provided in well-controlled environments that ensure, in the context of, for instance, the clinical trial setting, that patients receive the intervention.[3,4] In contrast, QI interventions are often designed to enhance the implementation of proven therapies and use data routinely collected in clinical practice. As a result, QI efforts are not always considered research[8]; in that case, an institutional review board may agree to waive *informed consent* and detailed review because the study exposes patients to minimal risks beyond those involved in standard clinical practice.[9]

Quality improvement interventions are frequently context dependent, complex, and iterative, seeking to address barriers to and facilitators of QI.[10] When high-quality *evidence* has securely established substantial net benefit of existing therapies, measuring the processes of care (ie, the incremental implementation of therapies) may be sufficient to establish the benefit of QI interventions. When the net benefit of therapies is less securely established, measurement of improved *patient-important outcomes* is necessary to establish the benefit of QI interventions.

Quality Improvement as a Science

Randomized clinical trials (RCTs) provide an optimal strategy to reduce *bias* associated with differences in *prognostic factors* among groups or with determinants of outcome that change over time (see Chapter 6, Why Study Results Mislead: Bias and Random Error). Publications in the QI field represent a heterogeneous literature[11] in which reports of local experience with a high *risk of bias* are much more frequent than reports of rigorously designed experiments.[12] Likely because of their lower risk of bias, rigorous RCTs are less likely to report significant improvements than are *observational studies*.[13]

Anecdotal QI reports can generate new hypotheses, fuel innovative changes, and motivate clinicians to change.[14] If no dissemination of a local QI intervention to other settings is planned, lower-quality evidence may be acceptable. However, when the apparent benefits of an intervention are widely publicized, spurious findings can result in *harm*, poor use of limited resources, or both. Therefore, QI studies must be rigorously designed, conducted, and evaluated.[14-16]

Some QI initiatives have prematurely implemented the dissemination of interventions based on randomized trials with important limitations. For example, the use of ß-blockers in noncardiac surgery was adopted as a target for QI efforts before evidence that this intervention may increase all-cause mortality and stroke.[17-19] Studies with both a low risk of bias and a high degree of applicability outside the original research setting are needed before QI interventions are widely disseminated.[12,16]

Link to Other Users' Guides

This chapter complements and enhances existing *Users' Guides* that address the effects of interventions— Chapter 7, Therapy (Randomized Trials); Chapter 11.6, Clinical Decision Support Systems; Chapter 14, Harm (Observational Studies); and Summarizing the Evidence—with an emphasis on issues specific to QI studies (Box 11.7-1). Furthermore, this

---

BOX 11.7-1

Users' Guide for an Article Assessing Quality Improvement (QI)

How serious is the risk of bias?

Did intervention and control groups start with the same prognosis?

Were patients randomized? If not, did the investigators use an alternative design that minimizes the risk of bias?

Was randomization concealed?

Were patients in the study groups similar with respect to known prognostic factors?

If the QI intervention primarily targeted clinicians, was the clinician or the clinician group the unit of analysis?

Was data quality acceptable?

Was prognostic balance maintained as the study progressed?

To what extent was the study blinded?

Aside from the experimental intervention(s), were the groups treated equally?

Was the initial prognostic balance maintained at the completion of the study?

Were patients analyzed in the groups to which they were randomized or allocated?

Was the trial stopped early?

Was follow-up complete?

What were the results?

How large was the treatment effect?

How precise was the estimate of the treatment effect?

How can I apply the results?

If the QI study focused on a process of care, what was the quality of evidence that the process improves patient-important outcomes?

Was follow-up sufficiently long?

Is the QI intervention exportable to my site?

Were all patient-important outcomes considered?

Are the likely benefits worth the potential hassles, harms, and costs?

guide focuses on individual *primary studies,* which should be interpreted in the context of all relevant high-quality evidence (see Chapter 2, What Is Evidence-Based Medicine?); it also complements the Standard for Quality Improvement Reporting Excellence (SQUIRE) guidelines.[20,21]

HOW SERIOUS IS THE RISK OF BIAS?

Were Patients Randomized? If Not, Did the Investigators Use an Alternative Design That Minimizes the Risk of Bias?

The observational design of most QI studies may reflect events outside the control of the researchers (eg, change caused by a new policy) or the impracticability of *randomization* (eg, unwillingness to participate in a *control group*).[13] Such observational designs make it difficult to determine whether the QI intervention is responsible for observed changes, therefore generating evidence regarding the effects of the intervention on the outcome that warrants only low confidence.[22]

Nonrandomized designs commonly used in QI studies include before-after studies (with and without concurrent controls), *time series designs* (interrupted or not), and *stepped wedge designs.*[23] Changes over time in patient populations or changes in practice unrelated to the QI intervention introduce risk of bias in uncontrolled before-after studies,[23] which often overestimate the magnitude of benefit.[23] For instance, investigators attributed an improvement in surgical outcomes in patients undergoing coronary artery bypass graft surgery in New York State to publicly reporting hospital and surgeon outcomes.[24] However, a subsequent investigation found that similar improvements occurred across the United States without any such intervention.[25]

Controlled before-after designs are infrequently used because of difficulty in identifying a suitable control group. However, even participants who appear well matched (eg, have similar demographic characteristics) at baseline may differ on important unmeasured factors (eg, adherence to the study intervention).

Another infrequently used but potentially even more powerful design involves introducing the intervention at different times in different settings, effectively conducting a series of before-after studies in the context of a single intervention. This design, which we refer to as an *interrupted time series design*, may increase confidence in the causal link between the intervention and outcome—or scupper a previous spurious conclusion about a causal link.

For example, a study of thoracic surgery addressed the effect of a clinical pathway for postoperative management. The authors compared outcomes during the baseline vs postintervention periods, reporting significant improvements.[26] However, reanalysis revealed a statistically significant preintervention trend, and time-series regression techniques revealed no significant differences after the intervention.[27]

The interrupted time series design does not, however, protect against the effects of other important events that may coincide with the study intervention. With this design, the study periods must be explicitly defined, and statistical techniques may be required to account for autocorrelation (ie, the same type of data collected at adjacent time points are likely more similar than data collected at widely spaced intervals) to avoid overestimating *treatment effects.*[23] *Statistical process control* is another common method used to analyze variations in the performance of a process over time. Variations may include improved performance in response to a QI intervention that, over time, will stabilize at a new, improved level.[28]

Studies using a stepped wedge design introduce the QI intervention to participants sequentially so that, by the end of the study, all participants are exposed to the intervention.[29] The order in which the intervention is introduced may be randomized, further reducing risk of bias.

For example, following a national UK recommendation to implement critical care outreach teams (CCOTs), one hospital undertook a

THERAPY

stepped wedge trial that evaluated the effects on hospital mortality and length of stay.[30] The CCOTs were introduced during 32 weeks, with pairing of wards to match important patient characteristics. One ward from each pair was randomized to earlier CCOT introduction, with usual care occurring in the other paired ward until subsequent CCOT introduction, allowing a matched comparison across 8 pairs of wards. The timing of CCOT initiation across ward pairs was randomly determined and phased in over time, with introduction of CCOTs in an additional ward pair at 4-month intervals. This study found that the CCOT intervention reduced in-hospital mortality vs usual care (*odds ratio*, 0.52; 95% *confidence interval* [CI], 0.32-0.85).

Some nonrandomized studies—if designed, conducted, and analyzed appropriately—may provide robust results.[16,31,32] Statistical methods (eg, *regression analysis*) to account for *confounding variables* (ie, prognostic factors that bias results because they are associated with both the QI intervention and the outcome) may strengthen observational studies.[32] When RCTs are used in QI, they are often pragmatic designs that evaluate whether the QI intervention is effective among broadly defined patient groups receiving care in real-world settings.[23,33]

For example, a study targeted at adult primary care patients with type 2 diabetes randomized 511 patients from 46 clinicians to receive usual care vs shared (patient-clinician) access to a Web-based, electronic diabetes tracker monitoring 13 indicators (eg, blood pressure, glycated hemoglobin [HbA_{1c}] level), as well as providing clinical advice to improve diabetes care.[34] This pragmatic RCT was conducted among community-based clinicians to evaluate effectiveness in the setting in which most patients with diabetes receive care. The intervention group had significantly more checks of

diabetic indicators than the usual care group at 6 months (difference, 1.27 more checks; 95% CI, 0.79-1.75) and experienced significant improvements in blood pressure and levels of HbA_{1c}. However, HbA_{1c} level may be a poor surrogate for patient-important outcomes (ie, randomized trials of intensive therapy to achieve low HbA_{1c} targets fail to reveal reductions in stroke or cardiovascular death[35]); improved blood pressure is a more reliable surrogate outcome, although it too may fail to reveal reductions for some outcomes.[36]

If the Intervention Primarily Targeted Clinicians, Was the Clinician or Clinician Group the Unit of Analysis?

Clinicians working in the same practice, ward, or hospital share a common environment that influences practice and outcomes. Quality improvement investigators must consider this issue in their analysis. For instance, if investigators randomized hospitals to receive an intervention to improve clinician practice, a significant result may occur if data on individual clinicians' practice are analyzed without considering that individual clinicians' results are clustered (ie, physicians working in a particular hospital may practice more similarly to one another than to physicians in other hospitals).[19] Failure to appropriately consider this *unit of analysis* or clustering issue is common in QI studies.[37]

For example, in an RCT that evaluated the effect of clinical reports encouraging use of peritoneal dialysis among patients with end-stage renal disease, 10 physicians who cared for 152 patients were randomized to the intervention or control groups.[38] The authors reported that a significantly greater number of patients started peritoneal dialysis in the group of physicians randomized to the intervention ($P = .04$). However, if the correct unit of analysis (ie, the 10 physicians rather than the 152 patients) was used or special statistical methods were used to account for clustering of patient outcomes by physician, this result is unlikely to have reached statistical significance.[37]

The typical solution is to randomize clinicians in groups to intervention and control, referred to as a *cluster randomized trial.*

Was Data Quality Acceptable?

Although the importance of methods to control data quality is well accepted in clinical research, the same is not true in many QI studies in which data are often collected as part of routine care, without additional resources or training in research methods.[32,39] Deficiencies in data quality can result in high risk of bias, and as a user of QI studies, you need to consider data quality in all study phases (Box 11.7-2).

For example, in a prospective, multicenter study (7688 patients) that evaluated the implementation of a surgical safety checklist on patient complications,[40] data collectors at 8 international sites (including resource-poor settings) received training and supervision from local researchers on the identification, classification, and recording of process-of-care measures and complications according to the National Surgical Quality Improvement Program (NSQIP) from the American College of Surgeons. However, this training occurred only at the beginning of the QI study, whereas standard NSQIP training occurs during a 1-year period, suggesting a potential limitation in training for data collectors. Furthermore, many of the complications evaluated (eg, deep venous thrombosis) require specific diagnostic tests for accurate detection, but the proportion of patients systematically evaluated for complications as part of routine care was not reported. Thus, data quality issues may have influenced the association between the surgical safety checklist and subsequent complications.

BOX 11.7-2

Data Quality Control Methods for Quality Improvement (QI)

Project Design

Were the aims of the QI project clearly stated?

Were appropriate definitions and measurement systems reported for all important data?

Data Collection

Were staff trained, with appropriate quality assurance review, regarding data collection?

Data Management

Was there appropriate review and reporting of missing and outlier/erroneous data?

Data Analysis

Was participant flow (eg, patients, clinicians, and hospitals) through the study explicitly reported (ie, number initially approached, participated, and dropped out)?

THERAPY

Was Follow-up Complete?

Given the resource constraints faced in conducting most QI research, missing data are common. Missing data should be explicitly reported because they can bias study results. If the magnitude of missing data and the potential for bias are both low in relation to the number of outcome events,[19] it may be appropriate to report the degree of missing data without explicitly addressing these data in the analysis.[32] In other situations, investigators may conduct *sensitivity analyses* to determine the potential effects of *loss to follow-up.* Results that do not change substantially with sensitivity analyses provide greater confidence.[32]

USING THE GUIDE

The use of an uncontrolled before-after design suggests a high risk of bias; an interrupted time series or stepped wedge (with randomization) study design would have less potential for bias. Quality assurance over data collection was, however, explicitly reported, with very few missing data. Moreover, the authors used regression methods to account for known imbalances between periods.[1]

WHAT WERE THE RESULTS?

How Large and Precise Are the Effects of the Quality Improvement Intervention?

Previous *Users' Guides* (see Chapter 9, Does Treatment Lower Risk? Understanding the Results) have described common ways of expressing the effect of an intervention (eg, *relative risk* and *risk difference*) and how to evaluate its precision via a CI (see Chapter 10, Confidence Intervals: Was the Single Study or Meta-analysis Large Enough?).[19]

USING THE GUIDE

Compared with the 2-month preintervention period, adherence to the guidelines in patients with sepsis improved for both the resuscitation bundle (5.3% vs 10.0%, $P < .001$) and the management bundle (10.9% vs 15.7%, $P = .001$) during the 4-month postimplementation period. Hospital mortality decreased (44.0% vs 39.7%, $P = .04$).[1] One-year follow-up in a subset of participating ICUs revealed that adherence to the resuscitation bundle returned to baseline, but management-bundle adherence and hospital mortality remained similar to those measures in the postintervention period.

HOW CAN I APPLY THE RESULTS?

If the QI Study Focused on a Process of Care, What Was the Quality of Evidence That the Process Improved Patient-Important Outcomes?

Quality improvement interventions appropriately focus on process-of-care measures when processes can be accurately and feasibly measured, and prior randomized trials have demonstrated that the processes improve outcomes that patients value. For instance, because RCTs have found decreased mortality with aspirin,[41] a QI intervention that increases the use of aspirin in patients with acute myocardial infarction leads to confidence that patients are better off, and QI researchers do not need to measure mortality.[19] When RCTs have not found the benefit of the interventions being encouraged by the QI intervention, QI investigators may strive to find improvement in patient-important outcomes within the QI study. Quality improvement interventions that result in more efficient or less expensive care with no effect on patient-important outcomes are also valuable. Broadly implementing interventions supported by insufficient evidence can be perilous.[16]

For example, a prospective study evaluated the implementation and refinement of a glucose control protocol using insulin infusion (targeting blood glucose levels of 80 to 120 mg/dL [to convert to mmol/L, multiply by 0.0555]) for patients with hyperglycemia and sepsis in a medical ICU. In 70 patients who received the protocol, 86 total hypoglycemic events were recorded, although incidence of hypoglycemia decreased from 7.6% (original protocol) to 0.3% (fourth protocol draft) as the protocol was progressively modified during the study.[42] However, a subsequent meta-analysis found a significant increase in the risk of hypoglycemia (*risk ratio*, 6.0; 95% CI, 4.5-8.0).[43] Importantly, moderate (*hazard ratio* [HR], 1.41; 95% CI, 1.21-1.62) or severe (HR, 2.10; 95% CI, 1.59-2.77) hypoglycemia is associated with a significantly increased risk of mortality.[44]

Was Follow-up Sufficiently Long?

Changes in practice may be short-lived, with many clinicians or organizations reverting to previously established routines (ie, drift in clinician behavior) once the stimulus for a new intervention is no longer present.[13] Furthermore, it often takes considerable time for groups or institutions to fully implement complex, *multifaceted interventions*. The median follow-up time for assessing the outcome of a QI intervention is less than 1 year in most studies,[13] which may be insufficient to determine the sustainability of the intervention. Follow-up studies of successful QI interventions should be performed to address sustainability. Widespread adoption of QI interventions may be unwise if the postintervention follow-up is less than 1 year.

For instance, a *cohort study* that examined the sustainability of a successful intervention to decrease catheter-related bloodstream infections found that infection rates remained low 36 months after the intervention.[45] In contrast, a study that evaluated the implementation of a multifaceted QI intervention (eg, development and dissemination of clinical guidelines supported by electronic registers, recall and reminder systems, staff education, and *audit and feedback*) to improve diabetes care and outcomes in Australia found a significant improvement in service delivery (eg, clinical examinations and laboratory investigations) at 1 year (from 40% to 49%), but there was a subsequent decrease in this outcome in years 2 and 3 (44% in each year).[46]

Is the Quality Improvement Intervention Exportable to My Site?

The context of a QI study is key to evaluating its applicability outside the original study site(s). Study context includes the local environment, processes, resources, leadership, culture, and traditions.[7] Quality improvement studies may involve clinicians or participants not typical of the real-world population. Deciding whether a QI study is generalizable requires an appreciation of the local barriers to and facilitators of QI.[10,47]

For example, despite recommendations from professional societies and national guidelines regarding selective use of routine preoperative

tests in patients with low anesthetic risk, a high number of tests were performed in a French academic hospital.[48] Previous studies found that most anesthesiologists at the hospital were not complying, despite familiarity with the recommendations. Clinicians adapted the national guidelines using strategies targeted at specific organizational barriers (eg, lack of preoperative anesthesia consultation). After this adaptation to local context, as well as active feedback regarding their practice and discussions about organizational changes, the hospital observed a sharp decrease in preoperative tests ordered for low-risk patients (80% vs 48%; $P < .05$).

The context of a QI study is also important in considering the acceptability and probability of success of the intervention in different settings. Local barriers (eg, alternative therapeutic protocols) and facilitators (eg, supportive *opinion leaders*) may differ. For instance, in an RCT that compared usual care vs clinician education by local opinion leaders coupled with performance feedback in elderly patients who had experienced acute myocardial infarction, the QI intervention significantly increased the use of aspirin (13% vs −3%, $P = .04$) and ß-blockers (31% vs 18%, $P = .02$).[47] In addition, an audit of local baseline practice may be required, because audit and feedback interventions may be most effective when baseline adherence to *evidence-based practice* is low.[49] Lastly, successful implementation and evaluation of a QI intervention in a number of settings (ie, replication) may help increase confidence in its *generalizability*. Hence, a clear understanding of context-related issues is required to understand the exportability and acceptability of the QI intervention to local practice.

Were All Patient-Important Outcomes Considered?

In reviewing the results of QI studies, one must consider whether important potential effects of the intervention were not measured.[50] Quality

TABLE 11.7-1

Unintended Consequences of Quality Improvement (QI)

Unintended Consequence	Potential Problems	Potential Solutions
Resources	Increased costs to medical system that result from increased direct costs of additional interventions Increased costs of data collection and information management during and after QI implementation Decreased resources allocated to other activities	Assess costs and cost-effectiveness of intervention as part of QI study Anticipate and monitor potential increased costs of the QI process; collect only essential data/information
Clinicians	Decreased attention to areas not subject to measurement in the QI intervention (ie, "crowding out" behavior) Inappropriate application of the QI intervention to ineligible patients in an effort to achieve broad success of the initiative	Consider monitoring other outcomes and clinician practices for any negative effect Ensure that the clinical area chosen for a QI intervention is the one most in need of improvement
Patients and policymakers	Access to biased or imprecise QI results impairs appropriate decision making The QI process measure may improve without change in the key patient-centered outcome QI measures or goals are inconsistent with patient preferences	Appropriate design, analysis, and reporting of QI interventions Ensure that quality measures closely match (or are good surrogate for) the desired outcome Monitor satisfaction as part of QI implementation

improvement interventions may have unintended consequences. For example, attempts to increase adherence to guidelines for colorectal cancer screening in a hospital in which many patients declined *screening* (because of their own *values and preferences*) resulted in decreased patient and clinician satisfaction.[51] Unintended consequences also may include effects on resource use and clinician behavior (Table 11.7-1).[52]

An important unintended consequence is "crowding out" behavior, in which gains in quality in one area occur at the expense of another.[52]

For example, a QI study that evaluated the effect of enhanced education and resources for medication management in depression resulted initially in improved mental health but over time resulted in reduced mental health because of reduced coping with stress,

potentially attributable to a shift away from psychological coping strategies.[53] Sustained benefits may have been realized if coping strategies were not "crowded out" by the new emphasis on medication management.

Are the Likely Benefits Worth the Potential Hassles, Harms, and Costs?

There are different thresholds for action based on the probabilities of benefits, harms, financial costs, and *opportunity costs* of a QI intervention (Table 11.7-2). The cost of a QI intervention (including time and effort of staff working to change clinician behavior) may be important, especially if the intervention confers only a small benefit. Moreover, it also is important to consider potential harms and costs that result from not implementing a QI intervention and thus forgoing possible improvements in

TABLE 11.7-2

Examples of Quality Improvement (QI) Studies and Thresholds for Decision Making in Implementing QI Interventions

Decision-Making Threshold	Examples of QI Studies			
	Multifaceted Protocol to Streamline Urgent Cardiac Catheterization and Revascularization in <90 Minutes for Prehospital Patients With Acute ST-Segment Elevation MI	**Education and Computerized Reminders for Early Administration of Empirical Antibiotics for Patients With Suspected Community-Acquired Pneumonia in the Emergency Department**	**Multifaceted Protocol to Improve Adherence to a Bundle of Evidence-Based Practices for Central Catheter Insertion to Prevent Catheter-Related Bloodstream Infections**	**Removing High-Concentration Intravenous Potassium Supplements From ICU Medication Box to Avoid Human Errors**
Evidence of the efficacy of underlying intervention in QI study	High-quality evidence of benefit[56]	High-quality evidence of benefit[57]	Moderate- to high-quality evidence of benefit[57]	No direct evidence available
Anticipated costs and harm of implementing QI intervention	High costs, potential for harm, or both	Low to moderate cost, potential for harm, or both	Low cost and potential for harm	Low cost and potential for harm
Quality of QI evidence required	Require at least moderate-quality QI evidence	Require at least moderate-quality QI evidence	Require at least low-quality QI evidence	No QI study necessary
GRADE recommendation for widespread implementation of intervention[a]	Weak	Strong	Strong	No specific recommendation

Abbreviations: GRADE, Grading of Recommendations Assessment, Development and Evaluation; ICU, intensive care unit; MI, myocardial infarction.

[a]Based on GRADE system, evaluating the balance between desirable and undesirable effects, quality of evidence, patient values and preferences, and costs (resource allocation).[19]

patient-important outcomes. Knowing such cost issues is often necessary before an organization decides to invest in that intervention, and lack of such information may delay implementation of an effective QI intervention. However, few QI studies (12%) provide an *economic analysis*.[13]

Requiring larger, more precise (ie, narrower CIs) treatment effects and rigorously conducted studies may be prudent when the risks or costs of an intervention are high. When this is the case, only high confidence in an appreciable magnitude of effect can justify the intervention.[54] For QI interventions with relatively low cost and low risk, action may reasonably

be taken even if a QI study has a small benefit or is supported by evidence that warrants lower confidence.[54] Large-magnitude effects are unlikely for such QI interventions.

One example of a relatively low-cost and low-risk QI intervention is an observational study aimed at reducing catheter-related bloodstream infections in 103 ICUs in Michigan through use of relatively simple interventions (eg, a catheter insertion checklist and stocking chlorhexidine and other supplies together in a central cart) to in turn increase use of evidence-based practices. That study found a significant decrease in the mean and median infection rate, from 7.7 and 2.7 per 1000 catheter-days at baseline to 1.4 and 0 per 1000 catheter-days in the period from 15 to 18 months after implementation ($P \leq .002$ for both comparisons).[46]

CLINICAL SCENARIO RESOLUTION

As the ICU medical director, you are faced with 2 important and related questions: did the QI intervention truly lead to improvement in the setting in which it was initially implemented, and if so, will it have a similar effect in your setting? Your research reveals that the most recent (2008) iteration of the Surviving Sepsis Campaign guidelines,[2] on which the QI intervention of this study was based, was developed using the *GRADE (Grading of Recommendations Assessment, Development and Evaluation)* approach.[55] Although some of the bundled interventions received a weak recommendation (eg, hydrocortisone for fluid-unresponsive septic shock), the study found a consistent increase in interventions that received a strong recommendation (eg, fluid resuscitation and vasopressors targeting a mean arterial pressure of ≥ 65 mm Hg). Although the study indicates a statistically significant decrease in hospital mortality (4% *absolute risk reduction*) that was sustained at 1 year after implementation of the QI program, the weak study design decreases confidence in the causal association between the QI intervention and observed outcomes. Furthermore, you note that no data were reported on costs or unintended consequences. However, the substantial decrease in hospital mortality, if truly attributable to the intervention, suggests that any unintended consequences were likely small compared with the benefits.

With this *Users' Guide* to assist in your appraisal of this study, you decide that although confidence is low, the intervention actually improved mortality and has relatively low cost and low potential for harm. You believe the educational intervention might be successfully applied in your own hospital setting, and you will work with hospital administrators to collect data on processes of care and hospital mortality associated with this intervention in your hospital.

CONCLUSIONS

Clinicians frequently do not implement interventions with demonstrated net benefit. The risk of bias of studies that evaluate the effectiveness of QI interventions is frequently high. Given the potential for widespread implementation of QI interventions, robust study methods are no less important in QI studies than in other research. Clinicians and others considering implementation of QI interventions should be aware of the risk of bias in a QI study, consider whether the investigators measured appropriate outcomes, be concerned if there has been no replication of the findings, consider the likelihood of success of the QI intervention in their practice setting, and consider the costs and possibility of unintended effects of its implementation.

References

1. Ferrer R, Artigas A, Levy MM, et al; Edusepsis Study Group. Improvement in process of care and outcome after a multicenter severe sepsis educational program in Spain. *JAMA*. 2008;299(19):2294-2303.

2. Dellinger RP, Levy MM, Carlet JM, et al; International Surviving Sepsis Campaign Guidelines Committee; American Association of Critical-Care Nurses; American College of Chest Physicians; American College of Emergency Physicians; Canadian Critical Care Society; European Society of Clinical Microbiology and Infectious Diseases; European Society of Intensive Care Medicine; European Respiratory Society; International Sepsis Forum; Japanese Association for Acute Medicine; Japanese Society of Intensive Care Medicine; Society of Critical Care Medicine; Society of Hospital Medicine; Surgical Infection

Society; World Federation of Societies of Intensive and Critical Care Medicine. Surviving Sepsis Campaign: international guidelines for management of severe sepsis and septic shock: 2008. *Crit Care Med*. 2008;36(1):296-327.

3. Institute of Medicine. *Crossing the Quality Chasm: A New Health System for the 21st Century*. Washington, DC: National Academies Press; 2001.

4. Institute of Medicine. *To Err Is Human: Building a Safer Health System*. Washington, DC: National Academies Press; 2000.

5. McGlynn EA, Asch SM, Adams J, et al. The quality of health care delivered to adults in the United States. *N Engl J Med*. 2003;348(26):2635-2645.

6. de Vries EN, Ramrattan MA, Smorenburg SM, Gouma DJ, Boermeester MA. The incidence and nature of in-hospital adverse events: a systematic review. *Qual Saf Health Care*. 2008;17(3):216-223.

7. Batalden PB, Davidoff F. What is "quality improvement" and how can it transform healthcare? *Qual Saf Health Care*. 2007;16(1):2-3.

8. Lynn J, Baily MA, Bottrell M, et al. The ethics of using quality improvement methods in health care. *Ann Intern Med*. 2007;146(9):666-673.

9. Miller FG, Emanuel EJ. Quality-improvement research and informed consent. *N Engl J Med*. 2008;358(8):765-767.

10. Davidoff F, Batalden P, Stevens D, Ogrinc G, Mooney S; SQUIRE Development Group. Publication guidelines for quality improvement in health care: evolution of the SQUIRE project. *Qual Saf Health Care*. 2008;17(suppl 1):i3-i9.

11. Rubenstein LV, Hempel S, Farmer MM, et al. Finding order in heterogeneity: types of quality-improvement intervention publications. *Qual Saf Health Care*. 2008;17(6):403-408.

12. Thomson RG, Moss FM. QIR and SQUIRE: continuum of reporting guidelines for scholarly reports in healthcare improvement. *Qual Saf Health Care*. 2008;17(suppl 1):i10-i12.

13. Alexander JA, Hearld LR. What can we learn from quality improvement research? a critical review of research methods. *Med Care Res Rev*. 2009;66(3):235-271.

14. Pronovost P, Wachter R. Proposed standards for quality improvement research and publication: one step forward and two steps back. *Qual Saf Health Care*. 2006;15(3):152-153.

15. Landefeld CS, Shojania KG, Auerbach AD. Should we use large scale healthcare interventions without clear evidence that benefits outweigh costs and harms? no. *BMJ*. 2008;336(7656):1277.

16. Auerbach AD, Landefeld CS, Shojania KG. The tension between needing to improve care and knowing how to do it. *N Engl J Med*. 2007;357(6):608-613.

17. Bangalore S, Wetterslev J, Pranesh S, Sawhney S, Gluud C, Messerli FH. Perioperative beta blockers in patients having non-cardiac surgery: a meta-analysis. *Lancet*. 2008;372(9654):1962-1976.

18. Devereaux PJ, Yang H, Yusuf S, et al; POISE Study Group. Effects of extended-release metoprolol succinate in patients undergoing non-cardiac surgery (POISE trial): a randomised controlled trial. *Lancet*. 2008;371(9627):1839-1847.

19. Guyatt GH, Briel M, Glasziou P, Bassler D, Montori VM. Problems of stopping trials early. *BMJ*. 2012;344:e3863.

20. Ogrinc G, Mooney SE, Estrada C, et al. The SQUIRE (Standards for QUality Improvement Reporting Excellence) guidelines for quality improvement reporting: explanation and elaboration. *Qual Saf Health Care*. 2008;17(suppl 1):i13-i32.

21. Davidoff F, Batalden P, Stevens D, Ogrinc G, Mooney SE; SQUIRE development group. Publication guidelines for quality improvement studies in health care: evolution of the SQUIRE project. *BMJ*. 2009;338:a3152.

22. Li LC, Moja L, Romero A, Sayre EC, Grimshaw JM. Nonrandomized quality improvement intervention trials might overstate the strength of causal inference of their findings. *J Clin Epidemiol*. 2009;62(9):959-966.

23. Eccles M, Grimshaw J, Campbell M, Ramsay C. Research designs for studies evaluating the effectiveness of change and improvement strategies. *Qual Saf Health Care*. 2003;12(1):47-52.

24. Hannan EL, Kilburn H Jr, Racz M, Shields E, Chassin MR. Improving the outcomes of coronary artery bypass surgery in New York State. *JAMA*. 1994;271(10):761-766.

25. Ghali WA, Ash AS, Hall RE, Moskowitz MA. Statewide quality improvement initiatives and mortality after cardiac surgery. *JAMA*. 1997;277(5):379-382.

26. Zehr KJ, Dawson PB, Yang SC, Heitmiller RF. Standardized clinical care pathways for major thoracic cases reduce hospital costs. *Ann Thorac Surg*. 1998;66(3):914-919.

27. Ramsay CR, Matowe L, Grilli R, Grimshaw JM, Thomas RE. Interrupted time series designs in health technology assessment: lessons from two systematic reviews of behavior change strategies. *Int J Technol Assess Health Care*. 2003;19(4):613-623.

28. Thor J, Lundberg J, Ask J, et al. Application of statistical process control in healthcare improvement: systematic review. *Qual Saf Health Care*. 2007;16(5):387-399.

29. Brown C, Lilford R. Evaluating service delivery interventions to enhance patient safety. *BMJ*. 2008;337:a2764.

30. Priestley G, Watson W, Rashidian A, et al. Introducing Critical Care Outreach: a ward-randomised trial of phased introduction in a general hospital. *Intensive Care Med*. 2004;30(7):1398-1404.

31. Glasziou P, Chalmers I, Rawlins M, McCulloch P. When are randomised trials unnecessary? picking signal from noise. *BMJ*. 2007;334(7589):349-351.

32. Needham DM, Sinopoli DJ, Dinglas VD, et al. Improving data quality control in quality improvement projects. *Int J Qual Health Care*. 2009;21(2):145-150.

33. Treweek S, Zwarenstein M. Making trials matter: pragmatic and explanatory trials and the problem of applicability. *Trials*. 2009;10:37.

34. Holbrook A, Thabane L, Keshavjee K, et al; COMPETE II Investigators. Individualized electronic decision support and reminders to improve diabetes care in the community: COMPETE II randomized trial. *CMAJ*. 2009;181(1-2):37-44.

35. Ray KK, Seshasai SR, Wijesuriya S, et al. Effect of intensive control of glucose on cardiovascular outcomes and death in patients with diabetes mellitus: a meta-analysis of randomised controlled trials. *Lancet*. 2009;373(9677):1765-1772.

36. Chew EY, Ambrosius WT, Davis MD, et al; ACCORD Study Group; ACCORD Eye Study Group. Effects of medical therapies on retinopathy progression in type 2 diabetes. *N Engl J Med*. 2010;363(3):233-244.

37. Calhoun AW, Guyatt GH, Cabana MD, et al. Addressing the unit of analysis in medical care studies: a systematic review. *Med Care*. 2008;46(6):635-643.

THERAPY

38. Balas EA, Boren SA, Hicks LL, Chonko AM, Stephenson K. Effect of linking practice data to published evidence: a randomized controlled trial of clinical direct reports. *Med Care.* 1998;36(1):79-87.

39. Solberg LI, Mosser G, McDonald S. The three faces of performance measurement: improvement, accountability, and research. *Jt Comm J Qual Improv.* 1997;23(3):135-147.

40. Haynes AB, Weiser TG, Berry WR, et al; Safe Surgery Saves Lives Study Group. A surgical safety checklist to reduce morbidity and mortality in a global population. *N Engl J Med.* 2009;360(5):491-499.

41. Baigent C, Blackwell L, Collins R, et al; Antithrombotic Trialists' (ATT) Collaboration. Aspirin in the primary and secondary prevention of vascular disease: collaborative meta-analysis of individual participant data from randomised trials. *Lancet.* 2009;373(9678):1849-1860.

42. Clayton SB, Mazur JE, Condren S, Hermayer KL, Strange C. Evaluation of an intensive insulin protocol for septic patients in a medical intensive care unit. *Crit Care Med.* 2006;34(12):2974-2978.

43. Griesdale DE, de Souza RJ, van Dam RM, et al. Intensive insulin therapy and mortality among critically ill patients: a meta-analysis including NICE-SUGAR study data. *CMAJ.* 2009;180(8):821-827.

44. Finfer S, Liu B, Chittock DR, et al; NICE-SUGAR Study Investigators. Hypoglycemia and risk of death in critically ill patients. *N Engl J Med.* 2012;367(12):1108-1118.

45. Pronovost PJ, Goeschel CA, Colantuoni E, et al. Sustaining reductions in catheter related bloodstream infections in Michigan intensive care units: observational study. *BMJ.* 2010;340:c309.

46. Bailie RS, Si D, Robinson GW, Togni SJ, D'Abbs PH. A multifaceted health-service intervention in remote Aboriginal communities: 3-year follow-up of the impact on diabetes care. *Med J Aust.* 2004;181(4):195-200.

47. Soumerai SB, McLaughlin TJ, Gurwitz JH, et al. Effect of local medical opinion leaders on quality of care for acute myocardial infarction: a randomized controlled trial. *JAMA.* 1998;279(17):1358-1363.

48. Capdenat Saint-Martin E, Michel P, Raymond JM, et al. Description of local adaptation of national guidelines and of active feedback for rationalising preoperative screening in patients at low risk from anaesthetics in a French university hospital. *Qual Health Care.* 1998;7(1):5-11.

49. Jamtvedt G, Young JM, Kristoffersen DT, O'Brien MA, Oxman AD. Does telling people what they have been doing change what they do? A systematic review of the effects of audit and feedback. *Qual Saf Health Care.* 2006;15(6):433-436.

50. Guyatt G, Montori V, Devereaux PJ, Schünemann H, Bhandari M. Patients at the center: in our practice, and in our use of language. *ACP J Club.* 2004;140(1):A11-A12.

51. Walter LC, Davidowitz NP, Heineken PA, Covinsky KE. Pitfalls of converting practice guidelines into quality measures: lessons learned from a VA performance measure. *JAMA.* 2004;291(20):2466-2470.

52. Bardach NS, Cabana MD. The unintended consequences of quality improvement. *Curr Opin Pediatr.* 2009;21(6):777-782.

53. Wells KB, Tang L, Miranda J, Benjamin B, Duan N, Sherbourne CD. The effects of quality improvement for depression in primary care at nine years: results from a randomized, controlled group-level trial. *Health Serv Res.* 2008;43(6):1952-1974.

54. Berwick DM. The science of improvement. *JAMA.* 2008;299(10):1182-1184.

55. Jaeschke R, Guyatt GH, Dellinger P, et al; GRADE Working Group. Use of GRADE grid to reach decisions on clinical practice guidelines when consensus is elusive. *BMJ.* 2008;337:a744.

56. Le May MR, So DY, Dionne R, et al. A citywide protocol for primary PCI in ST-segment elevation myocardial infarction. *N Engl J Med.* 2008;358(3):231-240.

57. Houck PM, Bratzler DW, Nsa W, Ma A, Bartlett JG. Timing of antibiotic administration and outcomes for Medicare patients hospitalized with community-acquired pneumonia. *Arch Intern Med.* 2004;164(6):637-644.

12.1

ADVANCED TOPICS IN THE RESULTS OF THERAPY TRIALS

Hypothesis Testing

Romina Brignardello-Petersen, Gordon Guyatt,
Kameshwar Prasad, Roman Jaeschke, Deborah J. Cook,
Stephen D. Walter, and George Tomlinson

THERAPY

IN THIS CHAPTER

For every treatment, there is a true, underlying effect that any individual experiment can only estimate (see Chapter 6, Why Study Results Mislead: Bias and Random Error). Investigators use statistical methods to advance their understanding of this true effect. This chapter explores the logic underlying one approach to statistical inquiry: hypothesis testing. Readers interested in how to teach the *concepts* reviewed in this chapter to clinical learners may be interested in an interactive script we have developed for this purpose.[1]

The hypothesis-testing approach to statistical exploration is to begin with what is called a *null hypothesis* and try to disprove that hypothesis. Typically, the null hypothesis states that there is no difference between the interventions being compared. To start our discussion, we will focus on *dichotomous* (yes/no) *outcomes*, such as dead or alive or hospitalized or not hospitalized.

For instance, in a comparison of vasodilator treatment in 804 men with heart failure, investigators compared the proportion of enalapril-treated patients who died with the proportion of patients who received a combination of hydralazine and nitrates who died.[2] We start with the assumption that the treatments are equally effective, and we adhere to this position unless the results make it untenable. We could state the null hypothesis in the vasodilator trial more formally as follows: the true difference in the proportion of patients surviving between those treated with enalapril and those treated with hydralazine and nitrates is 0.

In this hypothesis-testing framework, the statistical analysis addresses the question of whether the observed data are consistent with the null hypothesis. Even if the treatment truly has no positive or negative effect on the outcome (ie, the *effect size* is 0), the results observed will rarely agree exactly with the null hypothesis. For instance, even if a treatment has no true effect on mortality, seldom will we see exactly the same proportion of deaths in treatment and *control groups*. As the results diverge farther and farther from the finding of "no difference," however, the null hypothesis that there is no true difference between the treatments becomes progressively less credible. If the difference between results of the treatment and control groups becomes large enough, we abandon belief in the null hypothesis. We further develop the underlying logic by describing the role of chance in clinical research.

THE ROLE OF CHANCE

In Chapter 6, Why Study Results Mislead: Bias and Random Error, we considered a balanced coin with which the true *probability* of obtaining either heads or tails in any individual coin toss is 0.5. We noted that if we tossed such a coin 10 times, we would not be surprised if we did not see exactly 5 heads and 5 tails. Occasionally, we would get results quite divergent from the 5:5 split, such as 8:2 or even 9:1. Furthermore, very infrequently, the 10 coin tosses would result in 10 heads or tails.

Chance is responsible for this variability in results. Certain recreational games illustrate the way chance operates. On occasion, the roll of 2 unbiased dice (dice with an equal probability of rolling any number between 1 and 6) will yield 2 ones or 2 sixes. On occasion (much to the delight of the recipient), the dealer at a poker game will deal a hand that consists of 5 cards of a single suit. Even less frequently, the 5 cards will not only belong to a single suit but also have consecutive face values.

Chance is not restricted to the world of coin tosses, dice, and card games. If we take a sample of patients from a community, chance may result in unusual and potentially misleading distributions of chronic disease, such as hypertension or diabetes. Chance also may be responsible for substantial imbalance in *event rates* in 2 groups of patients given different treatments that are, in fact, equally effective. Much statistical inquiry is geared toward determining the extent to which unbalanced distributions could be attributed to chance and the extent to which we should invoke other explanations (differential *treatment effects*, for instance). As we discuss in this chapter, the size of the study (determining, in turn, the number of events) to a large extent determines the conclusions of its statistical inquiry.

THE *P* VALUE

One error that an investigator can make is to conclude that an outcome differs between a treatment group and a control group when, in fact, no such difference exists. In statistical terms, making the mistake of concluding that treatment and control differ when, in truth, they do not is called a *type I error,* and the probability of making such an error is referred to as the α *level.*

Imagine a situation in which we are uncertain whether a coin is biased. We could construct a null hypothesis that the true proportions of heads and tails are equal (ie, the coin is unbiased). With this scenario, the probability of any given toss landing heads is 50%, as is the probability of any given toss landing tails. We could test this hypothesis by an experiment in which we conduct a series of coin tosses. Statistical analysis of the results of the experiment would address the question of whether the results observed were consistent with chance.

Let us conduct a hypothetical experiment in which the suspect coin is tossed 10 times, and on all 10 occasions, the result is heads. How likely is this to have occurred if the coin were indeed unbiased? Most people would conclude that it is highly unlikely that chance could explain this extremely unlikely result. We would therefore be ready to reject the hypothesis that the coin is unbiased (the null hypothesis) and conclude that the coin is biased toward a toss of heads.

Statistical methods allow us to be more precise by ascertaining just how likely such an unusual result is if the null hypothesis is true. The *law of multiplicative probabilities* for independent events (in which one event in no way influences the other) tells us that the probability of 10 consecutive heads can be found by multiplying the probability of a single head 10 times over; that is, $(1/2) \times (1/2) \times (1/2)$, and so on, which yields a value of slightly less than 1 in a 1000. A series of 10 consecutive tails would be equally unusual and would also cause us to doubt that the coin was unbiased. The probability of getting 10 heads or 10 tails is just under 2/1000.

In a journal article, we would likely see this probability expressed as a *P* value, such as $P = .002$ (if the value was rounded to the third decimal). What is the precise meaning of this *P* value? If the coin were unbiased (ie, if the null hypothesis were true) and we were to repeat the experiment of the 10 coin tosses many times, by chance alone, we would get either 10 heads or 10 tails in approximately 2 per 1000 of these repetitions.

The framework of hypothesis testing involves a yes/no decision. Are we willing to reject the null hypothesis? This choice involves a decision about how much risk or chance of making a type I error we are willing to accept. The reasoning implies a threshold value that demarcates a boundary. On one side of this boundary, we are unwilling to reject the null hypothesis; on the other side, we are ready to conclude that chance is no longer a plausible explanation for the results. The threshold chosen is the α level mentioned above.

To return to the example of 10 consecutive heads or tails, most people observing this distribution would be ready to reject the null hypothesis, which—it turns out—would be expected to occur by chance alone less than twice per 1000 experiments. What if we repeat the thought experiment, and this time we obtain 9 tails and 1 head? Once again, it is unlikely that the result is because of the play of chance alone. As shown in Figure 12.1-1 (which you will recognize from Chapter 6; the theoretical distribution of the distribution of results on an infinite number of repetitions of the 10-coin-flip experiment when the coin is unbiased), the *P* value is .02, or 2 in 100. That is, if the coin were unbiased and the null hypothesis were true, we would expect results as extreme as—or more extreme than—those observed (ie, 10 heads or 10 tails, 9 heads and 1 tail, or 9 tails and 1 head) to occur by chance alone 2 times per 100 repetitions of the experiment.

Where we set this threshold or boundary is a matter of judgment. Statistical convention suggests a threshold that demarcates the plausible from the implausible at 5 times per 100, which is represented by an α value of .05. Once we have chosen our threshold (of $\alpha = .05$, for example), we call a result that falls beyond this boundary (ie, the result gives $P \leq .05$) *statistically significant.* The meaning of statistically significant, therefore, is "sufficiently unlikely to be due to chance alone that we are ready to reject the null hypothesis."

Statistically significant findings occasionally happen by chance, and it is only convention that makes the .05 threshold sacrosanct. Suppose we set $\alpha = .01$, so we reject the null hypothesis if $P \leq .01$. A finding with a $P < .01$ will happen, simply by chance, 1% of the time if the null hypothesis is true; this means we would reject a true null hypothesis 1%

FIGURE 12.1-1

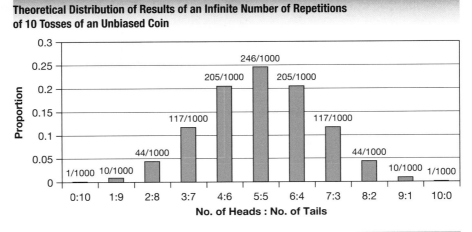

Theoretical Distribution of Results of an Infinite Number of Repetitions of 10 Tosses of an Unbiased Coin

of the time. If we wish to be more conservative (more sure when we reject the null hypothesis that chance cannot explain the difference observed), we might well choose a 1% threshold.

Let us repeat our experiment twice more, both times with a new coin. On the first repetition, we obtain 8 heads and 2 tails. Calculation of the P value associated with an 8/2 split tells us that, if the coin were unbiased, results as extreme as or more extreme than 8/2 (or 2/8) would occur solely as a result of the play of chance 11 times per 100 ($P = .11$) (Figure 12.1-1). We have crossed to the other side of the conventional boundary between what is plausible and what is implausible. If we accept the convention, the results are not statistically significant and we will not reject the null hypothesis.

On our final repetition of the experiment, we obtain 7 tails and 3 heads. Experience tells us that such a result, although not the most common, would not be unusual even if the coin were unbiased. The P value confirms our intuition: Results as extreme as, or more extreme than, this 7/3 split would occur under the null hypothesis 34 times per 100 ($P = .34$) (Figure 12.1-1). Again, we will not reject the null hypothesis.

When investigators compare 2 treatments, the question they ask is, how likely is it that the observed difference, or a larger one, could be a result of chance alone? If we accept the conventional boundary or threshold ($P \le .05$), we will reject the null hypothesis

and conclude that the treatment has some effect when the answer to this question is that repetitions of the experiment would yield differences as extreme as or more extreme than those we have observed less than 5% of the time. The 5% refers to both the observed difference and an equally large difference in the opposite direction because both results will be equally implausible (ie, this is a 2-sided significance test). Investigators sometimes conduct 1-sided significance tests where they consider differences in only 1 direction.

Let us return to the example of the randomized trial in which investigators compared enalapril and the combination of hydralazine and nitrates in 804 men with heart failure. The results of this study illustrate hypothesis testing using a dichotomous (yes/no) outcome, in this case, mortality.[2] During the *follow-up* period, which ranged from 6 months to 5.7 years, 132 of 403 patients (33%) assigned to receive enalapril died, as did 153 of 401 (38%) of those assigned to receive hydralazine and nitrates. Application of a statistical test that compares proportions (the χ^2 test) reveals that if there were actually no underlying difference in mortality between the 2 groups, differences as large as or larger than those actually observed would be expected 11 times per 100 ($P = .11$). Using the hypothesis-testing framework and the conventional threshold of $P < .05$, we would conclude that we cannot reject the null hypothesis and that the difference observed is compatible with chance.

TYPE I AND TYPE II ERRORS

Consider a woman who suspects she is pregnant and is undertaking a pregnancy test. The test has possible errors associated with its result. Figure 12.1-2 represents the 4 possible results: the woman is either pregnant or not pregnant, and the test result is either positive or negative. If the woman is pregnant, the test may be positive (*true positive*, cell a) or negative (*false negative*, cell b). If the woman is not pregnant, the test may be positive (*false positive*, cell c) or negative (*true negative*, cell d).

We can apply the same logic to the result of an experiment testing the effect of a treatment. The treatment either has an effect or it does not; the experiment is either positive ($P \le .05$) or negative ($P > .05$) (Figure 12.1-3). Here, a true-positive result occurs when there is a real treatment effect and the study results yield a $P \le .05$ (cell a), and a true-negative result occurs when treatment has no effect and the study yields a $P > .05$. We refer to a false-positive result (no true treatment effect, $P \le .05$, cell b) as a type I error. When we set our threshold α at .05, we fix the probability of a type I error at 5%: 1 in 20 times we will be misled and true null hypotheses will be rejected.

Another type of error that an investigator can make is to conclude that an effective treatment is useless. We refer to such a false-negative result (treatment truly effective, $P > .05$, cell c) as a *type II error*. A type II error occurs when we erroneously dismiss an actual treatment effect—and a potentially useful treatment. The likelihood of making a type II error is called the β level. We expand on this logic in the following discussion.

THE RISK OF A FALSE-NEGATIVE RESULT

A clinician might comment on the results of the comparison of treatment with enalapril with that of a combination of hydralazine and nitrates as follows: "Although I accept the 5% threshold and therefore agree that we cannot reject the null hypothesis, I am nevertheless still suspicious that enalapril results in a lower mortality than does the combination of hydralazine

FIGURE 12.1-2

Four Possible Results of a Pregnancy Test

	Pregnancy present	
	Yes	**No**
Test positive	*a* True positive	*b* False positive
Test negative	*c* False negative	*d* True negative

FIGURE 12.1-3

Four Possible Results of a Randomized Trial of an Experimental Intervention

	Treatment effect present	
	Yes	**No**
Study result positive	*a* True positive	*b* False positive type I error
Study result negative	*c* False negative type II error	*d* True negative

and nitrates. The experiment still leaves me in a state of uncertainty." In making these statements, the clinician is recognizing the possibility of a second type of error, the type II error, in hypothesis testing.

In the comparison of enalapril with hydralazine and nitrates in which we have failed to reject the null hypothesis ($P > .05$), the question is whether this is a true-negative result (cell d) or a false-negative result, a type II error (cell c). The investigators found that 5% fewer patients receiving enalapril died than those receiving the alternative vasodilator regimen. If the true difference in mortality really were 5%, we would readily conclude that patients will receive an important benefit if we prescribe enalapril. Despite this, we were unable to reject the null hypothesis. Why is it that the investigators observed an important difference between the mortality rates and yet were unable to conclude that enalapril is superior to hydralazine and nitrates?

Whenever we observe a large difference between treatment and control groups and yet cannot reject the null hypothesis, we should consider the possibility that the problem is failure to enroll enough patients. The likelihood of missing an important difference (and, therefore, of making a type II error) decreases as the sample size and thus the number of events get larger. We may think of our likelihood of avoiding a type II error; we refer to this likelihood as *power*. When a study is at high risk of making a type II error, we say it has inadequate power to detect an important difference. The larger the sample size, the lower the risk of type II error and the greater the power of the study.

Although the 804 patients recruited by the investigators conducting the vasodilator trial may sound like a substantial number, for dichotomous outcomes, such as mortality, even larger sample sizes are often required to detect small treatment effects. For example, researchers conducting the trials that established the optimal treatment of acute myocardial infarction with thrombolytic agents both anticipated and found *absolute differences* between treatment and control mortalities of less than 5%. Because of these small absolute differences between treatment and control, they required—and recruited—thousands of patients to ensure adequate power.

Whenever a trial has failed to reject the null hypothesis (ie, when $P > .05$), a possible interpretation is that the investigators may have missed a true treatment effect. In these negative studies, the larger the difference in effects in favor of the experimental treatment, the more likely it is that the investigators missed a true treatment effect.[3] Another chapter in this book describes how to decide whether a study is large enough to provide a secure basis for clinical decisions (see Chapter 10, Confidence Intervals: Was the Single Study or Meta-analysis Large Enough?).

Thus, it is important to bear in mind that when a trial fails to reject the null hypothesis, this only means that there is no evidence of a difference between the interventions under comparison. This is different from concluding that the effects of the 2 interventions are the same.[4]

NONINFERIORITY AND EQUIVALENCE TRIALS

Some studies are not designed to determine whether a new treatment is better than the current one, but rather whether a treatment that is less expensive, easier to administer, or less toxic is more or less as good, or at most only a little worse, than standard therapy. Such studies are often referred to as *equivalence trials* or *noninferiority trials* (see Chapter 8, How to Use a Noninferiority Trial).[5]

In hypothesis testing, we are aiming to disprove the null hypothesis. In equivalence and noninferiority trials, the null hypotheses are different from those in superiority trials. The null hypothesis of an equivalence trial states that there is a true difference between the 2 treatments, whereas the null hypothesis of a noninferiority trial states that one treatment is better than the other. As a consequence, the interpretation of type I error and type II error change.

Consider a noninferiority study of a new treatment that is in fact not worse than the standard. Consider further that the sample size (and thus the power) of the study is inadequate. If this is the case, the investigator runs the risk of a type II error: not rejecting the null hypothesis and thus failing to show that the new treatment is no worse than the previous standard. In these circumstances, patients who continue to receive standard therapy may miss important benefits of a noninferior and easier to administer, less expensive, or less toxic alternative.

CONTINUOUS MEASURES OF OUTCOME

To this point, our examples have used outcomes such as yes/no, heads or tails, and dying or not dying, all of which we can summarize as a proportion. Often, investigators compare the effects of 2 or more treatments using a variable, such as days in hospital or a score on a quality-of-life questionnaire. We call such variables, in which results can take a large number of values with small differences among those values, *continuous variables*. When we compare differences among groups using continuous outcomes, we typically ask whether we can exclude chance as the explanation of a difference in means.

The study of enalapril vs hydralazine and nitrates in patients with heart failure described previously[2] provides an example of the use of a continuous variable as an outcome in a hypothesis test. The investigators compared the effect of the 2 regimens on exercise capacity. In contrast to the effect on mortality, which favored enalapril, exercise capacity improved with hydralazine and nitrates but not with enalapril. Using a test appropriate for continuous variables (eg, the *t* test), the investigators compared the changes in exercise capacity from baseline to 6 months in the patients receiving hydralazine and nitrates with those changes in the enalapril group during the same period. Exercise capacity in the hydralazine group improved more, and the differences between the 2 groups are unlikely to have occurred by chance ($P = .02$).

MULTIPLE TESTS

Suppose we have assembled a set of all 5 Canadian coins (nickel, dime, quarter, dollar, 2-dollar) and want to test the hypothesis that these 5 coins are unbiased. As in the earlier example, we toss each coin 10 times and count the number of heads for each coin to be 4, 7, 5, 9, and 4. Using the results from 10 consecutive tosses of a single coin, we note that the 9 heads for the dollar coin are extremely unlikely if the coin is unbiased, so we conclude that the dollar coin is biased ($P = .02$, as before). If we had specified that we were going to focus on only the dollar coin and ignored the results for the others, this experiment would have been identical to the single coin-tossing experiment.

However, we tossed 5 coins and if any coin showed 9 or more heads or 9 or more tails, we would have considered this to be equally extreme unlikely. To calculate the *P* value for the observation that a single coin came up heads 9 times requires us to work out how unlikely it is, if all 5 coins are unbiased, to get at least 1 coin with 9 or more heads or 9 or more tails. Intuition tells us that 9 heads are more likely to happen when tossing 5 coins than when tossing only 1. Probability theory can tell us exactly how likely it is.

The chance of getting 9 or more identical results on 1 unbiased coin is 0.021 or 2.1%. This means that the chance of getting fewer than 9 identical results is $1 - 0.021 = 0.979$. The chance that all 5 coins will have fewer than 9 identical results is $0.979 \times 0.979 \times 0.979 \times 0.979 \times 0.979 = 0.90$. So there is a $1 - 0.90 = 0.10$ or 10% chance that at least 1 coin will have 9 or more identical results if all 5 coins are unbiased.

The example above illustrates that an outcome may be extremely unlikely in a single experiment but the same outcome would not be regarded as so unlikely in the context of repeated experiments. Consider a study that examined the effect of a treatment on 6 outcomes. To make the calculations easier, we will assume they are independent, meaning that one outcome on a patient does not depend in any way on the other outcomes.

Suppose we decided to test each outcome at the $\alpha = .05$ level. For any single outcome, if the treatment is completely ineffective, there is indeed only a 5% chance that we will cross the significance threshold and reject the null hypothesis; there is a 95% chance that we will not reject it. What happens when we examine 6 outcomes? The chance of not crossing the threshold for the first 2 outcomes is 0.95 multiplied by 0.95; for all 6 outcomes, the probability that not a single outcome would cross the 5% threshold is 0.95 to the sixth power, or 0.74. The probability that at least 1 outcome has a result that crosses the significance threshold is therefore $1.0 - 0.74 = 26\%$, or approximately 1 in 4, rather than 1 in 20. If we wished to maintain our overall type I error rate of 0.05, we could divide the threshold α by 6, so that each of the 6 tests would use a boundary value of approximately $0.05 / 6 = 0.0083$.[6]

Identifying the correct α level for a test that a hypothesis is testing is made appreciably more complicated if we are simultaneously considering more than 1 hypothesis. For instance, in the coin-tossing example above, we chose to use a single coin having 9 heads as our measure of how extremely unlikely the results were. Faced with the same set of outcomes, someone else might have chosen the coins with 7 and 9 heads and asked how extremely unlikely that was. And someone else might wonder how extreme the entire set of 4, 7, 5, 9, and 4 heads was. We also need to decide on the relevant hypothesis or hypotheses to test. Are we interested in testing hypotheses about the unbiased nature of each coin and calculating a *P* value for each coin? Or are we interested in the single global null hypothesis that all of the coins are unbiased? If that is our null hypothesis and we reject it, we simply conclude that at least 1 coin is biased, without saying which coin it is.

We find an example of the dangers of using multiple outcomes in a randomized trial of the effect of rehabilitation on quality of life after myocardial infarction, in which investigators randomly assigned patients to receive standard care, an exercise program, or a counseling program. They obtained patient reports of 10 outcomes: work, leisure, quality of work and leisure, sexual activity, adherence with advice, cardiac symptoms, psychiatric symptoms, general health, and satisfaction with outcome.[7] For almost all of these variables, there was no difference among the 3 groups. However, after 18 months of follow-up, patients were more satisfied with the exercise regimen than with the other 2 regimens, families in the counseling group were less protective than in the other groups, and patients participating in the counseling group worked more hours and had sexual intercourse more frequently.

Does this mean that both exercise and rehabilitation programs should be implemented because of the small number of outcomes that changed in their favor or that they should be rejected because most of the outcomes showed no difference? The authors themselves concluded that their results did not support the effectiveness of rehabilitation in improving quality of life. However, a program's advocate might argue that if even some of the ratings favored treatment, the intervention is worthwhile. The use of multiple instruments opens the door to such potential controversy.

We should be aware of multiple hypothesis testing that may yield misleading results. A number of statistical strategies exist for dealing with the issue of multiple hypothesis testing on the same data set. We have illustrated a useful strategy for clinicians in a previous example: dividing the *P* value by the number of tests. One also can specify, before the study is undertaken, a single primary outcome on which the major conclusions of the study will hinge. Another approach when conducting a study is to derive a single global test statistic that effectively combines the multiple outcomes into a single measure.

Finally, we might argue that in some situations, we can conduct several hypothesis tests without adjusting for multiple comparisons. When the hypotheses being tested represent distinct scientific questions, each of interest in its own right, it may be that interpretation of each hypothesis should not be influenced by the number of other hypotheses being tested.[6]

A full discussion of strategies for dealing with multiple outcomes is beyond the scope of the *Users' Guides to the Medical Literature*, but the interested reader can find a cogent discussion elsewhere.[8]

LIMITATIONS OF HYPOTHESIS TESTING

At this point, you may be entertaining a number of questions that leave you uneasy. Why use a single cut point for rejecting the null hypothesis when the choice of a cut point is somewhat arbitrary? Why dichotomize the question of whether a treatment is effective into a yes/no issue when it may be viewed more appropriately as a continuum (for instance, from "very unlikely to be effective" to "almost certainly effective")? See Chapter 10, Confidence Intervals: Was the Single Study or Meta-analysis Large Enough?, for an explanation of why we consider an alternative to hypothesis testing a superior approach.

References

1. Montori VM, Kleinbart J, Newman TB, et al. Tips for learners of evidence-based medicine, 2: measures of precision (confidence intervals). *CMAJ.* 2004;171:online-1 to online-12. http://www.cmaj.ca/cgi/data/171/6/611/DC1/1. Accessed February 10, 2014.

2. Cohn JN, Johnson G, Ziesche S, et al. A comparison of enalapril with hydralazine-isosorbide dinitrate in the treatment of chronic congestive heart failure. *N Engl J Med.* 1991;325(5):303-310.

3. Detsky AS, Sackett DL. When was a "negative" clinical trial big enough? how many patients you needed depends on what you found. *Arch Intern Med.* 1985;145(4):709-712.

4. Altman DG, Bland JM. Absence of evidence is not evidence of absence. *BMJ.* 1995;311(7003):485.

5. Kirshner B. Methodological standards for assessing therapeutic equivalence. *J Clin Epidemiol.* 1991;44(8):839-849.

6. Cook R, Dunnett C. Multiple comparisons. In: Armitage P, Colton T, eds. *Encyclopedia of Biostatistics*. New York, NY: Wiley; 1999:2736-2746.

7. Mayou R, MacMahon D, Sleight P, Florencio MJ. Early rehabilitation after myocardial infarction. *Lancet.* 1981;2(8260-61): 1399-1402.

8. Pocock SJ, Geller NL, Tsiatis AA. The analysis of multiple endpoints in clinical trials. *Biometrics.* 1987;43(3):487-498.

12.2

ADVANCED TOPICS IN THE RESULTS OF THERAPY TRIALS

Understanding the Results: More About Odds Ratios

Bram Rochwerg, Mahmoud Elbarbary, Roman Jaeschke, Stephen D. Walter, and Gordon Guyatt

THERAPY

IN THIS CHAPTER

ODDS IN ORDINARY LIFE

You might be most familiar with *odds* in the context of sporting events, when bookmakers or newspaper commentators quote the odds for and against a horse, a boxer, or a tennis player winning a particular event. In the context of games, suppose you have a typical die that has 6 faces. What is the *probability* (likelihood or

TABLE 12.2-1

The 2 × 2 Table

Exposure[a]	Outcome	
	Yes	**No**
Yes	*a*	*b*
No	*c*	*d*

Odds ratio $= \dfrac{a/b}{c/d} = \dfrac{ad}{cb}$

Relative risk (RR) $= \dfrac{a/(a+b)}{c/(c+d)}$

Relative risk reduction $= 1 - \text{RR} = \dfrac{c/(c+d) - a/(a+b)}{c/(c+d)}$

Risk difference (RD) $= \dfrac{c}{c+d} - \dfrac{a}{a+b}$

Number needed to treat $= 100/(\text{RD expressed as a \%})$

[a]The exposure may be a putatively beneficial therapy or a possibly harmful agent.

TABLE 12.2-2

Results From a Randomized Trial of Endoscopic Sclerotherapy Compared With Endoscopic Ligation for Bleeding Esophageal Varices[a]

Exposure	Outcome		Total
	Death	**Survival**	
Ligation	18	46	64
Sclerotherapy	29	36	65

Odds ratio = (18/46)/(29/36) = 0.39/0.80 = 0.49

Relative risk = (18/64)/(29/65) = 0.63

Relative risk reduction = 1 − 0.63 = 0.37

Risk difference = 0.455 − 0.28 = 0.165

Number needed to treat = 100%/16.5% = 7[b]

[a]Data from Stiegmann et al.[1]

[b]Actual number is 6.06, but number needed to treat is provided in nearest whole number.

chance) of rolling a 4 on a single throw? The answer is 1/6. What is the probability of rolling a number other than 4? The answer is 5/6.

Gamblers generally think in terms of odds. Odds refer to the probability of a particular event occurring vs the probability of that particular event not occurring. What are the odds of rolling a 4 on a single throw? The answer is (1/6)/(5/6), or 1:5. What are the odds of rolling a number other than 4? The answer is (5/6)/(1/6), which is 5:1.

THE 2 × 2 TABLE

As clinicians, we are interested less in rolling dice than in treating patients. We are also more accustomed to thinking in terms of probabilities than in terms of odds. Because odds vs probabilities provide certain advantages in statistical analyses, however, we frequently encounter odds in reading medical journal articles. Thus, we may read about the odds of experiencing vs avoiding a given outcome after a certain intervention.

Alternatively, in the context of *case-control studies*, we may be interested in knowing the odds of having a previous *exposure* vs not having that exposure. When we compare odds from 2 groups, we end up with the ratio of 2 odds, not surprisingly called an *odds ratio* (OR). In Chapter 9, Does Treatment Lower Risk? Understanding the Results, in which we discuss ways of presenting the magnitude of a *treatment effect*, such as the *relative risk* (RR), we introduced the concept of the OR. Compared with RR, which focuses on the risk (probability or likelihood) of an event among all exposed (ratio of events/total at risk of event), the OR is based on an estimate of odds of an event (ratio of having event/not having event). To help understand this concept, we present once again the 2 × 2 table (Table 12.2-1) and the results from ligation vs sclerotherapy of bleeding esophageal varices (Table 12.2-2), the example from Chapter 9.[1]

In this and other examples in this chapter, we focus on interventions that (we hope) reduce the probability of an adverse event. Thus, an OR less than 1.0 represents a decrease in the odds of an event happening (typically a benefit of treatment), an OR greater than 1 represents an increase in the odds of an event happening (typically, *harm*), and an OR equal to 1 denotes no effect.

In the example, the odds of dying in the ligation group are 18 (death) vs 46 (survival), or 18 to 46, or 18/46 (*a/b*), and the odds of dying in the sclerotherapy group are 29 to 36 (*c/d*). The formula for the ratio of these odds is (*a/c*)/(*b/d*) (Table 12.2-1); in our example, this yields (18/46)/(29/36), or 0.49. If one were formulating terms parallel to *risk* (in which we call a ratio of risks an RR), one would call the ratio of odds a *relative odds*. Epidemiologists have chosen RR as the preferred term for a ratio of risks and OR for a ratio of odds.

ODDS VS RISKS

Given that you will sometimes read studies in which investigators present RRs and others in which they present ORs, it may be informative to know the relationship between them (Table 12.2-3). Note that although odds are always greater than risks, when the risk is high there is a big difference between odds and risk. When the risk is low, the difference is small. When the risk is very low, the difference becomes vanishingly small. Odds ratios may appear in *randomized clinical trials* (RCTs) of treatment effects or, alternatively, in *observational studies* designed to assess the effect of either beneficial or, more typically, harmful exposures.

ODDS RATIOS IN STUDIES OF TREATMENT EFFECTS

As clinicians, we would like to be able to substitute the RR, which we intuitively understand, for the OR, which can be more difficult to grasp. The substitution will be appropriate when odds and risk are similar, which, it turns out, happens when risk is low (Table 12.2-3). The RR and OR diverge when risk and odds differ, which happens when risk is high (Table 12.2-3).

In most instances in medical investigation, adverse outcomes that we wish to prevent are, mercifully, rare. For instance, most patients who have experienced a myocardial infarction, who have had an exacerbation of chronic obstructive pulmonary disease, or who have undergone noncardiac surgery survive. Because the risk is low, the RR and OR will be very similar, and the substitution, although not exact, will not mislead. In some areas where the risk of bad outcomes is high (critically ill patients or those with metastatic cancer), the substitution may be misleading.

With both low event rates (in which OR is numerically close to RR) and with higher event rates (in which they may be farther apart), the OR will always make a treatment appear more effective than RR (ie, for the same results, the OR will be farther from 1.0 than the RR) (Table 12.2-4).

When event rates are high and treatment effects are large, there are ways of converting the OR to RR.[2,3] Fortunately, clinicians will rarely need them.

TABLE 12.2-3

Risks and Odds[a]

Risk	Odds
0.05	0.05/0.95 = 0.053
0.1	0.1/0.9 = 0.11
0.2	0.2/0.8 = 0.25
0.25	0.25/0.75 = 0.33
0.33	0.33/0.66 = 0.5
0.4	0.4/0.6 = 0.67
0.5	0.5/0.5 = 1.0
0.6	0.6/0.4 = 1.5
0.8	0.8/0.2 = 4.0

[a]Risk is equal to [odds/(1 + odds)]. Odds are equal to [risk/(1 − risk)].

TABLE 12.2-4

Comparison of Relative Risks and Odds Ratios

Risk Control	Risk Exposure	Odds Control	Odds Exposure	RR	OR
Undesirable Event					
4%	3%	0.042	0.031	0.75	0.74
40%	30%	0.67	0.43	0.75	0.65
Desirable Event					
10%	15%	0.11	0.18	1.5	1.59
30%	45%	0.43	0.82	1.5	1.91

Abbreviations: RR, relative risk; OR, odds ratio.

TABLE 12.2-5

Deriving the Number Needed to Treat From the Odds Ratio[a]

CER	Therapeutic Intervention (OR)								
	0.5	0.55	0.6	0.65	0.7	0.75	0.8	0.85	0.9
0.05	41	46	52	59	69	83	104	139	209
0.1	21	24	27	31	36	43	54	73	110
0.2	11	13	14	17	20	24	30	40	61
0.3	8	9	10	12	14	18	22	30	46
0.4	7	8	9	10	12	15	19	26	40
0.5	6	7	8	9	11	14	18	25	38
0.7	6	7	9	10	13	16	20	28	44
0.9	12	15	18	22	27	34	46	64	101

Abbreviations: CER, control event rate; NNT, number needed to treat; OR, odds ratio.

[a]The formula for determining the NNT is:

$$NNT = \frac{1 - CER(1 - OR)}{CER(1 - CER)(1 - OR)}$$

To see why, consider a *meta-analysis* of ligation vs sclerotherapy for esophageal varices[4] that demonstrated a (high) subsequent bleeding rate of 0.47 with sclerotherapy. The OR associated with ligation therapy was impressive: 0.52. The RR associated with ligation therapy was also impressive (0.67) but quite different from the OR. Despite the high event rate and large effect, the practical consequence of the difference is negligible. The 2 are close enough, and—this is the crucial point—choosing the RR or the OR is unlikely to have an important influence on treatment decisions.

Even when risk is high, the divergence between RR and OR will only occur when the treatment effect is substantial. Consider a treatment that is neither beneficial nor harmful. The RR is 1.0 and the OR is 1.0. When the effect is close to 1.0, any divergence between RR and OR will be small. This is why the OR will be misleading if interpreted as a RR only when there is both a high risk and a large effect.

The calculation of *number needed to treat* (NNT) and *number needed to harm* (NNH) provides another problem when investigators report ORs rather than RRs. When event rates are low, it is reasonable to assume that the RR will be very close to the OR. The higher the risk, the less secure this assumption.

For those who may run into the (unlikely) need for more precise information, Tables 12.2-5 and 12.2-6 provide a guide for making an accurate estimate of the NNT and NNH when you estimate the patient's *baseline risk* (*control event rate*) and the investigator has provided only an OR.

ODDS RATIOS IN CASE-CONTROL STUDIES OF PATIENT EXPOSURES

Up to now, our examples have come from RCTs. In these trials, we start with a group of patients who are *randomly allocated* to an intervention and a group of patients who are allocated to a control intervention. The investigators follow up the patients over time and record the frequency of events. The process is similar in observational studies termed *cohort studies*, although in this case the investigators do not control the exposure or treatment. For randomized trials and cohort studies, we can legitimately calculate risks, odds, *risk difference*, RRs, ORs, and even odds reductions.

In case-control studies, investigators select participants not according to whether they have been

TABLE 12.2-6

Deriving the Number Needed to Harm From the Odds Ratio[a]

CER	Therapeutic Intervention (OR)								
	1.1	1.2	1.3	1.4	1.5	2	2.5	3	3.5
0.05	212	106	71	54	43	22	15	12	9
0.1	112	57	38	29	23	12	9	7	6
0.2	64	33	22	17	14	8	5	4	4
0.3	49	25	17	13	11	6	5	4	3
0.4	43	23	16	12	10	6	4	4	3
0.5	42	22	15	12	10	6	5	4	4
0.7	51	27	19	15	13	8	7	6	5
0.9	121	66	47	38	32	21	17	16	14

Abbreviations: CER, control event rate; NNH, number needed to harm; OR, odds ratio.

[a]The formula for determining the NNH is:

$$NNH = \frac{CER\,(OR - 1) + 1}{CER\,(OR - 1)(1 - CER)}$$

exposed to the treatment or *risk factor* but according to whether they have already experienced a *target outcome*. At the start of the study, investigators identify participants who have experienced the outcome and those who have not, rather than identifying those with or without the exposure or intervention and following up those patients forward. Investigators then compare the proportion of case patients (eg, those with stroke, myocardial infarction, or cancer) who have had the exposure of interest (eg, radiation, sunlight, toxic chemical) with the proportion of control patients (eg, those without

stroke, myocardial infarction, or cancer) who have not had the exposure.

Note that the relative number of cases to controls is determined by the study investigators, who may choose to study one or more control patients per case patient. Therefore, case-control studies provide no information on the *prevalence* of disease. An example is the case-control study presented in 12.2-7. In this study, investigators examined the question of whether sunbeds or sunlamps increase the risk of skin melanoma.[5] The number of controls used for the exposure and nonexposure groups is

TABLE 12.2-7

Results of a Case-Control Study That Examined the Association of Cutaneous Melanoma and the Use of Sunbeds and Sunlamps[a]

Exposure to Sunbeds or Sunlamps	No. of Cases	No. of Controls in Scenario 1[b]	No. of Controls in Scenario 2[c]
Yes	67	41	82
No	210	242	484

Abbreviations: OR, odds ratio; RR, relative risk.

[a]Data from Walters et al.[5]

[b]Scenario 1: Apparent RR = (67/108)/(210/452) = 1.35; OR = (67/210)/(41/242) = 1.88.

[c]Scenario 2: Apparent RR = (67/149)/(210/694) = 1.49; OR = (67/210)/(82/484) = 1.88.

relatively arbitrary (scenario 1). In scenario 2, we have doubled the number of controls (and therefore decreased apparent prevalence of disease in this population). As seen, the apparent RR depends on prevalence and varies with the choice of number of controls to cases while the OR stays constant. Thus, the OR but not the RR is the acceptable measure of magnitude of association for case-control studies.[6]

THE MERITS OF THE ODDS RATIO

Historically, the OR, which has a number of other points in its favor (Box 12.2-1), has been the predominant measure of association.[2] With modern computing, the statistical advantages of the OR have become less salient.

CONCLUSION

ORs can express the relation between exposure and outcome. In cohort studies or RCTs, we investigate the ratio of odds of the occurrence of a particular outcome vs nonoccurrence between groups. In situations with low event rates, the OR and RR are numerically similar, but with high event rates, they are not. In case-control studies, we investigate the ratio of odds of prior exposure vs nonexposure between those with and without disease; OR (but not RR) can be used in such studies. In certain statistical models, OR is preferred as a measure of analyzing association. Despite the advantages of OR, the virtual impossibility of intuitive understanding that is relatively easy with RR leads us to prefer the latter statistic.

References

1. Stiegmann GV, Goff JS, Michaletz-Onody PA, et al. Endoscopic sclerotherapy as compared with endoscopic ligation for bleeding esophageal varices. *N Engl J Med*. 1992;326(23):1527-1532.

2. Davies HT, Crombie IK, Tavakoli M. When can odds ratios mislead? *BMJ*. 1998;316(7136):989-991.

3. Zhang J, Yu KF. What's the relative risk? A method of correcting the odds ratio in cohort studies of common outcomes. *JAMA*. 1998;280(19):1690-1691.

4. Laine L, Cook D. Endoscopic ligation compared with sclerotherapy for treatment of esophageal variceal bleeding. A meta-analysis. *Ann Intern Med*. 1995;123(4):280-287.

5. Walter SD, Marrett LD, From L, Hertzman C, Shannon HS, Roy P. The association of cutaneous malignant melanoma with the use of sunbeds and sunlamps. *Am J Epidemiol*. 1990;131(2):232-243.

6. Elbarbary M. Understanding and expressing "Risk." *J Saudi Heart Assoc*. 2010;22(3):159-164.

12.3

ADVANCED TOPICS IN THE RESULTS OF THERAPY TRIALS

What Determines the Width of the Confidence Interval?

Jan Brożek and Maicon Falavigna

IN THIS CHAPTER

SAMPLE SIZE DOES NOT DETERMINE THE WIDTH OF THE CONFIDENCE INTERVAL

Clinicians sometimes equate the size of a study or the number of participants in a study with the width of the *confidence interval* (CI) and thus with its precision. This chapter deals with issues of precision and the resulting CIs associated with *treatment effects* on *dichotomous* (yes/no) *outcomes,* such as death, stroke, or myocardial infarction. As it turns out, for the relative measures of *effect sizes* (eg, *relative risk* [RR] or *relative risk reduction* [RRR]), the number of patients in a study is a secondary determinant of the width of a CI, with the primary determinant being the absolute number of events.

SMALL SAMPLE SIZES CAN GIVE NARROWER CONFIDENCE INTERVALS THAN LARGE SAMPLE SIZES

Consider 2 hypothetical studies. Both show an RRR of 33% of some adverse outcome with an intervention A vs control. Study 1 has enrolled 100 patients in each of the experimental and *control groups*, and study 2 has enrolled 1000 patients in each group. Which of the 2 studies will generate a more precise estimate of treatment effect, represented by a narrower CI? The apparently obvious answer is study 2, with its sample size an order of magnitude larger than that of study 1.

Suppose, however, that study 2—the study with the larger sample size—generated its RRR of 33% on

the basis of 2 outcomes among 1000 people receiving intervention A vs 3 outcomes among 1000 people in the control group. Study 1 produced an RRR of 33% on the basis of 20 outcomes among 100 people receiving intervention A vs 30 outcomes in the control group.

Which RRR of 33% do you trust more? Which one is more precise? Which has the narrower associated CI? As shown in Table 12.3-1, study 1 yields the narrower CI because it is not the number of participants but rather the number of outcome events that matters most.

CONFIDENCE INTERVALS BECOME NARROWER AS THE NUMBER OF EVENTS INCREASES

In the following figures, we explore the association among sample size, number of events, and the precision of the study results by calculating CIs around the RRR from a set of hypothetical studies. The starting point is 100 patients per group, with 8 patients having an event in the treatment group and 12 patients having an event in the control group. The RRR is 33%, with a corresponding 95% CI ranging from 52% to 71%, which tells us that it is likely that, compared with the control therapy, treatment A reduces the risk of an event by no more than 71% and that it increases the risk of an event by no more than 52%—not very useful information.

Figure 12.3-1 shows that as the sample size increases while holding the event rate in both groups constant, the width of the CI decreases, eventually becoming narrow enough to be *statistically significant* and then even narrower, providing a very

TABLE 12.3-1

Sample Size, Event Rate, and the Width of the Confidence Interval

Study No.	No. of Events in Control Group	Total No. in Control Group	No. of Events in Experimental Group	Total No. in Experimental Group	RRR (95% CI)
1	30	100	20	100	33% (−8% to 59%)
2	3	1000	2	1000	33% (−233% to 87%)

Abbreviations: CI, confidence interval; RRR, relative risk reduction.

FIGURE 12.3-1

Sample Size and the Width of the Confidence Interval (Assuming Constant Event Rate)

Control events/total no.		Experimental events/total no.		Sample size multiplied by	RRR (95% CI)	Favors control	Favors treatment
12	100	8	100	1	33% (−52% to 71%)		
24	200	16	200	2	33% (−20% to 63%)		
36	300	24	300	3	33% (−8% to 59%)		
48	400	32	400	4	33% (−2% to 56%)		
60	500	40	500	5	33% (2% to 54%)		
120	1000	80	1000	10	33% (13% to 49%)		
240	2000	160	2000	20	33% (19% to 45%)		

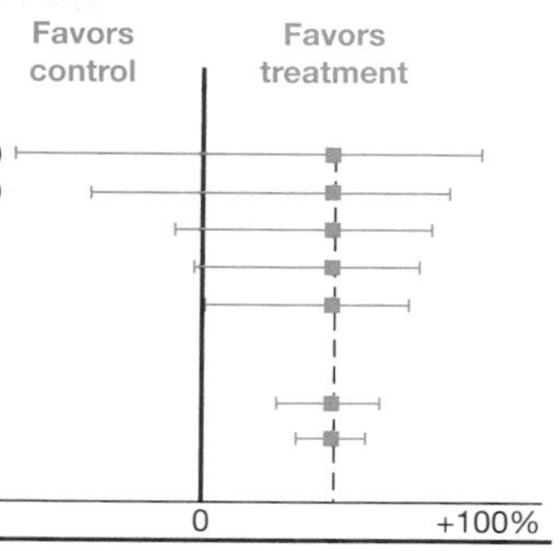

−100%　　　0　　　+100%

Abbreviation: RRR, relative risk reduction.

FIGURE 12.3-2

Event Rate and the Width of the Confidence Interval (With a Constant Sample Size)

Control events/total no.		Experimental events/total no.		Event rate multiplied by	RRR (95% CI)	Favors control	Favors treatment
12	100	8	100	1	33% (−52% to 71%)		
24	100	16	100	2	33% (−16% to 62%)		
36	100	24	100	3	33% (−2% to 57%)		
48	100	32	100	4	33% (6% to 53%)		

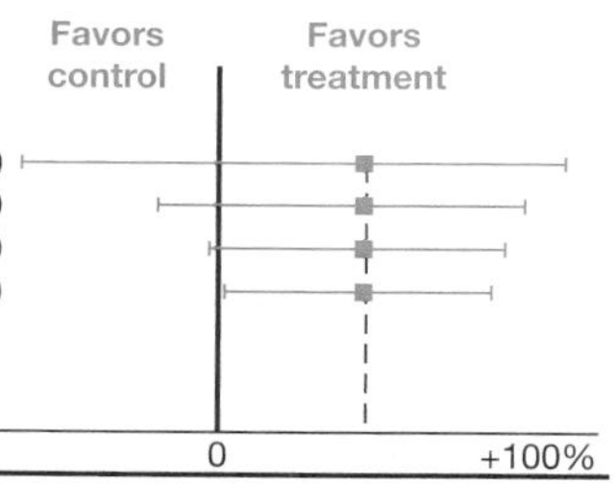

−100%　　　0　　　+100%

Abbreviation: RRR, relative risk reduction.

precise estimate of the effect. Figure 12.3-2 shows what would happen if we hold the sample size constant and increase the event rate. Investigators may achieve the former by enrolling more patients and the latter by a number of approaches, including extending the study duration, enrolling patients at higher risk of the outcome, using *composite outcomes*, or using *surrogate outcomes* with higher event rates. Use of composite and surrogate outcomes is, however, problematic: composite outcomes are often challenging to interpret and make treatment effects seem more important than they really are; surrogate end points are of uncertain value to patients (see Chapter 12.4, Composite End Points, and Chapter 13.4, Surrogate Outcomes).[1]

Closer inspection of these figures allows 2 additional observations. First, the width of the CI does not narrow linearly with the increase in sample size or event rate. In fact, it narrows proportionally to

their square root. So, for instance, increasing the sample size from 100 to 200 has more of an effect than increasing it from 200 to 300, and increasing the sample size from 200 to 300 has more effect than increasing it from 300 to 400.

Second, doubling the number of events by increasing the event rate (eg, enrolling participants who are more sick and whose risk of developing an outcome is therefore higher) while holding sample size constant decreases the width of the CI more than doubling the number of events by increasing the number of participants.

For example, a report from the Women's Health Study,[1] a *randomized clinical trial* in primary prevention of cardiovascular disease, which enrolled almost 20 000 women per group, found a barely significant benefit in stroke reduction with low-dose aspirin compared with *placebo* after 10 years of observation (RRR, 17%; 95% CI, 1%-31%). Despite the very large sample size, the estimate of the effect was imprecise—a wide CI allowing for an RRR of as much as 31% or as little as 1% relative reduction of strokes. This lack of precision was due to the low stroke event rate: 1.3% (266 of 19 942) in the placebo group vs 1.1% (221 of 19 934) in the aspirin group.

In contrast, the Scandinavian Simvastatin Survival Study (4S),[2] a smaller trial that evaluated simvastatin in secondary prevention of cardiovascular disease, which enrolled approximately 2200 per group (almost 10 times fewer than in the Women's Health Study), found an RRR of major coronary events of 34% (95% CI, 50%-25%) during a median follow-up period of 5.4 years. The width of the CI is slightly narrower than in the previous example because, despite a much smaller sample size, the risk of events in this population was high: 28% in the placebo group vs 19% in the simvastatin group.

WHAT HAPPENS IF WE THINK OF ABSOLUTE INSTEAD OF RELATIVE EFFECTS?

Think back to the example with which this chapter began: a study in which 2 in 1000 treated patients died, as did 3 in 1000 control patients. We decided that such a study, despite a large sample size, leaves us very uncertain about the apparent 33% RRR—indeed, the CI includes a more than 2-fold increase in RR and an 87% RRR.

But what if we asked a different question? What can we say about the absolute effect of the intervention? Not only does it appear small—only 1 in 1000—but the large denominator leaves us quite confident that the absolute risk reduction is small. Indeed, the upper boundary of the CI is a difference of 5.4/1000. So, the largest reduction in death compatible with the evidence is a reduction in deaths of fewer than 6 per 1000. Thus, although the RRR may still be large—87%—the data assure us that any absolute effect of the intervention is small.

BEWARE OF RANDOMIZED CLINICAL TRIALS WITH TOO FEW EVENTS

Studies with few events may produce CIs that indicate statistically significant results, if the event rate and the absolute difference are large. However, a small number of events may render the results fragile (ie, resulting in the loss of statistical significance with only a few additional events in the experimental or control group), decreasing our confidence in the results. Over and over again in this book, we caution you against trials with too few events and suggest you demand large numbers of events before you make strong inferences about treatment effects in the management of your patients[3] (see Chapter 11.3, Randomized Trials Stopped Early for Benefit, and Chapter 13.3, Misleading Presentations of Clinical Trial Results).

References

1. Ridker PM, Cook NR, Lee IM, et al. A randomized trial of low-dose aspirin in the primary prevention of cardiovascular disease in women. *N Engl J Med*. 2005;352(13):1293-1304.
2. Scandinavian Simvastatin Survival Study Group. Randomised trial of cholesterol lowering in 4444 patients with coronary heart disease: the Scandinavian Simvastatin Survival Study (4S). *Lancet*. 1994;344(8934):1383-1389.
3. Guyatt GH, Oxman AD, Kunz R, et al. GRADE guidelines 6. Rating the quality of evidence—imprecision. *J Clin Epidemiol*. 2011;64(12):1283-1293.

12.4

ADVANCED TOPICS IN THE RESULTS OF THERAPY TRIALS

Composite End Points

Ignacio Ferreira-González, Victor M. Montori, Jason W. Busse, Holger J. Schünemann, Roman Jaeschke, PJ Deveraux, Gaietà Permanyer-Miralda, and Gordon Guyatt

THERAPY

IN THIS CHAPTER

CLINICAL SCENARIO

You are an internist seeing a 65-year-old man with stress test–documented angina who—despite taking carefully titrated β-blockers, nitrates, aspirin, an angiotensin-converting enzyme (ACE) inhibitor, and a statin—is substantially restricted in his activities. The patient undergoes coronary angiography, which reveals 3-vessel severe coronary disease. You suggest to him the possibility of surgical revascularization with coronary artery bypass grafting (CABG). The patient expresses reluctance to undergo such an invasive procedure, and he asks if there is a less aggressive approach that might be almost as effective. You consider the possibility of a percutaneous coronary intervention (PCI) as an alternative.

FINDING THE EVIDENCE

You wonder what recent *evidence* might bear on the patient's dilemma. You ask the patient to join you in front of your computer, and you go to the online version of *ACP Journal Club*, which you can access through your library subscription (http://acpjc.acponline.org/gsa-search). To guide your search, you jot down your question in *PICO* format: In patients with 3-vessel coronary artery disease, what is the impact of PCI vs CABG on angina, major cardiovascular event, and overall mortality? (See Chapter 4, What Is the Question?) Because *ACP Journal Club* selects only a small subset of clinically relevant studies, you decide to start with a broad search (see Chapter 5, Finding Current Best Evidence). You therefore enter search terms describing only the patient population: those with multivessel coronary artery disease. The search yields 16 citations, the second of which is a *randomized clinical trial* (RCT) of PCI vs CABG called Synergy between PCI with Taxus and Cardiac Surgery (SYNTAX).[1] You tell the patient you will review this study carefully and discuss the results with him in a week.

In the SYNTAX study, you find that 1800 patients with 3-vessel or left main coronary artery disease were *randomized* to undergo CABG or PCI. The study found a significantly lower rate of the *composite end point*—death from any cause, stroke, myocardial infarction (MI), or subsequent revascularization—in the CABG arm (12.4%) than in the PCI group (17.8%) (*relative risk* [RR], 0.69; 95% *confidence interval* [CI], 0.55-0.87; $P = .002$). The authors concluded that CABG should remain the standard care for patients with severe coronary artery disease.

How should you interpret these results to best inform your patient's decision? Should you assume that the effect of treatment on the composite end point accurately captures the effect on its components (death, stroke, MI, and subsequent revascularization)? Or, rather, should you look more carefully at each component and draw the individual effects to your patient's attention?

In this chapter, we offer clinicians a strategy to interpret the results of clinical trials when investigators measure the effect of treatment on a composite of end points of varying importance, as was the case in the SYNTAX trial[1] in the clinical scenario.

COMPOSITE END POINTS

In the last 2 decades, as medical care has improved, the frequency with which patients with common conditions such as MI experience subsequent adverse events, including death, recurrent MI, or stroke, has decreased. Although welcome news for patients, the resultant low event rates provide challenges for clinical investigators who consequently require very large sample sizes and longer *follow-up* to test the incremental benefits of new therapies.

Clinical trialists have increasingly responded to these challenges by using composite end points that capture the number of patients experiencing any one of several adverse events—eg, death, MI, or hospitalization—as a primary study end point.[2] By increasing the number of events, such composite end points decrease the necessary sample size and also may reduce duration of follow-up. A paucity of events associated with any individual component and an understanding of the biology suggesting that treatment will act in more or less the same way across components provide the standard rationale for composite end points in contemporary clinical trials.[2]

Another benefit to justify the use of composite end points is to avoid competing *risks* in outcome assessment.[3] For example, one way to *prevent* stroke is to implement a treatment that increases mortality among patients who would otherwise have had a stroke. In this setting, a composite outcome of nonfatal stroke and mortality may avoid the potentially misleading result of a primary outcome focused on the individual outcome of stroke.

Finally, trialists may use composite end points to avoid the complexity of interpretation by providing a summary measure of potential risks and benefits associated with an intervention. For example, RCTs that evaluated the effects of warfarin vs acetylsalicylic acid among patients with atrial fibrillation all assessed the effect on the composite of ischemic stroke and hemorrhagic stroke.[4] These trials found a significant reduction in ischemic stroke with warfarin therapy (*hazard ratio* [HR], 0.48; 95% CI, 0.37-0.63); however, there was a nonsignificant trend toward excess hemorrhagic stroke with warfarin therapy (HR, 1.84; 95% CI, 0.87-3.87). This finding could leave the clinician and patient puzzled about the optimal course of action. To the extent that physicians and patients place similar weight on the importance of avoiding hemorrhagic and ischemic strokes, consideration of the effect on all strokes, ischemic or hemorrhagic (HR, 0.55; 95% CI, 0.43-0.71), may help resolve the issue.

The situations in which a composite end point is necessary to deal with competing risks are few and far between. The simplification of the previous paragraph is attractive but requires outcomes of virtually identical importance, also a rare situation. By far the most common use of composites is to decrease sample size. Indeed, approximately 50% of trials in the cardiovascular area now use composite end points.[5]

Unfortunately, as we shall see, choosing a composite end point to decrease sample size creates a challenge for anyone trying to interpret the results.

INTERPRETATION OF COMPOSITE END POINTS: WHAT ARE THE CLINICIAN'S OPTIONS?

Potentially, clinicians can assume that the relative effect of an intervention on the composite end point applies to each component of the composite end point. Applying this reasoning to the SYNTAX trial,[1] we would assume that the *relative risk reduction* (RRR) of 0.69 represents the effect of CABG on the outcomes of death, stroke, MI, and revascularization. Applying these RRRs to the event rate in the PCI arm, this would mean, in 1000 patients, approximately 12 fewer deaths, 2 fewer strokes, 13 fewer MIs, and 37 fewer revascularizations. As you will see subsequently when we take a more careful look at the results, such an assumption would be difficult to justify.

Alternatively, clinicians might consider the *treatment effect* on the combination of death, stroke, MI, and subsequent revascularization as just that, a combination, without making any inferences about the effect of treatment on each of the component end points. Adopting this interpretation, the clinician would answer the patient's question about the benefits of the CABG strategy by stating, "It will decrease your risk of serious cardiac events by about 31% in relative terms and by about 5.4% in absolute terms. In other words, in 1000 patients like you, there would be 54 who would have a serious cardiac event with PCI who would not have such an event with CABG."

For the clinicians and patients who want specific information about the magnitude of the RRR and *absolute risk reduction* (ARR) or *risk difference* (RD) among end points of differing importance, this interpretation is of limited utility. For instance, the patient in the scenario might ask, "Doctor, what serious cardiac events are you talking about?" and subsequently, "Given that I am much more interested in avoiding death and stroke than MI and serious MI than a subsequent revascularization with PCI, can

THERAPY

you please tell me the difference between CABG and PCI in terms of risk of death, stroke, and MI, and on subsequent revascularization?"

Adhering to an interpretation that the data allow no statements about treatment impact on components of the composite end point, the clinician can provide no assurance that the 31% decrease in RR applies to the most serious components: death and stroke. So, the clinician taking this approach would say to the patient, "I'm sorry, I cannot tell you about the individual components, just the overall effect."

A third approach focuses on the component end points of the SYNTAX trial (Table 12.4-1 and Figure 12.4-1).[1] Here we see a very different picture than in each of the first 2 approaches. Fewer patients (0.9% less) in the CABG arm died, but the results are compatible with chance (ie, CIs cross 1.0 and results do not exclude an increase in deaths of 1.0% with CABG) (see Chapter 10, Confidence Intervals: Was the Single Study or Meta-analysis Large Enough?). Similarly, with MI, 1.5% fewer patients had MI, but the results are compatible with an increase of approximately 3/1000 in MI with CABG. The revascularization result is much more definitive: 7.6% fewer patients needed to undergo subsequent revascularization, and at least 4.8% fewer needed to undergo subsequent revascularization (definitive

because the boundary of the CI, 4.8%, is a magnitude large enough that most patients would consider it an important reduction). Unfortunately, however, 1.6% more patients in the CABG group had a stroke, and the CI suggests the increase is at least 6/1000. This result—appreciable variability in absolute reductions in component end points, with the largest difference favoring the experimental treatment in the least important end point—is common in trials including composite end points.[5]

Both investigators and pharmaceutical companies would often prefer that clinicians focus on composite end points rather than the component end points. After all, a statement that CABG, relative to PCI, reduces the risk of a composite end point of death, stroke, MI, and subsequent revascularization is compelling because it gives us a sense of an important positive effect of the interventions on all 4 end points. On the other hand, stating that we can be confident that CABG decreases the risk of subsequent revascularizations but increases the risk of stroke and that its effects on death and MI are uncertain is a very different message.

Box 12.4-1 presents a set of questions to guide clinicians pondering whether to base a clinical decision on the effect of treatment on a composite end point or on the component end points. We will now describe how to apply these criteria.

TABLE 12.4-1

Results From the SYNTAX Trial[1]

End Points	PCI, No. (%) of Patients (n = 891)	CABG, No. (%) of Patients (n = 849)	Risk Difference, % (95% CI)	Relative Risk[a] (95% CI)
Patients with a composite end point[b]	159 (17.8)	105 (12.4)	5.4 (2.13-8.83)	0.69 (0.55-0.87)
Deaths	39 (4.4)	30 (3.5)	0.9 (−0.98 to 2.6)	0.8 (0.5-1.3)
Stroke	5 (0.6)	19 (2.2)	−1.6 (−2.8 to −0.57)	4 (1.5-10.6)
Myocardial infarctions	43 (4.8)	28 (3.3)	1.5 (−0.32 to 3.38)	0.68 (0.43-1.09)
Subsequent revascularization	120 (13.5)	50 (5.9)	7.6 (4.83-10.32)	0.44 (0.32-0.6)

Abbreviations: CABG, coronary artery bypass grafting; CI, confidence interval; PCI, percutaneous coronary intervention; SYNTAX, Synergy between PCI with Taxus and Cardiac Surgery.

[a]In this table, CABG is the reference category. In the original publication,[1] the reference category was PCI.

[b]The composite end point includes mortality, myocardial infarction, stroke, and subsequent revascularization.

FIGURE 12.4-1

Risk Difference in the SYNTAX Trial[1]

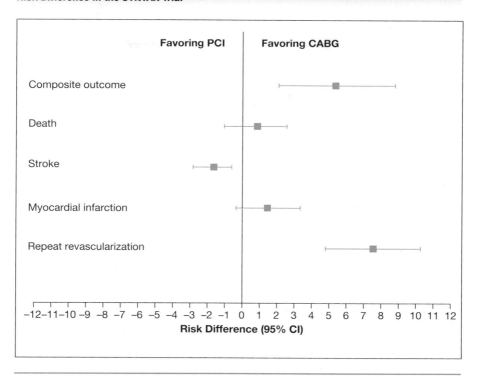

Abbreviations: CABG, coronary artery bypass grafting; CI, confidence interval; PCI, percutaneous coronary intervention; SYNTAX, Synergy between PCI with Taxus and Cardiac Surgery.

BOX 12.4-1

Users' Guides to Interpreting Composite End Points

Are the component end points of the composite end point of similar importance to patients?

Did the more and less important end points occur with similar frequency?

Can one be confident that the component end points share similar relative risk reductions?

Is the underlying biology of the component end points similar enough that one would expect similar relative risk reductions?

Are the point estimates of the relative risk reductions similar, and are the confidence intervals sufficiently narrow?

To the extent that one can answer yes to these questions, one can feel confident using the treatment effect on the combined end point as the basis for decision making.

To the extent that one answers no to these questions, one should look separately at the treatment effect on the component end points as the basis for decision making.

ARE THE COMPONENT END POINTS OF SIMILAR IMPORTANCE TO PATIENTS?

If all components of a composite end point are of equal importance to patients, the composite will accurately portray the net effect of treatment. If patients consider death, stroke, MI, and revascularization of equal importance, it does not much matter how a 5% ARR in the composite end point is distributed across a composite end point that includes these 4 components. Assuming similar effects across components will not adversely affect decision making, even if treatment effects actually differ substantially.

Patients almost invariably, however, assign varying degrees of importance to different *health outcomes*. As a result, ignoring a possible difference between effects of a treatment on different component end points on the assumption that they share identical patient importance will seldom be justified. The magnitude of the gradient in importance among end points therefore becomes the issue.

Consider an RCT of warfarin for the treatment of idiopathic pulmonary fibrosis.[6] The investigators chose a composite end point of death from any cause, hospitalization, and a 10% or greater absolute decline in functional vital capacity. Patients are likely to consider the decline in functional vital capacity without other adverse consequences of trivial importance in comparison with the need for hospitalization and the outcome of death. The large gradient in importance increases our skepticism about usefulness of the combined end point.

On the other hand, consider a trial that compares a new oral antithrombotic agent with the traditional vitamin K antagonist in patients with nonvalvular atrial fibrillation in which the primary composite end point comprised stroke and systemic embolism.[7-9] Most patients would consider stroke as more serious, but the gradient in importance is much smaller. This smaller gradient increases the credibility of the composite end point.

DID THE COMPONENT END POINTS OCCUR WITH SIMILAR FREQUENCY?

If the more patient-important component end points occur with far less frequency than the less patient-important component end points, the composite end point becomes uninformative, if not frankly misleading. Clinicians must look carefully at the specific results of each component to interpret the results of a study that presents a composite end point.

Consider the following statement: in patients with in-stent stenosis of CABGs, γ-radiation reduced the composite end point of death from cardiac causes, Q-wave MI, and revascularization of the target vessel. This result seems impressive because it suggests that γ-radiation reduces the incidence of death and MI, as well as the need for revascularization. The trial from which we draw this result randomized 120 patients with in-stent stenosis of a saphenous vein graft to γ-radiation (iridium 192) or *placebo*.[10] Of those in the iridium 192 arm, 32% experienced the primary composite end point of death from cardiac causes, Q-wave MIs, or revascularization of the target vessel at 12 months, as did 63% in the placebo arm (RRR, 50%; 95% CI, 25%-68%).

Although this result appears compelling, only 2 patients in the placebo arm (3.3%) and 1 patient in the iridium 192 arm (1.7%) sustained an MI (RD, 1.7%; 95% CI, −5.9% to 9.9%). The results are similar for cardiac death, which occurred in 4 patients (7%) in each arm (RD, 0%; 95% CI, −10.3% to 10.3%). Revascularizations constituted most of the events: 32 of 38 patients who experienced events in the placebo arm experienced only revascularization; the same was true of 14 of 19 who experienced events in the radiated group. Because of the very large discrepancy in the frequency of the more important and less important end points in this trial, the most reasonable conclusion is that the intervention reduced the RR of revascularization of the target vessel by 54% (95% CI, 29%-71%), an RD of 33% (95% CI, 16%-49%). However, the trial provides essentially no information about the effect of the intervention on MI or death.

Contrast this result with that of the Heart Outcomes Prevention Evaluation (HOPE) trial[11] that randomized 9297 patients at high risk of cardiac events to ramipril or placebo. Ramipril reduced cardiovascular deaths from 8.1% to 6.1% (RRR, 26%; 95% CI, 13%-36%), MI from 12.3% to 9.9% (RRR, 20%; CI, 10%-30%), and stroke from 4.9% to 3.4% (RRR, 32%; 95% CI, 16%-44%). Here, the difference in rates of death, MI, and stroke in the *control group* (8.1%, 12.3%, and 4.9%, respectively) is relatively small. The difference in events between treatment and control groups (2.0% for deaths, 2.4% for MI, and 1.5% for stroke) is even more similar. This similar frequency of occurrence of the more important and less important end points provides support for relying on the composite end point in clinical decision making.

CAN ONE BE CONFIDENT THAT THE COMPONENT END POINTS SHARE SIMILAR RELATIVE RISK REDUCTIONS?

Is the Underlying Biology of the Component End Points Similar Enough That One Would Expect Similar Relative Risk Reductions?

Comfort with using a composite end point of a study as the basis of clinical decision making rests in part on confidence that similar RRRs apply to the more important and less important components. Investigators should therefore construct composite end points in which the biology would lead us to expect similar effects across components.

For example, the Irbesartan Diabetic Nephropathy Trial[12] randomized 1715 patients with hypertension and nephropathy and type 2 diabetes to irbesartan, amlodipine, or placebo. The primary end point was the composite of a doubling of the baseline serum creatinine concentration, the onset of end-stage renal disease (serum creatinine >6.0 mg/dL, initiation of dialysis, or transplantation), or death from any cause. It is extremely plausible that, for 2 of these 3 components—doubling of creatinine and crossing the creatinine threshold of 6.0 mg/dL—the treatment effects would be similar. Indeed, one would be very surprised if results indicated otherwise. On the other hand, there are many contributors to all-cause mortality aside from renal failure (including, for instance, cardiac disease), and it might well be that treatments have different effects on these contributors. Thus, the biologic rationale that the treatments would have similar effects on all 3 components is weak. The relatively weak biologic rationale increases our reluctance to base treatment decisions on the composite end points, as opposed to its components. Indeed, in this instance, irbesartan lowered the incidence of both doubling of creatinine and end-stage renal disease but without apparent effect on all-cause mortality (Figure 12.4-2).

In contrast, the authors of the Clopidogrel versus Aspirin in Patients at Risk of Ischemic Events (CAPRIE) study, an RCT of aspirin vs clopidogrel in patients with a variety of manifestations of atherosclerosis, argued explicitly for the biologic rationale of their composite end point.[13] Citing results of prior trials of antiplatelet agents vs placebo, they note the similar biologic determinants of ischemic stroke, MI, and vascular death: "A meta-analysis of 142 trials … shows clearly that antiplatelet drugs reduce the incidence of a CEP [composite end point] of ischemic stroke, myocardial infarction, and vascular death, the odds reduction being 27%, which is consistent over a wide range of clinical manifestations."[13] Their argument strengthens the case for assuming, until evidence suggests otherwise, that RRRs are consistent across components of the trials' composite end point.

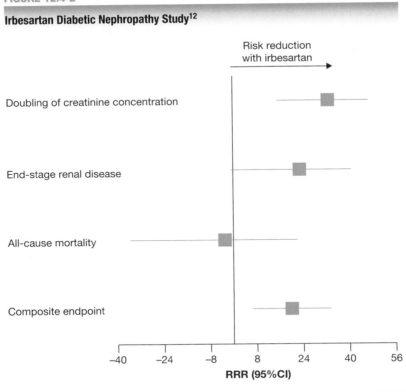

FIGURE 12.4-2

Irbesartan Diabetic Nephropathy Study[12]

Abbreviation: CI, confidence interval; RRR, relative risk reduction.

Are the Point Estimates of the Relative Risk Reductions Similar and Confidence Intervals Sufficiently Narrow?

No matter how compelling the investigators' biologic rationale, only similar RRRs can strongly increase our comfort with a composite end point.

For example, in the Trial to Assess Improvement in Therapeutic Outcomes by Optimizing Platelet Inhibition with Prasugrel–Thrombolysis in Myocardial Infarction (TRITON-TIMI) 38 trial,[14] investigators randomized 13 608 patients with moderately high-risk acute coronary syndrome and scheduled PCI to receive either prasugrel or clopidogrel for 6 to 15 months and recorded the effect of these medications on a primary composite end point of cardiovascular mortality, MI, and stroke. A reasonable biologic rationale suggests that if there is a difference between these 2 antiplatelet agents, the difference should be similar across the 3 outcomes. Figure 12.4-3, however, shows that this is not to the case. The RRR for the composite end point of 19% (95% CI, 10%-27%) does not apply to the individual components: RRRs of −2% for stroke, 24% for MI, and 11% for cardiovascular death. This variability suggests that clinicians should focus on individual

FIGURE 12.4-3

TRITON-TIMI 38 Trial[14]

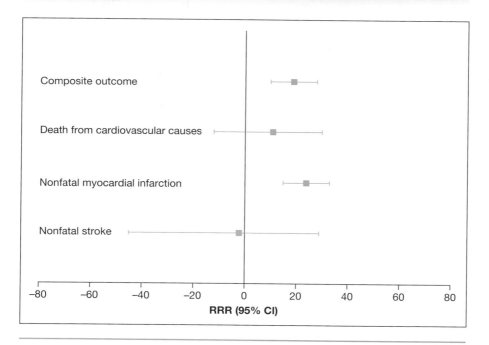

Abbreviations: CI, confidence interval; RRR, relative risk reduction; TRITON-TIMI, Trial to Assess Improvement in Therapeutic Outcomes by Optimizing Platelet Inhibition with Prasugrel–Thrombolysis in Myocardial Infarction.

end points. The TRITON-TIMI 38 trial suggests that a prasugrel-based regimen, compared with a regimen based on clopidogrel, may reduce the risk for MI but has uncertain effects on cardiovascular mortality and stroke in patients with acute coronary syndrome and scheduled PCI.[14]

The UK Prospective Diabetes Study (UKPDS) trial of intensive glycemic control vs conventional control in patients with type 2 diabetes provides another example.[15] This study reported that the primary end point of the trial was time to first diabetes-related end point (sudden death, death from hyperglycemia or hypoglycemia, fatal or nonfatal MI, angina, heart failure, stroke, renal failure,

amputation, vitreous hemorrhage, retinal photocoagulation, blindness in one eye, or cataract extraction); diabetes-related death (death from MI, stroke, peripheral vascular disease, renal disease, hyperglycemia or hypoglycemia, and sudden death); or all-cause mortality. Although the investigators reported a significant 12% reduction in the RR in the composite end point (95% CI, 1%-21%), the results do not exclude a harmful effect on diabetes-related deaths (RR, 0.90; 95% CI, 0.73-1.11) and all-cause mortality (RR, 0.94; 95% CI, 0.80-1.10).[15] Moreover, most of the apparent effect was a reduction (2.7% of the 3.2%, or 80% of the absolute reduction in risk of microvascular complications) in retinal photocoagulation.[15,16]

Reviewers typically summarize the results as showing a reduction in any of 21 diabetes-related end points with intensive glycemic control, and only 1 in 35 reviews of the UKPDS results highlighted the dominance on the overall effect of the reduction in the risk of photocoagulation.[17]

These results contrast with those of the HOPE trial of ramipril vs placebo in patients at high risk of vascular events that we described earlier.[11] Here, the RRRs in the same 3 end points were 26% (95% CI, 13%-36%) for cardiovascular death, 20% (95% CI, 10%-30%) for MI, and 32% (95% CI, 16%-44%) for stroke. For each of the 3 components of the composite end point, the clinician can be confident that treatment affects the component favorably.

Finally, consider the results of the Clopidogrel in Unstable Angina to Prevent Recurrent Events (CURE) trial, in which investigators randomized 12 562 patients with acute coronary syndrome to clopidogrel or placebo and examined the effect on the same composite end point as reported in the trial reviewed in our opening clinical scenario: cardiovascular death, MI, or stroke.[18] In this trial, there was a reduction in the RR of the composite outcome of 20%, with a reduction in the RR of MI, cardiovascular death, and stroke of 23%, 7%, and 14%, respectively. Here, although one could interpret the *point estimates* of the RRR as consistent with one another and with the composite, the range of the CIs should give us pause. Although the point estimate and 95% CI on the RRR leave us reasonably confident of an important treatment effect on MI (23%; 95% CI, 11%-33%), the same is not true of either cardiovascular death (7%; 95% CI, −8% to 21%), or stroke (14%; 95% CI, −18% to 37%). As a result, the statement that clopidogrel reduced a composite end point of cardiovascular death, stroke, and MI by 20% is potentially misleading, and use of the composite end point as a basis for clinical decision making is problematic.

Many of the examples we have presented highlight the typical situation. The number of events and magnitude of effect are typically greater (and often considerably greater) for the less important end points than for the more important. We have found that this is the case in randomized trials in cardiovascular interventions, in which components of greater importance to patients were associated with smaller treatment effects than less important ones (RRR of 8% for death and 33% for components of minor importance to patients).[5] In individual trials, wide CIs may leave us uncertain of the relative effect of the intervention on more and less important end points. Sometimes, however, when data accumulate from many trials, it becomes clear that skepticism about treatment effect on the most important outcomes, even in the presence of convincing evidence of impact on outcomes of lesser seriousness, was well warranted.

For example, consider that trials that compare drug-eluting stents with bare-metal stents indicate conclusively that the drug-eluting stent reduces the composite end point MACE (major adverse cardiac events—a composite of death, MI, and target lesion revascularization) compared with the bare-metal stent. The first RCT of drug-eluting stents found a nonconclusive effect at 1 year on the most important end points of death (RRR, 2%; 95% CI, −680% to 76%) and MI (RRR, 51%; 95% CI, −530% to 96%), whereas the drug-eluting stent had a large effect on reducing revascularization (RRR, 97%; 95% CI, 75%-99%).[19] These early results suggest a substantial difference in effects on the more important and less important end points, but the wide CIs around the former leave the issue in doubt. Subsequent systematic reviews have found that drug-eluting stents have no benefit in survival or Q-wave MI (in fact, there is an unfavorable trend for Q-wave MI), whereas there is a large benefit in reducing the need for revascularization.[20]

CLINICAL SCENARIO RESOLUTION

Let us return to the scenario with which our discussion began, that of the patient reluctant to undergo cardiac surgery to improve his prognosis and to control his angina. Is it reasonable to use the composite end point from the SYNTAX trial[1]—death, MI, stroke, and subsequent revascularization—to guide the decision, or should we focus on individual results of the 3 components?

To address this issue, we can ask the 3 questions in our *Users' Guides* (Box 12.4-1). Most patients will find death, stroke, and large MI with subsequent disability far more important than the need of a new revascularization. Subsequent revascularization occurred far more frequently than the 3 more important events (Table 12.4-1). Biologic rationale may support a presumption that the surgery strategy will

have similar effects on cardiac end points; however, one could also argue the opposite and make the case for a positive effect on MI and the need for new coronary revascularization but not on stroke. The relative effects on the 3 outcomes proved very different (Table 12.4-1). In the SYNTAX trial, the composite end point fails all 3 criteria, and the trial therefore requires focus on the component end points. In this case, the patient proved extremely stroke averse. "Doctor," he says, "that PCI is pretty simple, so the possibility that I might need a repeat is not a big deal to me. You tell me that although the CABG might reduce my risk of dying or having an MI, you are not sure. But it is very likely the CABG will increase my risk of stroke. To me, a stroke would be awful. I'll go with the PCI."

CONCLUSIONS

The widespread use of composite end points in RCTs reflects their utility as a solution to the problems of declining event rates, to better assess the effect in presence of competing risk, and to capture the net benefit of an intervention. Unfortunately, use of composite end points as major end points often makes the interpretation of the results of RCTs challenging.

At one extreme you may find trials in which (1) the component end points are of similar but not identical importance, (2) the end points that are more important occur with similar frequency to those that are less important, and (3) strong biologic rationale supports results that, across component end points, have similar RRRs with CIs excluding minimal effects. Under such circumstances clinicians can,

with confidence, use the composite end point as the primary basis for decision making.

At the other extreme, you may find trials in which (1) the component end points have very different levels of importance to patients, (2) the more important end points occur far less often than the less important end points, and (3) biologic rationale is weak, RRRs differ widely, and CIs for the more important end points include the possibility of harm. Under these circumstances, the point estimates and CIs for individual component end points should provide the basis for clinical decisions. Although situations between these extremes may leave reasonable people disagreeing about the most appropriate interpretation of the results, these *Users' Guides* will help clinicians appropriately interpret and apply the results of studies that present composite end points in clinical decisions.

References

1. Serruys PW, Morice MC, Kappetein AP, et al; SYNTAX Investigators. Percutaneous coronary intervention versus coronary-artery bypass grafting for severe coronary artery disease. *N Engl J Med*. 2009;360(10):961-972.
2. Freemantle N, Calvert M, Wood J, Eastaugh J, Griffin C. Composite outcomes in randomized trials: greater precision but with greater uncertainty? *JAMA*. 2003;289(19):2554-2559.
3. Ferreira-González I, Alonso-Coello P, Solà I, et al. Composite endpoints in clinical trials [in Spanish]. *Rev Esp Cardiol*. 2008;61(3):283-290.
4. van Walraven C, Hart RG, Singer DE, et al. Oral anticoagulants vs aspirin in nonvalvular atrial fibrillation: an individual patient meta-analysis. *JAMA*. 2002;288(19):2441-2448.

5. Ferreira-González I, Busse JW, Heels-Ansdell D, et al. Problems with use of composite end points in cardiovascular trials: systematic review of randomised controlled trials. *BMJ*. 2007;334(7597):786.

6. Noth I, Anstrom KJ, Calvert SB, et al; Idiopathic Pulmonary Fibrosis Clinical Research Network (IPFnet). A placebo-controlled randomized trial of warfarin in idiopathic pulmonary fibrosis. *Am J Respir Crit Care Med*. 2012;186(1):88-95.

7. Patel MR, Mahaffey KW, Garg J, et al; ROCKET AF Investigators. Rivaroxaban versus warfarin in nonvalvular atrial fibrillation. *N Engl J Med*. 2011;365(10):883-891.

8. Connolly SJ, Ezekowitz MD, Yusuf S, et al; RE-LY Steering Committee and Investigators. Dabigatran versus warfarin in patients with atrial fibrillation. *N Engl J Med*. 2009; 361(12):1139-1151.

9. Granger CB, Alexander JH, McMurray JJ, et al; ARISTOTLE Committees and Investigators. Apixaban versus warfarin in patients with atrial fibrillation. *N Engl J Med*. 2011;365(11): 981-992.

10. Waksman R, Ajani AE, White RL, et al. Intravascular gamma radiation for in-stent restenosis in saphenous-vein bypass grafts. *N Engl J Med*. 2002;346(16):1194-1199.

11. Yusuf S, Sleight P, Pogue J, Bosch J, Davies R, Dagenais G; The Heart Outcomes Prevention Evaluation Study Investigators. Effects of an angiotensin-converting-enzyme inhibitor, ramipril, on cardiovascular events in high-risk patients. *N Engl J Med*. 2000;342(3):145-153.

12. Lewis EJ, Hunsicker LG, Clarke WR, et al; Collaborative Study Group. Renoprotective effect of the angiotensin-receptor antagonist irbesartan in patients with nephropathy due to type 2 diabetes. *N Engl J Med*. 2001;345(12):851-860.

13. CAPRIE Steering Committee. A randomised, blinded, trial of clopidogrel versus aspirin in patients at risk of ischaemic events (CAPRIE). *Lancet*. 1996;348(9038):1329-1339.

14. Wiviott SD, Braunwald E, McCabe CH, et al; TRITON-TIMI 38 Investigators. Prasugrel versus clopidogrel in patients with acute coronary syndromes. *N Engl J Med*. 2007;357(20):2001-2015.

15. UK Prospective Diabetes Study (UKPDS) Group. Intensive blood-glucose control with sulphonylureas or insulin compared with conventional treatment and risk of complications in patients with type 2 diabetes (UKPDS 33). *Lancet*. 1998; 352(9131):837-853.

16. McCormack J, Greenhalgh T. Seeing what you want to see in randomised controlled trials: versions and perversions of UKPDS data. United Kingdom prospective diabetes study. *BMJ*. 2000;320(7251):1720-1723.

17. Shaughnessy AF, Slawson DC. What happened to the valid POEMs? A survey of review articles on the treatment of type 2 diabetes. *BMJ*. 2003;327(7409):266.

18. Yusuf S, Zhao F, Mehta SR, Chrolavicius S, Tognoni G, Fox KK; Clopidogrel in Unstable Angina to Prevent Recurrent Events Trial Investigators. Effects of clopidogrel in addition to aspirin in patients with acute coronary syndromes without ST-segment elevation. *N Engl J Med*. 2001;345(7):494-502.

19. Morice MC, Serruys PW, Sousa JE, et al; RAVEL Study Group. Randomized Study with the Sirolimus-Coated Bx Velocity Balloon-Expandable Stent in the Treatment of Patients with de Novo Native Coronary Artery Lesions: a randomized comparison of a sirolimus-eluting stent with a standard stent for coronary revascularization. *N Engl J Med*. 2002;346(23):1773-1780.

20. Garg S, Serruys PW. Coronary stents: current status. *J Am Coll Cardiol*. 2010;56(10)(suppl):S1-S42.

12.5

ADVANCED TOPICS IN THE RESULTS OF THERAPY TRIALS

Measuring Patients' Experience

Toshi A. Furukawa, Ian A. Scott, and Gordon Guyatt

IN THIS CHAPTER

TYPES OF INSTRUMENTS AND TESTS IN MEDICINE

Why do we offer treatment to patients? There are 3 reasons. We believe that our interventions increase longevity, decrease symptoms, or prevent future morbidity. Decreasing symptoms or feeling better includes avoiding discomfort (eg, pain, nausea, and breathlessness), distress (emotional suffering), and disability (loss of function).[2]

At least in part because of the difficulty in measurement, for many years, clinicians were willing to substitute physiologic or laboratory tests for the direct measurement of these *end points* or tended even to ignore them altogether. During the past 20 years, however, the increasing *prevalence* of chronic diseases has led clinicians to recognize the importance of direct measurement of how people are

feeling and the extent to which they are functioning in daily activities.

After reports that more than half of the disease *burden* in industrialized countries relates to disability[3] and a third of drug submissions to licensing authorities claim improvement in symptoms or function,[4,5] investigators have developed sophisticated methods to measure people's experience. Because, as clinicians, we are most interested in aspects of life that are directly related to health rather than issues such as financial solvency or the quality of the environment, we frequently refer to measurements of how people are feeling as *health-related quality of life* (HRQL). More recently, greater emphasis is placed on where the information comes from, and the term *patient-reported outcome* (PRO) has gained popularity.[6] In this chapter, we use the generic term PRO to refer to any report of the status of a patient's health condition that comes directly from the patient without interpretation of the patient's response by a clinician or anyone else.

Investigators measure HRQL by using self-report questionnaires that ask patients how they are feeling or what they are experiencing. Such questionnaires may use *dichotomous* response options, such as yes/no, or 5-point (or any other number) *Likert scales* (eg, feeling great, good, OK, bad, or terrible), or *visual analog scales*. Investigators aggregate responses to these questions into domains or dimensions that yield a single score for aspects of HRQL. For example, in the Chronic Respiratory Questionnaire (CRQ),[7] 5 questions yield a dyspnea score, and 7 different questions yield an emotional function score.

Clinicians often have limited familiarity with methods of measuring patients' experience. At the same time, they read articles that recommend administering or withholding treatment on the basis of its effect on patients' well-being. Poorly designed and reported investigations of patient experience within clinical trials can mislead clinical decision making.[8,9] This chapter is designed for clinicians asking the question: will this treatment make the patient feel better? This *Users' Guide* addresses 4 issues: whether you should or should not be concerned with measurement of how patients feel, the *validity* of the methods (eg, the extent of *risk of bias* and other concerns), interpreting the results, and applying the results to patients (Box 12.5-1).

IS MEASUREMENT OF HEALTH-RELATED QUALITY OF LIFE IMPORTANT?

Patients often will agree that, under most circumstances, prolonging their lives is a sufficient reason to accept a course of treatment. Under these circumstances, measurement of HRQL may be of little relevance.

Measurement of HRQL becomes important in 3 circumstances. First, although many of our

For instance, years ago, investigators found that 24-hour oxygen administration in patients with severe chronic airflow limitation reduced mortality.[10] The omission of HRQL data from the

---

BOX 12.5-1

Guidelines for Using Articles About Measures of Patient-Reported Outcomes

Is measurement of health-related quality of life (HRQL) important?

Are the results valid?[a]

Primary guides

Have the investigators measured aspects of patients' lives that patients consider important?

Is the instrument reliable (when measuring severity) or responsive (when measuring change)?

Does the instrument relate to other measurements in the way it should?

Secondary guides

Have the investigators omitted important aspects of patients' HRQL?

What are the results?

How can we interpret the scores?

How can I apply the results to patient care?

Has the information from the study addressed aspects of life that your patient considers important?

---

[a]Limitations of design of studies measuring patients' experience include issues beyond risk of bias. Thus, in this chapter, we continue to use the term "validity" to address both risk of bias and these additional issues.

---

original article ultimately was not considered important. Because the intervention prolongs life, our enthusiasm for continuous oxygen administration is not diminished by a subsequent report suggesting that more intensive oxygen therapy had little or no impact on HRQL.[11]

life-prolonging treatments have a negligible impact on HRQL, when they do lead to a deterioration in HRQL, patients may be concerned that small gains in life expectancy may not be worth the burden. For instance, patients may not accept toxic cancer chemotherapy that will provide marginal gains in longevity. In the extreme, an intervention such as mechanical ventilation may prolong the life of a patient in a vegetative state, but the patients' families may believe their loved ones would not want their lives prolonged under such circumstances.

Second, when the goal of treatment is to improve how people are feeling (rather than to prolong their lives) and reliable physiologic correlates of patients' experience are lacking, PRO measurement is imperative. For example, we would pay little attention to studies of antidepressant medications that failed to measure patients' mood or to trials of migraine medication that failed to measure pain.

Third, the more difficult decisions occur when the association between physiologic or laboratory measures and PRO is uncertain. Historically, clinicians tended to rely on *substitute end points* not because they were uninterested in making patients feel better, but because they assumed a strong link between physiologic measurements and patients' well-being. As we discuss in another chapter of this book (Chapter 13.4, Surrogate Outcomes), substitute end points or *surrogate outcomes*—such as bone density for fractures, cholesterol level for coronary artery disease deaths, and laboratory exercise capacity for ability to undertake day-to-day activities—have often proved misleading. Changes in these conventional measures of clinical status often show only weak to moderate correlations with changes in PRO[12] and fail to detect patient-important changes in PRO.[12] *Randomized trials* that measure both physiologic end points and PRO may find effects on one but not on the other. For example, trials in patients with chronic lung disease have found treatment effects on peak flow rate without improvement in PRO.[13] We therefore advocate great caution when relying on surrogate outcomes.

or second-generation or atypical antipsychotics), or perphenazine (a first-generation antipsychotic). Patients had a mean age of 41 years and had had the disease for a mean of 24 years.

Rates of discontinuation because of intolerable extrapyramidal adverse effects were greater among those receiving perphenazine than among those receiving newer antipsychotics. You therefore decide to focus your inquiry on comparisons of newer antipsychotics, and especially on olanzapine and risperidone, because the other 2 newer antipsychotics (quetiapine and ziprasidone) proved no better than the other 2 in any respect.

Half of the patients assigned to olanzapine kept receiving that medication for 3 months, whereas half of those assigned to risperidone had discontinued use of the medication after only 1 month. By 18 months, 64% of those assigned to olanzapine and 74% of those assigned to risperidone discontinued use of the study medication ($P = .002$). (Unfortunately, the authors did not report *confidence intervals* [CIs].[1])

During 1 to 3 months, olanzapine led to a 5-point to 7-point improvement in the Positive and Negative Syndrome Scale (PANSS), a standard measure to assess schizophrenia symptoms, with a possible score range of 30 to 210,[13] whereas risperidone resulted in improvements of approximately 3 or 4 points ($P = .002$). You wonder whether this represents an important clinical difference in the degree of improvement in the patient's psychiatric symptoms and, if so, whether adverse effects might outweigh the difference. The article itself provides no clue to the first question, and you set out to find the answers.

USING THE GUIDE

Referring to our opening scenario, in this landmark study of antipsychotics, called Clinical Antipsychotic Trials of Intervention Effectiveness (CATIE),[1] 1493 adults with chronic schizophrenia at 57 US clinical sites underwent *randomization* to receive 1 of the following 5 drugs: olanzapine, quetiapine, risperidone, ziprasidone (all newer

FINDING THE EVIDENCE

USING THE GUIDE

Definitively establishing a measurement instrument's usefulness requires several studies. As a result, critically appraising a PRO measure requires reading several articles. A good first step in addressing the instrument in our scenario is to identify the original report of the instrument, where you will usually find a detailed description and initial data about its measurement properties. You enter "PANSS" in PubMed, which yields 2441 articles. You jump to the last page of the retrieved studies, and identify the first reports of the PANSS.[14,15] For some well-established instruments, you may wish to purchase a published manual, if the instrument is very important for many of your patients. The manual for the PANSS is available from Multi-Health Systems Inc (http://www.mhs.com/product.aspx?gr=cli&id=overview&prod=panss).

Sometimes, initial studies may provide sufficient data for your critical appraisal. When they do not (as in the case of the PANSS, for which *responsiveness* was not evident in the first reports), we need to look for additional studies. To identify an article that deals with responsiveness or sensitivity to change, you enter "response OR sensitivity" as free text words and "PANSS" in the title field, and the search yields 23 citations. The title of 1 article (What Does the PANSS Mean?)[16] looks like it will provide the data you need.

ARE THE RESULTS VALID?

Limitations of design of studies that measure patients' experience include issues beyond risk of bias. Thus, in this chapter, we continue to use the term "validity" to address both risk of bias and these additional issues.

Have the Investigators Measured Aspects of Patients' Lives That Patients Consider Important?

We have described how investigators often substitute end points that make intuitive sense to them for those that patients value. Clinicians can recognize these situations by asking themselves the following question: if the end points measured by the investigators were the only thing that changed, would patients be willing to take the treatment? In addition to changes in clinical or physiologic variables, patients would require that they feel better or live longer. For instance, if a treatment of osteoporosis increased bone density without preventing back pain, loss of height, or fractures, patients would not be interested in risking the adverse effects—or incurring the costs and inconvenience—of treatment. The extent to which all relevant concepts or dimensions of health status important to patients are comprehensively sampled by the HRQL instrument reflects its *content validity.*

How can clinicians be sure that investigators have measured aspects of life that patients value? Investigators may find that the outcomes they have measured are important to patients by asking them directly.

For example, in a study that examined PROs in patients with chronic airflow limitation who were recruited from a secondary care respirology clinic, the investigators used a literature review and interviews with clinicians and patients to identify 123 items that reflected possible ways that patients' illness might affect their quality of life.[7] The investigators then asked 100 patients to identify the items that were relevant to them and to indicate how important those items were. They found that the most important problem areas for patients were their dyspnea during day-to-day activities and their chronic fatigue. An additional area of difficulty was emotional function, including feelings of frustration and impatience.

If the authors do not present direct *evidence* that their outcome measures are important to patients, they may cite previous work. For example, researchers conducting a randomized trial of respiratory rehabilitation in patients with chronic lung disease used a PRO measure based on the responses of patients in the study described just above, and they referred to that study.[17] Ideally, the report will

THERAPY

include enough information about the questionnaire to obviate the need to review previous reports.

Another alternative is to describe the content of the outcome measures in detail. An adequate description of the content of a questionnaire allows clinicians to use their own experience to decide whether what is being measured is important to patients.

For instance, the authors of an article describing a randomized trial of surgery vs watchful waiting for benign prostatic hyperplasia assessed the degree to which urinary difficulties bothered the patients or interfered with their activities of daily living, sexual function, social activities, and general well-being.[18] Few would doubt the importance of these items and the need to include them in the results of the trial.

USING THE GUIDE

The PANSS, used in the study of antipsychotics for chronic schizophrenia, covers a wide range of psychopathologic symptoms that patients with schizophrenia may experience, including the so-called positive symptoms (7 items for delusions, hallucinations, and so on), the so-called negative symptoms (7 items for blunted affect, withdrawal, and so on), and the general psychopathology (16 items for anxiety, depression, and so on).[14] These items can capture the overall picture of the patient's symptoms well but may miss more general aspects of HRQL, such as a sense of well-being or satisfaction with life.

Is the Instrument Reliable (When Measuring Severity) or Responsive (When Measuring Change)?

There are 2 ways in which investigators use PROs. They may wish to help clinicians distinguish between people who have a better or worse level of HRQL or to measure whether people are feeling better or worse over time.[19]

For instance, suppose a trial of a new drug for patients with heart failure finds that it works best in patients with the New York Heart Association (NYHA) functional classification class III and IV symptoms. We could use the NYHA classification for 2 purposes. First, for treatment decisions, we might use it as a tool by which to discriminate between patients who do and do not warrant therapy. We might also want to determine whether the drug was effective in improving an individual patient's functional status and, in so doing, monitor changes in the patient's NYHA functional class. However, for this purpose, the NYHA classification, which has only 4 levels, would likely not perform adequately.

Measuring Severity

If, when we are trying to discriminate among people with differing levels of disease severity at a single point in time, everyone gets the same score, we will not be able to separate the severely diseased from those with minor disease. The differences in disease severity we are trying to detect—the signal—come from cross-sectional differences in scores among patients. The bigger these differences are, the better the instrument is in discriminating among patients with different levels of disease severity (ie, the better its performance).

At the same time, if scores recorded from the same stable patients on repeated measurements fluctuate wildly—we call this fluctuation the noise—we will not be able to determine, with any sense of certainty, the patients' relative well-being.[20] The greater the noise, which comes from variability within patients, the more difficulty we will have detecting the signal.

The technical term usually used to describe the ratio of variability between patients—the signal—to the total variability—the signal plus the noise—is *reliability*. If patients' scores change little over time (when in fact patients' statuses are not changing) but are very different from patient to patient in accordance with the differences in disease severity of each patient, reliability will be high. If the changes in score within patients are high in relation to differences among patients, reliability will be low.

The mathematical expression of reliability is the *variance* (or variability) among patients divided by the variance among patients and the variance within patients. One index of reliability measures *homogeneity* or internal consistency of scores recorded for questionnaire items, constituting a scale expressed by *Cronbach α coefficient*. Cronbach α ranges from 0 to 1, and values of at least 0.7 are desirable.

A more useful measure, expressed as test-retest reliability, refers to reproducibility of measurements when the same instrument is applied to the same stable patients. Preferred mathematical expressions of this type of reliability are κ, when the scale is dichotomous or categorical (see Chapter 19.3, Measuring Agreement Beyond Chance), and *intraclass correlation coefficients* (ICCs), when the scale is continuous. Both measures vary between -1 and 1. As a rough rule of thumb, values of κ or ICC should exceed 0.7.

Measuring Change

In patients with chronic heart failure, we might want to determine whether a new drug was effective in improving patients' functional status, and to achieve this goal we might monitor changes in patients' NYHA functional class. When we use instruments to evaluate change over time, the instruments must be able to detect any important changes in the way patients are feeling, even if those changes are small. In this case, the signal comes from the difference in scores among patients whose status has improved or deteriorated, and the noise comes from the variability in scores among patients whose status has not changed. The term we use for the ability to detect change in the *signal-to-noise ratio* over time is responsiveness. It is sometimes also referred to as sensitivity to change.

An unresponsive instrument can result in false-negative results, in which the intervention improves how patients feel, yet the instrument fails to detect the improvement. This problem may be particularly salient for questionnaires that have the advantage of covering all relevant areas of HRQL but the disadvantage of covering each area superficially. With only 4 categories, a crude instrument such as the NYHA functional classification may work well for stratifying patients according to their level of disability but is very unlikely to detect small but important improvements in health status that result from treatment.

There is no universally accepted mathematical expression for responsiveness. Some studies judge a scale to be responsive when it can find a *statistically significant* change after an intervention of known efficacy. For example, the CRQ was found to be responsive when all of the domain scores improved substantially after initiation or modification of treatment, despite only small improvements in spirometric values.[7] Despite this high responsiveness, one of the CRQ subscales was subsequently found to have a modest reliability (internal consistency = 0.53; test-retest reliability = 0.73).[21]

In studies that find no difference in change in PROs when patients are in a treatment group vs a *control group*, clinicians should look for evidence that the instruments have been able to detect small but important effects in previous investigations. In the absence of this evidence, instrument unresponsiveness becomes a plausible reason for the failure to detect differences in PROs between the treatment and the control groups.

For example, researchers who conducted a randomized trial of a diabetes education program reported no changes in 2 measures of well-being, attributing the result to, among other factors, lack of integration of the program with standard therapy.[22] However, those patients involved in the education program, in comparison with those in a control group who did not receive the education, had an improvement in knowledge and self-care, along with a decrease in feelings of dependence on physicians. Given these changes, another explanation for the negative result—no difference between treatments in well-being—is inadequate responsiveness of the 2 well-being measures the investigators used.

USING THE GUIDE

In the report of the CATIE trial,[1] the authors do not address the responsiveness of the PANSS. A prior comparison of the PANSS with an independent global assessment of change, however, persuasively demonstrated its responsiveness.[16]

Does the Instrument Relate to Other Measurements in the Way It Should?

Validity has to do with whether the instrument is measuring what it is intended to measure. The absence of a *reference standard* for HRQL creates a challenge for anyone hoping to measure patients' experience. We can be more confident that an instrument is doing its job if the items appear to measure what is intended (the instrument's *face validity*), although face validity alone is of limited help. Empirical evidence that it measures the domains of interest allows stronger inferences.

To provide such evidence, investigators have borrowed validation strategies from psychologists, who for many years have thought carefully about how to best determine whether questionnaires that assess intelligence and attitudes really measure what is intended.

Establishing validity involves examining the logical associations that should exist among assessment measures. For example, we would expect that patients with a lower treadmill exercise capacity generally will have more dyspnea in daily life than those with a higher exercise capacity, and we would expect to see substantial correlations between a new measure of emotional function and existing emotional function questionnaires.

When we are interested in evaluating change over time, we examine correlations of changes in scores. For example, patients who deteriorate in their treadmill exercise capacity should, in general, experience increases in dyspnea, whereas those whose exercise capacity improves should experience less dyspnea, and a new emotional function measure should reveal improvement in patients who improve on existing measures of emotional function. The technical term for this process is testing an instrument's *construct validity*.

Clinicians should look for evidence of the validity of PRO measures used in clinical studies. Reports of randomized trials that used PRO measures seldom review evidence of the validity of the instruments they use, but clinicians can gain some reassurance from statements (backed by citations) that the questionnaires have been validated previously. In the absence of evident face validity or empirical evidence of construct validity, clinicians

are entitled to skepticism about the study's measurement of HRQL.[23]

A final concern arises if the measurement instrument is used in a culturally and linguistically different environment than the one in which it was developed—typically, use of a non-English version of an English-language questionnaire. Ideally, these non–English-language versions have undergone a translation process that ensures that the new version of the questionnaire reflects the idiom and the attitudes of the local population, a process called linguistic and cultural validation.[24] At the very least, the translation of the instrument should follow a procedure known as back-translation, whereby a first group of researchers translates the original into a new language, a second group blindly back-translates it into English, and a third group ascertains the equivalence of the original and the back-translated versions and resolves any discrepancies. If investigators provide no reassurance of appropriate linguistic validation, the clinician has another reason for caution regarding the results. In a review of 44 different versions of the McGill Pain Questionnaire representing 26 different languages/cultures, regardless of the method of cross-cultural adaptation, clinimetric testing of the adapted questionnaires was generally poorly performed, with only 9 undertaking back-translation. For 18 versions, no testing at all had been undertaken.[25]

USING THE GUIDE

In the antipsychotics study,[1] the investigators provide no citation to support the validity of the PANSS. As noted above, a quick search of PubMed (entering "PANSS" with no restriction) identified 2441 articles, showing that it is a widely used measure in psychiatry. Two reports describe extensive validation of the instrument.[14,15]

Are There Important Aspects of Health-Related Quality of Life That Have Been Omitted?

Although investigators may have addressed HRQL issues, they may not have done so comprehensively. When measuring patients' discomfort, distress, and disability, one can think of a hierarchy that begins with symptoms, moves on to the functional consequences of the symptoms, and ends with more complex elements, such as emotional function. Exhaustive measurement may be important in some contexts but not others.

If, as a clinician, you believe your patients' sole interest is in whether a treatment relieves the primary symptoms and most important functional limitations, you will be satisfied with a limited range of assessments. Randomized trials in patients with migraine[26] and postherpetic neuralgia[27] were restricted primarily to the measurement of pain, and studies of patients with rheumatoid arthritis[28] and back pain[29] measured pain and physical function but not emotional or social function. Depending on the magnitude of effect on pain, the adverse effects of the medication, and the circumstances of the patient (degree of pain, concern about toxicity, degree of impairment of function, or emotional distress), lack of comprehensiveness of outcome measurement may or may not be important.

Thus, as a clinician, you can judge whether these omissions are important to you or, more to the point, to your patients. You should consider that although the omissions are unimportant to some patients, they may be critical to others (see Chapter 27, Decision Making and the Patient). We therefore encourage you to bear in mind the broader effect of disease on patients' lives.

Disease-specific HRQL measures that explore the full range of patients' problems and experience remind us of domains we might otherwise forget. We can trust these measures to be comprehensive if the developers have conducted a detailed survey of patients with the illness or condition.

For example, the American College of Rheumatology developed the 7-item core set of disease activity measures for rheumatoid arthritis, 3 of which represent patients' own reports of pain, global disease activity, and physical function.[30] Despite the extensive and intensive development process of the 7 core items, the data set, when presented to patients, failed to include an important aspect of disease activity: fatigue.[31]

If you are interested in going beyond the specific illness and comparing the effect of treatments on PROs across diseases or conditions, you will look for a more comprehensive assessment. These comparisons require *generic HRQL* measures, covering all relevant areas of HRQL, that are designed for administration to people with any kind of underlying health problems (or no problem at all).

One type of generic measure, a *health profile*, yields scores for all domains of HRQL (eg, mobility, self-care, and physical, emotional, and social function). The most popular health profiles are short forms of the instruments used in the Medical Outcomes Study.[32,33] Inevitably, such instruments cover each area superficially, which may limit their responsiveness. Indeed, generic instruments are less powerful in detecting treatment effects than specific instruments.[34] Ironically, generic instruments also may not be sufficiently comprehensive; in certain cases, they may completely omit patients' primary symptoms. Even when investigators use both disease-specific and generic measures, these may still fail to adequately address adverse effects or toxicity of therapy.

For example, in a study of methotrexate for patients with inflammatory bowel disease,[35] patients completed the Inflammatory Bowel Disease Questionnaire, which addresses patients' bowel function, emotional function, systemic symptoms, and social function. Coincidentally, it measures some adverse effects of methotrexate, including nausea and lethargy, because they also afflict patients with inflammatory bowel disease who are not taking methotrexate, but it fails to measure other adverse effects, such as rash or mouth ulcers.

The investigators could have administered a generic instrument to assess aspects of patients' health status not related to inflammatory bowel disease, but once again, such instruments also would fail to directly address issues such as rash or mouth ulcers. The investigators chose a checklist approach to elucidate adverse effects and documented the frequency of occurrence of adverse events that were both severe enough and not severe enough to warrant discontinuation of treatment, but such an approach provides limited information about the influence of adverse effects on patients' lives.

WHAT ARE THE RESULTS?

How Can We Interpret the Scores?

Understanding the results of a trial that involves PROs involves special challenges. For example, in a clinical trial of management of acute back pain, patients presented with a baseline mean score of 34.6 on the Oswestry Back-Disability Index, a measure that focuses on disease-specific functional status (with lower scores representing less disability).[29] Among the patients randomized to bedrest, the mean score decreased to 16.0, which, however, was 3.9 points higher (ie, worse) than that of control patients.[29] Another trial addressed the effects of exercise training for patients with chronic heart failure. The summary score of the Kansas City Cardiomyopathy Questionnaire, a disease-specific health status measure for patients with heart failure, improved from the baseline score of 65.9 to 71.1 (an improvement of 5.2) in the intervention group and from 66.5 to 69.8 (an improvement of 3.7) in the control group.[36] Are the differences in the changes between intervention and control trivial, small but important, of moderate magnitude, or large and very important differences in efficacy between treatments?

Such examples reveal that the interpretability of most PRO measures is not self-evident. When interpreting PROs, clinicians must bear in mind that patients are likely to differ in the value they place on the same level of improvement, or deterioration, in physical or emotional function. This often necessitates clinicians and patients trading off benefits and *harms* in a process that we describe as shared decision making (see Chapter 27, Decision Making and the Patient). For example, a patient may be desperate

for small improvements in a particular domain of PRO and will be willing to take drugs with a substantial risk of adverse effects to achieve that improvement. However, another patient may be indifferent to small improvements and unwilling to tolerate even a small risk of important toxicity. Eliciting these preferences is an integral part of practicing *evidence-based medicine* (see Chapter 1, How to Use the Medical Literature—and This Book—to Improve Your Patient Care; Chapter 2, What Is Evidence-Based Medicine? and Chapter 27, Decision Making and the Patient).

When advising patients, clinicians require estimates of the magnitude of *intervention effects* (if any) that patients might expect in a PRO. This requires understanding the significance of changes in PROs, such as the Oswestry Back-Disability Index or the Kansas City Cardiomyopathy Questionnaire—an understanding we refer to as the instrument's interpretability. One can classify ways to establish the interpretability of PRO measures as *anchor based* or *distribution based*. These strategies lead to estimates of change in PRO measures that, either for individual patients or for a group of patients, constitute trivial, small, medium, and large treatment effects. No approach is without its limitations, but they all contribute important information.

Anchor-Based Approaches to Establishing Interpretability of PRO Measures

Anchor-based methods require an independent standard, or anchor, that is itself interpretable and at least moderately correlated with the instrument being assessed. This anchor typically helps to establish a *minimal important difference* (MID) of PRO instruments. The MID is the smallest change in score in the domain of interest that patients would perceive as beneficial and that would mandate, in the absence of troublesome adverse effects and excessive cost, a change in the patient's health care.[30] This concept also has been labeled "minimum clinically important difference" or "minimum important change."

The typical single anchor used in this approach is a global assessment of change corresponding to "no change," "small but important change," "moderate change," and "large change." The score on the PRO instrument in question corresponding with "small but important change" would be regarded as the

MID of that instrument. For instance, investigators asked patients with chronic respiratory disease or heart failure about the extent to which their dyspnea, fatigue, and emotional function had changed over time. To establish the MID, they focused on patients whose global rating suggested they had experienced a small but important change. They discovered, for all 3 domains, that the MID was approximately 0.5 on a scale of 1 to 7, in which 1 denoted extremely disabled/distressed/symptomatic and 7 denoted no disability/distress/symptoms. Other studies of patients with chronic airflow limitation, asthma, or rhinoconjunctivitis, using scales of 1 to 7, have suggested that the MID is often approximately 0.5 per question.[30,31,37] A moderate difference may correspond to a change of approximately 1.0 per question, and changes greater than 1.5 are likely to be large.[38]

USING THE GUIDE

Leucht et al[16] gained insight into the interpretation of the PANSS by comparing it to the clinician-rated Clinical Global Impression of Improvement scale, which is a global transition rating that classifies patients into 7 categories, from 1 (very much improved) to 7 (very much worse). They found that, to be rated as minimally improved, the PANSS scores needed to decrease by 19% to 28%. Because the baseline PANSS score in the data set was 94 (score range, 30-210), this translates to approximately 12 to 18 PANSS points. Because the PANSS consists of 30 items for psychopathologic schizophrenia, each rated on a 7-point Likert scale, ranging from 1 (no symptoms) to 7 (extreme), this MID roughly corresponds with the 0.5-per-question guideline noted in the respiratory and heart failure instruments.

Distribution-Based Approaches to Establishing Interpretability of PRO Measures

Distribution-based methods interpret results in terms of the relation between the magnitude of observed effect and some measure of variability in instrument scores. The magnitude of effect may be the difference in patients' scores before and after treatment or the difference in end point scores. As a measure of variability, investigators may choose

between-patient variability (eg, the SD of scores measured in patients at baseline) or within-patient variability (eg, the SD of change in scores that patients experienced during a study).

One *effect size* compares the mean of change scores divided by the SD of baseline scores. Some studies have suggested that an effect size of 0.5 thus calculated roughly corresponds with the MID as determined by the anchor-based approach.[39,40] Other investigators suggest this rule may be excessively simple, and further studies are necessary to determine its usefulness. If one believed this finding, for the Oswestry Back-Disability Index with a baseline SD of 16,[29] the MID would be $16 \times 0.5 = 8$.

How Can We Interpret Trials Reporting PRO Scores?

Reviewing anchor-based and distribution-based findings, investigators established that a 10-point change on the Oswestry Back-Disability Index signifies the MID.[41] Because the MID refers to changes in status in patients, knowing the MID still leaves problems in how to interpret differences between groups in clinical trials. Consider, in the example previously presented, that the group carrying on normal activities improved by 3.9 points more on the Oswestry Back-Disability Index than the group assigned to bedrest. Can we infer from the difference of 3.9, considerably less than the MID, that the treatment is unimportant to patients? Not necessarily, because not everyone in the trial experienced the mean effect. Although some patients may have experienced no benefit from treatment, it may have resulted in important improvement for others.

Investigators have gained insight into this issue by examining the distribution of change in PRO in individual patients and by calculating the proportions of responders (ie, those who improved by the MID or greater in the intervention and control groups). The difference in the proportions of those who responded in the 2 groups is the percentage that benefit and is also called the *risk difference* (see Chapter 9, Does Treatment Lower Risk? Understanding the Results).[41] The inverse of the percentage of participants who benefit (100/percentage benefiting) is the *number needed to treat* (NNT). The percentage of patients achieving a particular degree of benefit and the corresponding NNT to ensure that a single person obtains that benefit, if reported by the investigators of a trial using a PRO, provide useful information.

When investigators do not report the difference between treatment and control groups in the proportions who have some response over time or the corresponding NNT, we can compare the mean difference between the treatment and control groups in the PRO measure of interest against the MID. In so doing, we have to be careful not to necessarily dismiss the effect when the between-group difference is smaller than the MID.

For instance, in trials of asthma medication, mean differences among treatment groups of 0.9, 0.5, 0.3, and 0.2 on a 1-point to 7-point scale with an MID of 0.5 yielded differences in response rates of approximately 30%, 30%, 20%, and 5%, corresponding to NNTs of 3, 3, 5, and 20, respectively.[42] Note that in the last 2 cases, the mean differences are smaller than the MID, yet patients will almost certainly consider a 20% chance of important improvement with medication worthwhile and may even consider a 5% chance worthwhile. As a rule of thumb, if the mean difference among groups is less than 20% of the MID, the difference in the response rates among them is likely to be very small.

The investigators who conducted the trial of exercise training for chronic heart failure indicate the helpful reporting of PRO results.[36] The mean improvements on the Kansas City Cardiomyopathy Questionnaire (KCCQ) within the exercise group and the control group were 5.2 and 3.3 points, respectively, resulting in a difference between groups of 1.9 points (95% CI, 0.8-3.0; $P < .001$). The authors explained that KCCQ is a 23-item, self-administered, disease-specific questionnaire that is scored from 0 to 100, with higher scores representing better health status, and that its MID is approximately 5 according to a well-conducted study applying the anchor-based method.[43] Because the mean difference is less than half the MID, clinicians and patients might intuitively think that this change is likely unimportant. However, the investigators explicitly reported the proportions

of participants with 5 or greater improvements on the KCCQ as 54% in the exercise group and 29% in the usual care group, resulting in a difference in response rates of 25% and an NNT of 4.

What If We Don't Know the MID?

What if the authors did not report the numbers of responders, or patients achieving MID or greater changes, in their report? Many PRO measures do not have a well-established MID, and even when they do, trial reports often do not refer to them. For example, 75% of trials using PRO measures in oncology fail to discuss the size of their effects or its significance to patients.[44]

One possible approach is to compare the observed between-group difference with the total range of scores of that instrument. If the difference is less than 5% (eg, 5 points or fewer on a 1-point to 100-point scale or 3 points or fewer on a scale of 0 to 60 points), it is unlikely to be important; if the difference is greater than 10%, it is likely to be important.

Another approach is to attend to the effect size if it is reported, or if it is not reported, to calculate it yourself. The effect size is the difference between groups in mean end point scores (or mean changes) divided by the SD of the control group (or the pooled SD of the treatment and control groups). This measure is also called the *standardized mean difference* (SMD). Cohen provided a rough rule of thumb to interpret the magnitude of effect sizes. An SMD in the range of 0.2 represents a small effect, in the range of 0.5 a moderate effect, and in the range of 0.8 a large effect.[45]

A more sophisticated approach is to further transform an effect size into a NNT. Table 12.5-1 presents the conversion table from effect size into NNT for approximate effect sizes and response rates in the control group or in the treatment group.[46] We can use the effect size as reported in the study and the response rate we would expect to see in the control or treatment group based on our clinical knowledge. Several real-world examples have indicated that this conversion works relatively well for response rates between 20% and 80%.[47-49] Table 12.5-1 provides NNTs for typical effect sizes and typical response rates only, but an Excel spreadsheet is available

TABLE 12.5-1

From Effect Size Into Number Needed to Treat

Response rate in control group, %	20	30	40	50	60	70	80
Response rate in treatment group, %	80	70	60	50	40	30	20
ES = 0.2	16.5	13.7	12.7	12.6	13.4	15.2	19.5
ES = 0.5	6.0	5.3	5.1	5.2	5.7	6.8	9.1
ES = 0.8	3.5	3.2	3.3	3.5	3.9	4.8	6.7
ES = 1.0	2.8	2.6	2.7	2.9	3.4	4.2	6.0

Abbreviation: ES, effect size.

that can calculate NNT for any effect size and any response rate (see NNT Calculator2 at http://ebmh.med.kyoto-u.ac.jp/toolbox.html).

Investigators who conducted a trial of rheumatoid arthritis did not help clinicians interpret the magnitude of difference in PROs.[50] They reported that the mean difference in the disability scores between the treatment and control groups was −0.28 (95% CI, −0.43 to −0.13; $P < .001$). We do not know the MID for this disability scale; how then can we interpret the results? First, we could compare this 0.28 difference to the possible range of scores on that scale, 0 to 3 in the article. So the difference corresponds with approximately 10% of the total score and is likely to be important.

Second, we can calculate the SMD: 0.28 (the difference between treatment and control arms)/0.50 (the SD of the control group), or 0.56. Applying Cohen's guide, we interpret this as a moderate effect. We could go one step further by assuming the response rate in the control group. The article described that 16% of the patients in the control group had overall improvement in terms of both symptoms and functions. If we assume the approximate response rate in the disability domain to be 20%, then the NNT corresponding to an effect size of 0.56 would be between 3.5 and 6 (Table 12.5-1).

These calculations leave us considerably less confident than if investigators had reported the MID and calculated the proportion of intervention and control groups achieving the MID. Although there is some suggestion of improvement in the reports of PRO measures in oncology trials,[51] there is still great room for improvement in which measures to use,[52] how to report them, and how to interpret them.[9] Until such standards are achieved in the medical literature, clinicians need to resort to the strategies suggested here to make the results interpretable to themselves and to their patients.

USING THE GUIDE

The CATIE trial revealed that, by 3 months, olanzapine produced a reduction of approximately 7 points on the PANSS, whereas risperidone resulted in smaller reductions of approximately 3 points, a difference between groups of 4 points (these numbers are derived from graphs, where the overall difference is statistically significant at $P = .002$).[1] Because the MID of the PANSS is approximately 12 to 18, we are tempted to conclude that no antipsychotic could produce tangible changes, but, as we discussed above, this can be a misleading conclusion.

The trial report provides no indication of the proportion of patients who improved, remained unchanged, or deteriorated, and we therefore use

THERAPY

our other criteria. The difference is approximately 25% of the MID but less than 5% of the total score range of 180, reinforcing the impression that the difference is unimportant and may be trivial. The difference in the PANSS scores between olanzapine and risperidone is, on average, approximately 4 points at 3 months, and the SD of the PANSS at baseline is 18, which would then give a between-group effect size of $4/18 = 0.22$. This between-group effect size can be characterized as small, according to Cohen's guideline, further reinforcing the impression that any differences may be unimportant. The absolute percentage of patients achieving important improvement must be small among this group of patients with chronic schizophrenia, probably approximately 20%. Therefore, cells in Table 12.5-1 correspond with an effect size of 0.2 at 3 months and a response rate in the treatment group of 20%, indicating an NNT of 19.5 to produce an additional patient with a small but important change. Or, if we enter an effect size of 0.22 at 3 months and a response rate of 20% in the corresponding Excel calculator, available at http://ebmh.med.kyoto-u.ac.jp/toolbox.html (see NNT Calculator2), we obtain an NNT of approximately 18.

HOW CAN I APPLY THE RESULTS TO PATIENT CARE?

Has the Information From the Study Addressed Aspects of Life That Your Patient Considers Important?

Before answering the question about how the treatment would affect patients' lives, the clinician must be cognizant of the problems patients are experiencing, the importance they attach to those problems, and the value they might attach to having the problems ameliorated (see Chapter 27, Decision Making and the Patient). Instruments that measure PRO that focus on specific aspects of patients' function and

their symptoms may be of more use than global measures or measures that tell us simply about patients' satisfaction or well-being. For instance, patients with chronic lung disease may find it more informative to know that other patients who accepted treatment became less dyspneic and fatigued in daily activity, rather than simply that they judged their quality of life to be improved. Measures of PRO will be most useful when results facilitate their practical use by you and the patients in your practice.

USING THE GUIDE

The patient asked you 2 specific questions: what is the nature of the adverse effects he might experience, and how much better will he feel while taking alternative medications? Aside from his tremor, the patient is not too concerned about his current extrapyramidal adverse effects, but his family is concerned. The CATIE study found that the neurologic effects of olanzapine and risperidone were very similar, with approximately 8% experiencing some extrapyramidal signs.[1] The study also informs us about additional adverse effects—olanzapine will result in additional weight gain (body weight gain greater than 7% was observed in 30% who were taking olanzapine vs 14% taking risperidone; $P < .001$) and an increase in glycosylated hemoglobin—but it does not report whether there were any patient-important consequences of the increased blood glucose level. The study also reported that there was a greater increase in plasma prolactin for patients taking risperidone than for those taking other medications ($P < .001$), but again, it does not inform us if this led to any patient-important consequences. The patient is concerned about his current symptoms of insomnia, fearfulness, and hearing voices. The study does not report changes in those particular symptoms separately but, given changes in the PANSS, one would anticipate small average effects and a low likelihood of important improvement with olanzapine vs risperidone.

THERAPY

CLINICAL SCENARIO RESOLUTION

Returning to our opening clinical scenario, in light of the available information, you inform the patient that he is less likely to experience intolerable extrapyramidal adverse effects with newer antipsychotics, and given his concern about tremor and his family's concern about his looking ill, you recommend a switch to one of the newer agents. The patient concurs. Among the newer antipsychotics, olanzapine produced a greater reduction in symptoms, but the probability that your patient will benefit is small: 1 in 20 patients experienced a small but important change in symptoms when taking olanzapine that he or she would not have experienced if taking risperidone. Therefore, considering the tradeoff between a small likelihood of benefit in terms of decreased symptoms with olanzapine and the probability of increased weight gain and an increase in blood glucose of uncertain significance, the patient decides to try olanzapine first while being ready to switch to risperidone soon if significant adverse effects (such as substantial weight gain or polydipsia or polyuria as a result of hyperglycemia) develop.

CONCLUSION

We encourage clinicians to consider the effects of their treatments on patients' HRQL and to look for information regarding such effects in clinical trials.

Responsive, valid, and interpretable instruments that measure experience of importance to most patients should increasingly help guide our clinical decisions.

References

1. Lieberman JA, Stroup TS, McEvoy JP, et al; Clinical Antipsychotic Trials of Intervention Effectiveness (CATIE) Investigators. Effectiveness of antipsychotic drugs in patients with chronic schizophrenia. *N Engl J Med*. 2005;353(12):1209-1223.

2. Fletcher RH, Fletcher SW, Wagner EH. *Clinical Epidemiology*. Baltimore, MD: Williams & Wilkins; 1996.

3. Murray CJ, Vos T, Lozano R, et al. Disability-adjusted life years (DALYs) for 291 diseases and injuries in 21 regions, 1990-2010: a systematic analysis for the Global Burden of Disease Study 2010. *Lancet*. 2012;380(9859):2197-2223.

4. Szende A, Leidy NK, Revicki D. Health-related quality of life and other patient-reported outcomes in the European centralized drug regulatory process: a review of guidance documents and performed authorizations of medicinal products 1995 to 2003. *Value Health*. 2005;8(5):534-548.

5. Willke RJ, Burke LB, Erickson P. Measuring treatment impact: a review of patient-reported outcomes and other efficacy endpoints in approved product labels. *Control Clin Trials*. 2004;25(6):535-552.

6. Patrick DL, Guyatt GH, Acquadro C. Patient-reported outcomes. In: Higgins JPT, Green S, eds. *Cochrane Handbook for Systematic Reviews of Interventions*. Version 5.0.1. Oxford, England: The Cochrane Collaboration; 2008. http://handbook.cochrane.org/. Accessed January 15, 2014.

7. Guyatt GH, Berman LB, Townsend M, Pugsley SO, Chambers LW. A measure of quality of life for clinical trials in chronic lung disease. *Thorax*. 1987;42(10):773-778.

8. Kvam AK, Fayers P, Hjermstad M, Gulbrandsen N, Wisloff F. Health-related quality of life assessment in randomised controlled trials in multiple myeloma: a critical review of methodology and impact on treatment recommendations. *Eur J Haematol*. 2009;83(4):279-289.

9. Scott IA. Cautionary tales in the clinical interpretation of trials assessing therapy-induced changes in health status. *Int J Clin Pract*. 2011;65(5):536-546.

10. Nocturnal Oxygen Therapy Trial Group. Continuous or nocturnal oxygen therapy in hypoxemic chronic obstructive lung disease: a clinical trial. *Ann Intern Med*. 1980;93(3):391-398.

11. Heaton RK, Grant I, McSweeny AJ, Adams KM, Petty TL. Psychologic effects of continuous and nocturnal oxygen therapy in hypoxemic chronic obstructive pulmonary disease. *Arch Intern Med*. 1983;143(10):1941-1947.

12. Juniper EF, Svensson K, O'Byrne PM, et al. Asthma quality of life during 1 year of treatment with budesonide with or without formoterol. *Eur Respir J*. 1999;14(5):1038-1043.

13. Jaeschke R, Guyatt GH, Willan A, et al. Effect of increasing doses of beta agonists on spirometric parameters, exercise capacity, and quality of life in patients with chronic airflow limitation. *Thorax*. 1994;49(5):479-484.

14. Kay SR, Fiszbein A, Opler LA. The positive and negative syndrome scale (PANSS) for schizophrenia. *Schizophr Bull*. 1987;13(2):261-276.

15. Kay SR, Opler LA, Lindenmayer JP. Reliability and validity of the positive and negative syndrome scale for schizophrenics. *Psychiatry Res*. 1988;23(1):99-110.

16. Leucht S, Kane JM, Kissling W, Hamann J, Etschel E, Engel RR. What does the PANSS mean? *Schizophr Res*. 2005;79(2-3):231-238.

17. Goldstein RS, Gort EH, Stubbing D, Avendano MA, Guyatt GH. Randomised controlled trial of respiratory rehabilitation. *Lancet*. 1994;344(8934):1394-1397.

18. Wasson JH, Reda DJ, Bruskewitz RC, Elinson J, Keller AM, Henderson WG; The Veterans Affairs Cooperative Study Group on Transurethral Resection of the Prostate. A comparison of transurethral surgery with watchful waiting for moderate symptoms of benign prostatic hyperplasia. *N Engl J Med*. 1995;332(2):75-79.

19. Kirshner B, Guyatt G. A methodological framework for assessing health indices. *J Chronic Dis*. 1985;38(1):27-36.

20. Guyatt GH, Kirshner B, Jaeschke R. Measuring health status: what are the necessary measurement properties? *J Clin Epidemiol*. 1992;45(12):1341-1345.

21. Wijkstra PJ, TenVergert EM, Van Altena R, et al. Reliability and validity of the chronic respiratory questionnaire (CRQ). *Thorax*. 1994;49(5):465-467.

22. de Weerdt I, Visser AP, Kok GJ, de Weerdt O, van der Veen EA. Randomized controlled multicentre evaluation of an education programme for insulin-treated diabetic patients: effects on metabolic control, quality of life, and costs of therapy. *Diabet Med*. 1991;8(4):338-345.

23. Marshall M, Lockwood A, Bradley C, Adams C, Joy C, Fenton M. Unpublished rating scales: a major source of bias in randomised controlled trials of treatments for schizophrenia. *Br J Psychiatry*. 2000;176:249-252.

24. Guillemin F, Bombardier C, Beaton D. Cross-cultural adaptation of health-related quality of life measures: literature review and proposed guidelines. *J Clin Epidemiol*. 1993;46(12):1417-1432.

25. Menezes Costa LdaC, Maher CG, McAuley JH, Costa LO. Systematic review of cross-cultural adaptations of McGill Pain Questionnaire reveals a paucity of clinimetric testing. *J Clin Epidemiol*. 2009;62(9):934-943.

26. Mathew NT, Saper JR, Silberstein SD, et al. Migraine prophylaxis with divalproex. *Arch Neurol*. 1995;52(3):281-286.

27. Tyring S, Barbarash RA, Nahlik JE, et al; Collaborative Famciclovir Herpes Zoster Study Group. Famciclovir for the treatment of acute herpes zoster: effects on acute disease and postherpetic neuralgia: a randomized, double-blind, placebo-controlled trial. *Ann Intern Med*. 1995;123(2):89-96.

28. Kirwan JR; The Arthritis and Rheumatism Council Low-Dose Glucocorticoid Study Group. The effect of glucocorticoids on joint destruction in rheumatoid arthritis. *N Engl J Med*. 1995;333(3):142-146.

29. Malmivaara A, Häkkinen U, Aro T, et al. The treatmet of acute low back pain—bed rest, exercises, or ordinary activity? *N Engl J Med*. 1995;332(6):351-355.

30. Jaeschke R, Singer J, Guyatt GH. Measurement of health status: ascertaining the minimal clinically important difference. *Control Clin Trials*. 1989;10(4):407-415.

31. Juniper EF, Guyatt GH, Griffith LE, Ferrie PJ. Interpretation of rhinoconjunctivitis quality of life questionnaire data. *J Allergy Clin Immunol*. 1996;98(4):843-845.

32. Tarlov AR, Ware JE Jr, Greenfield S, Nelson EC, Perrin E, Zubkoff M. The Medical Outcomes Study: an application of methods for monitoring the results of medical care. *JAMA*. 1989;262(7):925-930.

33. Ware JE Jr, Kosinski M, Bayliss MS, McHorney CA, Rogers WH, Raczek A. Comparison of methods for the scoring and statistical analysis of SF-36 health profile and summary measures: summary of results from the Medical Outcomes Study. *Med Care*. 1995;33(4)(suppl):AS264-AS279.

34. Wiebe S, Guyatt G, Weaver B, Matijevic S, Sidwell C. Comparative responsiveness of generic and specific quality-of-life instruments. *J Clin Epidemiol*. 2003;56(1):52-60.

35. Feagan BG, Rochon J, Fedorak RN, et al; The North American Crohn's Study Group Investigators. Methotrexate for the treatment of Crohn's disease. *N Engl J Med*. 1995;332(5):292-297.

36. Flynn KE, Piña IL, Whellan DJ, et al; HF-ACTION Investigators. Effects of exercise training on health status in patients with chronic heart failure: HF-ACTION randomized controlled trial. *JAMA*. 2009;301(14):1451-1459.

37. Juniper EF, Guyatt GH, Willan A, Griffith LE. Determining a minimal important change in a disease-specific Quality of Life Questionnaire. *J Clin Epidemiol*. 1994;47(1):81-87.

38. Guyatt GH, Juniper EF, Walter SD, Griffith LE, Goldstein RS. Interpreting treatment effects in randomised trials. *BMJ*. 1998;316(7132):690-693.

39. Norman GR, Sloan JA, Wyrwich KW. Interpretation of changes in health-related quality of life: the remarkable universality of half a standard deviation. *Med Care*. 2003;41(5):582-592.

40. Sloan JA. Assessing the minimally clinically significant difference: scientific considerations, challenges and solutions. *COPD*. 2005;2(1):57-62.

41. Ostelo RW, de Vet HC. Clinically important outcomes in low back pain. *Best Pract Res Clin Rheumatol*. 2005;19(4):593-607.

42. Samsa G, Edelman D, Rothman ML, Williams GR, Lipscomb J, Matchar D. Determining clinically important differences in health status measures: a general approach with illustration to the Health Utilities Index Mark II. *Pharmacoeconomics*. 1999;15(2):141-155.

43. Spertus J, Peterson E, Conard MW, et al; Cardiovascular Outcomes Research Consortium. Monitoring clinical changes in patients with heart failure: a comparison of methods. *Am Heart J*. 2005;150(4):707-715.

44. Bridoux V, Moutel G, Lefebure B, et al. Reporting on quality of life in randomised controlled trials in gastrointestinal surgery. *J Gastrointest Surg*. 2010;14(1):156-165.

45. Cohen J. *Statistical Power Analysis in the Behavioral Sciences*. Hillsdale, NJ: Erlbaum; 1988.

46. Furukawa TA. From effect size into number needed to treat. *Lancet*. 1999;353(9165):1680.

47. Furukawa TA, Leucht S. How to obtain NNT from Cohen's d: comparison of two methods. *PLoS One*. 2011;6(4):e19070.

48. da Costa BR, Rutjes AW, Johnston BC, et al. Methods to convert continuous outcomes into odds ratios of treatment response and numbers needed to treat: meta-epidemiological study. *Int J Epidemiol*. 2012;41(5):1445-1459.

49. Samara MT, Spineli LM, Furukawa TA, et al. Imputation of response rates from means and standard deviations in schizophrenia. *Schizophr Res*. 2013;151(1-3):209-214.

50. Tugwell P, Pincus T, Yocum D, et al; The Methotrexate-Cyclosporine Combination Study Group. Combination therapy with cyclosporine and methotrexate in severe rheumatoid arthritis. *N Engl J Med*. 1995;333(3):137-141.

51. Efficace F, Osoba D, Gotay C, Sprangers M, Coens C, Bottomley A. Has the quality of health-related quality of life reporting in cancer clinical trials improved over time? towards bridging the gap with clinical decision making. *Ann Oncol*. 2007;18(4):775-781.

52. Hayes JA, Black NA, Jenkinson C, et al. Outcome measures for adult critical care: a systematic review. *Health Technol Assess*. 2000;4(24):1-111.

13.1

ADVANCED TOPICS IN APPLYING THE RESULTS OF THERAPY TRIALS

Applying Results to Individual Patients

Antonio L. Dans, Leonila F. Dans, Thomas Agoritsas, and Gordon Guyatt

THERAPY

IN THIS CHAPTER

A 66-year-old man of Chinese ethnicity visits you at your clinic for a periodic health examination. He is a retired professor from a local university, regularly wins games at the local chess club, and is physically active. However, his medical history reveals that he experienced a mild stroke 2 years ago. He still feels some heaviness in his left arm and lower extremities, but his speech has returned to normal and he is independent in his daily activities. He is even able to jog 2 km daily at a slow pace. He has never smoked. He drinks 2 to 3 glasses of wine every day. Further inquiry reveals that he has primary hypertension and type 2 diabetes mellitus and that he was diagnosed as having atrial fibrillation (AF) a year before his stroke.

The physical examination findings are unremarkable except for a blood pressure of 130/90 mm Hg and an irregular heart rate of 64/min. An electrocardiogram confirms that he indeed has AF.

The patient is taking 500 mg of metformin twice a day for his diabetes and 10 mg of ramipril once a day for his hypertension. Both the diabetes and hypertension have been well controlled for the past year. His only drug for stroke *prevention* is aspirin, 325 mg once a day.

Because the patient has a high risk for a recurrent embolic stroke, you consider prescribing an oral anticoagulant. You have used mostly warfarin in your practice, but in the past year, you have been discussing dabigatran etexilate, a novel anticoagulant recently approved by the US Food and Drug Administration for stroke prevention in AF, with some of your patients. Recently, you have heard concerns about the safety of warfarin among Asians, so you wonder if dabigatran would be a better choice for this patient.

evening, you decide to get an overview of current best evidence of using dabigatran etexilate in Asian patients with AF. Using the federated search engine ACCESSSS (http://plus.mcmaster.ca/accessss), you enter the 2 search terms "dabigatran" and "Asia," which retrieves available *evidence* from all levels of the pyramid of *evidence-based medicine* resources (see Chapter 5, Finding Current Best Evidence). Starting with the summaries at the top, you find general chapters in Best Practice and UpToDate but are not satisfied with the applicability of the evidence to Asian patients. On the level of preappraised research, you notice that no sound *systematic reviews* of studies are found in any resource searched (eg, *ACP Journal Club*, DARE, Cochrane, or MacPLUS). You then look at the bottom of the pyramid, where nonpreappraised research from PubMed is shown. Under the section filtered for reviews, you find a guideline entitled "Asian Venous Thromboembolism Guidelines: Prevention of Venous Thromboembolism," published in *International Angiology* in 2012, but it is unfortunately not retrievable through your institution. Under PubMed's section filtered for therapy, you find 3 studies, 1 of which seems relevant, entitled "Dabigatran Versus Warfarin: Effects on Ischemic and Hemorrhagic Strokes and Bleeding in Asians and Non-Asians With Atrial Fibrillation," published in *Stroke* in July 2013.[1] PubMed informs you that this is a secondary analysis from a trial entitled "Dabigatran Versus Warfarin in Patients with Atrial Fibrillation" published in the *New England Journal of Medicine* in August 2009.[2] You retrieve both articles.

FINDING THE EVIDENCE

You send the patient for some blood tests and promise to discuss therapeutic options for stroke prevention when he returns. That

INTRODUCTION

Clinicians looking at *randomized clinical trials* (RCTs) to guide medical decisions must decide how to apply results to individual patients. Chapter 7, Therapy (Randomized Trials), suggests 2 criteria for deciding on applicability: (1) Can I apply the results of the study to my patient? and (2) Are the benefits worth the *risks* and costs? In this chapter, we discuss these guidelines in greater detail.

Clinical trialists typically spend considerable effort ensuring comparability of treatment and *control groups* through strategies such as *randomization*, *blinding*, and *intention-to-treat analyses*. They often spend less effort on ensuring, through strategies such as population sampling, the representativeness of trial patients to typical patients in the community.[3] This is because the main focus of trials has been to answer the question, "Can the drug work in a controlled study setting?" rather than the question, "Will it apply to typical patients in the community?"

Nevertheless, published trials provide information that helps clinicians decide on the applicability of the results to individual patients. *Inclusion criteria* and *exclusion criteria*, for example, help us decide whether our patients would have been eligible to participate in the trial. *Subgroup analyses* may elucidate the effects of treatment on specific populations of interest as we apply the results (see Chapter 25.2, How to Use a Subgroup Analysis). In clinical practice, however, we face myriad patient subtypes, and trials typically are underpowered to address subgroup hypotheses.

Physicians, therefore, need to become skilled in applying trial results to individual patients. Box 13.1-1 summarizes criteria that will help you strike a balance between hasty generalizations and imprudent hesitation in the application of trial results. Sometimes, the *Users' Guides* may lead to clear decisions about whether to apply the results. At other times, they will at least increase or decrease your level of confidence in applying the results. For example, in the *GRADE (Grading of Recommendations Assessment, Development and Evaluation)* approach to rating confidence in estimates of intervention effects, the issue of applicability is partly addressed by the *indirectness* domain (see Chapter 23, Understanding and Applying the Results of a Systematic Review and Meta-analysis). Although directness addresses relevance of the entire research question to a specific situation, this chapter focuses mainly on applicability across different populations.

The *relative risk reductions* (RRRs) estimated in trials reflect the mean response of a population to a treatment. Because biologic and socioeconomic

---

BOX 13.1-1

Users' Guides for Applying Study Results to Individual Patients

Can I apply the results to my patients?

1. Have biologic factors that might modify the treatment response been excluded?
2. Can the patients adhere to treatment requirements?
3. Can the clinicians adhere to treatment requirements?

Are the benefits worth the risks and costs?

---

characteristics of individual patients sometimes modulate the *treatment effect*, the mean response may not always be the same in different patient subgroups. Here, we review the biologic and socioeconomic characteristics that may modify treatment response.

In reviewing the factors that may modulate effects, we present examples of apparent subgroup effects. Such apparent effects may, however, be the result of the play of chance rather than reflecting true differences. We have, in each case, applied the criteria for when to believe a subgroup analysis (see Chapter 25.2, How to Use a Subgroup Analysis). The *credibility* of any subgroup analysis varies on a continuum between surely real to surely spurious. Although we do not review the criteria here for each of our subgroup examples, we use language to describe the examples appropriate to the associated strength of inference.

CAN I APPLY THE RESULTS OF THE STUDY TO MY PATIENT?

Have Biologic Factors That Might Modify the Treatment Response Been Excluded?

Table 13.1-1 lists 5 biologic factors that sometimes lead us to hesitate in applying results to a particular patient. SCRAP is a mnemonic to remember these 5 factors, which include a patient's sex, presence of *comorbidity*, race or ethnicity, age, and pathology of the disease. The following examples illustrate how these factors may modify treatment effects in individual patients.

THERAPY

TABLE 13.1-1

Biologic Factors That May Modulate an Individual's Response to Therapy

Biologic Factor	Examples
Sex	Aspirin for prevention of atherosclerosis: the relative risk reduction for stroke and coronary disease is greater in women than in men[4]
	Use of stents after angioplasty: the risk reduction for bypass surgery is smaller among women[5,6]
Comorbidities	Measles vaccination: the degree of antibody response to vaccines has been observed to be lower in the presence of malnutrition[7,8]
	Treatment of hypertension: a target diastolic pressure of 80 mm Hg or less reduces events in patients with diabetes but not in the general population[9]
Race	Diuretics for hypertension: better response in blacks compared with whites[10]
	Proton pump inhibitors for peptic ulcer disease: more effective in Asians compared with non-Asians[11]
Age	Influenza vaccine for flu prevention: lower immune response in elderly patients[12]
	Dual therapy for peptic ulcer disease: higher *Helicobacter pylori* eradication rates in elderly patients[13]
Pathology	Influenza vaccine for flu prevention: effectiveness depends on viral strain used[14]
	Breast cancer chemotherapy: response dependent on certain gene expressions[15]

Sex

Investigators have identified apparent differences in response to interventions for prevention of cardiovascular disease between men and women.[4] For example, a *meta-analysis* that addresses the use of aspirin in primary prevention suggested that administration of aspirin to healthy women did not decrease the incidence of myocardial infarction as it did in men[5,16] (Figure 13.1-1). In contrast, aspirin reduced the incidence of stroke in women but not in men.

Another example of differences in treatment response involves the use of drug-eluting stents vs bare metal stents in men and women with coronary artery disease and similarly sized coronary arteries. A study by Hansen et al[6] found that, compared with bare metal stents, drug-eluting stents significantly reduced major adverse cardiac events in both men and women. However, the treatment effect was greater in women (*hazard ratio* [HR], 0.25; 95% *confidence interval* [CI], 0.13-0.46) than in men (HR, 0.60; 95% CI, 0.42-0.84).

Comorbidity

Comorbidities can modify the safety profile of an intervention. For example, one would ordinarily not consider warfarin in a patient with a recent gastrointestinal bleed. However, comorbidity can either decrease or increase the magnitude of treatment effects. Measles prevention is an example where comorbidities can decrease the effectiveness of prophylaxis. Cohort studies have found that comorbidities such as malnutrition, malaria, or human immunodeficiency virus infection can potentially reduce treatment response to vaccination as measured by immunogenicity.[7]

Table 13.1-2 presents an example where comorbidity apparently enhanced the effectiveness of treatment. The Hypertension Optimal Treatment study[8] suggested that target diastolic blood pressures below 80 mm Hg reduced cardiovascular events in patients with diabetes but not in the general population. Because of these findings, most hypertension guidelines recommend lower target blood pressures for patients with diabetes.

FIGURE 13.1-1

Meta-analysis of Aspirin in the Primary Prevention of Myocardial Infarction and Stroke in Men and Women

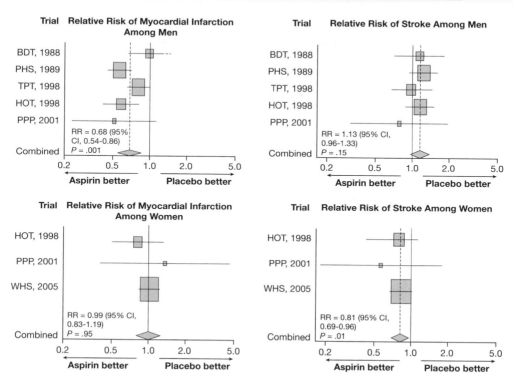

TABLE 13.1-2

Effect of Various Levels of Target Blood Pressure on the Incidence of Major Cardiovascular Events, Comparing Patients With Diabetes and the General Population[9]

Target DBP, mm Hg	No. of Events	Events per 1000 Patient-years	P for Trend	Comparison	RR (95% CI)
Patients With Diabetes					
≤90	45	24.4		≤90 vs ≤85	1.32 (0.84-2.06)
≤85	34	18.6		≤85 vs ≤80	1.56 (0.91-2.67)
≤80	22	11.9	.005	≤90 vs ≤80	2.06 (1.24-3.44)
General Population					
≤90	232	9.9		≤90 vs ≤85	0.99 (0.83-1.19)
≤85	234	10.0		≤85 vs ≤80	1.08 (0.89-1.29)
≤80	217	9.3	.5	≤90 vs ≤80	1.07 (0.89-1.28)

Abbreviations: CI, confidence interval; DBP, diastolic blood pressure; RR, relative risk.

TABLE 13.1-3

Meta-analyses of PPIs for Ulcer Bleeding, Comparing RCTs With Asians and Non-Asians

	Rate With PPI, %	Rate With Control, %	OR (95% CI)	NNT (95% CI)
Mortality				
Asian	1.5	4.7	0.35 (0.16-0.74)	31 (20-100)
Non-Asian	4.8	3.6	1.36 (0.94-1.96)	Incalculable
Additional Bleeding				
Asian	6.8	22.5	0.24 (0.16-0.36)	6 (5-8)
Non-Asian	11.9	15.5	0.72 (0.58-0.89)	27 (17-100)
Surgery				
Asian	2.9	9.2	0.29 (0.16-0.53)	16 (11-33)
Non-Asian	7.5	9.8	0.74 (0.56-0.97)	43 (20-100)

Abbreviations: CI, confidence interval; NNT, number needed to treat; OR, odds ratio; PPI, proton pump inhibitor; RCT, randomized clinical trial.

Reproduced from Leontiadis et al,[11] with permission from Wiley-Blackwell. Copyright © 2005.

Race

Racial or ethnic differences may sometimes modify response to treatment. In the treatment of hypertension, for example, blacks have proved more responsive to diuretics and less responsive to β-blockers than whites.[9] In peptic ulcer disease, a recent meta-analysis of patients with acute gastrointestinal bleeding suggests that proton pump inhibitors (PPIs) are more effective in Asians than whites in reducing mortality and preventing additional bleeding and surgical intervention (Table 13.1-3).[11] Potential explanations include a lower parietal cell mass, a higher *Helicobacter pylori* infection rate, or a slower metabolism rate for PPIs among Asians.

Age

Age can affect the response to some treatments. For example, compared with younger adults, older patients vaccinated against influenza have lower risk reductions in the incidence of flu,[12] perhaps because of a diminished immune response to the antigenic stimulus (Table 13.1-4). Sometimes, age increases the therapeutic response. A study found that the *H pylori* eradication rate with PPIs and antibiotics was approximately 2.5 times higher among patients older than 50 years than any patients younger than 50 years (63.6% vs 24%).[13] The mechanism for this difference is unclear, but investigators have theorized that, because *H pylori* infection has persisted longer in older patients, time-related alterations in the function or structure of the gastric mucosa might contribute to a more effective local drug action. Age-related decline in renal function also may lead to changes in pharmacokinetics that modulate the treatment effect.[14]

Pathology

Finally, diseases we refer to by the same name sometimes differ in the underlying pathology and, consequently, in response to treatment.

TABLE 13.1-4

Influence of Age on Effect Size Estimates of Trials Evaluating the Efficacy of Vaccination in Preventing Influenza in Healthy Adults

Median Age of Patients, y	Clinically Confirmed Cases		Laboratory Confirmed Cases	
	No. of Trials	RR (95% CI)[a]	No. of Trials	RR (95% CI)[a]
<33	15	0.54 (0.44-0.67)	5	0.22 (0.13-0.37)
≥33	23	0.89 (0.85-0.94)	16	0.43 (0.33-0.57)

Abbreviations: CI, confidence interval; RR, relative risk.
[a]RR pooled estimate (random-effects model and DerSimonian and Laird method).
Reproduced with permission from Belshe.[15]

In influenza vaccination, for example, effectiveness depends on whether the influenza strains in the coming year are the same as those contained in the vaccine.[15] Another example of differences in disease pathology that can modify a treatment effect is breast cancer, where response to chemotherapy depends on certain gene expressions.[17]

A Caution Against Overcaution

Deciding when to apply results to an individual patient can be challenging. Although our examples illustrate instances in which treatment effect may be modified by biologic factors, readers must be cautious in becoming overly restrictive in applying results of trials or systematic reviews. In general, we would suggest assuming applicability of results to individuals unless there is strong evidence that biologic differences will significantly enhance or attenuate the treatment response. There are many instances in which treatments have been withheld unnecessarily because of perceived biologic problems that affect applicability. Many apparent subgroup effects have proved spurious, and authors continue to claim subgroup effects despite failure to meet credibility criteria[18] (see Chapter 25.2, How to Use a Subgroup Analysis).

Women, for example, have generally received inferior care in the treatment and prevention of cardiovascular disease.[4] Although recent findings suggest sex differences in response to treatments, most of these differences do not warrant withholding therapy. As we have mentioned, in the case of stroke prevention, women seem to benefit even more than men from use of aspirin.

Another example of unjustified withholding of therapy was the use of diuretics for hypertension in patients with diabetes. Because diuretics increased blood sugar, many specialty societies did not recommend them as first-line therapy for patients with diabetes, despite convincing evidence that diuretics reduce cardiovascular events in the general population.[19] A long-term study has found that despite the metabolic effects, diuretics reduced serious morbid and mortal events in patients with diabetes.[20]

Similarly, because of their particular lipid profiles, statins were initially not recommended as first-line therapy for patients with diabetes and dyslipidemia, despite overwhelming proof of reductions in cardiovascular events in the general population. Fibrates were recommended as the drug of choice in patients with diabetes and hyperlipidemia until a systematic review found that statins work as well in patients with diabetes as in others.[21]

In our example comparing Asians and non-Asians with AF, the main study results regarding the efficacy outcome of stroke favored dabigatran at 150 mg twice a day over warfarin (*relative risk*, 0.64; 95% CI, 0.51-0.81).[2] Subgroup analyses found that the therapeutic advantage was maintained regardless of sex, comorbidity (previous stroke, myocardial infarction, diabetes, hypertension, heart failure, or need for concomitant antiplatelets), race, or age. There also seems to be no reason to suspect a difference in the pathology of stroke in this population because there were equal proportions of ischemic and hemorrhagic stroke between Asians and non-Asians.

However, in terms of the main safety outcome of major bleeding, the article by Hori et al[1] reports a potential subgroup effect according to ethnicity, which is of moderate credibility. A reduction in major bleeding was observed among Asians (HR, 0.57; 95% CI, 0.38-0.84) that was not seen in non-Asians (HR, 1.00; 95% CI, 0.87-1.16).[1]

Can the Patients Adhere to Treatment Requirements?

When satisfied that biologic differences do not compromise treatment applicability, clinicians must examine constraints related to the social environment that may modify the effectiveness and safety of treatments. This issue is important not just in disadvantaged populations but also in settings in which patients are privileged.

Because trials normally recruit patients with unusually high levels of *adherence*, trial patients tend to be systematically different from those in the general population. Investigators have documented these differences in situations such as management of hypertension[22] and asthma.[23] To the extent that groups of people exhibit different levels of adherence to treatment, clinicians may expect variation in treatment effectiveness. Variability in adherence between populations may stem from obvious resource limitations or from less obvious attitudinal or behavioral characteristics. Community studies reporting lower adherence rates from those reported in a clinical trial should raise suspicion that additional factors, such as specific attitudes and beliefs, might affect adherence.[22] Sociologic or anthropologic studies can further help identify these factors (see Chapter 13.5, Qualitative Research).

In the Philippines, for example, an attitude called "bahala na" connotes a lack of capacity or will to control one's fate.[24] In English, a near-equivalent statement would be "Let's just wait and see; there's really nothing much we can do about the situation." This external locus of control[25] may have an adverse effect on patient adherence.

Adherence is a major problem when it comes to oral anticoagulants, which are to be taken for long periods, often for the rest of a patient's life. This is an even greater problem with warfarin, which requires monthly blood tests so that the dose can be titrated to maintain an international normalized ratio (INR) between 2.0 and 3.0. The main measure of successful titration is the time in therapeutic range (TTR), that is, the percentage of time that a patient's INR lies in the range of 2.0 to 3.0, which should be greater than 65% to attain the full therapeutic potential of warfarin.[26]

The study by Hori et al[1] found that Asian patients taking warfarin attained a mean TTR of 54.5%, whereas non-Asian patients attained a TTR of 66.2%. This finding suggests an adherence problem among Asian patients who decide to use warfarin. An alternative explanation may be limited expertise of physicians in titrating the dose of warfarin. We deal with issue of clinicians' adherence in the next section.

Can the Clinicians Adhere to Treatment Requirements?

Clinicians' adherence comprises a host of diagnostic tests, monitoring equipment, interventional capabilities, skills, and other technical specifications needed to administer a treatment safely and effectively. The ability of clinicians to comply with these requirements may influence treatment effectiveness. This is especially true in trials of invasive interventions in which clinicians' skill becomes an important criterion for involvement in the clinical trial. When clinicians in the general population are not as skilled as those in a study, you should seriously question applicability of that study.

For example, in a meta-analysis of randomized trials of carotid endarterectomy for asymptomatic carotid stenosis, patients at relatively low risk of stroke benefited from surgery.[27] However, the surgery-associated stroke rate may have been low because of the high level of expertise of surgeons from the centers that participated in the trial. The net effect in other centers in the community may be an increase in adverse outcomes.[28] This is particularly concerning because surgical teams with complication rates and operative volumes that would have rendered them ineligible for the trial perform most endarterectomies.[29]

Like constraints in patient adherence, limitation in clinician adherence is likely to influence the critical balance between effectiveness and safety, possibly leading to nonapplicability of the results of an otherwise valid trial.

USING THE GUIDE

As discussed in the previous section, TTR can reflect not only patient adherence but also physician adherence or technical expertise in titration of the dose of warfarin. This would affect the efficacy of warfarin administration. Safety is influenced by the likelihood of elevated INRs, but it is also affected by the ability to cope with bleeding emergencies when they do occur. Thus, applicability of evidence regarding the consequences of bleeding events would entail consideration of access to emergency facilities and availability of expertise in using those facilities. The fact that rates of fatal bleeding were similar among Asians and non-Asians suggests that there were no major differences in this regard.

Are the Likely Benefits Worth the Potential Risks and Costs?

When you are satisfied that biologic and socioeconomic differences do not compromise applicability of the risks and benefits estimated in a trial, the next step in applying results is to estimate the patient-specific absolute benefit. This is reflected, for instance, in the *absolute risk reduction* (ARR) or its arithmetic inverse, the *number needed to treat* (NNT). Using the example of hypothetical drug A that reduces the incidence of stroke by 25% (RRR), Table 13.1-5 lists

TABLE 13.1-5

Effect of Baseline Risk of Stroke on the ARR and the NNT, Using Hypothetical Treatment A That Can Reduce Events by 25%[a]

Baseline Risk of Stroke Without Treatment (Rc), %	RRR, %	Risk of Stroke With Treatment (Rt), %	ARR, %	NNT
20	25	15	5	20
16	25	12	4	25
12	25	9	3	33
8	25	6	2	50
4	25	3	1	100

Abbreviations: ARR, absolute risk reduction; NNT, number needed to treat; RRR, relative risk reduction.

[a]Estimating NNT takes 5 easy steps: (1) estimate the baseline risk of your patient for the event (Rc); (2) estimate the RRR using the trial results; (3) calculate the new risk of an event with treatment (Rt) by reducing Rc by 25% (the RRR for treatment); (4) calculate the ARR by getting the difference between Rc and Rt; and (5) divide 100 by the ARR (expressed as a percentage) to estimate the patient-specific NNT.

the 5 steps in making the calculation. Given varying *baseline risks* among individuals, the resulting risk difference or ARR may vary. As a result, the NNT may vary as well from patient to patient.

Clinicians can derive estimates of the patient's baseline risk from various sources. First, they can use their intuition, which may sometimes be accurate—at least in terms of the extent to which risk is increased or decreased relative to the typical patient in a trial.[30] Second, if the randomized trials or meta-analyses report risks in patient subgroups, clinicians can choose the subgroup that best applies to the patient. For example, investigators pooled the individual patient data from all of the randomized trials testing antithrombotic therapy in nonvalvular AF and were able to provide estimates of prognosis for patients in subgroups with appreciable differences in risk.[31] Unfortunately, most trials and meta-analyses fail to report estimates of baseline risk in patient subgroups. Third, clinicians can find information about baseline risks in subgroups of patients in studies on *prognosis* (see Chapter 20, Prognosis). Sometimes, investigators use data from such prognostic studies to construct models that incorporate a large number of variables to create clinically helpful risk strata (see Chapter 19.4, Clinical Prediction Rules). When prospectively validated in new populations, these risk stratification systems can provide accurate patient-specific estimates of prognosis. A popular example is the Framingham risk calculator that estimates the risk of a coronary event for an individual according to age, sex, serum lipid levels, blood pressure, body mass index, use of tobacco, and blood glucose level.[32] Similar calculators estimate the risk of various outcomes, such as fracture based on bone mass density[33] and stroke in patients with AF.[34]

ESTIMATING PATIENT-SPECIFIC NUMBER NEEDED TO TREAT: AN EXAMPLE

Let us now consider as an example the decision about whether to offer alendronate for hip fracture prevention to a 64-year-old asymptomatic woman from the Philippines whose hip bone density T-score is −2.5. To estimate the baseline risk of hip fracture (step 1), we use the FORE 10-year Fracture Risk Calculator,[33] which tells us that such a patient faces a risk of approximately 0.20% per year (based on age, height of 62 in, weight of 113 lb, bone mineral density T score of −2.5 for the hip, Asian ethnicity, and absence of other *risk factors,* such as smoking, alcohol consumption, corticosteroid intake, prior fractures, or a family history of fracture).

As an estimate of RRR (step 2), we use the results of a Cochrane meta-analysis on the use of alendronate in preventing hip fractures in postmenopausal women.[35] This study found that alendronate can reduce the risk of hip fractures by approximately 40%.

To estimate the absolute risk of a hip fracture with treatment (step 3), we reduce the patient's baseline risk of 0.20% by 40%. This gives us an absolute risk of hip fracture with treatment of 0.12%. In step 4, we estimate the ARR as the difference between baseline risk and the risk with treatment, which is 0.20% − 0.12%, or 0.08%. Finally, in step 5, we get the arithmetic inverse of the ARR to estimate the patient-specific NNT. In this case, it turns out to be 100/0.08, or 1250 patients.

For those who prefer to avoid the arithmetic of the final step, a *nomogram* allows the clinician armed only with a ruler (or any other straight edge) to proceed from the patient's baseline risk, through the RRR (or RR increase), to the NNT or *number needed to harm.*[36]

Whatever strategy one chooses, varying patient risk will affect benefit regardless of the environment in which you practice. Even if you work in a Western tertiary care environment in which investigators conducted their original studies, you will still face high-risk and low-risk patients. The critical trade-off between risk and benefit may vary in these patient groups, mandating different treatment decisions (see Chapter 26, How to Use a Patient Management Recommendation: Clinical Practice Guidelines and Decision Analyses).

USING THE GUIDE

Returning to our decision about the administration of 150 mg of dabigatran twice a day instead of warfarin to our patient with AF and a previous stroke, we use the same 5 steps to generate a patient-specific NNT.

Step 1: Estimating baseline risk. To estimate baseline risk for stroke without treatment in our patient, we used the CHADSVASC score,[31] which considers the presence of congestive heart failure; hypertension; age older than 75 years or between 65 and 74 years; diabetes mellitus; previous stroke, transient ischemic attack, or thromboembolism; vascular disease; and sex. Because of his history of diabetes, hypertension, previous stroke, and age of 66 years, our patient's CHADSVASC score is 5. This means his risk of stroke is approximately 6.7% per year without any treatment. With warfarin titrated to an INR of 2.0 to 3.0, his risk would decrease by 68%[1] to approximately 2.1%. However, a final adjustment needs to be made in this estimate. The study by Hori et al[1] found that the risk of stroke among Asians is approximately twice the risk of stroke in non-Asians. Applying this finding to this patient, who is Chinese, results in an increase of his baseline risk from 2.1% to 4.2%.

To estimate the baseline risk for major bleeding on warfarin, we used the HAS-BLED score.[37] This scoring system considers uncontrolled hypertension, abnormal liver function, abnormal renal function, stroke, bleeding, labile INRs, being elderly (older than 65 years), and drug and alcohol intake.

Because of the previous stroke, his age (older than 65 years), and a history of alcohol consumption, our patient's HAS-BLED score is 2. This means his risk of bleeding while taking warfarin is approximately 1.9% per year.

Step 2: Estimating the treatment effect. On the basis of the Randomized Evaluation of Long-Term Anticoagulation Therapy study,[2] administration of dabigatran, 150 mg twice daily, instead of warfarin would reduce the risk of stroke by approximately 36% in addition to the risk reduction achieved with warfarin. Because the patient is Asian, the risk of major bleeding can be expected to decrease by 43%.

Step 3. Calculating the posttreatment risk. The posttreatment risk is derived by reducing the baseline risk of stroke by 36% and the baseline risk of bleeding by 43%. Thus, with treatment, the risk of stroke would decrease from 4.2% to 2.7%, and major bleeding would decrease from 1.88% to 1.07%.

Step 4. Calculating the ARR. The ARR is simply calculated as the baseline risk (step 1) minus the posttreatment risk (step 3). For stroke, this would mean 4.2% – 2.7%, or an ARR of 1.5%. For major bleeding, this would mean 1.88% – 1.07%, or an ARR of 0.81%. All of these apply to a 1-year time frame.

Step 5. Calculating the patient-specific NNT for this scenario. The final individualized NNT is the arithmetic inverse of the ARR. For stroke, the NNT would be 100/1.5, or 67. For major bleeding, the NNT would be 100/0.81, or 124.

CLINICAL SCENARIO RESOLUTION

What should we recommend regarding the use of 150 mg of dabigatran twice a day for the 66-year-old man of Chinese ethnicity presenting with AF and a history of ischemic stroke?

In analyzing biologic factors that may affect applicability of the trial results, we found studies that suggested that race or ethnicity may influence the balance between risks and benefits of the drug. Compared with warfarin, 150 mg of dabigatran twice a day reduced the risk of stroke to a similar extent in

both Asians and non-Asians. However, the reduction in major bleeds was only seen in Asians.

We also noted that Asian patients taking warfarin had lower TTR, although this may be due to problems in patient or clinician adherence with regimens to titrate the dose of warfarin.

Finally, we noted that baseline risk of stroke was approximately twice as high among Asians than among non-Asians. This led to adjustments in our estimates of the ARR in stroke and NNT.

THERAPY

Should we recommend 150 mg of dabigatran twice a day over warfarin for this patient? The drug seems to reduce strokes compared with warfarin in both Asians and non-Asians. The additional advantage in Asians is the reduction in major bleeding. In any patient, the treatment is simpler to take than warfarin because there is no need to monitor the INR. The main disadvantage is the cost of treatment, which is very high. The benefits of dabigatran appear substantial. In the Philippines, this patient would be paying out of pocket for the medication and would have to decide whether the cost is worth the benefits based on individual *values and preferences*.

CONCLUSION

Although the inspiration for this chapter came from a clinical scenario among Asian patients, the guidance is relevant to all situations in which clinicians must make decisions regarding applicability. By breaking down the problem into specific questions, we have provided guidance for clinicians' daily attempts to strike a balance between making unjustifiably broad decisions about *generalizability* and being too conservative in their conclusions.

One should not consider this guidance as absolute rules on whether to apply the results of a trial to a particular patient. In instances in which there is overwhelming proof of benefits in the general population, clinicians should insist on strong evidence of a differential response before deciding not to apply the evidence. When the evidence of benefit is less certain, however, doubt raised by considering these biologic factors may be enough to dissuade clinicians from recommending treatment.

When clinicians suspect limited applicability, what can they do? This will depend on whether the anticipated differences are important and, if they are important, whether they are remediable. Biologic differences often can be addressed by altering administration of a treatment (ie, adjusting the dose of a drug). Patient and clinician adherence problems, on the other hand, can be addressed by strategies such as education, training, and provision of necessary reminders or equipment.

Finally, as we have indicated, clinicians can estimate differences in baseline risk to generate patient-specific estimates of ARR (or increase in the context of harm). They may then use these estimates in shared decision making to provide patients with an estimate of the trade-off among benefits, risks, and costs (see Chapter 27, Decision Making and the Patient).

References

1. Hori M, Connolly SJ, Zhu J, et al; RE-LY Investigators. Dabigatran versus warfarin: effects on ischemic and hemorrhagic strokes and bleeding in Asians and non-Asians with atrial fibrillation. *Stroke*. 2013;44(7):1891-1896.

2. Connolly SJ, Ezekowitz MD, Yusuf S, et al; RE-LY Steering Committee and Investigators. Dabigatran versus warfarin in patients with atrial fibrillation. *N Engl J Med*. 2009;361(12):1139-1151.

3. Rothwell PM. External validity of randomised controlled trials: "to whom do the results of this trial apply?" *Lancet*. 2005;365(9453):82-93.

4. Crawford BM, Meana M, Stewart D, Cheung AM. Treatment decision making in mature adults: gender differences. *Health Care Women Int*. 2000;21(2):91-104.

5. Berger JS, Roncaglioni MC, Avanzini F, Pangrazzi I, Tognoni G, Brown DL. Aspirin for the primary prevention of cardiovascular events in women and men: a sex-specific meta-analysis of randomized controlled trials. *JAMA*. 2006;295(3):306-313.

6. Hansen KW, Kaiser C, Hvelplund A, et al; BASKET PROVE Investigators. Improved two-year outcomes after drug-eluting versus bare-metal stent implantation in women and men with large coronary arteries: importance of vessel size. *Int J Cardiol*. 2013;169(1):29-34.

7. Kizito D, Tweyongyere R, Namatovu A, et al. Factors affecting the infant antibody response to measles immunisation in Entebbe-Uganda. *BMC Public Health*. 2013;13:619. doi:10.1186/1471-2458-13-619.

8. Hansson L, Zanchetti A, Carruthers SG, et al; HOT Study Group. Effects of intensive blood-pressure lowering and low-dose aspirin in patients with hypertension: principal results of the Hypertension Optimal Treatment (HOT) randomised trial. *Lancet*. 1998;351(9118):1755-1762.

9. Falkner B, Kushner H. Effect of chronic sodium loading on cardiovascular response in young blacks and whites. *Hypertension*. 1990;15(1):36-43.

10. Wilson TW. History of salt supplies in West Africa and blood pressures today. *Lancet*. 1986;1(8484):784-786.

11. Leontiadis GI, Sharma VK, Howden CW. Systematic review and meta-analysis: enhanced efficacy of proton-pump inhibitor therapy for peptic ulcer bleeding in Asia: a post hoc analysis from the Cochrane Collaboration. *Aliment Pharmacol Ther*. 2005;21(9):1055-1061.

12. Villari P, Manzoli L, Boccia A. Methodological quality of studies and patient age as major sources of variation in efficacy estimates of influenza vaccination in healthy adults: a meta-analysis. *Vaccine*. 2004;22(25-26):3475-3486.

13. Treiber G, Ammon S, Klotz U. Age-dependent eradication of *Helicobacter pylori* with dual therapy. *Aliment Pharmacol Ther*. 1997;11(4):711-718.

14. Ammon S, Treiber G, Kees F, Klotz U. Influence of age on the steady state disposition of drugs commonly used for the eradication of *Helicobacter pylori*. *Aliment Pharmacol Ther*. 2000;14(6):759-766.

15. Belshe RB. Current status of live attenuated influenza virus vaccine in the US. *Virus Res*. 2004;103(1-2):177-185.

16. Ridker PM, Cook NR, Lee IM, et al. A randomized trial of low-dose aspirin in the primary prevention of cardiovascular disease in women. *N Engl J Med*. 2005;352(13):1293-1304.

17. Trock BJ, Leonessa F, Clarke R. Multidrug resistance in breast cancer: a meta-analysis of MDR1/gp170 expression and its possible functional significance. *J Natl Cancer Inst*. 1997;89(13):917-931.

18. Sun X, Briel M, Busse JW, et al. Credibility of claims of subgroup effects in randomised controlled trials: systematic review. *BMJ*. 2012;344:e1553. doi:10.1136/bmj.e1553.

19. Staessen JA, Wang JG, Thijs L. Cardiovascular prevention and blood pressure reduction: a quantitative overview updated until 1 March 2003. *J Hypertens*. 2003;21(6):1055-1076.

20. Kostis JB, Wilson AC, Freudenberger RS, Cosgrove NM, Pressel SL, Davis BR; SHEP Collaborative Research Group. Long-term effect of diuretic-based therapy on fatal outcomes in subjects with isolated systolic hypertension with and without diabetes. *Am J Cardiol*. 2005;95(1):29-35.

21. Vijan S, Hayward RA; American College of Physicians. Pharmacologic lipid-lowering therapy in type 2 diabetes mellitus: background paper for the American College of Physicians. *Ann Intern Med*. 2004;140(8):650-658.

22. Cardinal H, Monfared AA, Dorais M, LeLorier J. A comparison between persistence to therapy in ALLHAT and in everyday clinical practice: a generalizability issue. *Can J Cardiol*. 2004; 20(4):417-421.

23. Kennedy WA, Laurier C, Malo JL, Ghezzo H, L'Archevêque J, Contandriopoulos AP. Does clinical trial subject selection restrict the ability to generalize use and cost of health services to "real life" subjects? *Int J Technol Assess Health Care*. 2003;19(1):8-16.

24. Bulatao J. *Split-Level Christianity*. Manila, Philippines: University of St. Tomas Press; 1966.

25. Raja SN, Williams S, McGee R. Multidimensional health locus of control beliefs and psychological health for a sample of mothers. *Soc Sci Med*. 1994;39(2):213-220.

26. Connolly SJ, Pogue J, Eikelboom J, et al; ACTIVE W Investigators. Benefit of oral anticoagulant over antiplatelet therapy in atrial fibrillation depends on the quality of international normalized ratio control achieved by centers and countries as measured by time in therapeutic range. *Circulation*. 2008;118(20):2029-2037.

27. Chambers BR, You RX, Donnan GA. Carotid endarterectomy for asymptomatic carotid stenosis. *Cochrane Database Syst Rev*. 2000;(2):CD001923.

28. Barnett HJ, Eliasziw M, Meldrum HE, Taylor DW. Do the facts and figures warrant a 10-fold increase in the performance of carotid endarterectomy on asymptomatic patients? *Neurology*. 1996;46(3):603-608.

29. Tu JV, Hannan EL, Anderson GM, et al. The fall and rise of carotid endarterectomy in the United States and Canada. *N Engl J Med*. 1998;339(20):1441-1447.

30. Grover SA, Lowensteyn I, Esrey KL, Steinert Y, Joseph L, Abrahamowicz M. Do doctors accurately assess coronary risk in their patients? preliminary results of the coronary health assessment study. *BMJ*. 1995;310(6985):975-978.

31. Atrial Fibrillation Investigators. Risk factors for stroke and efficacy of antithrombotic therapy in atrial fibrillation: analysis of pooled data from five randomized controlled trials. *Arch Intern Med*. 1994;154(13):1449-1457.

32. Sheridan S, Pignone M, Mulrow C. Framingham-based tools to calculate the global risk of coronary heart disease: a systematic review of tools for clinicians. *J Gen Intern Med*. 2003;18(12):1039-1052.

33. Ettinger B, Hillier TA, Pressman A, Che M, Hanley DA. Simple computer model for calculating and reporting 5-year osteoporotic fracture risk in postmenopausal women. *J Womens Health (Larchmt)*. 2005;14(2):159-171.

34. Van Staa TP, Setakis E, Di Tanna GL, Lane DA, Lip GY. A comparison of risk stratification schemes for stroke in 79,884 atrial fibrillation patients in general practice. *J Thromb Haemost*. 2011;9(1):39-48.

35. Wells GA, Cranney A, Peterson J, et al. Alendronate for the primary and secondary prevention of osteoporotic fractures in postmenopausal women. *Cochrane Database Syst Rev*. 2008;(1):CD001155.

36. Chatellier G, Zapletal E, Lemaitre D, Menard J, Degoulet P. The number needed to treat: a clinically useful nomogram in its proper context. *BMJ*. 1996;312(7028):426-429.

37. Pisters R, Lane DA, Nieuwlaat R, de Vos CB, Crijns HJ, Lip GY. A novel user-friendly score (HAS-BLED) to assess 1-year risk of major bleeding in patients with atrial fibrillation: the Euro Heart Survey. *Chest*. 2010;138(5):1093-1100.

THERAPY

ADVANCED TOPICS IN APPLYING THE RESULTS OF THERAPY TRIALS

Numbers Needed to Treat

Gerard Urrutia, Ignacio Ferreira-González, Gordon Guyatt, and PJ Devereaux

THERAPY

IN THIS CHAPTER

HOW CAN WE SUMMARIZE BENEFITS AND RISKS?

Evidence-based practice (EBP) requires that clinicians summarize and consider both the benefits and *risks* of treatment for patients. Furthermore, clinicians must consider patient *values and preferences* related to these competing benefits and risks to determine which management strategies are in patients' best interests (see Chapter 27, Decision Making and the Patient).

These activities require clear summaries of the magnitude of *treatment effect*. The *relative risk reduction* (RRR; the *control event rate* minus the treatment event rate divided by the control event rate), the *absolute risk reduction* (ARR; the control event rate minus the treatment event rate), and the *number needed to treat* (NNT) represent alternative ways of summarizing the effect of treatment (see Chapter 9, Does Treatment Lower Risk? Understanding the Results). In this chapter, we provide examples of trials that have reported NNT and discuss how best to interpret this measure and apply it in clinical decision making.

THE NUMBER NEEDED TO TREAT IN WEIGHING BENEFIT AND HARM

The NNT, the number of patients the clinician must treat for a particular period to *prevent* 1 adverse *target event* (such as a stroke) or to create a positive outcome (such as a patient free of dyspepsia), may be the most attractive single measure. Arithmetically, the NNT is the inverse of the ARR. Clinicians could therefore simply take the ARR from a *randomized clinical trial* (RCT), calculate its inverse, and derive an NNT for their patients. However, because patients often begin with very different risks of adverse outcomes, such an approach can be profoundly misleading.

Consider, for instance, the GUSTO (Global Utilization of Streptokinase and Tissue Plasminogen Activator for Occluded Coronary Arteries) trial,[1] which reported the mortality within 30 days of hospital admission for approximately 20 000 patients who received streptokinase and approximately 10 000 who received tissue plasminogen activator (tPA). In the patients receiving tPA, the risk of dying was 6.3%; in those receiving streptokinase, the risk was 7.3%. The relative risk of dying with tPA is therefore 6.3/7.3 (86%), the RRR is 1.0 − 0.86 (14%), the ARR is 7.3 − 6.3 (1%), and the NNT is 100/1 (100). When deciding on whether an individual patient required tPA, we could assume that we might treat 100 patients to prevent a single death.

Such an approach ignores the fact that in the acute phase of ST-elevation myocardial infarction, patients have very different risks of dying. The Thrombolysis in Myocardial Infarction risk score estimates that in the month after ST-elevation myocardial infarction, the likelihood of dying in low-risk patients (ie, those who are younger, with noncomplicated Killip I inferior wall myocardial infarction and absence of other adverse *prognostic factors*) is 4.4%, whereas 36% of high-risk patients (ie, older patients and those with Killip III-IV anterior wall myocardial infarction) will die.[2] Thus, the impact of tPA assessed by NNT will vary broadly, depending on the *baseline risk* (Table 13.2-1).

APPLICATION OF NUMBERS NEEDED TO TREAT

Table 13.2-1 provides different scenarios of the uses of the NNT in weighting benefit and harm. The time frame should be considered to properly evaluate the NNT in every scenario. For example, the effects of different blood pressure–lowering regimens on major cardiovascular events have been assessed in a systematic review.[15] During a 1-year period, the

TABLE 13.2-1

Examples of Numbers Needed to Treat Generated From Reports of Randomized Clinical Trials and Meta-analyses

Condition or Disorder	Intervention vs Control	Outcome During 1 Year[a]	Risk Groups[a]	RRR (95% CI)[a]	ARR Across Risk Groups	NNT
Acute phase of ST-elevation myocardial infarction[b]	Thrombolysis with tPA vs streptokinase	Total mortality at 1 mo	Low = 0.8%-4.4% Medium = 4.5%-16% High = 16.1%-36%	14% (5.9%-21.3%)[1]	0.1%-0.6% 0.6%-2.2% 2.25%-5%	1000-166 166-44 44-20
Acute phase of ST-elevation myocardial infarction[b]	Primary angioplasty vs thrombolysis	Total mortality or myocardial infarction or stroke at 1 mo	Low = 0.8%-4.4% Medium = 4.5%-16% High = 16.1%-36%	42% (22%-59%)[3]	0.34%-1.8% 1.8%-6.7% 6.7%-15%	294-55 55-15 15-7
Survivors of myocardial infarction[c,d]	ACE inhibitor therapy vs placebo	Total mortality	Low = 4% Medium = 19.8% High = 28.8%	17% (3%-29%)[4]	0.68% 3.3% 4.8%	147 30 20
Persons without diagnosed cardiovascular disease[e,f]	Statin therapy vs placebo	Major cardiovascular event[g]	Low = <2% Moderate = 6.5% High = 12.5% Very High = 20%	10% (4%-15%)[5]	0.2% 0.65% 1.25% 2%	500 154 80 50
Persons without diagnosed cardiovascular disease[e,f]	Aspirin vs placebo	Any important vascular event over 5 years[h]	Low = <2% Moderate = 6.5% High = 12.5% Very High = 20%	15% (0%-28%)[6]	0.3% 1% 1.9% 2.25%	333 100 53 44
Persons without diagnosed cardiovascular disease[e]	Aspirin vs placebo	Major bleeding episodes (fatal and nonfatal)	Not available	RRI = 75% (31%-130%)[7]	0.21%	NNH = 476
Congestive heart failure[i]	Spironolactone vs placebo	Total mortality	Low = 8% Medium = 21% High = 33%	30% (18%-40%)[8]	2.40% 6.30% 9.90%	42 16 10

(Continued)

THERAPY

TABLE 13.2-1

Examples of Numbers Needed to Treat Generated From Reports of Randomized Clinical Trials and Meta-analyses *(Continued)*

Condition or Disorder	Intervention vs Control	Outcome During 1 Year[a]	Risk Groups[a]	RRR (95% CI)[a]	ARR Across Risk Groups	NNT
Congestive heart failure[j]	ACE inhibitor vs placebo	Total mortality	Low = 8% Medium = 21% High = 33%	23% (12%-33%)[9]	1.84% 4.83% 7.59%	54 21 13
Congestive heart failure[j]	β-Blocker vs placebo	Total mortality	Low = 8% Medium = 21% High = 33%	35% (20%-47%)[10]	2.8% 7.35% 11.55%	36 14 9
Congestive heart failure[j]	Resynchronization therapy plus optimal medical therapy vs optimal medical therapy alone	Total mortality	Low = 8% Medium = 21% High = 33%	27% (15%-38%)[10]	2.2% 6.7% 9%	45 15 11
History of coronary event[i]	Implantation of cardioverter/defibrillator	Risk of sudden cardiac death	Low = 5% Medium = 20% High = 27% Very high = 35%	53% (48%-74%)[11]	2.65% 10.6% 14.3% 18.5%	38 9 7 5
Nonvalvular atrial fibrillation[k]	Warfarin vs placebo	Stroke	Low = 1.9% Low-medium = 2.8% Medium = 3.6% Medium-high = 6.4% High = 8% Very high = 44%	62% (48%-72%)[12]	1.1% 1.7% 2.2% 4% 5% 27%	85 58 45 25 20 4
Nonvalvular atrial fibrillation[k]	Oral anticoagulant vs aspirin	Stroke	Low = 1.9% Low-medium = 2.8% Medium = 3.6% Medium-high = 6.4% High = 8% Very high = 44%	45% (29%-57%)[13]	0.85% 1.26% 1.62% 2.9% 3.6% 19.8%	117 79 62 35 28 5

Condition	Treatment	Outcome	Baseline risk	RRR	ARR	NNT
Nonvalvular atrial fibrillation[k]	New oral anticoagulant (rivaroxaban, dabigatran, apixaban) vs warfarin	Stroke or systemic embolism	Low = 1.9% Low-medium = 2.8% Medium = 3.6% Medium-high = 6.4% High = 8% Very high = 44%	22% (8%-33%)[14]	0.42% 0.6% 0.8% 1.4% 1.8% 9.7%	238 166 125 71 55 10
Hypertension[l]	ACE inhibitor vs placebo	Fatal or nonfatal stroke or fatal or nonfatal myocardial infarction	Low risk = <1.5% High risk = >3%	22% (17%-27%)[15]	0.33 % 0.66 %	303 151
Hypertension[l]	Calcium-antagonist vs placebo	Fatal or nonfatal stroke or fatal or nonfatal myocardial infarction	Low risk = <1.5% High risk = >3%	18% (5%-29%)[15]	0.27 % 0.54%	370 185
HIV infection[m]	Ritonavir vs placebo	AIDS-defining illness	Low = 0.7% High = 2.1%	42% (29%-52%)[16]	0.29% 0.9%	340 113
HIV infection[m]	Triple vs dual antiretroviral regimen	AIDS-defining illness	Low = 0.7% High = 2.1%	25% (19%-48%)[17]	0.17% 0.52%	571 190
Survivors of curative resection for colorectal cancer[n]	Intensive follow-up vs usual care	Total mortality	Low = 2% Med = 6% High = 11%	19% (6%-30%)[18]	0.38% 1.1% 2.1%	263 88 48
Survivors of curative resection for colorectal cancer[n]	Adjuvant chemotherapy with fluorouracil and folinic acid vs usual care	Total mortality	Low = 2% Med = 6% High =11%	16% (4%-28%)[19]	0.32% 1.9% 3.8%	312 53 26
Symptomatic carotid stenosis[o]	Carotid endarterectomy vs optimal medical care, including antiplatelet therapy	Stroke	Low = 3.5% High = 6%	PRRI = 20% (range, 0%-44%) RRR = 27% (range, 5%-44%) RRR = 48% (range, 27%-73%)	ARI = 3.7% ARR = 1.6% ARR = 2.9%	NNH = 27 NNT = 62 NNT = 35

(Continued)

THERAPY

TABLE 13.2-1

Examples of Numbers Needed to Treat Generated From Reports of Randomized Clinical Trials and Meta-analyses *(Continued)*

Condition or Disorder	Intervention vs Control	Outcome During 1 Year[a]	Risk Groups[a]	RRR (95% CI)[a]	ARR Across Risk Groups	NNT
Rheumatoid arthritis treated with nonsteroidal anti-inflammatory drugs[q]	Concurrent misoprostol vs placebo	Development of serious upper gastrointestinal tract complications	Low = 0.8% Medium = 2.0% High = 18%	40% (1.8%-64%)[20]	0.32% 0.80% 7.20%	312 125 14
One or more unprovoked seizure[r]	Immediate treatment with antiepileptic drugs vs treatment only after seizure reoccurrence	Recurrent seizures	Low = 13.5% Medium = 30% High = 34%	60% (40%-70%)[21]	8.1% 18.3% 20.1%	12 6 4
Breast cancer[s]	Radiotherapy plus tamoxifen vs tamoxifen alone	Any recurrence	Low = 4.3% High = 7.8%	22% (13%-29%)[22]	0.94% 1.7%	106 59
Breast cancer[s]	10 years vs 5 years of tamoxifen	Any recurrence	Low = 4.3% High = 7.8%	13% (4%-22%)[23]	0.56% 1%	178 100

Abbreviations: ACE, angiotensin-converting enzyme; ARI, absolute risk increase; ARR, absolute risk reduction; CI, confidence interval; HIV, human immunodeficiency virus; NNH, number needed to harm; NNT, number needed to treat; RRI, relative risk increase; RRR, relative risk reduction; tPA, tissue plasminogen activator.

[a]Unless otherwise specified, all calculations performed have been standardized during 1 year, assuming both a constant baseline risk and a constant risk reduction through the time frame of the corresponding study.

[b]Risk according to the Thrombolysis in Myocardial Infarction risk scale for the ST-elevation myocardial infarction. Strata risk have been defined as follows: low risk, less than 4 points; medium risk, 4 to 6 points; high risk, more than 6 points, where each point corresponds to the presence of any of the following 30-day mortality predictors in the acute phase of the event: age (<65 years, 1 point; 65-74 years, 2 points; >74 years, 3 points), systolic blood pressure less than 100 mm Hg (3 points), heart rate greater than 100/min (2 points), Killip II-IV (2 points), anterior ST-elevation or left bundle-branch block (1 point), diabetes mellitus (1 point), weight less than 67 kg (1 point), and time to treatment less than 4 hours (1 point).[2]

[c]After 1 week of the index episode.

[d]Low indicates 1 to 10 premature ventricular beats (PVBs) per hour and no congestive heart failure (CHF); medium, 1 to 10 PVBs per hour and CHF; and high, more than 10 PVBs per hour and CHF. The PVBs were analyzed from Holter recordings performed between the first week and the first month after the index episode.[24]

[e]More than 90% of patients studied did not have diagnosed cardiovascular disease.

[f]One-year risk of fatal cardiovascular disease. Risk varies according to a patient's sex, cholesterol levels, smoking status, and age. For example, low risk indicates patients aged 40 to 49 years with systolic blood pressure (SBP) of 120 to 140 mm Hg, who do not smoke and with total cholesterol levels below 200 mg/dL; moderate risk, patients 50 years and older with SBP of 140 to 160 mm Hg, who may have total cholesterol levels higher than 300 mg/dL, and who do not smoke; high risk, patients 60 years and older with SBP of 160 to 180 mm Hg, who may have total cholesterol levels higher than 250 mg/dL, and who do not smoke; and very high risk, patients 70 years and older with SBP of 180 mm Hg, who may have total cholesterol level levels higher than 300 mg/dL, and who do not smoke. Modified from Conroy.[25] Please refer to Conroy[25] to identify the various combinations of factors that determine a patient's risk category.

[g]"Major cardiovascular event" is defined as major coronary event (nonfatal myocardial infarction or death related to coronary artery disease), nonfatal or fatal stroke, or coronary revascularization.

[h]Any important vascular event is the composite of vascular death, nonfatal myocardial infarction, or nonfatal stroke.[6]

[i]Low risk indicates New York Heart Association (NYHA) functional class II; medium risk, NYHA functional class III; and high risk, NYHA functional class IV.[26]

[j]Risk of sudden cardiac death according to the following risk groups: low-risk group, history of coronary event; medium-risk subgroup, history of coronary event and ejection fraction less than 30%; high-risk subgroup, out-of-hospital cardiac arrest survivor secondary to acute coronary event; and very high-risk subgroup, sustained ventricular tachycardia or ventricular fibrillation episodes in the convalescent phase after coronary event (usually after the first 48 hours of the index episode). Modified from Myerburg and Castellanos.[27]

[k]Adjusted stroke rate. Every risk stratum is defined from a score scale risk, in which each of the following adds 1 point: recent congestive heart failure, hypertension, age of at least 75 years, or diabetes mellitus. Prior stroke or transient ischemic attack adds 2 points. The score defines each risk stratum as follows: low risk (0 points), low-medium risk (1 point), medium risk (2 points), medium-high risk (3 points), high risk (4 points), and very high risk (6 points).[28]

[l]Low risk: SBP of 140 to 159 mm Hg or diastolic blood pressure (DBP) of 90 to 99 mm Hg without any other cardiovascular risk factor. Medium risk: SBP of 140 to 159 mm Hg or DBP of 90 to 99 mm Hg with 1 to 2 additional risks factors or SBP of 160 to 179 mm Hg or DBP of 100 to 109 mm Hg with 0, 1, or 2 additional risk factors. High risk: SBP of 140 to 159 mm Hg or DBP of 90 to 99 mm Hg with 3 or more risk factors, SBP of 160 to 179 mm Hg or DBP of 100 to 109 mm Hg with 3 or more risk factors, or SBP greater than 180 mm Hg or DBP greater than 110 mm Hg. Modified from Whitworth et al.[29]

[m]Baseline human immunodeficiency virus 1 RNA level: low, 501 to 3000 copies/mL; medium, 3001 to 10000 copies/mL; high, 10001 to 30000 copies/mL; and very high, more than 30000 copies/mL.[30]

[n]1.5 Years' mortality of colorectal cancer according to Duke stages.

[o]Low indicates less than 50% stenosis; medium, 50% to 69% stenosis; and high, more than 70% stenosis.[31]

[p]Because the effects of carotid endarterectomy vary with the degree of stenosis, 3 different benefits or risks of surgery are presented.

[q]Low risk indicates patients with none of the following risk factors: age of 75 years or older, history of peptic ulcer, history of gastrointestinal bleeding, or history of cardiovascular disease. Medium risk indicates patient with any single factor. High risk indicates patients with all 4 factors.[20]

[r]Low risk indicates first seizure; medium risk, second seizure; and high risk, third seizure.[21]

[s]Low indicates no nodes affected; medium, 1 to 3 affected nodes; and high, more than 3 nodes affected.[22]

NNT for prevention of stroke or myocardial infarction with angiotensin-converting enzyme inhibitors in low-risk and high-risk hypertensive patients is 303 and 151, respectively (Table 13.2-1). However, if a time frame of 20 years is considered, the corresponding NNTs are 27 and 13. These figures indicate how the form of NNT data presentation can determine the effect of the information for clinicians and patients.

CONCLUSION

Clinicians can use data from the table in making treatment decisions with patients. More important, the results illustrate the importance of considering individual patients' baseline risk and the RRR associated with treatment before advising patients about the optimal management of their health problems.

References

1. The GUSTO investigators. An international randomized trial comparing four thrombolytic strategies for acute myocardial infarction. *N Engl J Med*. 1993;329(10):673-682.

2. Morrow DA, Antman EM, Charlesworth A, et al. TIMI risk score for ST-elevation myocardial infarction: a convenient, bedside, clinical score for risk assessment at presentation: an intravenous nPA for treatment of infarcting myocardium early II trial substudy. *Circulation*. 2000;102(17):2031-2037.

3. Andersen HR, Nielsen TT, Rasmussen K, et al; DANAMI-2 Investigators. A comparison of coronary angioplasty with fibrinolytic therapy in acute myocardial infarction. *N Engl J Med*. 2003;349(8):733-742.

4. Domanski MJ, Exner DV, Borkowf CB, Geller NL, Rosenberg Y, Pfeffer MA. Effect of angiotensin converting enzyme inhibition on sudden cardiac death in patients following acute myocardial infarction: a meta-analysis of randomized clinical trials. *J Am Coll Cardiol*. 1999;33(3):598-604.

5. Baigent C, Keech A, Kearney PM, et al; Cholesterol Treatment Trialists' (CTT) Collaborators. Efficacy and safety of cholesterol-lowering treatment: prospective meta-analysis of data from 90,056 participants in 14 randomised trials of statins. *Lancet*. 2005;366(9493):1267-1278.

6. Eidelman RS, Hebert PR, Weisman SM, Hennekens CH. An update on aspirin in the primary prevention of cardiovascular disease. *Arch Intern Med*. 2003;163(17):2006-2010.

7. Hansson L, Zanchetti A, Carruthers SG, et al; HOT Study Group. Effects of intensive blood-pressure lowering and low-dose aspirin in patients with hypertension: principal results of the Hypertension Optimal Treatment (HOT) randomised trial. *Lancet*. 1998;351(9118):1755-1762.

8. Pitt B, Zannad F, Remme WJ, et al; Randomized Aldactone Evaluation Study Investigators. The effect of spironolactone on morbidity and mortality in patients with severe heart failure. *N Engl J Med*. 1999;341(10):709-717.

9. Garg R, Yusuf S; Collaborative Group on ACE Inhibitor Trials. Overview of randomized trials of angiotensin-converting enzyme inhibitors on mortality and morbidity in patients with heart failure. *JAMA*. 1995;273(18):1450-1456.

10. Brophy JM, Joseph L, Rouleau JL. Beta-blockers in congestive heart failure: a Bayesian meta-analysis. *Ann Intern Med*. 2001;134(7):550-560.

11. Ezekowitz JA, Armstrong PW, McAlister FA. Implantable cardioverter defibrillators in primary and secondary prevention: a systematic review of randomized, controlled trials. *Ann Intern Med*. 2003;138(6):445-452.

12. Hart RG, Benavente O, McBride R, Pearce LA. Antithrombotic therapy to prevent stroke in patients with atrial fibrillation: a meta-analysis. *Ann Intern Med*. 1999;131(7):492-501.

13. van Walraven C, Hart RG, Singer DE, et al. Oral anticoagulants vs aspirin in nonvalvular atrial fibrillation: an individual patient meta-analysis. *JAMA*. 2002;288(19):2441-2448.

14. Miller CS, Grandi SM, Shimony A, Filion KB, Eisenberg MJ. Meta-analysis of efficacy and safety of new oral anticoagulants (dabigatran, rivaroxaban, apixaban) versus warfarin in patients with atrial fibrillation. *Am J Cardiol*. 2012;110(3):453-460.

15. Turnbull F; Blood Pressure Lowering Treatment Trialists' Collaboration. Effects of different blood-pressure-lowering regimens on major cardiovascular events: results of prospectively-designed overviews of randomised trials. *Lancet*. 2003;362(9395):1527-1535.

16. Cameron DW, Heath-Chiozzi M, Danner S, et al; The Advanced HIV Disease Ritonavir Study Group. Randomised placebo-controlled trial of ritonavir in advanced HIV-1 disease. *Lancet*. 1998;351(9102):543-549.

17. Yazdanpanah Y, Sissoko D, Egger M, Mouton Y, Zwahlen M, Chêne G. Clinical efficacy of antiretroviral combination therapy based on protease inhibitors or non-nucleoside analogue reverse transcriptase inhibitors: indirect comparison of controlled trials. *BMJ*. 2004;328(7434):249.

18. Renehan AG, Egger M, Saunders MP, O'Dwyer ST. Impact on survival of intensive follow up after curative resection for colorectal cancer: systematic review and meta-analysis of randomised trials. *BMJ*. 2002;324(7341):813.

19. Gray R, Barnwell J, McConkey C, Hills RK, Williams NS, Kerr DJ; Quasar Collaborative Group. Adjuvant chemotherapy versus observation in patients with colorectal cancer: a randomised study. *Lancet*. 2007;370(9604):2020-2029.

20. Silverstein FE, Graham DY, Senior JR, et al. Misoprostol reduces serious gastrointestinal complications in patients with rheumatoid arthritis receiving nonsteroidal anti-inflammatory drugs: a randomized, double-blind, placebo-controlled trial. *Ann Intern Med*. 1995;123(4):241-249.

21. Hauser WA, Rich SS, Lee JR, Annegers JF, Anderson VE. Risk of recurrent seizures after two unprovoked seizures. *N Engl J Med*. 1998;338(7):429-434.

22. Overgaard M, Jensen MB, Overgaard J, et al. Postoperative radiotherapy in high-risk postmenopausal breast-cancer patients given adjuvant tamoxifen: Danish Breast Cancer Cooperative Group DBCG 82c randomised trial. *Lancet*. 1999;353(9165):1641-1648.

23. Davies C, Pan H, Godwin J, et al; Adjuvant Tamoxifen: Longer Against Shorter (ATLAS) Collaborative Group. Long-term effects of continuing adjuvant tamoxifen to 10 years versus stopping at 5 years after diagnosis of oestrogen receptor-positive breast cancer: ATLAS, a randomised trial. *Lancet.* 2013;381(9869):805-816.

24. Maggioni AP, Zuanetti G, Franzosi MG, et al. Prevalence and prognostic significance of ventricular arrhythmias after acute myocardial infarction in the fibrinolytic era. GISSI-2 results. *Circulation.* 1993;87(2):312-322.

25. Conroy RM, Pyörälä K, Fitzgerald AP, et al; SCORE project group. Estimation of ten-year risk of fatal cardiovascular disease in Europe: the SCORE project. *Eur Heart J.* 2003; 24(11):987-1003.

26. Matoba M, Matsui S, Hirakawa T, et al. Long-term prognosis of patients with congestive heart failure. *Jpn Circ J.* 1990;54(1):57-61.

27. Myerburg RJ, Castellanos A. Cardiac arrest and sudden death. In: Saunders WB, ed. *Heart Disease: A Textbook of Cardiovascular Medicine.* Philadelphia, PA: Saunders; 1997:742-779.

28. Gage BF, Waterman AD, Shannon W, Boechler M, Rich MW, Radford MJ. Validation of clinical classification schemes for predicting stroke: results from the National Registry of Atrial Fibrillation. *JAMA.* 2001;285(22):2864-2870.

29. Whitworth JA; World Health Organization, International Society of Hypertension Writing Group. 2003 World Health Organization (WHO)/International Society of Hypertension (ISH) statement on management of hypertension. *J Hypertens.* 2003;21(11):1983-1992.

30. Mellors JW, Muñoz A, Giorgi JV, et al. Plasma viral load and CD4+ lymphocytes as prognostic markers of HIV-1 infection. *Ann Intern Med.* 1997;126(12):946-954.

31. Barnett HJ, Taylor DW, Eliasziw M, et al; North American Symptomatic Carotid Endarterectomy Trial Collaborators. Benefit of carotid endarterectomy in patients with symptomatic moderate or severe stenosis. *N Engl J Med.* 1998;339(20):1415-1425.

THERAPY

13.3

ADVANCED TOPICS IN APPLYING THE RESULTS OF THERAPY TRIALS

Misleading Presentations of Clinical Trial Results

Alonso Carrasco-Labra, Victor M. Montori, John P. A. Ioannidis, Roman Jaeschke, PJ Devereaux, Michael Walsh, Holger J. Schünemann, Mohit Bhandari, and Gordon Guyatt

IN THIS CHAPTER

Introduction

Seven Guides to Avoid Being Misled

1. Read Only Methods and Results; Bypass the Discussion

2. Read the Summary Structured Abstract Published in Evidence-Based Secondary Publications (Preappraised Resources)

3. Beware Large Treatment Effects in Trials With Only a Few Events

4. Beware Faulty Comparators

5. Beware Small Treatment Effects and Extrapolation to Very Low-Risk Patients

6. Beware Uneven Emphasis on Benefits and Harms

7. Wait for the Overall Results to Emerge; Do Not Rush

Conclusion

INTRODUCTION

Science is often not objective.[1] The choice of research questions, the methods to collect and analyze data, and the interpretation of results all reflect the perspective of the investigator.[2] Try as they may to be objective and impartial, investigators' intellectual and/or emotional investment in their own ideas and their personal interest in academic success and advancement may further compromise scientific objectivity. Investigators often overemphasize the importance of their findings and the quality of their work. Scrutiny of the work of the authors of this chapter will reveal we are not immune to these lapses.

In addition, *conflicts of interest* arise when for-profit organizations, such as device, biotechnology, and pharmaceutical companies, provide funds for research, consulting, and attending scientific meetings. In recent years, there has been a large increase in the number of trials for which authors declare industry affiliation.[3] Investigators accepting industry funds

may have conflicts of interest. Even more problematic, they may cede their right to directly supervise data collection, participate in or supervise data analysis, and write the research reports to which their names are attached.[4-6] Finally, clinical studies funded by for-profit companies are more likely to report results and conclusions that favor the intervention being tested than are trials funded by nonprofit bodies.[7-9]

Extensive publicity highlighting these problems has caught the attention of many clinicians, who are therefore well aware of their vulnerability to biased and potentially misleading presentations of *randomized clinical trial* (RCT) results. This book describes, in some detail, guides to help recognize methodologic weaknesses that may introduce *bias*. These criteria, however, do not protect readers against misleading interpretations of apparently methodologically sound studies. Indeed, all of the studies we use as examples in this chapter satisfy minimal *risk of bias* criteria, and most are exceptionally strong. In this chapter, we go beyond issues of risk of bias to present a set of *Users' Guides* to address biased presentation and interpretation of data to aid clinicians in optimally applying research findings (Box 13.3-1). We illustrate these guides with real-world examples, not to adversely criticize investigators, but to raise awareness of the dangers that the medical literature currently presents to unwary clinicians.

There are some *Users' Guides* to avoid being misled that are at least as important as those we present here, so important that we have allocated them their own chapters (see Chapter 8, How to Use a Noninferiority Trial; Chapter 11.3, Randomized Trials Stopped Early for Benefit; Chapter 12.4, Composite End Points; Chapter 13.4, Surrogate Outcomes; and Chapter 25.2, How to Use a Subgroup Analysis). Attention to those issues, and the 7 guides below, will help you negotiate the minefield of sophisticated clinical trial reports that may serve interests beyond those of your patients.

BOX 13.3-1

Users' Guides to Avoid Being Misled by Biased Presentation and Interpretation of Data

1. Read methods and results; bypass the discussion section

2. Read the summary structured abstract published in evidence-based secondary publications (ie, preappraised resources)

3. Beware large effects in trials with only a few events

4. Beware faulty comparators

5. Beware small treatment effects and extrapolation to very low-risk patients

6. Beware uneven emphasis on benefits and harms

7. Wait for the overall results to emerge; do not rush

Montori Victor M, Jaeschke Roman, Schünemann Holger J, Bhandari Mohit, Brozek Jan L, Devereaux P J et al. Users' guide to detecting misleading claims in clinical research reports BMJ 2004; 329:1093. Adapted with permission from the BMJ Publishing Group.

SEVEN GUIDES TO AVOID BEING MISLED

1. Read Only Methods and Results; Bypass the Discussion

The Discussion—and to some extent the Introduction and the Conclusion sections of the published research articles—often offer inferences that differ from those that a dispassionate reader would draw from the Methods and Results sections of such articles.[10]

Consider, for example, 2 *systematic reviews* with *meta-analyses* published in 2001 that summarized randomized trials that assessed the effect of albumin use for fluid resuscitation. One review, funded by the Plasma Proteins Therapeutic Association, pooled 42 short-term trials reporting mortality and found no significant difference in mortality with albumin vs crystalloid solutions across all groups of patients (*relative risk* [RR], 1.11; 95% *confidence interval* [CI], 0.95-1.28) and in patients with burns (RR, 1.76; 95% CI, 0.97-3.17).[11] The other review, funded by the UK National Health Service, pooled 31 short-term trials that reported mortality and found a significantly higher mortality with albumin in all patient groups (RR, 1.52; 95% CI, 1.17-1.99) and in patients with burns (RR, 2.40; 95% CI, 1.11-5.19).[12]

Although these 2 systematic reviews included a slightly different set of trials (eg, the former included an additional trial in patients with burns), both yield *point estimates* that suggest that albumin may increase mortality and CIs that include the possibility of a considerable increase in mortality. The trials were small, many had a high risk of bias, and the results were *heterogeneous*. The authors of the first review concluded, in their discussion, that their results "should serve to allay concerns regarding the safety of albumin." In contrast, the discussion section of the second review recommended banning the use of albumin outside the context of a rigorously conducted RCT.

Authors of an editorial accompanying the first systematic review[13] suggested that the funding source may have been, at least in part, responsible for the different interpretations. At that time, the Plasma Proteins Therapeutic Association was promoting access to and reimbursement for the use of albumin, an expensive intervention; on the other hand, the National Health Service paid for albumin use in the United Kingdom.

Examples of potential conflicts of interest that apparently drive conclusions abound. Systematic examinations of the association between funding and conclusions have found that trial investigators have greater enthusiasm for the *experimental treatment* when funded by for-profit than nonprofit interests.[14-17] Even after adjusting for magnitude of *treatment effect* and adverse events, for-profit funding has been reported to be associated with a 5-fold increase in the odds of recommending an experimental drug as treatment of choice (*odds ratio* [OR], 5.3; 95% CI, 2.0-14.4) compared with nonprofit funding.[14]

These issues also extend to systematic reviews of RCTs. Industry-supported systematic reviews that address drug treatments, although reporting similar treatment effect, provide more favorable conclusions compared with Cochrane reviews that address the same question.[18] Industry influence also extends to *cost-effectiveness analyses* and *clinical practice guidelines*.[19]

To apply this first guide and thereby bypass the Discussion section of research reports, clinicians must be able to make sense of the methods and results.

2. Read the Summary Structured Abstract Published in Evidence-based Secondary Publications (Preappraised Resources)

Secondary journals, such as *ACP Journal Club, Evidence-Based Medicine,* and *Evidence-Based Mental Health,* publish *structured abstracts* and commentary that summarize research articles published elsewhere. These materials are produced by a team of clinicians and methodologists and often in collaboration with the authors of the original articles. These abstracts often include critical information about research conduct (eg, *allocation concealment; blinding* of patients, clinicians, data collectors, data analysts, and outcome adjudicators; and complete *follow-up*) that may have been omitted from the original reports.[20] They also may diminish some of the "spin" that distorts the abstracts of the original publications.[21] The structured abstracts do not include the Introduction or the Discussion sections of the original report or the conclusions of the original study. The title and the conclusions of this secondary abstract are typically the product of critical appraisal by individuals for whom competing financial or personal interests will be minimal or absent.

Compare, for example, the *ACP Journal Club* abstract and commentary with that of the full publication of an important trial[22] that addressed the prevention of stroke.[23] The title of the original publication describes the study as testing "a perindopril-based blood pressure lowering regimen," and the article reports that the perindopril-containing regimen resulted in a 28% *relative risk reduction* (RRR) in the risk of recurrent stroke (95% CI, 17%-38%).[23]

The *ACP Journal Club* abstract and its accompanying commentary identified the publication as describing 2 parallel but separate randomized *placebo*-controlled trials, including approximately 6100 patients with a history of stroke or transient ischemic attack. In the first trial, patients were randomized to receive perindopril or placebo; active treatment had no appreciable effect on stroke (RRR, 5%; 95% CI, −19% to 23%). In the second trial, patients were allocated to receive perindopril plus indapamide or double placebo. Combined treatment resulted in a 43% RRR (95% CI, 30%-54%) in recurrent stroke. The *ACP Journal Club* commentary notes that the authors, in communication with the editors, refused to accept the interpretation of the publication as reporting 2 separate RCTs (which explains why it is difficult for even the knowledgeable reader to get a clear picture of the design from the original publication).

The objectivity and methodologic sophistication of those preparing the independent structured abstracts may provide additional value for clinicians. We suggest reviewing the structured abstract of any article that appears in high-quality preappraised secondary publications. We do not claim perfection of this methodologic review: residual hidden bias or misleading presentation may elude the methodologists. Nevertheless, the resource is certain, on occasion, to help.

3. Beware Large Treatment Effects in Trials With Only a Few Events

Clinicians should be skeptical of large treatment effects from trials that are stopped early with few events (see Chapter 11.3, Randomized Trials Stopped Early for Benefit). In addition, clinicians should be cautious about an unusually large effect (eg, an RRR >50%) from a study with few events (eg, <100). One reason to be cautious is that investigators may not have had a formal *stopping rule* applied to *stopped early trials* but may have been taking repeated looks at their data and chose to stop early when they saw a large effect. If this is the case, neither the nominal *P* value nor the CI is valid.

Very large effects are implausible because multiple mechanisms underlie most diseases, and therapies typically address only 1 or 2 of those mechanisms.[24] The complementary success of angiotensin-converting enzyme (ACE) inhibitors, antiplatelet agents, lipid-lowering agents, and β-blockers in reducing cardiac events in patients with myocardial infarction (MI) illustrates this multiplicity of disease mechanisms. Predictably, each agent offers only a modest magnitude of risk reduction (from 20% to 33%).

An empirical evaluation of more than 85 000 meta-analytic *forest plots* from 3082 systematic reviews indicates that in almost 10% of the analyses, the first trial had *statistically significant* results and a very large effect, but the conduct of subsequent studies almost always revealed a much smaller treatment effect.[25]

For example, a study conducted in 1997 aimed to determine the efficacy and safety of an angiotensin II receptor blocker (ARB) compared with an ACE inhibitor in patients with heart failure.[26] This trial randomized 772 patients and found a 46% RRR in death when receiving ARB treatment (*P* = .03). However, only 49 events were observed. Subsequently, a large RCT that recruited 3152 participants found no benefit on mortality for the same comparison.[27] A larger trial of 5477 patients with congestive heart failure was unable to find statistically significant higher mortality with ARB treatment (RR, 1.13; 95% CI, 0.99-1.28; *P* = .07).[28] Finally, a Cochrane systematic review that included 22 studies and more than 17 000 patients found that ARBs, compared with ACEs, have a similar effect on mortality (RR, 1.05; 95% CI, 0.91-1.22; *P* = .48).[29] Thus, evidence of promising large treatment effects from small—or even not so small—RCTs should be used cautiously. The possibility that further and larger trials or meta-analyses can contradict early results cannot be discarded.[24]

Consider another RCT that assessed the effects of β-blockers in 112 participants undergoing surgery for peripheral vascular diseases that was stopped early.[30] Of 59 patients who received the intervention, 2 had a major event (perioperative mortality or nonfatal MI) compared with 18 of 53 patients who received standard care (RR, 0.10; 95% CI, 0.02-0.41). With only 20 events in total, the study results suggested a large treatment effect—a 90% RRR.

Although the CI is precise, conclusions derived from this very large treatment effect estimated from a trial that was stopped early with a small sample size and only 20 events warrant extreme caution (see Chapter 11.3, Randomized Trials Stopped Early for Benefit). Another reason for questioning the trial results emerged subsequently because the trial was identified as a possible case of research misconduct.[30] Box 13.3-2 presents 6 reasons to be cautious about adopting new treatments on the basis of initial promising results, including the possibility of subsequent discovery of research misconduct.

It is not only individual trials that sometimes provide potentially misleading large estimates of effect on the basis of relatively small numbers of events—this is also true of systematic reviews and meta-analyses. Consider a systematic review of RCTs that evaluated antibiotic prophylaxis in neutropenic patients and concluded that prophylaxis with fluoroquinolones reduces the risk of infection-related mortality by an impressive 62% (RR, 0.38; 95% CI, 0.21-0.69; $P = .001$).[31] In total, 1022 patients were included in this meta-analysis with only 47 events. If a trialist were planning to conduct an RCT to answer the same clinical question, a minimum sample size of 6400 participants would be required to detect a 25% RRR in infection-related mortality (assuming $\alpha = 0.05$, $\beta = 0.20$, and a *control event rate* of 7%). We call the sample size required for a single trial anticipating a modest treatment effect the *optimal information size* (OIS). The fact that the total sample size in this meta-analysis (n = 1022) is substantially smaller than the OIS (n = 6400), the remarkable 62% RRR in mortality and the relatively small number of events (n = 47) all support skepticism regarding the results.

One final consideration is the concept of fragility, which refers to how the inferences from a clinical trial might differ if one changed just a few events to nonevents or vice versa. One can apply the fragility concept to the second Leicester Intravenous Magnesium Intervention Trial (LIMIT-2), which assessed the effect of intravenous magnesium in 2316 participants with suspected acute MI.[32] Of 1159 patients receiving the intervention, 90 died, compared with 118 of 1157 in the placebo group (RRR, 24%; 95% CI, 1%-43%). Although in this trial the treatment effect is relatively modest with quite a few events (ie, >100 events), the results still can be misleading,

---

BOX 13.3-2

Reasons for Being Cautious in Adopting New Interventions

1. Initial studies may be biased by inadequacies in concealment, blinding, loss to follow-up, or stopping early.

2. Initial studies are particularly susceptible to reporting bias.

3. Initial studies are particularly susceptible to dissemination bias; markedly positive studies are likely to receive disproportionate attention.

4. Initial studies may overestimate effects by chance (particularly if effects are large and the number of events is small).

5. There is a substantial probability (20%) that serious adverse effects will emerge subsequently (cyclooxygenase 2 inhibitors provide a notable example).

6. On rare occasions, research results will prove to have been fraudulent.

---

as a subsequent trial has demonstrated (Fourth International Study of Infarct Survival).[33]

If one considers how the results of LIMIT-2 might change if only a few events were missed in the intervention group (eg, due to losses to follow-up, assessor bias, or chance), the CI would quickly move toward the null. In LIMIT-2, if only 2 events were missed in the intervention group, the results would lose their statistical significance. Therefore, when the number of events required to move the P value past the conventional threshold for statistical significance is small, one should be cautious of believing that a treatment effect truly exists.

The implication is clear: beware of large effects with a small number of events because the results are likely to be misleading. Be careful even with larger events and a modest sample size because study results can still be fragile. Statistical simulations suggest that—in the face of substantial adverse effects, burden, or cost—changes in practice should generally wait until at least 1 replication has been reported with at least 300 events across the available studies (see also Guide 7 in this chapter).[34]

THERAPY

4. Beware Faulty Comparators

Industry-funded studies typically yield larger treatment effects than studies funded by nonprofit organizations.[3,16,17,35,36] One major explanation is choice of comparators.[37] The use of a placebo and no treatment as comparators is common, even when RCTs have established the effectiveness of active treatments.[38]

This frequent use of placebo/no-treatment comparators when effective treatments are available results in very limited availability of head-to-head comparisons of what are otherwise considered first-choice treatments.[39] The biased choice of comparators extends to meta-analyses of randomized trials, where the focus may be on trying to make a case to promote specific agents.[40] Box 13.3-3 lists the types of faulty comparators in studies to which clinicians should be alert.

A study of 136 trials new treatments for multiple myeloma provides an illustration of likely industry bias in the choice of comparators. Of the trials funded by for-profit entities, 60% compared their new interventions against placebo or no treatment; this was true of only 21% of trials funded by nonprofit organizations.[35]

In another example, 3 important trials of ARBs for patients with diabetic nephropathy used placebo—rather than ACE inhibitors, which have demonstrated

effectiveness—as the control management strategy.[41-43] The accompanying editorial suggested that the economic interests of the sponsor dictated that choice of comparator. The sponsors may have avoided an ACE inhibitor control group because "…sales of angiotensin-receptor blockers would be lower if the 2 classes of drugs proved equally effective."[44]

Choice of dose and administration regimen also can result in misleading comparisons,[45] such as would result if less effective or more toxic agents rather than the best ones available were included in a study or if a trial included the best available agent but in excessively small or excessively large doses.

For example, Safer[45] identified 8 trials sponsored by 3 drug companies that compared newer second-generation neuroleptic agents with a fixed high dose (20 mg/d; optimal dosing, <12 mg/d[46]) of haloperidol. Not surprisingly, these trials found that patients who used the new agents had fewer extrapyramidal adverse effects. Safer[45] offers another example in which a study compared paroxetine against amitriptyline, a sedating tricyclic antidepressant. The trial administered amitriptyline twice daily, possibly leading to excessive daytime somnolence.[47] In a separate example, Johansen and Gotzsche[48] noted the use of an ineffective comparator (nystatin) and the use of an inadequate and unusual administration route (oral amphotericin B, poorly absorbed in the gastrointestinal tract) as comparators in RCTs of the efficacy of antifungals in patients with cancer and neutropenia.

When reading reports of RCTs with active comparators, clinicians should ask whether the comparator should have been another active agent rather than placebo. If the comparator was an active agent, the question is whether the dose, formulation, and administration regimen was optimal.

5. Beware Small Treatment Effects and Extrapolation to Very Low-Risk Patients

Pharmaceutical companies are conducting very large RCTs to be able to exclude chance as an explanation for small treatment effects. Results are consistent with small treatment effects when either the point estimate is very close to no effect (an RRR or *absolute risk reduction* [ARR] close to 0; an RR or OR close to 1) or the CI includes values close to no effect.

BOX 13.3-3
Faulty Comparators

- Comparison with placebo when effective agents are available
- Comparison with less effective agents when more effective comparators are available
- Comparison with more toxic agents when less toxic comparators are available
- Comparison with too low a dose (or inadequate dose titration) of an otherwise effective comparator, leading to misleading claims of effectiveness
- Comparison with a too high (and thus toxic) dose (or inadequate dose titration) of an otherwise safe comparator, leading to misleading claims of lower toxicity

For example, in a very large trial of antihypertensive regimens, investigators randomly allocated more than 6000 individuals to receive ACE inhibitor therapy vs diuretic agents and concluded "initiation of antihypertensive treatment involving ACE inhibitors in older subjects ... appears to lead to better outcomes than treatment with diuretic agents...."[49] In absolute terms, however, the difference between the regimens was small: there were 4.2 events per 100 patient-years and 4.6 events per 100 patient-years in the ACE inhibitor and diuretic groups, respectively. The corresponding RRR of 11% had an associated 95% CI of −1% to 21%.

In this case, we have 2 reasons to doubt the importance of the apparent difference between treatment groups. First, the point estimate suggests a small *absolute difference* (0.4 events per 100 patient-years), and second, the CI suggests it may have been even smaller. Indeed, there may have been no true difference at all.

There are a variety of strategies that investigators and sponsors use to create a spurious impression of a large treatment effect (Box 13.3-4). When the absolute risk of adverse events in untreated patients—the *baseline risk*—is low, you are likely to see a presentation that focuses on RRR and deemphasizes or ignores ARR. The focus on RRR conveys a spurious sense of the importance of the result.

For instance, the European Trial on the Reduction of Cardiac Events with Perindopril in Stable Coronary Artery Disease (EUROPA) found a reduction in MI with perindopril in patients who survived a previous MI and was hailed as a breakthrough. The RRR in MI of 22% (95% CI, 10%-33%) translates into an ARR of 1.4% during 4 years. Thus, clinicians must treat approximately 70 patients for 4 years to prevent a single MI. In particular, when one considers that most of these patients may already be ingesting aspirin or warfarin, a statin, and a β-blocker to reduce their MI risk, one may question the characterization of the incremental benefit as a breakthrough.

Other techniques complement the use of RRRs in making treatment effects appear large. For visual presentations, beware of *survival curves* in which the x-axis intersects the y-axis much above the 0 level, giving the visual impression of a large effect.[50] Another technique relates to choice of time span for

---

BOX 13.3-4

Strategies for Making a Treatment Effect Appear Larger Than It Is

1. Use relative rather than absolute risk; a 50% relative risk reduction may mean a decrease in risk from 1% to 0.5%.

2. Express risk during a long period; the reduction in risk from 1% to 0.5% may occur during 10 years.

3. For visual presentations, make sure the x-axis intersects the y-axis well above 0; if the x-axis intersects the y-axis at 60%, you can make an improvement from 70% to 75% appear as a 33% increase in survival.

4. Include a few high-risk patients in a trial of predominantly low-risk patients; even though most events occur in high-risk individuals, claim important benefits for a large number of low-risk patients in the general population.

5. Ignore the lower boundary of the confidence interval (CI); when the lower boundary of the CI around the relative risk reduction approaches 0, declare significance and henceforth focus exclusively on the point estimate.

6. Focus on statistical significance; when a result achieves statistical significance but both relative and absolute effects are small, highlight the statistical significance and downplay or ignore the magnitude.

---

presenting treatment effect: long periods for effects that investigators or sponsors wish to make appear large and short ones for those they wish to make appear small.

For instance, McCormack and Greenhalgh[51] pointed out that report 33 of the UK Prospective Diabetes Study trial[52] expressed the risk of severe hypoglycemia as the percentage of participants per year (eg, 2.3% per year for patients receiving insulin). This contrasts with the expression of the benefits as the percentage of participants during 10 years (eg, 3.2% absolute reduction in the risk of any diabetes-related *end points*). By choosing to express harms during a short period (per year) and benefits during a long

THERAPY

period (a decade), the presentation obscures the fact that the absolute increase in frequency of hypoglycemia with intensive glycemic control is approximately 7 times the absolute reduction in diabetes complications.

A shift of the target study population to include very low-risk patients means a potentially major expansion in market size for the agent and a consequently larger effect on health care costs associated with small and possibly marginal gains in health. In the past few years, several professional societies have decreased the threshold for diagnosis and treatment of hypertension, diabetes, and hyperlipidemia, which has increased the proportion of people eligible for treatment.[53,54] Even if RCTs reveal benefits in populations that include such very low-risk patients, the number of events in very low-risk patients is typically few, and the results of such trials are driven entirely by a few higher-risk patients.[55]

Whenever relative or absolute benefits are small or the lower boundary of the CI approaches no effect, the treatment benefits and the potential *harm*, inconveniences, and costs are likely to be, at best, finely balanced. Judicious rather than routine administration of new drugs under these circumstances is likely to best serve patient needs and represent prudent allocation of health care resources.

6. Beware Uneven Emphasis on Benefits and Harms

Clinical decision making requires a balanced interpretation of both benefits and harms associated with any intervention. Unfortunately, many clinical trials neglect even the minimal reporting of harm.[56,57] In an analysis of trials from 7 areas, investigators found that the space allocated to harms was slightly less than the space allocated to the names of authors and their affiliations.[56] Even when investigators report some information regarding harms, failure to present event rates in treatment and control groups, omission of severity of the events, or inappropriate combining of disparate events can compromise sensible interpretation. Despite some improvement in reporting of harms over time in some areas, most fields continue to devote suboptimal attention to intervention harms.[58]

For example, a trial of intravenous immunoglobulin in advanced human immunodeficiency virus infection that was stopped early because of efficacy failed to mention any adverse events.[59] In this trial, omission of harm data compounds problems associated with early discontinuation (see Chapter 11.3, Randomized Trials Stopped Early for Benefit). In another example, a placebo-controlled trial of nabumetone for rheumatoid arthritis stated that "the adverse experience profiles were similar for both treatment groups," with no further information concerning the nature of the adverse effects.[60]

7. Wait for the Overall Results to Emerge; Do Not Rush

Many clinical specialties move at a high speed in terms of introducing new treatments, diagnostics, and other interventions. Although this is exciting and often may improve patient outcomes, problems will arise if clinicians adopt interventions prematurely. The most common problem is that early claims of efficacy or efficiency are exaggerated. As clinical studies accumulate, it is more common for effects to shrink than to increase.[25,61-63]

An initial study may reveal a very large effect, and when the next study reveals a negligible or even negative effect, the result is controversy. This scenario is most commonly observed in molecular medicine studies, in which turnaround of information can be fast and proposed hypotheses can be rejected rapidly. Subsequent studies of the same question may reveal intermediate results between these 2 extremes.[64,65]

For example, an article in 1994 reported that a variant of the vitamin D receptor gene explains most of the population risk for having low bone-mineral density (ie, weak bones prone to fracture).[66] The finding made the cover page of *Nature*, which heralded the "osteoporosis gene." Other subsequent studies revealed an opposite effect with the same variant predisposing to stronger bones. A subsequent large-scale analysis of 100-fold more participants than the original *Nature* study revealed that there is no effect at all.[67]

Another reason to wait for more evidence is that RCTs do not enroll sufficient patients or have sufficiently long follow-up to permit detection of relatively uncommon, serious adverse events, particularly if those adverse events occur not uncommonly in the absence of the intervention (such as MIs that occur without exposure to cyclooxygenase 2 inhibitors).[68] For example, approximately 20% of drugs that the US Food and Drug Administration (FDA) licenses are either withdrawn from the market or have major safety warnings added to the drug labels within 25 years of initial licensing.[69]

In 2006, the DREAM (Diabetes Reduction Assessment with Ramipril and Rosiglitazone Medication) study reported that the use of rosiglitazone at 8 mg/d for 3 years, compared with placebo, "reduces incident type 2 diabetes (HR, 0.38; 95% CI, 0.33 to 0.44) and increases the likelihood of regression to normoglycemia in adults with impaired fasting glucose or impaired glucose tolerance, or both." The study also reported, however, a higher although nonsignificant increased risk of MI (*hazard ratio* [HR], 1.66; 95% CI, 0.73-3.80).[70] Two subsequent systematic reviews[70,71] that included more than 35 000 patients provided additional evidence that rosiglitazone increases the risk of MI events (OR, 1.43; 95% CI, 1.03-1.98; $P = .03$[72]; and OR, 1.28; 95% CI, 1.02-1.63; $P = .04$[73]).

A final reason to wait is that evidence of serious misrepresentation of results may emerge. For instance, the original published report of a trial that investigated the toxicity of anti-inflammatory drugs contained 6-month data and indicated that celecoxib caused fewer symptomatic ulcers and ulcer complications than diclofenac or ibuprofen.[74] However, when the FDA reviewed the 12-month data from both trials, the result was inconclusive: the RR for ulcer complications in patients receiving celecoxib and in patients receiving ibuprofen or diclofenac was 0.83 (95% CI, 0.46-1.50).[75] The authors explained their omission on the basis of large differential loss to follow-up, particularly of high-risk patients in the diclofenac arm, after 6 months.[76] Fortunately, such egregious instances of misleading presentations of evidence are rare.

Box 13.3-2 provides a number of reasons for caution in adopting new interventions. In every case in which new promising interventions are available, the clinician should balance the risk of offering potentially suboptimal management by using the established intervention vs prematurely offering the new intervention that may be less effective than advertised or may be associated with as yet undisclosed or unknown toxicity. The decision is not easy, particularly because clinicians face both marketing pressures and peer pressure to be up-to-date according to what is reported in scientific meetings and medical journals. Indeed, many may perceive themselves as practicing *evidence-based medicine* when they adopt the newest therapy tested in a recently published RCT.

CONCLUSION

We have presented 7 guides for users that can help clinicians protect themselves and their patients from potentially misleading presentations and interpretations of data in the medical literature. These strategies are unlikely to be foolproof. Decreasing the dependence of the research endeavor and regulatory agencies on industry funding, improving adherence with complete registration of clinical trials and disclosure of the results, and instituting more structured approaches to the peer review and reporting of research[77,78] may decrease the magnitude of misleading reporting to which clinicians must be alert. At the same time, potentially misleading reporting will always be present, and prudent clinicians need critical appraisal tools, including the 7 guides outlined in this chapter.

THERAPY

References

1. Horton R. The rhetoric of research. *BMJ*. 1995;310(6985):985-987.
2. Trotter G. Why were the benefits of tPA exaggerated? *West J Med*. 2002;176(3):194-197.
3. Buchkowsky SS, Jewesson PJ. Industry sponsorship and authorship of clinical trials over 20 years. *Ann Pharmacother*. 2004;38(4):579-585.
4. LaRosa SP. Conflict of interest: authorship issues predominate. *Arch Intern Med*. 2002;162(14):1646.
5. Davidoff F, DeAngelis CD, Drazen JM, et al. Sponsorship, authorship, and accountability. *N Engl J Med*. 2001;345(11):825-827.
6. Bodenheimer T. Uneasy alliance: clinical investigators and the pharmaceutical industry. *N Engl J Med*. 2000;342(20): 1539-1544.
7. Yank V, Rennie D, Bero LA. Financial ties and concordance between results and conclusions in meta-analyses: retrospective cohort study. *BMJ*. 2007;335(7631):1202-1205.

8. Brignardello-Petersen R, Carrasco-Labra A, Yanine N, et al. Positive association between conflicts of interest and reporting of positive results in randomized clinical trials in dentistry. *J Am Dent Assoc.* 2013;144(10):1165-1170.

9. Safer DJ. Design and reporting modifications in industry-sponsored comparative psychopharmacology trials. *J Nerv Ment Dis.* 2002;190(9):583-592.

10. Bero LA, Rennie D. Influences on the quality of published drug studies. *Int J Technol Assess Health Care.* 1996;12(2):209-237.

11. Wilkes MM, Navickis RJ. Patient survival after human albumin administration: a meta-analysis of randomized, controlled trials. *Ann Intern Med.* 2001;135(3):149-164.

12. Alderson P, Bunn F, Lefebvre C, et al. Human albumin solution for resuscitation and volume expansion in critically ill patients. *Cochrane Database Syst Rev.* 2002;(1):CD001208.

13. Cook D, Guyatt G. Colloid use for fluid resuscitation: evidence and spin. *Ann Intern Med.* 2001;135(3):205-208.

14. Als-Nielsen B, Chen W, Gluud C, Kjaergard LL. Association of funding and conclusions in randomized drug trials: a reflection of treatment effect or adverse events? *JAMA.* 2003;290(7):921-928.

15. Bhandari M, Busse JW, Jackowski D, et al. Association between industry funding and statistically significant pro-industry findings in medical and surgical randomized trials. *CMAJ.* 2004;170(4):477-480.

16. Lexchin J, Bero LA, Djulbegovic B, Clark O. Pharmaceutical industry sponsorship and research outcome and quality: systematic review. *BMJ.* 2003;326(7400):1167-1170.

17. Bekelman JE, Li Y, Gross CP. Scope and impact of financial conflicts of interest in biomedical research: a systematic review. *JAMA.* 2003;289(4):454-465.

18. Jørgensen AW, Hilden J, Gøtzsche PC. Cochrane reviews compared with industry supported meta-analyses and other meta-analyses of the same drugs: systematic review. *BMJ.* 2006;333(7572):782.

19. Stamatakis E, Weiler R, Ioannidis JP. Undue industry influences that distort healthcare research, strategy, expenditure and practice: a review. *Eur J Clin Invest.* 2013;43(5):469-475.

20. Devereaux PJ, Manns BJ, Ghali WA, Quan H, Guyatt GH. Reviewing the reviewers: the quality of reporting in three secondary journals. *CMAJ.* 2001;164(11):1573-1576.

21. Boutron I, Dutton S, Ravaud P, Altman DG. Reporting and interpretation of randomized controlled trials with statistically nonsignificant results for primary outcomes. *JAMA.* 2010;303(20):2058-2064.

22. Tirschwell D. Combined therapy with indapamide and perindopril but not perindopril alone reduced the risk for recurrent stroke. *ACP J Club.* 2002;136(2):51.

23. PROGRESS Collaborative Group. Randomised trial of a perindopril-based blood-pressure-lowering regimen among 6,105 individuals with previous stroke or transient ischaemic attack. *Lancet.* 2001;358(9287):1033-1041.

24. Devereaux PJ, Yusuf S. The evolution of the randomized controlled trial and its role in evidence-based decision making. *J Intern Med.* 2003;254(2):105-113.

25. Pereira TV, Horwitz RI, Ioannidis JP. Empirical evaluation of very large treatment effects of medical interventions. *JAMA.* 2012;308(16):1676-1684.

26. Pitt B, Segal R, Martinez FA, et al. Randomised trial of losartan versus captopril in patients over 65 with heart failure (Evaluation of Losartan in the Elderly Study, ELITE). *Lancet.* 1997;349(9054):747-752.

27. Pitt B, Poole-Wilson PA, Segal R, et al. Effect of losartan compared with captopril on mortality in patients with symptomatic heart failure: randomised trial: the Losartan Heart Failure Survival Study ELITE II. *Lancet.* 2000;355(9215):1582-1587.

28. Dickstein K, Kjekshus J; OPTIMAAL Steering Committee of the OPTIMAAL Study Group. Effects of losartan and captopril on mortality and morbidity in high-risk patients after acute myocardial infarction: the OPTIMAAL randomised trial. Optimal Trial in Myocardial Infarction with Angiotensin II Antagonist Losartan. *Lancet.* 2002;360(9335):752-760.

29. Heran BS, Musini VM, Bassett K, Taylor RS, Wright JM. Angiotensin receptor blockers for heart failure. *Cochrane Database Syst Rev.* 2012;4(4):CD003040. doi:10.1002/14651858.CD003040.pub2.

30. Poldermans D, Boersma E, Bax JJ, et al; Dutch Echocardiographic Cardiac Risk Evaluation Applying Stress Echocardiography Study Group. The effect of bisoprolol on perioperative mortality and myocardial infarction in high-risk patients undergoing vascular surgery. *N Engl J Med.* 1999;341(24):1789-1794.

31. Gafter-Gvili A, Fraser A, Paul M, Leibovici L. Meta-analysis: antibiotic prophylaxis reduces mortality in neutropenic patients. *Ann Intern Med.* 2005;142(12, pt 1):979-995.

32. Woods KL, Fletcher S, Roffe C, Haider Y. Intravenous magnesium sulphate in suspected acute myocardial infarction: results of the second Leicester Intravenous Magnesium Intervention Trial (LIMIT-2). *Lancet.* 1992;339(8809):1553-1558.

33. ISIS-4 (Fourth International Study of Infarct Survival) Collaborative Group. ISIS-4: a randomised factorial trial assessing early oral captopril, oral mononitrate, and intravenous magnesium sulphate in 58,050 patients with suspected acute myocardial infarction. *Lancet.* 1995;345(8951):669-685.

34. Guyatt GH, Oxman AD, Kunz R, et al. GRADE guidelines 6: rating the quality of evidence–imprecision. *J Clin Epidemiol.* 2011;64(12):1283-1293.

35. Djulbegovic B, Lacevic M, Cantor A, et al. The uncertainty principle and industry-sponsored research. *Lancet.* 2000;356(9230):635-638.

36. Bero L, Oostvogel F, Bacchetti P, Lee K. Factors associated with findings of published trials of drug-drug comparisons: why some statins appear more efficacious than others. *PLoS Med.* 2007;4(6):e184.

37. Mann H, Djulbegovic B. *Biases Due to Differences in the Treatments Selected for Comparison (Comparator Bias).* Oxford, UK: James Lind Library: Library and Information Services Department of the Royal College of Physicians of Edinburgh; 2003.

38. Tonelli AR, Zein J, Ioannidis JP. Geometry of the randomized evidence for treatments of pulmonary hypertension. *Cardiovasc Ther.* 2013;31(6):e138-e146.

39. Kappagoda S, Ioannidis JP. Neglected tropical diseases: survey and geometry of randomised evidence. *BMJ.* 2012;345:e6512. doi:10.1136/bmj.e6512.

40. Haidich AB, Pilalas D, Contopoulos-Ioannidis DG, Ioannidis JP. Most meta-analyses of drug interventions have narrow scopes and many focus on specific agents. *J Clin Epidemiol.* 2013;66(4):371-378.

41. Parving H-H, Lehnert H, Bröchner-Mortensen J, Gomis R, Andersen S, Arner P; Irbesartan in Patients with Type 2 Diabetes and Microalbuminuria Study Group. The effect of irbesartan on the development of diabetic nephropathy in patients with type 2 diabetes. *N Engl J Med.* 2001;345(12):870-878.

42. Brenner BM, Cooper ME, de Zeeuw D, et al; RENAAL Study Investigators. Effects of losartan on renal and cardiovascular outcomes in patients with type 2 diabetes and nephropathy. *N Engl J Med.* 2001;345(12):861-869.

43. Lewis EJ, Hunsicker LG, Clarke WR, et al; Collaborative Study Group. Renoprotective effect of the angiotensin-receptor antagonist irbesartan in patients with nephropathy due to type 2 diabetes. *N Engl J Med.* 2001;345(12):851-860.

44. Hostetter TH. Prevention of end-stage renal disease due to type 2 diabetes. *N Engl J Med.* 2001;345(12):910-912.

45. Safer DJ. Design and reporting modifications in industry-sponsored comparative psychopharmacology trials. *J Nerv Ment Dis.* 2002;190(9):583-592.

46. Geddes J, Freemantle N, Harrison P, Bebbington P. Atypical antipsychotics in the treatment of schizophrenia: systematic overview and meta-regression analysis. *BMJ.* 2000;321(7273):1371-1376.

47. Christiansen PE, Behnke K, Black CH, Ohrström JK, Bork-Rasmussen H, Nilsson J. Paroxetine and amitriptyline in the treatment of depression in general practice. *Acta Psychiatr Scand.* 1996;93(3):158-163.

48. Johansen HK, Gotzsche PC. Problems in the design and reporting of trials of antifungal agents encountered during meta-analysis. *JAMA.* 1999;282(18):1752-1759.

49. Wing LM, Reid CM, Ryan P, et al; Second Australian National Blood Pressure Study Group. A comparison of outcomes with angiotensin-converting—enzyme inhibitors and diuretics for hypertension in the elderly. *N Engl J Med.* 2003;348(7):583-592.

50. Pocock SJ, Clayton TC, Altman DG. Survival plots of time-to-event outcomes in clinical trials: good practice and pitfalls. *Lancet.* 2002;359(9318):1686-1689.

51. McCormack J, Greenhalgh T. Seeing what you want to see in randomised controlled trials: versions and perversions of UKPDS data. United Kingdom prospective diabetes study. *BMJ.* 2000;320(7251):1720-1723.

52. UK Prospective Diabetes Study (UKPDS) Group. Intensive blood-glucose control with sulphonylureas or insulin compared with conventional treatment and risk of complications in patients with type 2 diabetes (UKPDS 33). *Lancet.* 1998;352(9131):837-853.

53. Thorpe KE. The rise in health care spending and what to do about it. *Health Aff (Millwood).* 2005;24(6):1436-1445.

54. Thorpe KE, Florence CS, Howard DH, Joski P. The rising prevalence of treated disease: effects on private health insurance spending. *Health affairs (Project Hope).* Jan-Jun 2005;Suppl Web Exclusives:W5-317-w315-325.

55. Ioannidis JP, Lau J. The impact of high-risk patients on the results of clinical trials. *J Clin Epidemiol.* 1997;50(10):1089-1098.

56. Ioannidis JP, Lau J. Completeness of safety reporting in randomized trials: an evaluation of 7 medical areas. *JAMA.* 2001;285(4):437-443.

57. Ioannidis JP, Evans SJ, Gøtzsche PC, et al; CONSORT Group. Better reporting of harms in randomized trials: an extension of the CONSORT statement. *Ann Intern Med.* 2004;141(10):781-788.

58. Ioannidis JP. Adverse events in randomized trials: neglected, restricted, distorted, and silenced. *Arch Intern Med.* 2009;169(19):1737-1739.

59. Kiehl MG, Stoll R, Broder M, Mueller C, Foerster EC, Domschke W. A controlled trial of intravenous immune globulin for the prevention of serious infections in adults with advanced human immunodeficiency virus infection. *Arch Intern Med.* 1996;156(22):2545-2550.

60. Lanier BG, Turner RA Jr, Collins RL, Senter RG Jr. Evaluation of nabumetone in the treatment of active adult rheumatoid arthritis. *Am J Med.* 1987;83(4B):40-43.

61. Ioannidis JP. Contradicted and initially stronger effects in highly cited clinical research. *JAMA.* 2005;294(2):218-228.

62. Pereira TV, Ioannidis JP. Statistically significant meta-analyses of clinical trials have modest credibility and inflated effects. *J Clin Epidemiol.* 2011;64(10):1060-1069.

63. Trikalinos TA, Churchill R, Ferri M, et al; EU-PSI project. Effect sizes in cumulative meta-analyses of mental health randomized trials evolved over time. *J Clin Epidemiol.* 2004;57(11):1124-1130.

64. Ioannidis JP, Trikalinos TA. Early extreme contradictory estimates may appear in published research: the Proteus phenomenon in molecular genetics research and randomized trials. *J Clin Epidemiol.* 2005;58(6):543-549.

65. Ioannidis J, Lau J. Evolution of treatment effects over time: empirical insight from recursive cumulative metaanalyses. *Proc Natl Acad Sci U S A.* 2001;98(3):831-836.

66. Morrison NA, Qi JC, Tokita A, et al. Prediction of bone density from vitamin D receptor alleles. *Nature.* 1994;367(6460):284-287.

67. Uitterlinden AG, Weel AE, Burger H, et al. Interaction between the vitamin D receptor gene and collagen type Ialpha1 gene in susceptibility for fracture. *J Bone Miner Res.* 2001;16(2):379-385.

68. Hippisley-Cox J, Coupland C. Risk of myocardial infarction in patients taking cyclo-oxygenase-2 inhibitors or conventional non-steroidal anti-inflammatory drugs: population based nested case-control analysis. *BMJ.* 2005;330(7504):1366.

69. Lasser KE, Allen PD, Woolhandler SJ, Himmelstein DU, Wolfe SM, Bor DH. Timing of new black box warnings and withdrawals for prescription medications. *JAMA.* 2002;287(17):2215-2220.

70. Gerstein HC, Yusuf S, Bosch J, et al; DREAM (Diabetes REduction Assessment with ramipril and rosiglitazone Medication) Trial Investigators. Effect of rosiglitazone on the frequency of diabetes in patients with impaired glucose tolerance or impaired fasting glucose: a randomised controlled trial. *Lancet.* 2006;368(9541):1096-1105.

71. Psaty BM, Furberg CD. The record on rosiglitazone and the risk of myocardial infarction. *N Engl J Med.* 2007;357(1):67-69.

72. Nissen SE, Wolski K. Effect of rosiglitazone on the risk of myocardial infarction and death from cardiovascular causes. *N Engl J Med.* 2007;356(24):2457-2471.

73. Nissen SE, Wolski K. Rosiglitazone revisited: an updated meta-analysis of risk for myocardial infarction and cardiovascular mortality. *Arch Intern Med.* 2010;170(14):1191-1201.

74. Silverstein FE, Faich G, Goldstein JL, et al. Gastrointestinal toxicity with celecoxib vs nonsteroidal anti-inflammatory drugs for osteoarthritis and rheumatoid arthritis: the CLASS study:

THERAPY

a randomized controlled trial. Celecoxib Long-term Arthritis Safety Study. *JAMA.* 2000;284(10):1247-1255.

75. Hrachovec JB, Mora M. Reporting of 6-month vs 12-month data in a clinical trial of celecoxib. *JAMA.* 2001;286(19):2398-2400.

76. Silverstein F, Simon LS, Faich G. Reporting of 6-month vs 12-month data in a clinical trial of celecoxib. *JAMA.* 2001; 286(19):2399-2400.

77. Docherty M, Smith R. The case for structuring the discussion of scientific papers. *BMJ.* 1999;318(7193):1224-1225.

78. Moher D, Schulz KF, Altman DG. The CONSORT statement: revised recommendations for improving the quality of reports of parallel-group randomised trials. *Lancet.* 2001; 357(9263):1191-1194.

13.4

ADVANCED TOPICS IN APPLYING THE RESULTS OF THERAPY TRIALS

Surrogate Outcomes

Heiner C. Bucher, Deborah J. Cook, Anne M. Holbrook, and Gordon Guyatt

THERAPY

IN THIS CHAPTER

You are an internist treating an overweight 56-year-old woman who was diagnosed as having type 2 diabetes mellitus 8 years ago. Her glycosylated hemoglobin (HbA_{1c}) level has not been well controlled (typically at 8.3%) during the past 12 months, despite the fact that she is receiving metformin therapy and you have been providing her with repeated counseling regarding weight and exercise. Her low-density lipoprotein cholesterol (LDL-C) and blood pressure (99 mg/dL and <135/80 mm Hg, respectively) are managed with statin therapy and an angiotensin-converting enzyme (ACE) inhibitor combined with a thiazide diuretic. You are aware that your patient's blood glucose level is too high, but on the basis of previous discussions, you are also aware that she is reluctant to take more medications and that she is opposed to insulin, which may increase her struggles with her weight. Your patient is very astute, and she has asked you about the effect of the medication on complications related to diabetes, including stroke and myocardial infarction.

A colleague has been talking to you about exenatide, a once-weekly injectable glucagon-like peptide 1 receptor agonist, lauding its better control of HbA_{1c} in patients with inadequately controlled type 2 diabetes. He mentions the drug has essentially no *risk* of hypoglycemia and has beneficial effects on weight compared with dipeptidyl peptidase-4 (DPP-4) inhibitors, sulfonylureas, thiazolidinediones, and insulin. Wondering if your patient would agree to an injectable drug in light of the expected advantages, you are optimistic that if improved glucose control with exenatide is also associated with a reduction in macrovascular complications of diabetes, then shared decision making may lead her to try the drug. You, therefore, conduct a literature search to determine what *evidence* is available that addresses this issue.

FINDING THE EVIDENCE

You are aware that research that addresses antidiabetic therapies is voluminous and complex because investigators have tested many treatments, dosages, and combinations of treatments against each other. For a rapid overview, you start with a resource that will summarize existing evidence at a topic-level (see Chapter 5, Finding Current Best Evidence). You opt for UpToDate, type "exenatide," and find the chapter title, "Glucagon-like peptide-1 (GLP-1) based therapies for the treatment of type 2 diabetes mellitus." Among several studies that partially inform your question, the chapter cites a Cochrane *systematic review* on GLP-1 that included 17 *randomized clinical trials* (RCTs) comparing different regimens.[1] Accessing the full review, you browse through included studies for a head-to-head-comparison between exenatide plus metformin vs metformin alone that reports *patient-important outcomes*, such as cardiovascular events. Failing to find such a trial, you identify another one that is rated as having a low *risk of bias* and that compared the glucose-lowering effect of exenatide when added to metformin vs sitagliptin and pioglitazone with HbA_{1c} being the *end point* of interest.[2]

WHAT IS A SURROGATE OUTCOME?

Ideally, clinicians making treatment decisions should refer to methodologically strong RCTs examining the effect of therapy on patient-important outcomes, such as stroke, myocardial infarction, *health-related quality of life* (HRQL), and death. Often, however, conducting these trials requires such a large sample size or extended patient *follow-up* that researchers or drug companies look for alternatives. Substituting laboratory or physiologic measures that are associated with patient-important outcomes (*surrogate end points*) permits researchers to conduct smaller and shorter trials, thus offering a seemingly efficient solution to the dilemma.[3]

Surrogate end points—outcomes that substitute for direct measures of how a patient feels, functions, or survives[4]—may include physiologic or functional variables (eg, HbA_{1c} as a surrogate end point for outcomes related to type 2 diabetes, such as cardiovascular disease; blood pressure as a surrogate end point for stroke; or laboratory exercise capacity as a surrogate end point for HRQL) or measures of subclinical disease (such as degree of atherosclerosis on coronary angiography as a surrogate end point for future myocardial infarction or cardiac death).

The substitution of surrogate end points for patient-important outcomes is attractive when the surrogate can be measured earlier, more easily, more frequently, with higher precision, or with less confounding by competing risks or other therapies. To allow trustworthy inferences about what matters to patients, however, the marker not only has to be statistically correlated with the relevant patient-important outcomes but also must capture, to the greatest extent possible, the net effect of the intervention on those outcomes.[3]

USE OF SURROGATE OUTCOMES: GOOD, BAD, OR INDIFFERENT?

Reliance on surrogate end points may be beneficial or harmful. On the one hand, use of the surrogate end point may lead to rapid and appropriate access to new treatments. For example, the decision and practice of the US Food and Drug Administration to approve new antiretroviral drugs based on information from trials using surrogate end points recognized the need for effective therapies for patients with human immunodeficiency virus (HIV) infection. The first generation of protease inhibitors proved effective in RCTs that focused on patient-important outcomes.[5] More recent trials of antiretroviral drugs from different classes have found effects on surrogate markers of HIV infection, whereas results from cohort studies suggest associated reduction of AIDS and AIDS-related morbidity.[6]

On the other hand, reliance on surrogate end points can be misleading and thus result in excess morbidity and mortality. For instance, flosequinan, milrinone, ibopamine, vesnarinone, and xamoterol all improve surrogate outcomes of hemodynamic function in ambulatory patients with heart failure, but RCTs have found that each of these agents leads to excess mortality (see Chapter 11.2, Surprising Results of Randomized Trials).

How are clinicians to distinguish between valid surrogate markers—those in which a therapy-induced improvement in the surrogate consistently predicts an improvement in a patient-important outcome—and those of questionable *validity*? The approach described in this chapter to critically appraise studies using surrogate end points will help clinicians apply the results of studies that use surrogate end points to the management of individual patients.

Crucial to this determination, clinicians need to assess more than a single study to decide on the adequacy of a surrogate end point. Evaluation may require a systematic review, preferably with a meta-analysis, of *observational studies* of the association between the surrogate end point and the *target end point,* along with the much more important review of some or all of the RCTs that have evaluated treatment effect on both end points. Although most clinicians will not have the time to conduct such an investigation, our guidelines will allow them to evaluate the arguments of experts—or those of the pharmaceutical industry—for prescribing treatments on the basis of their effect on surrogate end points. Our guides, as presented in Box 13.4-1, bear directly on criteria that help clinicians judge whether they can trust results from trials that focus on surrogate end points.

Is There a Strong, Independent, Consistent Association Between the Surrogate Outcome and the Patient-Important Outcome?

To function as a valid substitute for an important target outcome, the surrogate end point must be associated with that target outcome. Often, researchers choose surrogate end points because they have found a *correlation* between a surrogate outcome and a target outcome in observational studies. Their understanding of biologic characteristics gives them confidence that changes in the surrogate will lead to changes in the important outcome. The stronger the association, the more likely it is that there is a link between the surrogate and the target. The strength of an association is reflected in statistical measures such as the *relative risk* (RR) or the *odds ratio* (OR) (see Chapter 9, Does Treatment Lower Risk? Understanding the Results).

Many biologically plausible surrogates are associated only weakly with patient-important outcomes. For example, measures of respiratory function in patients with chronic lung disease—or conventional exercise tests in patients with heart and lung disease—are correlated weakly with the capacity to undertake activities of daily living.[7,8] When correlations are low, the surrogate is likely to be a poor substitute for the target outcome.

In addition to the strength of the association, one's confidence in the validity of the association depends on whether it is consistent across different studies and after adjustment for known *confounding variables*. For example, ecologic studies such as the Seven Countries Study[9] suggested a strong correlation between serum cholesterol levels and coronary heart disease mortality even after adjusting for other predictors such as age, smoking, and systolic blood pressure. When a surrogate is associated with an outcome after adjusting for multiple other potential *prognostic factors*, the association is an *independent association*—although that does not necessarily mean it is causal (see Chapter 15.1, Correlation and Regression). Subsequent large observational studies have confirmed the association between cholesterol and coronary disease mortality in individuals from all continents.[10]

Similarly, cohort studies have consistently revealed that a single measurement of plasma viral load predicts the subsequent risk of AIDS or death in patients with HIV infection.[11-17] For example, in one study, the proportions of patients who progressed to AIDS after 5 years in the lowest through the highest quartiles of viral load were 8%, 26%, 49%, and 62%, respectively.[17] Moreover, this association retained its predictive power after adjustment for other potential predictors, such as CD4 cell count.[11-16] Such strong, consistent, independent associations establish a measure as a potentially useful surrogate.

USING THE GUIDE

For the patient with type 2 diabetes, the question is whether we can substitute HbA_{1c} for the patient-important outcome of a cardiovascular event (fatal or nonfatal myocardial infarction or stroke). Ideally, to establish the association between HbA_{1c} and having a cardiovascular event in type 2 diabetes would require a large cohort in which patients with type 2 diabetes have been followed up from the onset of diabetes to—for some patients—the development of a cardiovascular event. Large cohort studies do reveal an association between the extent of blood glucose control and macrovascular complications.[18,19] In a *meta-analysis* of 13 cohort studies, an absolute increase in HbA_{1c} of 1% was consistently associated with an increased risk for a cardiovascular event of approximately 18% (RR, 1.18; 95% CI, 1.10-1.26).[20] Thus, there is good evidence for an independent and consistent association between increases in HbA_{1c} and unfavorable cardiovascular outcomes.

Have Randomized Trials of the Same Drug Class Shown That Improvement in the Surrogate End Point Has Consistently Led to Improvement in Patient-Important Outcomes?

Meeting the first criterion—a strong, independent association between the surrogate and the patient-important outcome—is necessary, but it is not sufficient to support reliance on a surrogate outcome. Not only must the surrogate outcome be in the causal pathway of the disease process, but also we must be confident that any change in the surrogate with treatment captures all critical effects on patient-important outcomes.[3] This condition will fail if our understanding of the surrogate is limited (eg, the relation is causal in one circumstance but not in the context of the treatment under consideration) or if the treatment either positively or negatively affects morbidity or mortality independent of its effect on the surrogate. Clinical trial history is full of examples of drugs and surgical therapies that had a striking, apparently beneficial effect on a surrogate strongly and independently associated with a patient-important outcome but failed to improve that outcome when tested in RCTs—or indeed, made the outcome worse (see Chapter 11.2, Surprising Results of Randomized Trials).

Because surrogates are so seductive, we review 2 additional striking examples.

Higher levels of high-density lipoprotein cholesterol (HDL-C) are strongly, independently, and consistently associated with a lower incidence of myocardial infarction and cardiovascular death. It logically follows that a drug that increases HDL-C will reduce cardiovascular events. Torcetrapib achieved the desired effect on HDL-C but, despite the satisfactory effect on the surrogate outcome, increased the number of deaths.[21]

Class I antiarrhythmic agents[22] effectively prevented ventricular ectopic beats that are strongly associated with adverse *prognosis* in patients with myocardial infarction.[23] In this case, the clinical community did not wait for the RCTs, and the drugs were widely used in clinical practice. When finally—with considerable delay—an RCT was launched to evaluate the effect of the drugs on morbidity and mortality, the agents increased mortality.[24] Inappropriate reliance on the surrogate end point of suppression of nonlethal arrhythmias is likely to have led to the deaths of thousands of patients.

Before offering an intervention on the basis of effects on a surrogate outcome, clinicians should note a consistent association between surrogate and patient-important outcomes in RCTs. Clinicians are in a stronger position to trust surrogate end points if a new drug belongs to a class of drugs in which RCTs have verified a strong association between surrogate end point and target outcome for all drugs of that class. For example, several large trials of primary and secondary prevention of coronary heart disease with statins have found reductions in adverse cardiovascular outcomes (although even here the results are not completely consistent—see Chapter 28.4, Understanding Class Effects).[25,26] With some hesitation, we may therefore assume a *class effect*—that is, that a new statin such as rosuvastatin with a similar or even more powerful LDL-C–lowering potency also may reduce patient-important outcomes. Even putting aside reservations regarding the consistency of the association, however, the recent experience in observational studies of a 10-fold increase in severe rhabdomyolysis associated with cerivastatin, another statin that had been approved solely on the basis of its lipid-lowering activities,[27] reminds us that reliance on a surrogate for benefit still leaves the issue of toxicity open to serious question.

We would, for 2 reasons, be reluctant to easily generalize these results to another class of lipid-lowering agents. First, the biologic association between the surrogate outcome and the patient-important outcome that exists with one class of agents may not exist with another. For example, bone density is consistently and independently associated with fracture reduction. Furthermore, increased bone density appears to be an important mechanism of fracture reduction with one class of antiosteoporosis drugs, bisphosphonates. Sodium fluoride therapy, however, resulted in treatment-induced increased bone density but to an increase, not decrease, in fractures.[28,29] Generalizing the relation between bone density and fractures with bisphosphonates to another class of drugs, as this example shows, would be a serious mistake.[30]

There is a second reason to hesitate to generalize the association of change in the surrogate outcome and change in the patient-important outcome in one class of drugs to a second class. There may be effects of an agent unrelated to those mediated by the surrogate that influence the patient-important outcome. Consider, for instance, trials that found that a class of anticholesterol agents (fibrates) produced a significant reduction of myocardial infarction but an increased risk of mortality from other causes (gastrointestinal disease) that counteracted this benefit and led to no effect on overall mortality.[25]

This criterion is complicated by various interpretations of the term "drug class." A manufacturer will naturally argue for a broad definition of "class" when its drug fits in a class of agents with a consistent positive association between surrogate and target end points (such as β-blockers in patients who have sustained a myocardial infarction or ACE inhibitors for preventing progression of proteinuric kidney disease). If substances are related to drugs with known or suspected adverse effects on target events (eg, clofibrate or some cyclooxygenase 2 inhibitors), manufacturers are more likely to argue that the chemical or physiologic connection is not sufficiently close for the new drug to be relegated to the same class as the harmful agent (see Chapter 28.4, Understanding Class Effects).

In any case, if there is no relevant evidence that plausibly comes from other drugs of a new class, clinicians must rely on evidence on the association between the surrogate end point and target outcome from between-class comparisons. Inferences from such evidence will be substantially weaker than within-class evidence; conservative, wise practice would delay use of the new drug until evidence of an effect on patient-important outcomes is available.

USING THE GUIDE

Returning to the opening scenario, we have established from observational studies that HbA_{1c} holds the characteristics of a potentially reliable surrogate marker for cardiovascular events. However, there is no evidence that addresses the effect on patient-important outcomes in RCTs comparing GLP-1 agonists and other antidiabetic drugs as an adjunct to metformin. In meta-analyses of RCTs with add-on therapy to metformin, long-acting exenatide and liraglutide led to a greater reduction in HbA_{1c} and body weight in patients with type 2 diabetes with poor HbA_{1c} control than the add-on therapy with sitagliptin, a DPP-4 inhibitor, or pioglitazone.[1,31] Therefore, as the next step, you have to examine the consistency of evidence for a class effect of HbA_{1c} and cardiovascular end points in other contexts.

Have Randomized Trials of Different Drug Classes Shown That Improvement in the Surrogate End Point Has Consistently Led to Improvement in the Patient-Important Outcome?

When evidence on patient-important outcomes within a new class of drugs—as in our example of GLP-1 agonists—is lacking, we must examine the consistency of the change in a surrogate and a patient-important end point across drug classes.

We have already presented the example of the inconsistent association between changes in bone density and fracture reduction in osteoporosis with bisphosphonates vs sodium fluoride.[28] The treatment of heart failure provides a second instructive example. Trials of ACE inhibitors in patients with heart failure have revealed parallel increases in exercise capacity[32-35] and reduction in mortality,[36] suggesting that clinicians may be able to rely on exercise capacity as a valid surrogate. Milrinone (a phosphodiesterase inhibitor[37]) and epoprostenol (a prostaglandin[38]), drugs from different classes, have improved exercise tolerance in patients with symptomatic heart failure. When these drugs were evaluated in RCTs, however, both increased cardiovascular mortality—which in the first case was statistically significant[39] and in the second case led to the trial *stopping early*.[40] Thus, exercise tolerance is inconsistent in predicting improved mortality and is therefore an invalid substitute.

Other suggested surrogate end points in patients with heart failure have included ejection fraction, heart rate variability, and markers of autonomic function.[41] The dopaminergic agent ibopamine positively influences all 3 surrogate end points, yet an RCT found that the drug increases mortality in patients with heart failure, mainly due to ibopamine-induced tachyarrhythmias.[42] Again, the evidence indicates that we cannot rely on ejection fraction, heart rate variability, or markers of autonomic function as trustworthy surrogates.

There is, however, at least one example of appropriate surrogates that have produced consistent effects of within-class and between-class changes for surrogate and patient-important outcomes. For instance, therapy trials in patients with HIV have consistently found that modification of CD4 cell count and complete suppression of HIV-1 RNA plasma viral load are associated with improved patient-important outcomes (Table 13.4-1). Trials that compare different classes of antiretroviral therapies have found that patients randomized to more potent drug regimens had higher CD4 cell counts and higher rates of suppression of HIV-1 viral load and were less likely to progress to AIDS or death.[5,43] Subsequently conducted large cohort studies that investigated new, different antiretroviral drugs have found substantial reductions in AIDS and AIDS-related morbidity.[44] Even though there is no guarantee that the next trial that uses a different class of drugs will reveal the same pattern, these results strengthen our confidence that, for example, a new integrase inhibitor for HIV infection that increases the CD4 cell count and effectively suppresses HIV-1 viral load will result in a reduction in AIDS-related morbidity and mortality.

We must bear in mind, however, that convincing evidence of the validity of the surrogate does not obviate concern about initially inapparent long-term drug toxicity. For instance, the first-generation protease inhibitors lopinavir and indinavir appear to be associated with an increased risk of myocardial infarction, an association not found with the use of nonnucleoside reverse transcriptase inhibitors.[45]

USING THE GUIDE

Returning to our opening clinical scenario, aside from insulin, there are now substances from 6 different classes available for the treatment of type 2 diabetes that are known to lower HbA_{1c} levels.[46] Results of RCTs that addressed patient-important end points are available for metformin, the thiazolidinediones rosiglitazone and pioglitazone, and for saxagliptin and alogliptin, 2 DPP-4 inhibitors.[47,48] These drugs have been compared to different control groups. A systematic review found that monotherapy with metformin was associated with a reduced risk of diabetes-associated and myocardial infarction–related mortality and with a reduced overall mortality.[49] In the UK Prospective Diabetes Study, the early add-on therapy of metformin to sulfonylureas, however, was associated with a relative increase in diabetes-related mortality of 96%.[50] In a systematic review of RCTs that added metformin to insulin, compared with insulin alone, no improved cardiovascular outcomes in type 2 diabetes were found.[51] In another systematic review of RCTs, rosiglitazone was superior in HbA_{1c} reduction compared with the control, but it also was associated with an increased risk of myocardial infarction and congestive heart failure.[52] In yet another systematic review with different inclusion criteria, both rosiglitazone and pioglitazone were associated with increased risk for congestive heart failure—suggesting a class effect due to increased fluid retention.[53] In 2 large *placebo*-controlled RCTs, saxagliptin and alogliptin did not reduce the composite of cardiovascular death, myocardial infarction, or ischemic stroke, and saxagliptin was associated with a higher risk of hospitalization due to congestive heart failure.[47,48] Supporting the results of these studies with specific drugs, a number of trials of tighter vs less tight glucose control in patients with type 2 diabetes, each of which used different strategies for achieving tight control, found that tight control lowers HbA_{1c} levels with no discernible effect on mortality, cardiovascular mortality, or stroke and only a small *relative risk reduction* in myocardial infarction. Thus, there is no consistent

THERAPY

evidence that changes in HbA$_{1c}$ lead to a consistent reduction in cardiovascular events across different antidiabetic drug classes. Indeed, the evidence suggests the contrary.

In Table 13.4-1, we apply our validity criteria to our example of GLP-1 agonists and a number of more recent controversial examples of the use of surrogate end points.

TABLE 13.4-1

Selected Controversial Examples of Applied Validity Criteria for the Critical Evaluation of Studies Using Surrogate End Points

Types of Intervention	Surrogate End Point	Target End Point	Criterion 1	Criterion 2	Criterion 3
			Is there a strong, independent, consistent association between the surrogate end point and the clinical end point?	Is there evidence from randomized trials in the same drug class that improvement in the surrogate end point has consistently led to improvement in the target outcome?	Is there evidence from randomized trials in other drug classes that improvement in the surrogate end point has consistently led to improvement in the target outcome?
Glucagon-like peptide 1 receptor agonist exenatide[2]	HbA$_{1c}$	Cardiovascular event	Yes[18,9]	No[1,31]	No[50-53]
Antilipidemic drug dalcetrabid[57]	HDL-C	Cardiovascular event†	Yes[58,59]	No[57]	No[60,61]
Antilipidemic drug rosuvastatin[62,63]	Cholesterol reduction or LDL-C reduction	Myocardial infarction or death from myocardial infarction	Yes[9,64]	Yes[25]	No[25]
Folic acid plus vitamins B$_6$ and B$_{12}$[65]	Homocysteine	Cardiovascular event[b]	Yes[66-69]	No [65,70,71]	No[72c]
Proteinase inhibitor[a] atazanavir[73]	HIV-1 viral plasma load	AIDS or death	Yes[11-16]	Yes[5,43]	Yes[74]
Proteinase inhibitor[a] atazanavir[73] or darunavir[75]	CD4 cell count	AIDS or death	Yes[11-16]	Yes[5,43]	Yes[74]

Abbreviations: HbA$_{1c}$, glycosylated hemoglobin; HDL-C, high-density lipoprotein cholesterol; HIV, human immunodeficiency virus; LDL-C, low-density lipoprotein cholesterol.

[a]In combination therapy with 2 reverse-transcription inhibitors.

[b]Death from coronary heart disease, nonfatal myocardial infarction, ischemic stroke, unstable angina, or cardiac arrest with resuscitation.

[c]Comparator intervention of interest: vitamins B$_6$ and B$_{12}$.

WHAT ARE THE RESULTS?

How Large, Precise, and Lasting Was the Treatment Effect?

When considering results of intervention studies, we are interested not only in whether an intervention alters a surrogate end point but also in the magnitude, precision, and duration of the effect. If an intervention results in large reductions in the surrogate end point, if the 95% CIs around those large reductions are narrow, and if the effect persists for a sufficiently long period, our confidence that the target outcome will be favorably affected increases. Positive effects that are smaller, with wider CIs and shorter duration of follow-up, leave us less confident.

We have already cited evidence suggesting that CD4 cell counts may be an acceptable surrogate end point for mortality in patients with HIV infection.[11-16] Before the successful introduction of potent antiretroviral therapy, an RCT of immediate vs delayed zidovudine therapy in asymptomatic patients with HIV infection reported a positive result for immediate therapy, largely on the basis of the existence of a greater proportion of treated patients with CD4 cell counts above 350/μL at a median follow-up of 1.7 years.[54] Subsequently, the Concorde trial addressed the same question in an RCT with a median follow-up of 3.3 years.[55] The Concorde investigators found a continuous decrease in CD4 cell counts in the treatment and control groups, but the median difference of 30/μL in favor of treated patients at study termination was statistically significant. Nevertheless, the study found no effect of zidovudine in terms of reduced progression to AIDS or death. The Concorde authors concluded that the small but highly significant and persistent difference in CD4 cell count between the groups was not translated into a significant clinical benefit and it "called into question the uncritical use of CD4 cell counts as a surrogate endpoint."[55] Thus, in the rare instances when a surrogate is judged valid, the effect of an intervention on that surrogate end point must be large, robust, and of sufficient duration before inferences about patient-important effects become credible.

USING THE GUIDE

Returning to our scenario and the RCT we retrieved, 170 patients with type 2 diabetes who had a baseline HbA_{1c} of 8.5% and who were treated with metformin were randomized to receive, in addition, once-weekly injectable exenatide (2 mg) plus placebo vs oral sitagliptin (100 mg) or oral pioglitazine (45 mg) with placebo injections for 26 weeks.[2] Treatment with exenatide reduced HbA_{1c} levels by 1.5% (95% CI, 1.4%-1.7%) compared with sitagliptin (0.9%; 95% CI, 0.7%-1.1%) or pioglitazone (1.2%; 95% CI, 1.0%-1.4%). The treatment differences were −0.6% (95% CI, −0.9% to −0.4%; $P < .0001$) for exenatide vs sitagliptin and −0.3% (95% CI, −0.6% to −0.1%; $P = .0165$) for exenatide vs pioglitazone. We have already established serious doubts about the use of HbA_{1c} as a surrogate for patient-important outcomes. Even without such concerns, the modest effect of exenatide vs the other drugs on the surrogate would leave reservations about its superiority with respect to patient-important outcomes.

Are the Likely Treatment Benefits Worth the Potential Harms and Costs?

The 3 questions clinicians should ask themselves in applying the results of studies with surrogate outcomes are the same ones we have suggested for any issue of therapy or prevention (see Chapter 7, Therapy [Randomized Trials]): Were the study patients similar to my patient? Were all patient-important outcomes considered? Are the likely benefits worth the potential harms and costs? The third criterion—balancing the benefits against the treatment harms—presents particular challenges when investigators have focused only on surrogate end points.

Before offering a treatment to patients, clinicians need to know the magnitude of the likely benefit. Estimating this magnitude becomes a challenging endeavor when knowledge of benefit is limited to the effect of the intervention on a surrogate end point. One approach is to look for one or more RCTs in a similar patient population that assess a related intervention using both surrogate and target end points and extrapolate from those data. When this is unavailable, we are left extrapolating from prognostic models that relate the surrogate marker to the target clinical outcome. Empirical evidence, however, indicates that such extrapolations from surrogate end point efficacy data are prone to bias and likely to result in an overestimation of roughly 50% of the *treatment effect* seen when relying on patient-important end points.[56]

CLINICAL SCENARIO RESOLUTION

How can we ascertain the risk reduction of the long-acting GLP-1 agonist exenatide vs competing drugs on cardiovascular events in patients already taking metformin for type 2 diabetes if all we know is the effect on HbA$_{1c}$? The short answer is that we cannot. Given that we have no confidence that the greater reduction in HbA$_{1c}$ will lead to a reduction in macrovascular adverse events, we can have no confidence at all in modeling exercises to estimate the magnitude of effect.

We have found a strong, more or less consistent, independent, and biologically plausible association between HbA$_{1c}$ and cardiovascular events in type 2 diabetes. The evidence that different antidiabetic compounds that consistently reduce HbA$_{1c}$ also consistently reduce cardiovascular events in type 2 diabetes is, at best, insufficient. Thus, extrapolation from the HbA$_{1c}$-lowering effects in obese patients with type 2 diabetes from metformin monotherapy—the only evidence so far for an effect in lowering the HbA$_{1c}$ level and the number of cardiovascular events—to other antidiabetic drugs or metformin-based combination therapy is not appropriate.

Clinicians and patients also must consider potential harm and adverse effects when making treatment decisions. Most patients tolerate exenatide well; however, the incidences of nausea (24%), diarrhea (18%), and vomiting (11%) were considerably higher than with comparator drugs in the trial of interest.[2] Furthermore, any new drug is at risk for the emergence of rare but serious adverse effects after treatment of large numbers of patients.

What can we tell our patient? If she wishes to minimize her risk for a cardiovascular event further, RCT evidence warranting high confidence suggests she should continue with her statin and blood pressure treatments. The patient is concerned about the relative high rate of nausea associated with GLP-1 agonists and the need to inject the drug and is particularly struck that you can give her no assurance that adding exenatide rather than other agents she has already rejected would decrease her likelihood of macrovascular complications of her diabetes. She, therefore, declines use of exenatide.

CONCLUSION

When we use surrogate end points to make inferences about expected benefit of treatments, we are making assumptions regarding the link between the surrogate end point and patient-important outcomes. In this chapter, we outline criteria that you can use to decide when these assumptions might be appropriate. Very seldom do surrogates meet all of the criteria we suggest—indeed, viral load in HIV is the only compelling example of which we are aware. Even when criteria are met, the magnitude of the effect on the surrogate must be substantial, consistent, and prolonged to leave us confident of patient-important benefit.

These considerations suggest that waiting for results from RCTs that investigate the effect of the intervention on outcomes of unequivocal importance to patients is the only definitive solution to the surrogate outcome dilemma. The large number of instances in which reliance on surrogate end points has led clinicians astray argues for the wisdom of this conservative approach (see Chapter 11.2, Surprising Results of Randomized Trials). On the other hand, when a patient's risk of serious morbidity or mortality is high, this wait-and-see strategy may pose problems for patients and their physicians. Whether patients are ready to gamble on an uncertain benefit in the face of certain *burden*, toxic effects, and cost is an issue for shared decision making (see Chapter 27, Decision Making and the Patient).

We encourage clinicians to critically question therapeutic interventions in which the only proof of efficacy is from surrogate end point data. When the

surrogate end point meets all of our validity criteria, when the effect of the intervention on the surrogate end point is large, when the patient's risk of the target outcome is high, when the patient places a high value on avoiding the target outcome, and when there are no satisfactory alternative therapies, clinicians may choose to recommend therapy on the basis of RCTs that evaluate only surrogate end points. In all situations, clinicians must carefully consider the known and potential adverse effects and the costs of therapy before recommending an intervention solely on the basis of surrogate end points.

References

1. Shyangdan DS, Royle P, Clar C, Sharma P, Waugh N, Snaith A. Glucagon-like peptide analogues for type 2 diabetes mellitus. *Cochrane Database Syst Rev.* 2011;(10):CD006423. doi:10.1002/14651858.CD006423.pub2.

2. Bergenstal RM, Wysham C, Macconell L, et al; DURATION-2 Study Group. Efficacy and safety of exenatide once weekly versus sitagliptin or pioglitazone as an adjunct to metformin for treatment of type 2 diabetes (DURATION-2): a randomised trial. *Lancet.* 2010;376(9739):431-439.

3. Biomarkers Definitions Working Group. Biomarkers and surrogate endpoints: preferred definitions and conceptual framework. *Clin Pharmacol Ther.* 2001;69(3):89-95.

4. Temple RJ. A regulatory authority's opinion about surrogate endpoints. In: Nimmo WS, Tucker GT, eds. *Clinical Measurement in Drug Evaluation.* New York, NY: J Wiley; 1995:3-22.

5. Hammer SM, Squires KE, Hughes MD, et al. A controlled trial of two nucleoside analogues plus indinavir in persons with human immunodeficiency virus infection and CD4 cell counts of 200 per cubic millimeter or less. AIDS Clinical Trials Group 320 Study Team. *N Engl J Med.* 1997;337(11):725-733.

6. Olsen CH, Gatell J, Ledergerber B, et al; EuroSIDA Study Group. Risk of AIDS and death at given HIV-RNA and CD4 cell count, in relation to specific antiretroviral drugs in the regimen. *AIDS.* 2005;19(3):319-330.

7. Guyatt GH, Thompson PJ, Berman LB, et al. How should we measure function in patients with chronic heart and lung disease? *J Chronic Dis.* 1985;38(6):517-524.

8. Mahler DA, Weinberg DH, Wells CK, Feinstein AR. The measurement of dyspnea: contents, interobserver agreement, and physiologic correlates of two new clinical indexes. *Chest.* 1984;85(6):751-758.

9. Verschuren WM, Jacobs DR, Bloemberg BP, et al. Serum total cholesterol and long-term coronary heart disease mortality in different cultures: twenty-five-year follow-up of the seven countries study. *JAMA.* 1995;274(2):131-136.

10. Yusuf S, Hawken S, Ounpuu S, et al; INTERHEART Study Investigators. Effect of potentially modifiable risk factors associated with myocardial infarction in 52 countries (the INTERHEART study): case-control study. *Lancet.* 2004; 364(9438):937-952.

11. Mellors JW, Rinaldo CR Jr, Gupta P, White RM, Todd JA, Kingsley LA. Prognosis in HIV-1 infection predicted by the quantity of virus in plasma. *Science.* 1996;272(5265):1167-1170.

12. Mellors JW, Kingsley LA, Rinaldo CR Jr, et al. Quantitation of HIV-1 RNA in plasma predicts outcome after seroconversion. *Ann Intern Med.* 1995;122(8):573-579.

13. Ruiz L, Romeu J, Clotet B, et al. Quantitative HIV-1 RNA as a marker of clinical stability and survival in a cohort of 302 patients with a mean CD4 cell count of 300 x 10(6)/l. *AIDS.* 1996;10(11):F39-F44.

14. O'Brien TR, Blattner WA, Waters D, et al. Serum HIV-1 RNA levels and time to development of AIDS in the Multicenter Hemophilia Cohort Study. *JAMA.* 1996;276(2):105-110.

15. Hammer SM, Katzenstein DA, Hughes MD, et al; AIDS Clinical Trials Group Study 175 Study Team. A trial comparing nucleoside monotherapy with combination therapy in HIV-infected adults with CD4 cell counts from 200 to 500 per cubic millimeter. *N Engl J Med.* 1996;335(15):1081-1090.

16. Yerly S, Perneger TV, Hirschel B, et al. A critical assessment of the prognostic value of HIV-1 RNA levels and CD4+ cell counts in HIV-infected patients: The Swiss HIV Cohort Study. *Arch Intern Med.* 1998;158(3):247-252.

17. Ho DD. Viral counts count in HIV infection. *Science.* 1996;272(5265):1124-1125.

18. Khaw KT, Wareham N, Bingham S, Luben R, Welch A, Day N. Association of hemoglobin A_{1c} with cardiovascular disease and mortality in adults: the European prospective investigation into cancer in Norfolk. *Ann Intern Med.* 2004; 141(6):413-420.

19. Kuusisto J, Mykkänen L, Pyörälä K, Laakso M. NIDDM and its metabolic control predict coronary heart disease in elderly subjects. *Diabetes.* 1994;43(8):960-967.

20. Selvin E, Marinopoulos S, Berkenblit G, et al. Meta-analysis: glycosylated hemoglobin and cardiovascular disease in diabetes mellitus. *Ann Intern Med.* 2004;141(6):421-431.

21. Barter PJ, Caulfield M, Eriksson M, et al; ILLUMINATE Investigators. Effects of torcetrapib in patients at high risk for coronary events. *N Engl J Med.* 2007;357(21):2109-2122.

22. McAlister FA, Teo KK. Antiarrhythmic therapies for the prevention of sudden cardiac death. *Drugs.* 1997;54(2):235-252.

23. Bigger JT Jr, Fleiss JL, Kleiger R, Miller JP, Rolnitzky LM. The relationships among ventricular arrhythmias, left ventricular dysfunction, and mortality in the 2 years after myocardial infarction. *Circulation*. 1984;69(2):250-258.

24. Echt DS, Liebson PR, Mitchell LB, et al. Mortality and morbidity in patients receiving encainide, flecainide, or placebo. The Cardiac Arrhythmia Suppression Trial. *N Engl J Med*. 1991;324(12):781-788.

25. Studer M, Briel M, Leimenstoll B, Glass TR, Bucher HC. Effect of different antilipidemic agents and diets on mortality: a systematic review. *Arch Intern Med*. 2005;165(7):725-730.

26. Mihaylova B, Emberson J, Blackwell L, et al; Cholesterol Treatment Trialists' (CTT) Collaborators. The effects of lowering LDL cholesterol with statin therapy in people at low risk of vascular disease: meta-analysis of individual data from 27 randomised trials. *Lancet*. 2012;380(9841):581-590.

27. Furberg CD, Pitt B. Withdrawal of cerivastatin from the world market. *Curr Control Trials Cardiovasc Med*. 2001; 2(5):205-207.

28. Riggs BL, Hodgson SF, O'Fallon WM, et al. Effect of fluoride treatment on the fracture rate in postmenopausal women with osteoporosis. *N Engl J Med*. 1990;322(12):802-809.

29. Haguenauer D, Welch V, Shea B, Tugwell P, Adachi JD, Wells G. Fluoride for the treatment of postmenopausal osteoporotic fractures: a meta-analysis. *Osteoporos Int*. 2000;11(9):727-738.

30. Guyatt GH, Cranney A, Griffith L, et al. Summary of meta-analyses of therapies for postmenopausal osteoporosis and the relationship between bone density and fractures. *Endocrinol Metab Clin North Am*. 2002;31(3):659-679, xii.

31. Deacon CF, Mannucci E, Ahrén B. Glycaemic efficacy of glucagon-like peptide-1 receptor agonists and dipeptidyl peptidase-4 inhibitors as add-on therapy to metformin in subjects with type 2 diabetes: a review and meta analysis. *Diabetes Obes Metab*. 2012;14(8):762-767.

32. Drexler H, Banhardt U, Meinertz T, Wollschläger H, Lehmann M, Just H. Contrasting peripheral short-term and long-term effects of converting enzyme inhibition in patients with congestive heart failure: a double-blind, placebo-controlled trial. *Circulation*. 1989;79(3):491-502.

33. Lewis GR. Comparison of lisinopril versus placebo for congestive heart failure. *Am J Cardiol*. 1989;63(8):12D-16D.

34. Giles TD, Fisher MB, Rush JE. Lisinopril and captopril in the treatment of heart failure in older patients: comparison of a long- and short-acting angiotensin-converting enzyme inhibitor. *Am J Med*. 1988;85(3B):44-47.

35. Riegger GA. Effects of quinapril on exercise tolerance in patients with mild to moderate heart failure. *Eur Heart J*. 1991;12(6):705-711.

36. Garg R, Yusuf S; Collaborative Group on ACE Inhibitor Trials. Overview of randomized trials of angiotensin-converting enzyme inhibitors on mortality and morbidity in patients with heart failure. *JAMA*. 1995;273(18):1450-1456.

37. DiBianco R, Shabetai R, Kostuk W, Moran J, Schlant RC, Wright R. A comparison of oral milrinone, digoxin, and their combination in the treatment of patients with chronic heart failure. *N Engl J Med*. 1989;320(11):677-683.

38. Sueta CA, Gheorghiade M, Adams KF Jr, et al; Epoprostenol Multicenter Research Group. Safety and efficacy of epoprostenol in patients with severe congestive heart failure. *Am J Cardiol*. 1995;75(3):34A-43A.

39. Packer M, Carver JR, Rodeheffer RJ, et al; The PROMISE Study Research Group. Effect of oral milrinone on mortality in severe chronic heart failure. *N Engl J Med*. 1991;325(21):1468-1475.

40. Califf RM, Adams KF, McKenna WJ, et al. A randomized controlled trial of epoprostenol therapy for severe congestive heart failure: The Flolan International Randomized Survival Trial (FIRST). *Am Heart J*. 1997;134(1):44-54.

41. Yee KM, Struthers AD. Can drug effects on mortality in heart failure be predicted by any surrogate measure? *Eur Heart J*. 1997;18(12):1860-1864.

42. Hampton JR, van Veldhuisen DJ, Kleber FX, et al; Second Prospective Randomised Study of Ibopamine on Mortality and Efficacy (PRIME II) Investigators. Randomised study of effect of ibopamine on survival in patients with advanced severe heart failure. *Lancet*. 1997;349(9057):971-977.

43. Cameron DW, Heath-Chiozzi M, Danner S, et al; The Advanced HIV Disease Ritonavir Study Group. Randomised placebo-controlled trial of ritonavir in advanced HIV-1 disease. *Lancet*. 1998;351(9102):543-549.

44. Sterne JA, Hernán MA, Ledergerber B, et al; Swiss HIV Cohort Study. Long-term effectiveness of potent antiretroviral therapy in preventing AIDS and death: a prospective cohort study. *Lancet*. 2005;366(9483):378-384.

45. Worm SW, Sabin C, Weber R, et al. Risk of myocardial infarction in patients with HIV infection exposed to specific individual antiretroviral drugs from the 3 major drug classes: the data collection on adverse events of anti-HIV drugs (D:A:D) study. *J Infect Dis*. 2010;201(3):318-330.

46. Nathan DM. Finding new treatments for diabetes—how many, how fast... how good? *N Engl J Med*. 2007;356(5):437-440.

47. Scirica BM, Bhatt DL, Braunwald E, et al; SAVOR-TIMI 53 Steering Committee and Investigators. Saxagliptin and cardiovascular outcomes in patients with type 2 diabetes mellitus. *N Engl J Med*. 2013;369(14):1317-1326.

48. White WB, Cannon CP, Heller SR, et al; EXAMINE Investigators. Alogliptin after acute coronary syndrome in patients with type 2 diabetes. *N Engl J Med*. 2013;369(14):1327-1335.

49. Saenz A, Fernandez-Esteban I, Mataix A, Ausejo M, Roque M, Moher D. Metformin monotherapy for type 2 diabetes mellitus. *Cochrane Database Syst Rev*. 2005;(3):CD002966.

50. UK Prospective Diabetes Study (UKPDS) Group. Effect of intensive blood-glucose control with metformin on complications in overweight patients with type 2 diabetes (UKPDS 34). *Lancet*. 1998;352(9131):854-865.

51. Hemmingsen B, Christensen LL, Wetterslev J et al. Comparison of metformin and insulin versus insulin alone for type 2 diabetes: systematic review of randomised clinical trials with meta-analyses and trial sequential analyses. *BMJ*. 2012;344:e1771. doi:10.1136/bmj.e1771.

52. Singh S, Loke YK, Furberg CD. Long-term risk of cardiovascular events with rosiglitazone: a meta-analysis. *JAMA*. 2007;298(10):1189-1195.

53. Lago RM, Singh PP, Nesto RW. Congestive heart failure and cardiovascular death in patients with prediabetes and type 2 diabetes given thiazolidinediones: a meta-analysis of randomised clinical trials. *Lancet*. 2007;370(9593):1129-1136.

54. Cooper DA, Gatell JM, Kroon S, et al; The European-Australian Collaborative Group. Zidovudine in persons with asymptomatic HIV infection and CD4+ cell counts greater than 400 per cubic millimeter. *N Engl J Med*. 1993;329(5):297-303.

55. Concorde Coordinating Committee. Concorde: MRC/ANRS randomised double-blind controlled trial of immediate and deferred zidovudine in symptom-free HIV infection. *Lancet.* 1994;343(8902):871-881.

56. Ciani O, Buyse M, Garside R, et al. Comparison of treatment effect sizes associated with surrogate and final patient relevant outcomes in randomised controlled trials: meta-epidemiological study. *BMJ.* 2013;346:f457. doi:10.1136/bmj.f457.

57. Schwartz GG, Olsson AG, Abt M, et al; dal-OUTCOMES Investigators. Effects of dalcetrapib in patients with a recent acute coronary syndrome. *N Engl J Med.* 2012; 367(22):2089-2099.

58. Miller NE, Thelle DS, Forde OH, Mjos OD. The Tromsø heart-study: high-density lipoprotein and coronary heart-disease: a prospective case-control study. *Lancet.* 1977;1(8019):965-968.

59. Gordon T, Castelli WP, Hjortland MC, Kannel WB, Dawber TR. High density lipoprotein as a protective factor against coronary heart disease: The Framingham Study. *Am J Med.* 1977;62(5):707-714.

60. Boden WE, Probstfield JL, Anderson T, et al; AIM-HIGH Investigators. Niacin in patients with low HDL cholesterol levels receiving intensive statin therapy. *N Engl J Med.* 2011;365(24):2255-2267.

61. Nissen SE, Tardif JC, Nicholls SJ, et al; ILLUSTRATE Investigators. Effect of torcetrapib on the progression of coronary atherosclerosis. *N Engl J Med.* 2007;356(13):1304-1316.

62. Jones PH, Davidson MH, Stein EA, et al; STELLAR Study Group. Comparison of the efficacy and safety of rosuvastatin versus atorvastatin, simvastatin, and pravastatin across doses (STELLAR* Trial). *Am J Cardiol.* 2003;92(2):152-160.

63. Brown WV, Bays HE, Hassman DR, et al; Rosuvastatin Study Group. Efficacy and safety of rosuvastatin compared with pravastatin and simvastatin in patients with hypercholesterolemia: a randomized, double-blind, 52-week trial. *Am Heart J.* 2002;144(6):1036-1043.

64. Law MR, Wald NJ, Thompson SG. By how much and how quickly does reduction in serum cholesterol concentration lower risk of ischaemic heart disease? *BMJ.* 1994;308(6925): 367-372.

65. Lonn E, Yusuf S, Arnold MJ, et al; Heart Outcomes Prevention Evaluation (HOPE) 2 Investigators. Homocysteine lowering with folic acid and B vitamins in vascular disease. *N Engl J Med.* 2006;354(15):1567-1577.

66. Boushey CJ, Beresford SA, Omenn GS, Motulsky AG. A quantitative assessment of plasma homocysteine as a risk factor for vascular disease: probable benefits of increasing folic acid intakes. *JAMA.* 1995;274(13):1049-1057.

67. Wald DS, Law M, Morris JK. Homocysteine and cardiovascular disease: evidence on causality from a meta-analysis. *BMJ.* 2002;325(7374):1202.

68. Homocysteine Studies Collaboration. Homocysteine and risk of ischemic heart disease and stroke: a meta-analysis. *JAMA.* 2002;288(16):2015-2022.

69. Eikelboom JW, Lonn E, Genest J Jr, Hankey G, Yusuf S. Homocyst(e)ine and cardiovascular disease: a critical review of the epidemiologic evidence. *Ann Intern Med.* 1999; 131(5):363-375.

70. Bønaa KH, Njølstad I, Ueland PM, et al; NORVIT Trial Investigators. Homocysteine lowering and cardiovascular events after acute myocardial infarction. *N Engl J Med.* 2006; 354(15):1578-1588.

71. Liem A, Reynierse-Buitenwerf GH, Zwinderman AH, Jukema JW, van Veldhuisen DJ. Secondary prevention with folic acid: effects on clinical outcomes. *J Am Coll Cardiol.* 2003; 41(12):2105-2113.

72. Myung SK, Ju W, Cho B, et al; Korean Meta-Analysis Study Group. Efficacy of vitamin and antioxidant supplements in prevention of cardiovascular disease: systematic review and meta-analysis of randomised controlled trials. *BMJ.* 2013;346:f10. doi:10.1136/bmj.f10.

73. Johnson M, Grinsztejn B, Rodriguez C, et al. Atazanavir plus ritonavir or saquinavir, and lopinavir/ritonavir in patients experiencing multiple virological failures. *AIDS.* 2005;19(2):153-162.

74. Montaner JS, Reiss P, Cooper D, et al. A randomized, double-blind trial comparing combinations of nevirapine, didanosine, and zidovudine for HIV-infected patients: the INCAS Trial. Italy, The Netherlands, Canada and Australia Study. *JAMA.* 1998;279(12):930-937.

75. Orkin C, DeJesus E, Khanlou H, et al. Final 192-week efficacy and safety of once-daily darunavir/ritonavir compared with lopinavir/ritonavir in HIV-1-infected treatment-naïve patients in the ARTEMIS trial. *HIV Med.* 2013;14(1):49-59.

THERAPY

13.5

ADVANCED TOPICS IN APPLYING THE RESULTS OF THERAPY TRIALS

Qualitative Research

Mita Giacomini and Deborah J. Cook

THERAPY

IN THIS CHAPTER

Walking out of the hospital on Friday night, you reflect on your week of rounds with all of the patients for whom you provide care. You are a hospitalist and most of your patients are elderly, have multiple comorbidities, and live independently in a retirement home, apartment, or house. Although you strive to move them along the trajectory of their illness toward recovery, minimizing complications, and maintaining their prehospital function, some patients do not return home. This week, you admitted 3 patients whose hospitalization you predict is a terminal event. In conversations, a family member of one of these patients acknowledged that possibility. You pledge in the coming week to engage in advance care planning more directly, beginning by exploring your patients' awareness that they may not survive this hospital stay.

FINDING THE EVIDENCE

It is Monday at noon and you are attending grand medical rounds in your hospital. The speaker visiting from a nearby institution is presenting the results of some recent studies on end-of-life care for hospital inpatients. A major message in her presentation is the importance of attending to language in patient encounters, and your interest is piqued. One slide summarizing an article seems directly relevant to your concerns because it describes the results of a qualitative study of physician-patient communication about serious illness and, in particular, how conversations "dance around death."[1] You record the author, journal, and year of publication in your smartphone and look it up later that afternoon in your office. Accessing the single citation matcher of PubMed (http://www.ncbi.nlm.nih.gov/pubmed/citmatch), you type the author's name and journal, quickly find the article, then download and read it.

INTRODUCTION

Qualitative research addresses social rules and meanings germane to the "social" sciences rather than the natural and physical laws of the "natural" sciences. Qualitative research aims to discover, describe, and understand rather than to test or evaluate. Qualitative and quantitative studies address fundamentally different phenomena and questions about them. They are not interchangeable with respect to either goals or methods.

What are social phenomena, and how do they differ from natural or biomedical phenomena? Imagine you have never encountered a wristwatch before and want to research what it does. If you are a natural scientist approaching the watch as a natural phenomenon, you might observe its mechanics and discover what causes its arms to move. You would find that the watch, like all things, obeys immutable laws of physics. But can this evidence help you understand the watch's effect on human social life? No, because approaching it as a natural object cannot reveal the powerful social forces associated with a watch's function. Understanding these aspects requires meaningful description and interpretation of those descriptions. For instance, what do the numbers on the face of the watch do? Their power lies in their symbolic nature: they represent agreed-on times of the day, which in turn relate to social conventions (eg, lunch). By virtue of social rules, those hands and numbers move people. Interestingly, the watch works the same way with the numbers missing because we also share tacit understandings of how the hands and numbers relate. A qualitative researcher would explore and discover these social meanings and rules. Social rules change with context and can prevail even when being violated. They will require careful description and interpretations to detect and understand.[2] Qualitative research methods offer descriptive and qualitative tools for investigation.

In *quantitative research*, critical appraisal of individual studies focuses on *risk of bias* in assessments of *intervention effect*, *prognosis*, or diagnostic test performance. In qualitative research, critical appraisal focuses on the truth value of descriptions or interpretations in relation to the research setting and the user's own setting. Many qualitative researchers reject terms such as *validity* in favor of terms such as *credibility* or *trustworthiness.* Users need to have confidence that qualitative researchers conducted careful, sensitive work behind the scenes, beyond their brief methods descriptions. Descriptions of methods should indicate that the researchers know and followed the procedures of their chosen methods. Readers can assess this indirectly through authors' reference to terms and procedures appropriate to their specific methods, reference to procedures standard to most qualitative methods, and authors' reference to more detailed methods texts. Here, we focus on the last 2 criteria, which readers can readily apply to critical appraisal (mention of generally conventional procedures and reference to a text). The first criterion (sophisticated use of methodologic language) would be appropriate for readers trained in the specific qualitative method. To represent the criterion of overall rigor and believability, we will use the term "credibility." Users also need to have confidence in the quality of the findings themselves. Poor-quality qualitative findings tend to be not so much false (it is difficult to prove an interpretation entirely wrong) as shallow or uninsightful. High-quality findings from well-performed qualitative studies are worthy of consideration.[3]

The social science and professional disciplines have developed myriad qualitative methods. Each method focuses on different kinds of research questions, and each has distinctive disciplinary and philosophic assumptions about the nature of social reality and how to learn about it.[4] Readers will find overviews and comparisons of specific methods elsewhere.[5-8] Differences among specific qualitative methods matter to researchers and for evaluating whether a study makes a strong contribution to scientific knowledge in a given discipline (as opposed to user knowledge in a practice setting). Some academics object to the relevance of standard criteria across methods or even across individual studies.[9,10] The variety of qualitative methods explains in part the absence of widely accepted standards for the critical appraisal of "all" qualitative research.[11]

For the clinical user, however, appraisal focuses pragmatically on whether a peer-reviewed, published study offers credible and useful insights for a problem at hand. Proposed guidelines for appraising qualitative studies typically address the basic issues outlined in Box 13.5-1. Limitations of study design of qualitative studies include issues beyond risk of bias. Thus, in this chapter, we use the term "credibility" to

---

BOX 13.5-1

Users' Guides for an Article Reporting the Results of Qualitative Research in Health Care

Is the qualitative research relevant?

Are the results credible?[a]

Is a specific qualitative method cited?

Was the choice of participants or observations explicit and comprehensive?

Was research ethics approval obtained?

Was data collection sufficiently comprehensive and detailed?

Were the data analyzed appropriately and the findings corroborated adequately?

What are the results?

How can I apply the results to patient care?

Does the study offer helpful theory?

Does the study help me understand the context of my practice?

Does the study help me understand social phenomena in my practice?

---

[a]Limitations of study design of qualitative studies include issues beyond risk of bias. Thus, in this chapter, we use the term "credibility" to address both risk of bias and these additional issues.

---

address both risk of bias and these additional issues. We focus on understanding and using qualitative research information for clinical practice. We refer readers elsewhere for introductions to the design and conduct of qualitative research[12-14] or critical appraisal for the scientific purposes of peer review or for evaluating the credibility of individual studies that contribute to *systematic reviews.*[9,15,16]

IS THE QUALITATIVE RESEARCH RELEVANT?

To be relevant for clinicians, qualitative research must not only be relevant to the clinician's question but also fulfill 2 other criteria. First, the clinical problem must concern social phenomena. For example, a qualitative study will not tell you whether an intervention improves outcomes (a *randomized clinical trial* would). However, it could help you discover how people experienced the intervention, how they accommodated or reacted to it, or what outcomes they most valued and why. Second, the research must offer theoretical or conceptual insights into the problem. Whereas quantitative research makes inferences to populations, qualitative research makes inductive, descriptive inferences to *theory* about social phenomena.[17]

Qualitative studies may generate simple or elaborate theories. Findings may contribute to knowledge in the social sciences, or they may prove useful for lay, professional, or interdisciplinary audiences. For clinicians, qualitative findings may provide understanding and explanation of unrecognized, poorly understood, or unfamiliar phenomena. They also may provide new insight into familiar patterns and problems, such as communication barriers. Although armchair hypothesizing has its place, qualitative research can offer a more rigorous and empirically grounded source of insight into what might be going on.

Beyond aiming for qualitative evidence when it is relevant in general (ie, for questions of social or personal meaning), users should assess the specific relevance of the articles they find to the problems or questions they face. In qualitative research, researchers express the focus of their study as a research question or research objective. Readers should find a clear statement of these in terms that relate closely to the topic of concern.

USING THE GUIDE

Anderson et al[1] clearly describe their study objectives, which relate directly to your concern: "We aimed to describe initial communications about serious illness between hospitalists and patients, and to identify patterns that led to sensitive and honest discussions of death and dying, even at a first meeting."[1] As you seek to understand how best to address the topic of dying with patients and families, you have a sense that an understanding of these dynamics might help you develop sharper hypotheses about possible solutions to the problem.

ARE THE RESULTS CREDIBLE?

Qualitative research is not a single method but a large family of methods, including, for example, *grounded theory, ethnography, phenomenology, case study, critical theory,* and *historiography.*[4] These methods originated from different disciplines, and each approaches social reality somewhat differently, with distinct methods and procedures. We focus on general features of credibility and usefulness that apply across most methods common in the clinical literature.

The methods section of a qualitative study should describe several aspects of the research design, including the specific methodologic tradition followed, how researchers targeted and sampled study participants or other phenomena, how they generated and recorded the data, the comprehensiveness of data collection, and procedures for analyzing the data and validating the findings.

Is a Specific Qualitative Method Cited?

To critique or use a qualitative research report, clinicians do not require expertise in qualitative methods, although they do confidence in the researchers' expertise. Authors should indicate their specific qualitative method and their commitment to its guiding assumptions and procedures. Readers should look in the introduction or methods sections for a named method (eg, grounded theory or ethnography). A given qualitative method may have variants, so authors should also cite a relevant and authoritative methods text. Given a named method and cited standard text, users can be more confident that researchers followed conventions. Without a stated method and text, confidence in the credibility of the results diminishes.

Was the Choice of Participants or Observations Explicit and Comprehensive?

Readers of qualitative studies should look for sound reasoning describing and justifying sample selection strategies. The units sampled should be appropriate to the research question, and the extent of sampling should be sufficient to generate a thorough

USING THE GUIDE

Anderson et al[1] state at the outset of their Methods section that they will use a grounded theory approach, citing Charmaz[18] as a reference for the application of grounded theory. This distinguishes their method from 2 earlier schools of grounded theory, which followed slightly different aims and procedures. Within this tradition, the researchers also describe a technique called *dimensional analysis* to guide data analysis; they give several citations to this approach as well. To learn more methodologic details, readers can go to these sources. Otherwise, they may assume that the researchers followed the conventions of their cited methods.

USING THE GUIDE

Anderson et al[1] sampled admission encounters between hospitalists and patients during a 20-month period at 2 hospitals in the United States. In this study, the admission encounter (a social interaction), not the individual, is the unit of analysis. To purposively sample relevant encounters, they recruited all hospitalists at the 2 hospitals; 91% consented to participate. These physicians identified and invited patients "whose death or intensive care unit admission in the next year would not surprise them"[1]; 66% of the patients consented to participate. This purposive sampling process yielded 39 audiotaped admission encounters that involved 23 hospitalist physicians and 39 seriously ill patients. Researchers excluded encounters that involved non–English-speaking patients and any who could not grant informed consent; therefore, findings may miss special communication challenges or dynamics for these groups. The study was conducted in the western United States. Readers need to consider how communication and culture in that locale and health care system may differ from those of their own setting.

understanding and thus a complete analysis. The *unit of analysis* for a qualitative study is often, but not always, the participating individual. Sampling may focus on entities other than human participants (eg, interactions, observation periods, events, interviews, rituals, routines, and statements). Some studies use multiple units of analysis, calling for multiple data sources. Furthermore, the exploratory and inductive nature of qualitative research often prevents investigators from specifying a study sample in strict terms, lest they overlook important types of participants or other units of analysis that they did not anticipate at the outset.

In contrast to the imperative in quantitative research to select a large number of representative participants, qualitative researchers aim for a small number of participants (or observations) selected deliberately for features relevant to the analysis. This process is called *purposive sampling*. Purposive sampling aims for relevant diversity. Selection criteria evolve in parallel with analysis to explore emerging themes or perspectives. Depending on the questions, purposive sampling might seek any of the following: typical cases, unusual cases, critical cases, cases that reflect important political issues, or cases with connections to other cases.[19] *Convenience sampling* and *random sampling* are usually inadequate for a comprehensive investigation and require a compelling explanation.

Was Research Ethics Approval Obtained?

The ethical treatment of human research participants is a fundamental feature of the quality of any health research. In qualitative research, ethics protocols and their approval also reflect favorably on the ability of the investigators to approach participants with due respect and sensitivity, diligent attentiveness, empathy, engagement in the research process,[20] and attention to *reflexivity*.[16] Reflexivity is researchers' awareness of how they inevitably participate in the social setting they study and their consideration of how this can lead to understanding and influencing what they learn. Reflexivity differs from *bias* in quantitative research in that it cannot be removed; rather, its nature needs to be recognized and accounted for in both qualitative data collection and analysis.

Clear ethics procedures reflect favorably on— although do not alone determine—the credibility of the qualitative research findings.[20] Qualitative studies require the approval of a formal research ethics board to examine the protocol and informed consent process for potential risks to participants, including loss of confidentiality, interview burdens, incentives that may undermine voluntary consent, truthfulness in information provided to participants, researcher interference in care or other experiences, and the possibility of psychological trauma from participating. Standard practices include securing voluntary informed consent from individuals or their substitute decision makers, protecting the confidentiality of participants through discreet secure data collection, and ensuring anonymity of reported data. Qualitative reports should state that the study received formal ethics board approval, and readers can seek signs of sensitive engagement with participants in the ethical conduct of the study (eg, whether the approach to participants respected the social setting and participants' situation in it or how participants' vulnerabilities were characterized and addressed).

USING THE GUIDE

Anderson et al[1] report that the study protocol was approved by the research ethics board at the investigators' university. Duly considering the possible vulnerability of the severely ill patient participants, the authors describe modifications they made to the informed consent process to avoid harm (ie, not disclosing to potential participants that they were chosen because of their very poor prognosis).

Was Data Collection Sufficiently Comprehensive and Detailed?

To achieve a comprehensive, rich picture of participants' experiences and social dynamics, investigators must involve enough relevant types of participants or situations and enough individual instances to generate a robust analysis. Researchers usually choose from among 3 basic data collection strategies. *Field observation* involves witnessing and recording events as they occur. *Interviews* engage participants

in dialogue, allowing them to interpret events and experiences in their own terms. *Document analysis* involves the interpretive review of written material. The research topic determines the best strategy, including whether single or multiple types of data are needed. In some social settings, the best strategy may be unethical or infeasible; authors should explicitly state the reason for a less optimal approach.

Field Observation

Field observation means monitoring participants' actions in "real time." For *direct observation*, the investigator personally observes events and records detailed field notes within the social milieu. The investigator may be present as a participant or a nonparticipant in the studied interactions. For *participant observation*, the researcher assumes a social role beyond that of a researcher within the social setting (eg, clinician or committee member). In *nonparticipant observation*, the role remains that of a researcher who participates as little as possible in the studied interactions. For both nonparticipant and participant observation, readers should consider whether the researchers' presence and role allowed them access to candid and meaningful social interactions. Their involvement may allow extra insights or distort participants' behavior, depending on the context.

Finally, *indirect observation* through video or audio recordings removes researchers from the social dynamic while still capturing events as they unfold. The surveillance technology itself has a social presence, however, and may influence what participants say and do. Regardless of the observation method, observers will always have some effect on what they study. This is part of reflexivity in qualitative methods and should be considered and accounted for in the analysis.

Interviews

Qualitative researchers commonly use interviews to explore individuals' experiences and ideas, as well as to recount experiences or events in the past. Interviews may be more or less structured and may involve 1 or more individuals. Because of their exploratory nature, most qualitative interviews are either *semistructured,* meaning that they follow a general guide of topics while allowing the investigator to phrase questions in natural language and to follow the dialogue into unanticipated topics as they arise. *Open-ended questions* aim for more participant-driven responses during interviews, with little anticipated in advance, (eg, asking "Tell me what it's like…").

Standardized, structured interviews are usually inappropriate for qualitative research because they contrive the dialogue, presuppose the content of responses, and generally invite no content that could deviate from the researchers' expectations. Researchers interview participants either as individuals or in groups (or *focus groups*). For evoking personal experiences and perspectives, particularly on sensitive topics, individual interviews usually work best. Group dynamics may inhibit intimate personal disclosures, although they may facilitate disclosures for emotionally sensitive topics if participants feel empowered speaking in the presence of peers.[21] For capturing interpersonal dynamics, language, and culture, group interviews can provide invaluable data. Critical readers should examine researchers' rationale for choosing a particular approach and assess its appropriateness to the topic.

Document Analysis

Documents or material artifacts (eg, medical records, Web reports, or news media reports) can provide especially useful data for policy-related, historical, or organizational studies of health care.[22] Researchers must take into account the authorship, audience, and purposes of these sources and interpret their content accordingly. For example, some represent the perspectives of collective organizations rather than individuals. Beyond the content, rhetorical strategies, such as lines of argument, metaphors, or illustrations in documents, provide insights into authors' ideas or agendas.

Whether data are collected through observation, interviews, or documents, they must be adequate in quantity, quality, and diversity to address the research questions. Several aspects of a qualitative report indicate how extensively the investigators collected data: the number of observations, interviews, or documents; the duration of the observations; the duration of the study period; the diversity of units of analysis and data collection techniques; the number or diversity of investigators involved in collecting and analyzing data; and the degree of involvement of individual investigators in data collection and analysis.[23,24]

USING THE GUIDE

Anderson et al[1] used one type of highly relevant data: transcribed audiotapes of encounters. The transcripts included the entire exchange between patient and physician—not only the words spoken but also nuances of communication, such as silences, emphasis, and volume. Audiotapes miss visual communication, such as body language; however, collecting visual data through videotaping or direct observation would have been more intrusive and might have deterred participation or inhibited communication. The investigators kept their presence to a minimum to better learn what goes on in the intimacy of the clinical encounter between physician and patient. They thus collected extensive and fairly exhaustive data on each encounter.

Readers should ask next whether enough encounters and types of encounters were included. The sampling process yielded 39 encounters. Typically, grounded-theory studies use approximately 20 to 40 transcripts. This range provides a rough rule of thumb used for research planning and budgeting, but whether this is really enough will be determined in the analysis process (discussed below).

In a table, the authors list some indicators of participant types and diversity. Men and women were equally represented, and most participants were middle-aged and white. The researchers characterize ethnicity/race in a way that is conventional but not necessarily meaningful for understanding the association between race and health in the United States or in other countries with different sociodemographics.[25] Patients with cancer constituted slightly more than half of the participants, with 5 or fewer patients having other diagnoses, such as chronic disease; posttransplant, end-stage kidney or liver disease; or other conditions. Readers must consider how the mix of seriously ill patients (eg, their diagnoses and readiness to discuss such issues) in these 2 hospitals compares to the mix in their own. Self-evaluated patient health tells us something about patients' beliefs and any divergence between patient and physician perspectives at the outset of the clinical encounter. Although the physicians considered all of these patients terminally ill (a patient selection criterion), only 23% of patients saw themselves this way. Most patients (56%) considered themselves seriously but not terminally ill, and the rest (21%) considered themselves to be relatively healthy.

Did the Investigators Analyze the Data Appropriately and Corroborate the Findings Adequately?

Qualitative research is a cyclic rather than linear process. Qualitative researchers begin with an exploratory question and preliminary concepts that help identify whom to study and how to approach the setting. They then collect relevant data, observe patterns in the data, and organize these into *themes* (*concepts* and their relationships). Next, they resume data collection to explore and challenge these preliminary themes and revise or refine them. They may repeat this cycle several times and continue collecting data until the analysis is well developed and further observations yield no useful new information (a point commonly referred to as *theoretical saturation*[26] or *informational redundancy*,[27] depending on the method). Such analysis-stopping criteria are so basic to qualitative analysis that authors may omit stating this achievement in their report. Readers can be more confident of a thorough analysis, however, when authors state the point at which they stopped collecting data.

During analysis, investigators also corroborate key findings by using multiple sources of information, a process called *triangulation*. Triangulation is a metaphor and does not mean literally the use of 3 sources. The appropriate number and types of sources depend on the importance and controversy of the finding. Because no 2 qualitative data sources will generate exactly the same information or interpretations, investigators must still interpret the discrepancies or consistencies among sources.[28] This can lead not to resolution but to new research questions. For example, if a research participant reported in 1 qualitative interview that she uses intravenous

drugs but in a subsequent interview said that she has never used them, the question for analysis would become not only whether the participant is in fact a drug user but also how she sees herself and why her story changed (eg, misunderstanding the question, lying, boasting, or confusion). This example also indicates how the concepts investigated by qualitative analysis change, unlike the fixed variables of quantitative research. The task of corroborating a qualitative finding differs from, for example, establishing intrarater or interrater *reliability* in a quantitative study in which we assume a fixed fact and that deviation from this fact is an error.[29] To the qualitative researcher, the deviation is just new information.

Readers may encounter several triangulation techniques for corroborating qualitative findings.[3,30] Each has distinctive advantages and shortcomings. *Investigator triangulation* involves more than 1 investigator collecting and analyzing the data, and findings emerge through consensus among multiple investigators. Sometimes interdisciplinary teams bring richer perspectives. If, however, the investigators are not sufficiently engaged with each other the difficulties of interdisciplinary communication can limit findings to only those similarly understood concepts or common places.[31] Investigators external to the study could bring a fresh perspective but may have a limited or superficial understanding of the study setting and data.[3]

Member checking involves sharing draft findings with the participants to get feedback on whether the findings make sense to them, whether researchers interpreted their viewpoints faithfully, or whether they perceive errors of fact. Some question, however, whether researchers should appropriately expect analysis and critique from participants.[9] Finally, *theory triangulation* involves comparison of emergent findings with preexisting social science theory.[32]

Some qualitative research reports describe the use of qualitative analysis software packages; this is not required for a rigorous analysis but helps with managing large volumes of data and tracking the analysis. The quality of the analysis ultimately rests on investigators' judgments, regardless of whether they used software or which software they used.

For a qualitative analysis to be finished, the analysis must drive data collection. Requirements for developing and corroborating the findings determine the final sample size at the end (not the outset) of the project. As the study progresses, analysis focuses more on corroborating, challenging, and elaborating the emerging findings by revisiting the data in hand and collecting additional data specifically for these purposes. Researchers should indicate that data collection in part followed analysis in parallel or in iterative stages. Studies that collect all of the data before analysis may offer narrower or less robust findings.

health or death. The authors illustrate selected findings with excerpted quotes from the clinical encounters, allowing readers to see how the investigators made their interpretations. The quotations ring true to the authors' interpretations, which gives readers confidence in the interpretation of the rest of the data.

USING THE GUIDE

The article by Anderson et al[1] provides a thorough description of analytic methods and procedures, which is typical of research published in social science journals. This degree of methods description is less common in clinical journals, in part because of page limitations. Longer, more detailed methods and findings sections might allow readers to better appraise the credibility of the research. Anderson et al[1] report systematic data analysis procedures that follow the conventions of grounded theory and dimensional analysis, including coding the data in stages, from more open-ended interpretations to more focused theory formulation. They gave attention not only to identifying types of social interaction but also to characterizing complex processes and dynamics. Each analysis stage involved iteration among data collection, reading the data, and developing the dimensions, matrix, and metaphor that constituted the findings. The authors report data sufficiency by stating the criteria for stopping data collection: data redundancy and saturation for key findings. They took several measures to ensure that the results were meaningful from multiple perspectives. Investigator triangulation is implied by their use of a multi-investigator team and the review of preliminary findings by an external peer group of qualitative researchers. As a member-checking step, they conducted a focus group with hospitalists for feedback on the findings. They note that member-checking with patient participants was not possible because of their discharge from the hospital and very poor

WHAT ARE THE RESULTS?

Qualitative research produces descriptive theories about the way things are and interpretive theories about what things mean in a given social setting. Qualitative analysis concludes with the process of writing because authors construct sensible narratives and arguments, evocative metaphors, or meaningful terms and labels to summarize their insights. Ideally, participants, authors, and readers should find the narrative accounts compelling. Qualitative theories (ie, findings) consist of concepts and their relationships (commonly called themes).

A common, although sometimes simplistic,[33] structure for theoretical findings is a list of key concepts as major categories and subcategories. This kind of theory can offer readers meaningful labels for classifying and reflecting on phenomena in their own settings. For deeper understanding, however, readers often need richer theory that addresses the relationships among categories.[9,33] Key relationships may be more dynamic than hierarchical categories and subcategories (eg, processes over time, mutual influence, and symbolic relationships).

A good qualitative report provides enough narrative detail to evoke a vivid picture of the interactions or experiences of the research participants and what these mean. Authors typically illustrate key findings with data excerpts from field notes, interview transcripts, or documents. These excerpts offer the reader an opportunity to assess how the investigators interpreted the data. Illustrative data excerpts should clearly support the interpretation taken from them; if they do not, this may raise doubts about the interpretive skills of the investigators, the completeness of the analysis, or both.

THERAPY

USING THE GUIDE

Anderson et al[1] identify the conversation topics and dynamics in the clinical encounter that move discussions toward or away from acknowledging the possibility of death. Figure 13.5-1[1] summarizes the dynamics of communication. The physician and patient "dance" through their interactions to move their conversations either toward or away from acknowledging the possibility of dying. Each uses distinctive maneuvers to steer the discussion. To move discussion toward acknowledgment, patients may cue the physician for more information or disclose their emotions; physicians may explore patients' understanding of their illness or explore the emotions disclosed.

To steer discussion away from acknowledgment, the patient may focus narrowly on the acute concerns; the physician too may focus on acute or biomedical issues or defer further discussion to other physicians. The degree of acknowledgment reached through the encounter can fall anywhere along a continuum from no to full acknowledgment. The patient's diagnosis can affect the way communication unfolds, with the salient types being (1) terminal progressive illness (eg, metastatic cancer), (2) chronic illness (eg, diabetes), and (3) acute illness (eg, pulmonary embolism). Death was discussed in more direct terms (eg, "dying") with acutely or chronically ill patients and more in euphemisms (eg, "the end") with terminally ill patients. Patients' own prior suspicions that they may die also affected physicians' willingness to disclose the possibility of dying. This possibility was not raised with any patients who described themselves as "relatively healthy."

FIGURE 13.5-1

"Dancing Around Death:" Explanatory Matrix Describing Physician-Patient Communication About Serious Illness

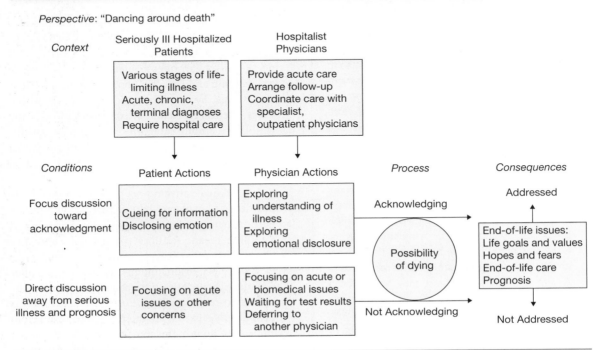

HOW CAN I APPLY THE RESULTS TO PATIENT CARE?

Does the Study Offer Helpful Theory?

Qualitative findings generalize to a theory rather than to a population.[17] Readers must use judgment to transfer this theory to other settings. *Transferability* will be different for each user of the research and requires the user to ask the following questions: Would it be reasonable for these findings—or a specific part of them—to apply in my own setting? How might things work similarly or differently in that setting? Answering these questions draws on additional sources of wisdom, including experience, training, or theoretical or empirical knowledge. Readers should compare the participants and the context of the research setting to their own, with attention not only to standard features, such as demographics or locale, but also to language, culture, and other social norms. Readers revisit the question of relevance at this point to consider whether the findings, as well as the research objectives, address key concerns.

Authors should express essential themes using common, clear language that translates well into action.[34] Readers can further gauge a theory's quality and usefulness by considering characteristics such as coherence, comprehensiveness, and relevance.[35] Coherence entails parsimony (invoking a minimal number of assumptions), consistency (according with what is already known and explains the unexpected), clarity (expressing ideas evocatively and sensibly), and fertility (suggesting directions for further investigation or action). Any illustrations, such as figures showing matrixes, models, or flow diagrams, should make sense with respect to both their component parts and relationships between them. An empirically developed theory need not agree with existing beliefs or social science theories. Whether it agrees or not, authors should critically discuss how their findings relate to prevailing knowledge.[36]

Does the Study Help Me Understand Social Phenomena in My Practice?

Interpretive qualitative research offers clinicians an understanding of social roles, interactions,

relationships, and experiences. Many qualitative studies of interest to clinicians focus on communication or behaviors among patients, families, and caregivers. They provide theory to aid understanding, not a definitive answer to a question. Qualitative findings must be applied with judgment to specific situations, which will always differ from the setting of the study. However, even when qualitative research findings do not reflect the reader's own experience, they may provide insight into what is really going on.

USING THE GUIDE

Anderson et al[1] summarize their findings in Figure 13.5-1, which illustrates typical topics of hospitalist-patient discussions and how specific topics draw conversations toward or away from acknowledging the possibility of dying. The figure and text express this dynamic clearly, in terms meaningful to clinical readers and social scientists and without requiring readers to make complex or dubious assumptions. The metaphor of "dancing" seems particularly illustrative. It invites readers to consider whether, and how, the "dance" might be done differently to achieve optimal communication and draws attention to how both physician and patient take steps—and respond to each other's steps—to steer the conversation. Readers can use these findings to reflect on their own interactions with patients in their own settings (hospital or elsewhere) by asking whether they see themselves "dancing around death" in encounters with patients. When and how do they do this, and is their style of "dancing" best for their patients? Might different patients need different approaches? Through these insights, intuitive moves may become more conscious and reasoned. To pursue acknowledgment more directly, Anderson et al[1] suggest clear steps for hospitalists based on their findings (eg, more routinely exploring patients' emotions or understandings of their illnesses).

THERAPY

USING THE GUIDE

The study by Anderson et al[1] helps readers distinguish and see more clearly different types of seriously ill patients, their typical attitudes toward discussing the possibility of dying, and the steps and countersteps that physicians and patients use to steer discussions about death. Both typically avoid the topic altogether if the patient sees himself/herself as essentially healthy, despite a very poor prognosis. Discussions with terminally ill patients tend to use euphemisms, whereas discussions with chronically and acutely ill patients use more direct language. Probing or expressing emotions moves discussions toward acknowledging the possibility of dying, whereas a focus on immediate biomedical issues moves discussions away. Although this study informs clinicians of how the dynamic works, it is primarily up to the individual clinician encountering a specific patient to decide whether and how to deliberately steer the dialogue toward or away from dying. Clinicians also may apply these findings—that is, the "dancing with death" theory about how conversations about dying work—to developing their own ideas for more harmonious communication. For example, one might consider whether conversations with family members might involve similar strategies to approach or avoid the topic of dying. They can try taking a step toward the discussion and see what step the family member takes in response. The image of a "dance" invites them generally toward or away from this topic gradually, sometimes responsive to or sometimes gently countering the other person. In discussions with family members or with patients different from those in this study's research setting, clinicians still may use these findings to address the needs and concerns of seriously ill patients more gracefully and respectfully.

CLINICAL SCENARIO RESOLUTION

As a physician striving to minister sensitive, compassionate, end-of-life care, you pause for some reflective thinking about conversational strategies to engage your 3 patients who you suspect may not leave the hospital. You first decide to broach the issue today with the most conversational among them, a 70-year-old retired social worker who seems to value direct dialogue and who has some familiarity with personal health care decision making. Your second patient is more reserved and stoic and has not yet made personal comments about his diagnosis of metastatic prostate cancer. You plan to probe his feelings about his illness, realizing that until now you have been avoiding the topic, focusing instead on test results while awaiting the oncologist's return visit. Your third patient has mild dementia, and it was her son who questioned you about whether his mother might be unable to return to her retirement home after rehabilitation following the stroke that precipitated the current hospitalization. You decide to telephone him today to request a family meeting later in the week, citing the need to follow up on the insightful question he posed when you first met.

References

1. Anderson WG, Kools S, Lyndon A. Dancing around death: hospitalist-patient communication about serious illness. *Qual Health Res*. 2013;23(1):3-13.
2. Geertz C. *Thick Description: Toward an Interpretive Theory of culture: The Interpretation of Cultures*. New York, NY: Basic Books; 1973:3-30.
3. Lincoln YS, Guba EG. Establishing trustworthiness. In: *Naturalistic Inquiry*. London, England: Sage Publications; 1985:289-331.
4. Giacomini M. Theory matters in qualitative research. In: Bourgeault I, DeVries R, Dingwall R, eds. *Handbook of Qualitative Health Research*. Thousand Oaks, CA: Sage Publications; 2010:125-156.

5. Creswell JW. *Qualitative Inquiry and Research Design: Choosing Among Five Approaches.* Thousand Oaks, CA: Sage Publications; 2007.

6. Hodges BD, Kuper A, Reeves S. Discourse analysis. *BMJ.* 2008;337:a879. doi:10.1136/bmj.a879.

7. Lingard L, Albert M, Levinson W. Grounded theory, mixed methods, and action research. *BMJ.* 2008;337:a567. doi:10.1136/bmj.39602.690162.47.

8. Reeves S, Kuper A, Hodges BD. Qualitative research methodologies: ethnography. *BMJ.* 2008;337:a1020. doi:10.1136/bmj.a1020.

9. Melia KM. Recognizing quality in qualitative research. In: Bourgeault I, DeVries R, Dingwall R, eds. *Handbook of Qualitative Health Research.* Thousand Oaks, CA: Sage Publications; 2010:559-574.

10. Rolfe G. Validity, trustworthiness and rigour: quality and the idea of qualitative research. *J Adv Nurs.* 2006;53(3):304-310.

11. Dixon-Woods M, Shaw RL, Agarwal S, Smith JA. The problem of appraising qualitative research. *Qual Saf Health Care.* 2004;13(3):223-225.

12. Bourgeault I, DeVries R, Dingwall R. *Handbook of Qualitative Health Research.* Thousand Oaks, CA: Sage Publications; 2010.

13. Denzin N, Lincoln Y. *The SAGE Handbook of Qualitative Research.* 4th ed. Thousand Oaks, CA: Sage Publications; 2011.

14. Creswell JW. *Qualitative Inquiry and Research Design.* 3rd ed. Thousand Oaks, CA: Sage Publications; 2012.

15. Crowe M, Sheppard L. A review of critical appraisal tools show they lack rigor: alternative tool structure is proposed. *J Clin Epidemiol.* 2011;64(1):79-89.

16. Kuper A, Lingard L, Levinson W. Critically appraising qualitative research. *BMJ.* 2008;337:a1035. doi:10.1136/bmj.a1035.

17. Yin RK. The case study method as a tool for doing evaluation. *Curr Sociol.* 1992;40(1):122-137.

18. Charmaz K. *Constructing Grounded Theory: A Practical Guide Through Qualitative Analysis.* Los Angeles, CA: Sage Publications; 2006.

19. Patton MQ. Designing qualitative studies. In: *Qualitative Evaluation and Research Methods.* 3rd ed. Thousand Oaks, CA: Sage Publications; 2002:209-257.

20. Davies D, Dodd J. Qualitative research and the question of rigor. *Qual Health Res.* 2002;12(2):279-289.

21. Steward DW, Shamdasani PN. Group dynamics and focus group research. In: *Focus Groups: Theory and Practice.* London, England: Sage Publications; 1990:33-50.

22. Hodder I. The interpretation of documents and material culture. In: Denzin N, Lincoln Y, eds. *Handbook of Qualitative Research.* 2nd ed. London, England: Sage Publications; 2000:703-716.

23. Kirk J, Miller ML. *Reliability and Validity in Qualitative Research.* London, England: Sage Publications; 1986.

24. Patton MQ. Fieldwork strategies and observation methods. In: *Qualitative Evaluation and Research Methods.* Thousand Oaks, CA: Sage Publications; 2002:259-338.

25. Krieger N. Methods for the scientific study of discrimination and health: an ecosocial approach. *Am J Public Health.* 2012;102(5):936-944.

26. Charmaz K. Theoretical sampling, saturation, and sorting. In: *Constructing Grounded Theory: A Practical Guide Through Qualitative Analysis.* Los Angeles, CA: Sage Publications; 2006:96-122.

27. Lincoln YS, Guba EG. Designing a naturalistic inquiry. In: *Naturalistic Inquiry.* London, England: Sage Publications; 1985:221-249.

28. Stake R. Triangulation. In: Stake R, ed. *The Art of Case Study Research.* London, England: Sage Publications; 1995:107-120.

29. Power EM. Toward understanding in postmodern interview analysis: interpreting the contradictory remarks of a research participant. *Qual Health Res.* 2004;14(6):858-865.

30. Patton MQ. Enhancing the quality and credibility of qualitative analysis. *Health Serv Res.* 1999;34(5, pt 2):1189-1208.

31. Giacomini M. Interdisciplinarity in health services research: dreams and nightmares, maladies and remedies. *J Health Serv Res Policy.* 2004;9(3):177-183.

32. Lincoln YS, Guba EG. Is being value-free valuable? In: *Naturalistic Inquiry.* London, England: Sage Publications; 1985:160-186.

33. Sandelowski M, Barroso J. Finding the findings in qualitative studies. *J Nurs Scholarsh.* 2002;34(3):213-219.

34. Sandelowski M, Leeman J. Writing usable qualitative health research findings. *Qual Health Res.* 2012;22(10):1404-1413.

35. Elder NC, Miller WL. Reading and evaluating qualitative research studies. *J Fam Pract.* 1995;41(3):279-285.

36. Charmaz K. Writing the draft. In: *Constructing Grounded Theory: A Practical Guide Through Qualitative Analysis.* Los Angeles, CA: Sage Publications; 2006:151-176.

THERAPY

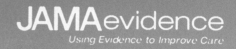
Using Evidence to Improve Care

HARM (OBSERVATIONAL STUDIES)

14

Harm (Observational Studies)

Mitchell Levine, John P. A. Ioannidis, Alfred Theodore Haines, and Gordon Guyatt

IN THIS CHAPTER

Does Soy Milk (or Soy Formula) Increase the Risk of Developing Peanut Allergy in Children?

You are a general practitioner examining a 29-year-old patient who is 8 months pregnant with her second child. Her first child, who is now 3 years old, had an intolerance to cow's milk as an infant. He was switched to soy formula and then soy milk, which he subsequently tolerated well. At 2 years of age, cow's milk was reintroduced without any problems, and he has been receiving cow's milk since. The mother was planning to start feeding her next child soy formula at birth but heard from a neighbor that it can increase the risk of peanut allergy in her child—a potentially serious and life-long problem. She asks for your advice on the topic. Because you are not familiar with this issue, you inform the patient that you will examine the *evidence* and discuss your findings with her when she returns for her next prenatal visit in 1 week.

FINDING THE EVIDENCE

You formulate the relevant question: In infants, is there an association between *exposure* to soy milk and the subsequent development of peanut allergy? You search a point-of-care clinician evidence synthesis tool with the term "peanut allergy." Under the subtopic "Causes and Risk Factors," you see that "consumption of soy milk or soy formula" is identified as a possible *risk factor* and a reference is provided. You click on the hypertext link to view the relevant article.[1]

The article describes a *case-control study* that used a geographically defined *cohort* of 13 971 preschool children. The investigators identified children with a convincing history of peanut allergy who reacted to a peanut challenge in which they were blind to whether they were being exposed to peanut protein or a "placebo." They collected detailed information from the children's parents and from 2 groups of control parents (a random sample from the geographically defined cohort and from a subgroup of children from the cohort who had eczema in the first 6 months of life and whose mothers had a history of eczema).

Box 14-1 presents our usual 3-step approach to using an article about *harm* from the medical

BOX 14-1

Users' Guides for an Article About Harm

How serious is the risk of bias?

In a cohort study, aside from the exposure of interest, did the exposed and control groups start and finish with the same risk for the outcome?

Were patients similar for prognostic factors that are known to be associated with the outcome (or did statistical adjustment address the imbalance)?

Were the circumstances and methods for detecting the outcome similar?

Was the follow-up sufficiently complete?

In a case-control study, did the cases and control group have the same risk for being exposed in the past?

Were cases and controls similar with respect to the indication or circumstances that would lead to exposure (or did statistical adjustment address the imbalance)?

Were the circumstances and methods for determining exposure similar for cases and controls?

What are the results?

How strong is the association between exposure and outcome?

How precise was the estimate of the risk?

How can I apply the results to patient care?

Were the study patients similar to the patient in my practice?

Was follow-up sufficiently long?

Is the exposure similar to what might occur in my patient?

What is the magnitude of the risk?

Are there any benefits that are known to be associated with exposure?

literature to guide your practice. You will find these criteria useful for a variety of issues that involve concerns of etiology or risk factors in which a potentially harmful exposure cannot be randomly assigned. These *observational studies* involve using cohort or case-control designs.

HOW SERIOUS IS THE RISK OF BIAS?

Clinicians often encounter patients who face potentially harmful exposures to either medical interventions or environmental agents. These circumstances give rise to common questions: Do cell phones increase the risk of brain tumors? Do vasectomies increase the risk of prostate cancer? Do changes in health care policies (eg, activity-based funding) lead to harmful *health outcomes*? When examining these questions, clinicians and administrators must evaluate the *risk of bias*, the strength of the association between the assumed cause and the adverse outcome, and the relevance to patients in their practice or domain.

In answering any clinical question, our first goal should be to identify whether there is an existing *systematic review* of the topic that can provide a summary of the highest-quality available evidence (see the Summarizing the Evidence section). Interpreting such a *review* requires an understanding of the rules of evidence for individual or *primary studies, randomized clinical trials* (RCTs), and observational studies. The tests for judging the risk of bias associated with results of observational studies will help you decide whether exposed and *control groups* (or cases and controls) began and completed the study with sufficient similarities that we can obtain a minimally biased assessment of the influence of exposure on outcome (see Chapter 6, Why Study Results Mislead: Bias and Random Error).

Randomized clinical trials provide less biased estimates of potentially harmful effects than other study designs because randomization is the best way to ensure that groups are balanced with respect to known and unknown determinants of the outcome (see Chapter 7, Therapy [Randomized Trials]). Although investigators conduct RCTs to determine whether therapeutic agents are beneficial, they also should look for harmful effects and may sometimes

make surprising discoveries about the adverse effects of the intervention on their primary outcomes (see Chapter 11.2, Surprising Results of Randomized Trials).

There are 4 reasons why RCTs may not be helpful for determining whether a putative harmful agent truly has deleterious effects. First, we may consider it unethical to randomize patients to exposures that might result in harmful effects without benefit (eg, smoking).

Second, we are often concerned about rare and serious adverse effects that may become evident only after tens of thousands of patients have consumed a medication for a period of years. For instance, even a very large RCT failed to detect an association between clopidogrel and thrombotic thrombocytopenic purpura,[3] which appeared in a subsequent observational study.[4] Randomized clinical trials that address adverse effects may be feasible for adverse event rates as low as 1%,[5,6] but the RCTs needed to explore harmful events occurring in fewer than 1 in 100 exposed patients are logistically difficult and often prohibitively expensive because of the huge sample size and lengthy *follow-up* required. *Meta-analyses* may be helpful when the event rates are very low.[7] However, availability of large-scale evidence on specific harms in systematic reviews is not common. For example, in a report of nearly 2000 systematic reviews, only 25 had large-scale data on 4000 or more randomized participants regarding well-defined harms that might be associated with the interventions under study.[8]

Third, RCT duration of follow-up is limited, yet not infrequently we are interested in knowing effects years, or even decades, after the exposure (eg, long-term consequences of chemotherapy in childhood).[9]

Fourth, even when events are sufficiently frequent and occur during a time frame feasible for RCTs to address, study reports often fail to adequately provide information on harm.[10]

Given that clinicians will not find RCTs to answer most questions about harm, they must understand the alternative strategies used to minimize *bias*. This requires a familiarity with observational study designs (Table 14-1).

There are 2 main types of observational studies: cohort and case-control. In a cohort study, investigators identify exposed and nonexposed groups

TABLE 14-1

Directions of Inquiry and Key Methodologic Strengths and Weaknesses for Different Study Designs

Design	Starting Point	Assessment	Strengths	Weaknesses
Randomized clinical trial	Exposure status	Outcome event status	Low susceptibility to bias	Feasibility and generalizability constraints
Cohort	Exposure status	Outcome event status	Feasible when randomization of exposure not possible, generalizability	Susceptible to bias
Case-control	Outcome event status	Exposure status	Overcomes temporal delays and the need for huge sample sizes to accumulate rare events	Susceptible to bias

of patients, each a cohort, and then follow them forward in time, monitoring the occurrence of outcomes of interest in an attempt to identify whether there is an association between the exposure and the outcomes. The cohort design is similar to an RCT but without randomization; rather, the determination of whether a patient received the exposure of interest results from the patient's or investigator's preference or from happenstance.

Case-control studies also assess associations between exposures and outcomes. Rare outcomes or those that take a long time to develop can threaten the feasibility not only of RCTs but also of cohort studies. The case-control study provides an alternative design that relies on the initial identification of cases—that is, patients who have already developed the target outcome—and the selection of controls—persons who do not have the outcome of interest. Using case-control designs, investigators assess the relative frequency of previous exposure to the putative harmful agent in the cases and the controls.

For example, in addressing the impact of nonsteroidal anti-inflammatory drugs (NSAIDs) on clinically apparent upper gastrointestinal tract hemorrhage, investigators needed a cohort study to deal with the problem of infrequent events. Bleeding among those taking NSAIDs has been reported to occur approximately 1.5 times per 1000 person-years of exposure, in comparison with 1.0 per 1000 person-years in those not taking NSAIDs.[11] Because the event rate in unexposed patients is so low (0.1%), an RCT to study an increase in risk of 50% would require huge numbers of patients (sample size calculations suggested approximately 75 000 patients per group) for adequate power to test the hypothesis that NSAIDs cause the additional bleeding.[12] Such an RCT would not be feasible, but a cohort study, in which the information comes from a large administrative database, would be possible.

Cohort Studies

Cohort studies may be prospective or retrospective. In prospective cohort studies, the investigator enrolls patients or participants, starts the follow-up, and waits for the outcomes (events of interest) to occur. Such studies may take many years to complete, and thus they are difficult to conduct. An advantage, however, is that the investigators can plan how to monitor patients and collect data.

In retrospective cohort studies, the data regarding both exposures and outcomes have been previously collected; the investigator obtains the data and determines whether participants with and without the outcome of interest have been exposed to the putative causal agent or agents. These studies are easier to perform because they depend on the availability of data on exposures and outcomes that have already happened. On the other hand, the investigator has less control over the quality and relevance of the available data. In the end, clinicians need not pay too much attention to whether studies are prospective or retrospective but should instead focus on the risk of bias criteria in Box 14-1.

In a Cohort Study, Aside From the Exposure of Interest, Did the Exposed and Control Groups Start and Finish With the Same Risk for the Outcome?

Were Patients Similar for Prognostic Factors That Are Known to Be Associated With the Outcome (Or Did Statistical Adjustment Level Address This Imbalance)?

Cohort studies will yield biased results if the group exposed to the putative harmful agent and the unexposed group begin with additional differences in baseline characteristics that give them a different prognosis (ie, a different risk of the target outcome) and if the analysis fails to deal with this imbalance. For instance, in the association between NSAIDs and the increased risk of upper gastrointestinal tract bleeding, age may be associated with exposure to NSAIDs and gastrointestinal bleeding. In other words, because patients taking NSAIDs will be older and because older patients are more likely to bleed, this variable makes attribution of an increased risk of bleeding to NSAID exposure problematic. When a variable with prognostic power differs in frequency in the exposed and unexposed cohorts, we refer to the situation as *confounding*.

There is no reason that patients who self-select (or who are selected by their physicians) for exposure to a potentially harmful agent should be similar to the nonexposed patients with respect to important determinants of the harmful outcome. Indeed, there are many reasons to expect they will not be similar. Physicians are appropriately reluctant to prescribe medications they perceive will put their patients at risk.

In one study, 24.1% of patients who were given a then-new NSAID, ketoprofen, had received peptic ulcer therapy during the previous 2 years compared with 15.7% of the control population.[13] The likely reason is that the ketoprofen manufacturer succeeded in persuading clinicians that ketoprofen was less likely to cause gastrointestinal bleeding than other agents. A comparison of ketoprofen to other agents would be subject to the risk of finding a spurious increase in bleeding with the new agent (compared with other therapies) because higher-risk patients would have been receiving the ketoprofen. This bias may be referred to as a selection bias or a bias due to confounding by indication.

The prescription of benzodiazepines to elderly patients provides another example of the way that selective physician prescribing practices can lead to a different distribution of risk in patients receiving particular medications, sometimes referred to as the *channeling bias*.[14] Ray et al[15] found an association between long-acting benzodiazepines and risk of falls (*relative risk* [RR], 2.0; 95% *confidence interval* [CI], 1.6-2.5) in data from 1977 to 1979 but not in data from 1984 to 1985 (RR, 1.3; 95% CI, 0.9-1.8). The most plausible explanation for the change is that patients at high risk for falls (those with dementia) selectively received these benzodiazepines during the earlier period. Reports of associations between benzodiazepine use and falls led to greater caution, and the apparent association disappeared when physicians began to avoid using benzodiazepines in those at high risk of falling.

Therefore, investigators must document the characteristics of the exposed and nonexposed participants and either demonstrate their comparability (very unusual in cohort studies) or use statistical techniques to adjust for these differences. Effective adjusted analyses for prognostic factors require the accurate measurement of those prognostic factors. For prospective cohorts, the investigators may take particular care of the quality of this information. For retrospective databases, however, one has to make use of what is available. Large administrative databases, although providing a sample size that may allow ascertainment of rare events, often have limited quality of data concerning relevant patient characteristics, health care encounters, or diagnoses. For example, in a cross-sectional study designed to measure the accuracy of electronic reporting of care practices compared with manual review, electronic reporting significantly underestimated rates of appropriate asthma medication and pneumococcal vaccination and overestimated rates of cholesterol control in patients with diabetes.[16]

Even if investigators document the comparability of potentially confounding variables in exposed and nonexposed cohorts, and even if they use statistical techniques to adjust for differences, important prognostic factors that the investigators do not know about or have not measured may be unbalanced between the groups and thus may be responsible for differences in outcome. We call this *residual confounding*.

Returning to our earlier example, it may be that the illnesses that require NSAIDs, rather than the NSAIDs themselves, contribute to the increased risk of bleeding. Thus, the strength of inference from a cohort study will always be less than that of a rigorously conducted RCT.

Were the Circumstances and Methods for Detecting the Outcome Similar?

In cohort studies, ascertainment of outcome is the key issue. For example, investigators have reported a 3-fold increase in the risk of malignant melanoma in individuals who work with radioactive materials. One possible explanation for some of the increased risk might be that physicians, concerned about a possible risk, search more diligently and therefore detect disease that might otherwise go unnoticed (or they may detect disease at an earlier point). This could result in the exposed cohort having an apparent, but spurious, increase in risk—a situation known as *surveillance bias*.[18]

The choice of outcome may partially address this problem. In one cohort study, for example, investigators assessed perinatal outcomes among infants of men exposed to lead and organic solvents in the printing industry by means of a cohort study that assessed all of the men who had been members of the printers' unions in Oslo, Norway.[19] The investigators used job classification to categorize the fathers as being exposed to lead and organic solvents or not exposed to those substances. Investigators' awareness of whether the fathers had been exposed to the lead or solvents might bias their assessment of the infant's outcome for minor birth defects or defects that required special investigative procedures. On the other hand, an outcome such as preterm birth would be unlikely to increase simply as a result of *detection bias* (the tendency to look more carefully for an outcome in one of the comparison groups) because prior knowledge of exposure is unlikely to influence whether an infant is considered preterm or not. The study found that exposure was associated with an 8-fold increase in preterm births but no increase in birth defects, so detection bias was not an issue for the results that were obtained in this study.

Was the Follow-up Sufficiently Complete?

As we pointed out in Chapter 7, Therapy (Randomized Trials), loss to follow-up can introduce bias because the patients who are lost may have different outcomes from those patients still available for assessment. This is particularly problematic if there are differences in follow-up between the exposed and nonexposed groups.

For example, in a well-executed study,[20] investigators determined the vital status of 1235 of 1261 white men (98%) employed in a chrysotile asbestos textile operation between 1940 and 1975. The RR for lung cancer death over time increased from 1.4 to 18.2 in direct proportion to the cumulative exposure among asbestos workers with at least 15 years since first exposure. In this study, the 2% missing data were unlikely to affect the results, and the loss to follow-up did not threaten the strength of the inference that asbestos exposure caused lung cancer deaths.

Case-Control Studies

Case-control studies are always retrospective in design. The outcomes (events of interest) have already happened and participants are designated to 1 of 2 groups: those with the outcomes (cases) and those where the outcome is absent (controls). Retrospectively, investigators ascertain prior exposure to putative causal agents. This design entails inherent risks of bias because exposure data require memory and recall or are based on a collection of data that were originally accumulated for purposes other than the intended study.

In a Case-Control Study, Did the Cases and Control Group Have the Same Risk (Chance) for Being Exposed in the Past?

Were Cases and Controls Similar With Respect to the Indication or Circumstances That Would Lead to Exposure (or Did Matching or Statistical Adjustment Address the Imbalance)?

As with cohort studies, case-control studies are susceptible to unmeasured confounding. For instance, in looking at the association between use of β-agonists and mortality among patients with asthma, investigators need to consider—and match or adjust for—previous hospitalization and use of other medications to avoid confounding by disease severity. Patients who use more β-agonists may have more severe asthma, and this severity, rather than β-agonist use, may be responsible for increased mortality. As in cohort studies, however, matching and adjustment cannot eliminate the risk of bias, particularly when exposure varies over time. In other words, matching or adjustment for hospitalization or use of other medications may not adequately capture all of the variability in underlying disease severity in asthma. In addition, the adverse lifestyle behaviors of patients with asthma who use large amounts of β-agonists could be the real explanation for the association.

To further illustrate the concern about unmeasured confounding, consider the example of a case-control study that was designed to assess the association between diethylstilbestrol

ingestion by pregnant women and the development of vaginal adenocarcinomas in their daughters many years later.[21] An RCT or prospective cohort study designed to test this cause-and-effect relationship would have required at least 20 years from the time when the association was first suspected until the completion of the study. Furthermore, given the infrequency of the disease, an RCT or a cohort study would have required hundreds of thousands of participants. By contrast, using the case-control strategy, the investigators delineated 2 relatively small groups of young women. Those who had the outcome of interest (vaginal adenocarcinoma) were designated as the cases (n = 8), and those who did not experience the outcome were designated as the controls (n = 32). Then, working backward in time, the investigators determined exposure rates to diethylstilbestrol for the 2 groups. They found a significant association between in utero diethylstilbestrol exposure and vaginal adenocarcinoma, and they found their answer without a delay of 20 years and by studying only 40 women.

An important consideration in this study would be whether the cases could have been exposed to diethylstilbestrol in any special circumstances that would not have affected women in the control group. In this situation, diethylstilbestrol had been prescribed to women at risk for miscarriages or premature births. Could either of these indications be a confounder? Before the introduction of diethylstilbestrol, vaginal adenocarcinoma in young women was uncommon, but miscarriages and premature birth were common. Thus, it would be unlikely that miscarriages and premature births were directly associated with vaginal adenocarcinoma, and in the absence of such an association, neither could be a confounder.

In another study, investigators used a case-control design relying on computer-record linkages between health insurance data and a drug insurance plan to investigate the possible association between use of β-adrenergic agonists and mortality rates in patients with asthma.[22] The database for the study included 95% of the population of the province of Saskatchewan, Canada. The investigators selected 129 patients who had experienced a fatal or near-fatal asthma attack to serve as cases and used a matching process to select another 655 patients who also had asthma but who had not had a fatal or near-fatal asthma attack to serve as controls.

The tendency of patients with more severe asthma to use more β-adrenergic medications could create a spurious association between drug use and mortality rate. The investigators attempted to control for the confounding effect of disease severity by measuring the number of hospitalizations in the 24 months before death (for the cases) or before the index date of entry into the study (for the control group) and by using an index of the aggregate use of medications. They found an association between the routine use of large doses of β-adrenergic agonists through metered-dose inhalers and death from asthma (*odds ratio* [OR], 2.6 per canister of inhaler per month; 95% CI, 1.7-3.9), even after correcting for measures of disease severity.

Were the Circumstances and Methods for Determining Exposure Similar for Cases and Controls?

In case-control studies, ascertainment of the exposure is a key issue. However, if case patients have a better memory for exposure than control patients, the result will be a spurious association.

For example, a case-control study found a 2-fold increase in risk of hip fracture associated with psychotropic drug use.[23] In this study, investigators established drug exposure by examining computerized claim files from the Michigan Medicaid program, a strategy that avoided selective memory of exposure—*recall bias*—and differential probing of cases and controls by an interviewer—*interviewer bias*.

Another example was a case-control study that evaluated whether the use of cell phones was associated with an increased risk of motor vehicle crash.[24] Suppose the investigators had tried to ask people who had a motor vehicle crash and control patients (who were in no crash at the same day and time) whether they were using their cell phone around the time of interest. People who were in a crash would have been more likely to recall such use because their memory might be heightened by the unfortunate circumstances. This would have led to a spurious association because of differential recall. Alternatively, they might specifically deny the use of a cell phone because of embarrassment or legal concerns, thus obscuring an association. Therefore, the investigators in this study used a computerized database of cell phone use instead of patient recall.[24] Moreover, the investigators used each person in a crash as his or her own control. The time of the crash was matched against corresponding times of the life of the same person when they were driving but when no crash occurred (eg, same time driving to work). This appropriate design established that use of cell phones was associated with an increased risk of having a motor vehicle crash.

Not all studies have access to unbiased information on exposure. For instance, in a case-control study of the association between coffee and pancreatic cancer, the patients with cancer may be more motivated to identify possible explanations for their problem and provide a greater recounting of coffee use.[25] Also, if the interviewers are not blinded to whether a patient is a case or a control patient, the interviewer may probe deeper for exposure information from cases. In this particular study, there were no objective sources of data regarding exposure. Recall or interviewer bias might have explained the apparent association.

As it happened, another bias provided an even more likely explanation for what turned out to be a spurious association. The investigators chose control patients from the practices of the physicians treating the patients with pancreatic cancer. These control patients had a variety of gastrointestinal problems, some of which were exacerbated by coffee ingestion. The control patients had learned to avoid coffee, which explains the investigators' finding of an association between coffee (which the patients with pancreatic cancer consumed at general population levels) and pancreatic cancer. Subsequent investigations, using more appropriate controls, refuted this association.[26]

In addition to a biased assessment of exposure, *random error* in exposure ascertainment is also possible. In random misclassification, exposed and unexposed patients are misclassified, but the rates of misclassification are similar in cases and controls. Such nondifferential misclassification dilutes any association (ie, the true association will be larger than the observed association). Fortunately, unless the misclassification is extremely large, the reduction in the true association will not be important.

What Is the Risk of Bias in Cross-sectional Studies?

Like the cohort and the case-control study, the *cross-sectional study* is also an observational study design. Like a cohort study, a cross-sectional study is based on an assembled population of exposed and unexposed participants. However, in the cross-sectional study, the exposure and the existing or prevalent outcome are measured at the same point in time. Accordingly, the direction of association may be difficult to determine. Another important limitation is that the outcome or the threat of experiencing an adverse outcome may have led patients assigned as cases to leave the study, so a measure of association may be biased against the association. However, cross-sectional studies are relatively inexpensive and quick to conduct and may be useful in generating and exploring hypotheses that will be subsequently investigated using other observational designs or RCTs.

What Is the Risk of Bias in Case Series and Case Reports?

Case series (descriptions of a series of patients) and case reports (descriptions of individual patients) do not provide any comparison groups, so it is impossible to determine whether the observed outcome would likely have occurred in the absence of the exposure. Although descriptive studies have been reputed to have significant findings mandating an immediate change in clinician behavior, this is rarely justified, and without availability of evidence from stronger study designs, there are potentially undesirable consequences when actions are taken in response to evidence warranting very low confidence. Recall the consequences of case reports of specific birth defects occurring in association with thalidomide exposure.[27]

Consider the case of the drug Bendectin (a combination of doxylamine, pyridoxine, and dicyclomine used as an antiemetic in pregnancy), whose manufacturer withdrew it from the market as a consequence of case reports suggesting that it was teratogenic.[28] Later, although a number of comparative studies reported the drug's relative safety,[29] they could not eradicate the prevailing litigious atmosphere—which prevented the manufacturer from reintroducing Bendectin. Thus, many pregnant women who might have benefited from the drug's availability were denied the symptomatic relief it could have offered.

For some interventions, registries of adverse events may provide the best possible initial evidence. For example, there are vaccine registries that record adverse events among people who have received the vaccine. These registries may signal problems with a particular adverse event that would be very difficult to capture from prospective studies limited by sample sizes that were too small. Even retrospective studies might be too difficult to conduct if people who receive the vaccine differ substantially from those who do not and if adjustment or matching cannot deal with the differences. In this situation, investigators might conduct a *before-after study* using the general population before the introduction of the new vaccine occurred. Such comparisons using historical controls are, however, prone to bias because many other factors may have changed in the same period. If, however, changes in the incidence of an adverse event are very large, the signal may be real. An example is the clustering of intussusception cases among children receiving a particular type of rotavirus vaccine,[30] resulting in a decision to withdraw the vaccine. The association was subsequently supported by a case-control study.[31] Eventually, another type of rotavirus vaccine was developed that did not cause this adverse event.

In general, clinicians should not draw conclusions about relationships from case series, but rather, they should recognize that the results may generate questions, or even hypotheses, that clinical investigators can address with studies that have optimal safeguards against risk of bias. When the immediate risk of exposure outweighs the benefits (and outweighs the risk of stopping an exposure), the clinician may have to make a management decision with less than optimal data.

How Serious Is the Risk of Bias: Summary

Just as it is true for the resolution of questions of therapeutic effectiveness, clinicians should first look to RCTs to resolve issues of harm. They will often be disappointed in the search and must make use of studies of weaker design. Regardless of the design, however, they should look for an appropriate control population. For cohort studies, the control group should have a similar baseline risk of outcome, or investigators should have used statistical techniques to adjust for differences. In case-control studies, the cases and the controls should have had a similar opportunity to have been exposed, so that if a difference in exposure is observed, one might legitimately conclude that the association could be due to a link between the exposure and the outcome and not due to a confounding factor. Nevertheless, investigators should routinely use statistical techniques to match cases and controls or adjust for differences.

Even when investigators have taken all of the appropriate steps to minimize bias, clinicians should bear in mind that residual differences between groups still may bias the results of observational studies.[32]

Because evidence, clinician preferences, and patient *values and preferences* determine the use of interventions in the real world, exposed and unexposed patients are likely to differ in prognostic factors.

USING THE GUIDE

Returning to our earlier discussion, the study that we retrieved investigating the association between soy milk (or soy formula) and the development of peanut allergy used a case-control design.[1] Those with peanut allergy (cases) appeared to be similar to controls with respect to the indication or circumstances leading to soy exposure, but there were a few potentially important imbalances. In the peanut allergy group, a family history of peanut allergy and an older sibling with a history of milk intolerance were more common and could have biased the likelihood of a subsequent child's being exposed to soy. To avoid confounding, the investigators conducted an *adjusted analysis.*

The methods for determining exposure were similar for cases and controls because the data were collected with the interviewers and parents unaware of the hypothesis that related soy exposure to peanut allergy (thus avoiding interviewer bias and perhaps recall bias). With regard to access to soy, all of the children came from the same geographic region, although this does not ensure that cultural and economic factors that might determine soy access were similar in cases and controls. Overall, protection from risk of bias seemed adequate.

WHAT ARE THE RESULTS?

How Strong Is the Association Between Exposure and Outcome?

We describe options that can be used for expressing an association between an exposure and an outcome—the *risk ratio* or RR and the OR—in other chapters of this book (see Chapter 9, Does Treatment Lower

Risk? Understanding the Results, and Chapter 12.2, Understanding the Results: More About Odds Ratios).

For example, in a cohort study that assessed in-hospital mortality after noncardiac surgery in male veterans, 23 of 289 patients with a history of hypertension died compared with 3 of 185 patients without the condition.[34] The RR for mortality in hypertensive patients compared with normotensive patients (23/289 and 3/185, respectively) was 4.9 (95% CI, 1.5-16.1). The RR tells us that death after non-cardiac surgery occurs almost 5 times more often in patients with hypertension than in normotensive patients.

The estimate of the RR depends on the availability of samples of exposed and unexposed patients, where the proportion of the patients with the outcome of interest can be determined. The RR is not applicable to case-control studies in which the number of cases and controls—and, therefore, the proportion of individuals with the outcome—is chosen by the investigator. For case-control studies, instead of using a ratio of risks, the RR, we use a ratio of odds, the OR, specifically the odds of a case patient being exposed divided by the odds of a control patient being exposed. Unless the risk of the outcome in the relevant population is high (20% or more), you can think of the OR as providing a good estimate of the much easier to conceptualize RR.

How Precise Is the Estimate of the Risk?

Clinicians can evaluate the precision of the estimate of risk by examining the CI around that estimate (see Chapter 10, Confidence Intervals: Was the Single Study or Meta-analysis Large Enough?). In a study in which investigators have found an association between an exposure and an adverse outcome, the lower limit of the estimate of RR associated with the adverse exposure provides an estimate of the lowest possible magnitude of the association. Alternatively, in a negative study (in which the results are not *statistically significant*), the upper boundary of the CI

around the RR tells the clinician just how big an adverse effect still may be present, despite the failure to find a statistically significant association.

USING THE GUIDE

The investigators calculated an OR of 2.6 (95% CI, 1.3-5.2) for the risk of peanut allergy in those exposed to soy vs those not exposed.[1] These results were adjusted for skin manifestations of allergy (ie, atopy). The consumption of soy by the infants was independently associated with peanut allergy and could not be explained as a dietary response to other atopic conditions. It nevertheless remains possible that the association with soy was confounded by other, unknown factors. Unfortunately, the investigators did not evaluate the possibility of a dose-response relationship for soy exposure and the development of peanut allergy.

HOW CAN I APPLY THE RESULTS TO PATIENT CARE?

Were the Study Patients Similar to the Patient in My Practice?

If possible biases in a study are not sufficient to dismiss the study out of hand, you should consider the extent to which the results might apply to the patient in your practice. Would your patient have met the eligibility criteria? Is your patient similar to those described in the study with respect to potentially important factors, such as patient characteristics or medical history? If not, is the biology of the harmful exposure likely to be different for the patient for whom you are providing care?

Was Follow-up Sufficiently Long?

Studies can be pristine in terms of avoiding bias but of limited use if patients are not followed up for a sufficiently long period. That is, they may provide an unbiased estimate of the effect of an exposure during the short term, but the time frame in which we are interested is a substantially longer period. For example, most cancers take a decade or longer to develop from the original assault at the biologic level to the clinically detected malignant tumor. If the question is whether a specific exposure, say to an industrial chemical, is related to a subsequent cancer, one would not expect cancers detected in the first few years to reflect any of the effect of the exposure under question.

Is the Exposure Similar to What Might Occur in My Patient?

Clinicians should ask whether there are important differences in the exposures of a study (eg, dose and duration) between their patient and the patients in the study. For example, it should be clear that the risk of thrombophlebitis associated with oral contraceptive use described in the 1970s may not be applicable to the patient in the 21st century because of the lower estrogen dose in oral contraceptives currently used. Another example of questionable applicability comes from a study that found that workers employed in a chrysotile asbestos textile operation between 1940 and 1975 had an increased risk of lung cancer death, a risk that increased from 1.4 to 18.2 in direct relation to cumulative exposure among asbestos workers with at least 15 years since first exposure.[18] The study does not provide trustworthy information regarding what might be the risks associated with only brief or intermittent exposure to asbestos (eg, a person working for a few months in an office located in a building subsequently found to have abnormally high asbestos levels).

What Is the Incremental Risk?

The RR and OR do not tell us how frequently the problem occurs; they tell us only that the observed effect occurs more or less often in the exposed group vs the unexposed group. Even when we observe a large and statistically significant relative difference between the 2 groups, the results still may not be important if the adverse event is rare. Thus, we need a method for assessing the absolute impact of the exposure. In our discussion of therapy (see Chapter 7, Therapy [Randomized

Trials], and Chapter 9, Does Treatment Lower Risk? Understanding the Results), we describe how to calculate the *risk difference* and the number of patients whom clinicians must treat to prevent an adverse event (*number needed to treat*). When the issue is harm, we can use data from a randomized trial or cohort study (but not a case-control study) in a similar way to calculate the number of patients who would have to be exposed to result in an additional harmful event. However, this calculation requires knowledge of the *absolute risk* in unexposed individuals in our population.

For example, during a mean of 10 months of follow-up, investigators conducting the Cardiac Arrhythmia Suppression Trial, an RCT of anti-arrhythmic agents,[35] found that the mortality rate was 3.0% for placebo-treated patients and 7.7% for those treated with either encainide or flecainide. The absolute risk increase was 4.7%, the reciprocal of which (100/4.7) tells us that, on average, for every 21 patients treated with encainide or flecainide for approximately a year, there would be 1 excess death.

This contrasts with our example of the association between NSAIDs and upper gastrointestinal tract bleeding. Of 2000 unexposed patients in that study, 2 will have a bleeding episode each year. Of 2000 patients taking NSAIDs, 3 will have such an episode each year. Thus, if we treat 2000 patients with NSAIDs, we can expect a single additional bleeding event.[11]

Are There Any Benefits That Offset the Risks Associated With Exposure?

Even after evaluating the evidence that an exposure is harmful and establishing that the results are potentially applicable to the patient in your practice, determining subsequent actions may not be simple. In addition to considering the magnitude of the risk, one must consider the adverse consequences of reducing or eliminating exposure to the harmful agent (ie, the magnitude of any potential benefit that patients will no longer receive).

Clinical decision making is simple when harmful consequences are unacceptable and benefit is absent. For example, because the evidence of increased mortality from encainide and flecainide came from an RCT with low risk of bias,[35] we can be at least moderately confident of a substantial increase in risk of death. Because treating only 21 people would result in an excess death, it is no wonder that clinicians quickly curtailed their use of these antiarrhythmic agents when the study results became available.

The clinical decision is also made easier when an acceptable alternative for avoiding the risk is available. Even if the evidence warrants low confidence, the availability of an alternative substance can result in a clear decision.

CLINICAL SCENARIO RESOLUTION

You determine that the patient's unborn child, once he or she reaches early childhood, would likely fulfill the eligibility criteria in the study. Also relevant to the clinical scenario, but perhaps unknown, is whether the soy products discussed in the study are similar to the ones that the patient is considering using. With regard to the magnitude of risk, the prevalence of peanut allergy is approximately 4 per 1000 children. An approximate calculation would suggest that, if the OR with exposure to soy is truly 2.6, 10 children per 1000 would be affected by peanut allergy, an additional 6 children in every 1000. In other words, the number of children needed to be exposed to soy to result in 1 additional child having peanut allergy is 167 (1000/6). Finally, there are no data regarding the negative consequences of withholding soy formula or soy milk products, and the use of these products would clearly be dependent on how severe and sustained an intolerance to cow's milk was in a particular child.

To decide on your course of action, you proceed through 3 steps of using the medical literature to guide your clinical practice. First, you consider the risk of bias in the study before you. Adjustments of known confounders did not diminish the association between soy exposure as a neonate and the development of peanut allergy. Also, the design of the study provides adequate safeguards against recall or interviewer bias. You conclude that, with the obvious limitations of the observational design (generally only warranting low confidence in estimates of effect), the study is at low risk of bias.

Turning to the results, you note a moderate association between soy exposure and the development of peanut allergy (moderate typically being considered ORs greater than 2 and less than 5) that is strong enough, despite the limitations of the observational design, that it leaves you moderately confident of an association between exposure to soy and peanut allergy. The lower boundary of the CI (1.3) and the uncertainty around the baseline risk estimate of 4 per 10 000 children lead you to conclude that you have only low confidence in your estimate of the incremental harm of peanut allergy of 6 in 1000.

You proceed to the third step, and consider the implications of the study results for your patient. The study would appear to apply to a future child of your patient. Although the best estimate of the absolute increase in risk is only 6 in 1000, and you have only low confidence in this estimate, the consequences of peanut allergy can be a serious health threat to a patient and quite disruptive for a family because of the required precautions and food restrictions. You discuss the situation with the mother, who elects to start feedings with milk products. Together you agree that, given the limited confidence in estimates and the small absolute risk, should the child appear to have distressing milk allergy, she will probably switch to soy.

References

1. Lack G, Fox D, Northstone K, Golding J; Avon Longitudinal Study of Parents and Children Study Team. Factors associated with the development of peanut allergy in childhood. *N Engl J Med*. 2003;348(11):977-985.

2. CAPRIE Steering Committee. A randomised, blinded, trial of clopidogrel versus aspirin in patients at risk of ischaemic events (CAPRIE). *Lancet*. 1996;348(9038):1329-1339.

3. Bennett CL, Connors JM, Carwile JM, et al. Thrombotic thrombocytopenic purpura associated with clopidogrel. *N Engl J Med*. 2000;342(24):1773-1777.

4. Silverstein FE, Graham DY, Senior JR, et al. Misoprostol reduces serious gastrointestinal complications in patients with rheumatoid arthritis receiving nonsteroidal anti-inflammatory drugs. A randomized, double-blind, placebo-controlled trial. *Ann Intern Med*. 1995;123(4):241-249.

5. Bombardier C, Laine L, Reicin A, et al; VIGOR Study Group. Comparison of upper gastrointestinal toxicity of rofecoxib and naproxen in patients with rheumatoid arthritis. *N Engl J Med*. 2000;343(21):1520-1528.

6. Langman MJ, Jensen DM, Watson DJ, et al. Adverse upper gastrointestinal effects of rofecoxib compared with NSAIDs. *JAMA*. 1999;282(20):1929-1933.

7. Papanikolaou PN, Ioannidis JP. Availability of large-scale evidence on specific harms from systematic reviews of randomized trials. *Am J Med*. 2004;117(8):582-589.

8. Geenen MM, Cardous-Ubbink MC, Kremer LC, et al. Medical assessment of adverse health outcomes in long-term survivors of childhood cancer. *JAMA*. 2007;297(24):2705-2715.

9. Ioannidis JP, Haidich AB, Pappa M, et al. Comparison of evidence of treatment effects in randomized and nonrandomized studies. *JAMA*. 2001;286(7):821-830.

10. Carson JL, Strom BL, Soper KA, West SL, Morse ML. The association of nonsteroidal anti-inflammatory drugs with upper gastrointestinal tract bleeding. *Arch Intern Med*. 1987;147(1):85-88.

11. Walter SD. Determination of significant relative risks and optimal sampling procedures in prospective and retrospective comparative studies of various sizes. *Am J Epidemiol*. 1977;105(4):387-397.

12. Leufkens HG, Urquhart J, Stricker BH, Bakker A, Petri H. Channelling of controlled release formulation of ketoprofen (Oscorel) in patients with history of gastrointestinal problems. *J Epidemiol Community Health*. 1992;46(4):428-432.

13. Joseph KS. The evolution of clinical practice and time trends in drug effects. *J Clin Epidemiol*. 1994;47(6):593-598.

14. Ray WA, Griffin MR, Downey W. Benzodiazepines of long and short elimination half-life and the risk of hip fracture. *JAMA*. 1989;262(23):3303-3307.

15. Kern LM, Malhotra S, Barrón Y, et al. Accuracy of electronically reported "meaningful use" clinical quality measures: a cross-sectional study. *Ann Intern Med*. 2013;158(2):77-83.

16. Hiatt RA, Fireman B. The possible effect of increased surveillance on the incidence of malignant melanoma. *Prev Med*. 1986;15(6):652-660.

17. Kristensen P, Irgens LM, Daltveit AK, Andersen A. Perinatal outcome among children of men exposed to lead and organic solvents in the printing industry. *Am J Epidemiol*. 1993;137(2):134-144.

18. Dement JM, Harris RL Jr, Symons MJ, Shy CM. Exposures and mortality among chrysotile asbestos workers. Part II: mortality. *Am J Ind Med*. 1983;4(3):421-433.

19. Herbst AL, Ulfelder H, Poskanzer DC. Adenocarcinoma of the vagina.Association of maternal stilbestrol therapy with tumor appearance in young women. *N Engl J Med*. 1971;284(15):878-881.

20. Spitzer WO, Suissa S, Ernst P, et al. The use of beta-agonists and the risk of death and near death from asthma. *N Engl J Med*. 1992;326(8):501-506.

21. Ray WA, Griffin MR, Schaffner W, Baugh DK, Melton LJ III. Psychotropic drug use and the risk of hip fracture. *N Engl J Med*. 1987;316(7):363-369.

22. Redelmeier DA, Tibshirani RJ. Association between cellular-telephone calls and motor vehicle collisions. *N Engl J Med*. 1997;336(7):453-458.

23. MacMahon B, Yen S, Trichopoulos D, Warren K, Nardi G. Coffee and cancer of the pancreas. *N Engl J Med*. 1981;304(11):630-633.

24. Baghurst PA, McMichael AJ, Slavotinek AH, Baghurst KI, Boyle P, Walker AM. A case-control study of diet and cancer of the pancreas. *Am J Epidemiol*. 1991;134(2):167-179.

25. Lenz W. Epidemiology of congenital malformations. *Ann N Y Acad Sci*. 1965;123:228-236.

26. Soverchia G, Perri PF. [2 cases of malformations of a limb in infants of mothers treated with an antiemetic in a very early phase of pregnancy]. *Pediatr Med Chir*. 1981;3(1):97-99.

27. Holmes LB. Teratogen update: bendectin. *Teratology*. 1983; 27(2):277-281.

28. Centers for Disease Control and Prevention (CDC). Intussusception among recipients of rotavirus vaccine--United States, 1998-1999. *MMWR Morb Mortal Wkly Rep*. 1999;48(27):577-581.

29. Murphy TV, Gargiullo PM, Massoudi MS, et al; Rotavirus Intussusception Investigation Team. Intussusception among infants given an oral rotavirus vaccine. *N Engl J Med*. 2001;344(8):564-572.

30. Kellermann AL, Rivara FP, Rushforth NB, et al. Gun ownership as a risk factor for homicide in the home. *N Engl J Med*. 1993;329(15):1084-1091.

31. Browner WS, Li J, Mangano DT; The Study of Perioperative Ischemia Research Group. In-hospital and long-term mortality in male veterans following noncardiac surgery. *JAMA*. 1992;268(2):228-232.

32. Echt DS, Liebson PR, Mitchell LB, et al. Mortality and morbidity in patients receiving encainide, flecainide, or placebo. The Cardiac Arrhythmia Suppression Trial. *N Engl J Med*. 1991;324(12):781-788.

15.1

ADVANCED TOPICS IN HARM

Correlation and Regression

Shanil Ebrahim, Stephen D. Walter, Deborah J. Cook,
Roman Jaeschke, and Gordon Guyatt

HARM (OBSERVATIONAL STUDIES)

IN THIS CHAPTER

INTRODUCTION

Investigators are sometimes interested in the relationship among different measures or variables. They may pose questions related to the correlation of these variables. For example, they might ask, "How well does the clinical impression of symptoms in a child with asthma relate to the parents' perception?" "How strong is the relationship between a patient's physical and emotional functions?"

By contrast, other investigators may be primarily interested in predicting individuals at high risk of having a subsequent event. For instance, can we identify patients with asthma who are at high risk for exacerbations that require hospitalization?

Still other investigators may seek the causal relations among biologic phenomena. For instance, they might ask, "What determines the extent to which a patient with asthma will experience dyspnea when exercising?" Finally, investigators also may pose causal questions that could directly inform patient management. For example, "Does use of long-acting β-agonists in asthma really increase the likelihood of dying?"

Clinicians may be interested in the answers to all 3 sorts of questions—those of correlation, prediction, and causation. To the extent that the relationship between child and parental perceptions is weak, clinicians must obtain both perspectives. If physical and emotional functions are only weakly related, then clinicians must probe both areas thoroughly. We may target patients at high risk of subsequent adverse events with prophylactic interventions. If clinicians know that hypoxemia is strongly related to dyspnea, they may be more inclined to administer oxygen to patients with dyspnea. The clinical implications of the causal questions are more obvious. We may avoid long-acting β-agonists if they really increase the likelihood of dying.

We refer to the degree of association among different variables or phenomena as *correlation*.[1] If we want to describe the relationship among different variables and subsequently use the value of a variable to predict another or make a causal inference, we use a technique called *regression*.[1] In this chapter, we provide examples to illustrate the use of correlation and regression in the medical literature.

CORRELATION

Correlation is a statistical tool that permits researchers to examine the strength of the relationship between 2 variables when neither variable is necessarily considered the *dependent variable*.

Traditionally, we perform laboratory measurements of exercise capacity in patients with cardiac and respiratory illnesses by using a treadmill or cycle ergometer. Approximately 30 years ago, investigators interested in respiratory disease began to use a simpler test that is related more closely to day-to-day activity.[2] In the walk test, patients are asked to cover as much ground as they can during a specified period (typically 6 minutes) walking in an enclosed corridor. For several reasons, we may be interested in the strength of the relationship between the walk test and conventional laboratory measures of exercise capacity. If the tests relate strongly enough to one another, we might be able to substitute one test for the other. In addition, the strength of the relationship might inform us of the potential of laboratory tests of exercise capacity to predict patients' ability to undertake physically demanding activities of daily living.

What do we mean by the strength of the relationship between 2 measures? One finds a strong positive relationship between 2 measures when patients who obtain high scores on the first also tend to obtain high scores on the second, when those in whom we find intermediate scores on the first also tend to have intermediate values on the second, and when patients who tend to score low on one measure score low on the other measure.[3] One also can have strong negative relationships: those who score high on one measure score low on the other.[3] If patients who score low on one measure are equally likely to score low or high on another measure, the relationship between the 2 variables is poor, weak, or nonexistent.[3]

We can gain a sense of the strength of the correlation by examining a visual plot relating patients' scores on the 2 measures. Figure 15.1-1 presents such a plot relating walk test results (on the x-axis) to the results of the cycle ergometer exercise test (on the y-axis). The data for this plot, and those for the subsequent analyses using walk test results, come from 3 studies of patients with chronic airflow limitation.[4-6] Each dot in Figure 15.1-1 represents an individual patient and presents 2 pieces of information: the patient's walk test score and cycle ergometer exercise time. Although the walk test results are truly continuous, the cycle ergometer results tend to take only certain values because patients usually stop the test at the end of a particular level rather than part way through a level.

Examining Figure 15.1-1, you can see that, in general, patients who score well on the walk test also tend to score well on the cycle ergometer exercise test, and patients who score poorly on the cycle ergometer tend to score poorly on the walk test. However, you can find patients who represent exceptions, scoring better than most other patients on one test but not as well on the other test. These data, therefore, represent a moderate relationship between 2 variables: the walk test and the cycle ergometer exercise test.

One can summarize the strength of a relationship between 2 continuous (also called interval) variables in a single number, the *Pearson correlation coefficient*. The Pearson correlation coefficient, which is denoted by *r*, can range from −1.0 to 1.0. A correlation of 1.0 or −1.0 occurs when there is a perfect linear relationship between the 2 scores, such that one is completely predictable from the other. A correlation coefficient of −1.0 corresponds to a perfect negative relationship, whereby higher scores on test A are associated with lower scores on test B. A correlation coefficient of 1.0 corresponds to a perfect positive relationship, whereby higher scores on test A are associated with higher scores on test B.

FIGURE 15.1-1

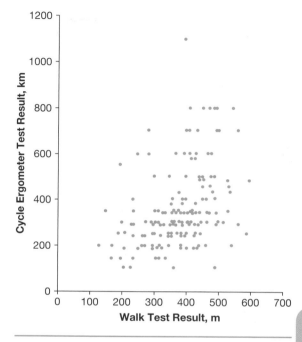

Relationship Between Walk Test Results and Cycle Ergometer Exercise Test Results

Reproduced from Guyatt et al,[1] by permission of the publisher. © 1995 Canadian Medical Association.

A correlation coefficient of 0 denotes no relationship between the 2 variables (ie, the scores on test A and the scores on test B fall in a random pattern). Typically, when calculating a correlation coefficient, a linear relationship between the variables is assumed. There may be a relationship between the variables, but it may not take the form of a straight line when viewed visually. For example, even if larger scores on the variables are found together, one may increase more slowly than the other for low values but will increase more quickly than the other for high values. If there is a strong relationship but it is not a linear one, the correlation coefficient may be misleading.

In the example depicted in Figure 15.1-1, the relationship appears to approximate a straight line, and the *r* value for the correlation between the walk test and the cycle ergometer is 0.50. Should the clinician be pleased and comfortable or displeased and uncomfortable with this moderately strong correlation? It depends on how we wish to apply the information. If we were thinking of using the walk test value as a substitute for the cycle ergometer—after all, the walk test is much simpler to perform— we would be disappointed. A correlation of 0.8 or higher (although the threshold is arbitrary) would be required for us to be confident in that kind of substitution. If the correlation were too low, there would be too much risk that a person with a high walk test score would have mediocre or low performance on the cycle ergometer test or that a person who did poorly on the walk test would do well on the cycle ergometer test. On the other hand, if we assume that the walk test gives a good indication of exercise capacity in daily life, the moderate correlation suggests that the cycle ergometer result tells us something (less than the walk test, but still something) about day-to-day exercise capacity.

In getting a sense of the magnitude of a correlation, in addition to the possibility of substituting one variable for another (requiring a very high correlation) or one variable giving us some indication of status on another (requiring a lower correlation), think of the proportion of variability in one variable that is explained by the other. The square of the correlation represents the proportion of variance explained (eg, if the correlation is 0.4, variable A explains 16% of the variance in variable B; if the correlation is 0.8, variable A explains 64% of the variance in variable B).

You often will see a P value in association with a correlation coefficient (see Chapter 12.1, Hypothesis Testing). When correlation coefficients are considered, the P value is usually associated with the typical *null hypothesis* that the true correlation between the 2 measures is 0. Thus, the P value represents the probability that, if the true correlation were 0, an apparent relationship as strong as or stronger than that actually observed would have occurred as a result of chance. The smaller the P value, the less likely it is that chance explains the apparent relationship between the 2 measures.

The P value depends not only on the strength of the relationship but also on the sample size. In this case, we had data on both the walk test and the cycle ergometer from 179 patients, and with a correlation of 0.50, the associated P value is less than .001. A relationship can be very weak, but if the sample size is sufficiently large, the P value may be small. For instance, with a sample size of 500, we reach the conventional threshold P value of .05 at a correlation of only 0.10. At the same time, for any given sample size, a stronger correlation will be associated with a lower P value.

In evaluating *treatment effects*, the size of the effect and the *confidence interval* (CIs) around the effect tend to be much more informative than P values (see Chapter 10, Confidence Intervals: Was the Single Study or Meta-analysis Large Enough?).[7] The same is true of correlations, in which the magnitude of the correlation and the CI around the correlation are the key parameters.

The 95% CI around the correlation between the walk test and laboratory exercise tests ranges from 0.38 to 0.60. A lower limit of 0.38 in the CI signifies a modest correlation.

REGRESSION

Regression examines the strength of a relationship between 1 or more predictor variables and a target variable. As clinicians, we are often interested in prediction. We would like to be able to predict which persons will develop a disease (such as coronary artery disease) and which persons will not; we would like to be able to predict which patient will do well and which patient will do poorly. We also are interested in making causal inferences in situations in which *randomized clinical trials* are not possible. Regression techniques are useful in addressing both sorts of issues.[8]

Regression Modeling With Continuous Target Variables

In any regression, we have a target outcome or response variable that we call the dependent variable because it is influenced or determined by other variables or factors. When this dependent variable is a continuous variable—such as a 6-minute walk test score that can take a large number of values—a *linear regression* is typically used.[9] Sometimes, individuals treat target variables that take 1 of a number of discrete values, such as the 10 or so levels that a patient might achieve on a conventional exercise test, as if they were continuous.

Regressions also involve explanatory or predictor variables that we suspect may be associated with, or causally related to, the dependent variable. These independent variables can be binary (either/or; also called dichotomous), such as sex (male or female). They may be categorical, with more than 2 categories, such as marital status (single, married, divorced, or widowed). Finally, they may be continuous, such as forced expiratory volume in 1 second (FEV_1).

When there is a single predictor variable and a single dependent variable, we call the regression approach a *bivariable* or *simple regression*.[10] When we are examining more than 1 independent variable, we call the regression approach a *multivariable* or *multiple regression*. The term univariable is reserved for descriptive statistical tests that involve only 1 variable and no independent variable, typically used to describe a sample or to expand a sample to a wider population.[11]

Let us assume we are trying to predict patients' walk test scores using easily measured variables: sex, height, and FEV_1 as a measure of lung function. Alternatively, we can think of the investigation as examining a causal hypothesis: to what extent are patients' walk test scores determined by sex, height, and pulmonary function? Either way, the dependent variable here is the walk test result, and the independent variables are sex, height, and FEV_1.

Figure 15.1-2, a histogram of the walk test scores of 219 patients with chronic lung disease, shows that walk test scores vary widely among patients. If we had to predict an individual's walk test score without any other information, our best guess would be the mean score of all patients (394 m). For many patients, however, this prediction would be well off the mark.

FIGURE 15.1-2

Distribution of Walk Test Results in the Total Sample of 219 Patients

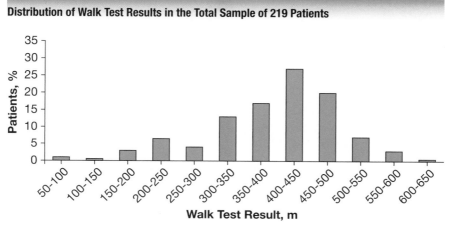

Walk Test Result, m

Figure 15.1-3 shows the relationship between FEV_1 and the walk test. Note that there is a relationship between the 2 variables, although the relationship is not as strong as the relationship between the walk test and the exercise test depicted in Figure 15.1-1. Thus, some of the differences, or variation, in walk test scores seems to be explained by, or attributable to, the patient's FEV_1. We can construct an equation using FEV_1 to predict walk test scores.

Generally, when we construct regression equations, we refer to the predictor (independent) variable as x and the target (dependent) variable as y. The regression equation in this example assumes a linear fit between the FEV_1 and the walk test data and specifies the point at which the straight line meets the y-axis (the intercept) and the steepness of the line (the slope). In this case, the regression is expressed as follows:

$$y = 298 + 108x$$

where y is the value of the walk test, 298 is the intercept, 108 is the slope of the line, and x is the value of the FEV_1 in liters. In this case, the intercept of 298 has little practical meaning; it predicts the walk test distance of a patient with an FEV_1 of 0. The slope of 108, however, has some meaning; it predicts that for every increase in FEV_1 of 1 L, the patient will walk 108 m farther. We show the regression line corresponding to this formula in Figure 15.1-3.

Having constructed the regression equation, we can examine the correlation between the 2 variables, and we can assess whether the correlation might be explained by chance. The correlation is 0.40, suggesting that chance is a very unlikely explanation ($P < .001$). Thus, we conclude that FEV_1 explains or accounts for a statistically significant proportion of the variability, or variance, in walk test scores.

We also can examine the relationship between the walk test score and patients' sex (Figure 15.1-4). Although there is considerable variability within the sexes, men tend to have higher walk test scores than women. If we had to predict a man's score, we would choose the mean score of the men (410 m); to predict a woman's score, we would choose the women's mean score of 363 m.

We can ask the question, "Does the apparent relationship between sex and walk test score result from chance?" One way of answering this question is to construct another simple regression equation with walk test as the dependent variable and patient's sex as the independent variable. As it turns out, chance is an unlikely explanation of the relationship between sex and the walk test ($P < .001$).

In Figure 15.1-5, we have separated the men from the women, and for each sex, we have divided them into groups with high and

FIGURE 15.1-3

Relationship Between FEV₁ and Walk Test Results in 219 Patients

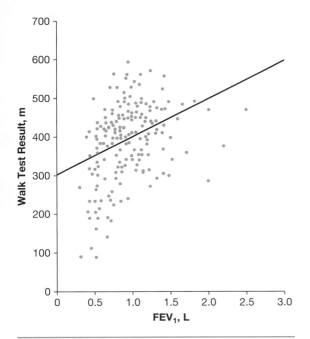

Abbreviation: FEV_1, forced expiratory volume in 1 second.

Reproduced from Guyatt et al,[1] by permission of the publisher. © 1995 Canadian Medical Association.

FIGURE 15.1-4

Distribution of Walk Test Results in Men and in Women (Sample of 219 Patients)

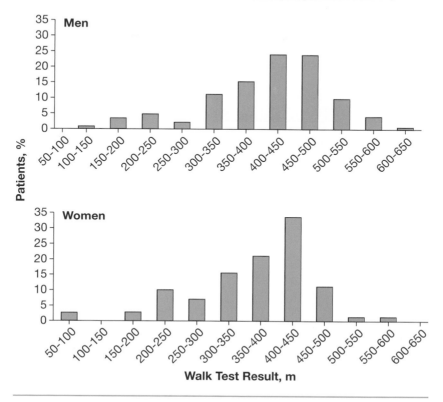

Reproduced from Guyatt et al,[1] by permission of the publisher. © 1995 Canadian Medical Association.

low FEV_1 results. Although there is a range of scores within each of these groups, the range is narrower than among all women or all men and even more so than all patients. When we use the mean of the men as our best guess of the walk test score of a man and the mean of the women as our best guess of the walk test score of a woman, we will, on average, be closer to the true value than if we had used the mean for all patients.

Figure 15.1-5 illustrates how we can take more than 1 independent variable into account at the same time in explaining or predicting the dependent variable. We can construct a mathematical model that explains or predicts the walk test score by simultaneously considering all of the independent variables, thus creating a multivariable regression equation.

Multivariable regression equations allow us to determine whether each of the variables that were associated with the dependent variable in the bivariable equations makes contributions to explaining the variation. Independent variables that are strongly associated with one another (such as age and year of birth) usually will not make strong separate contributions to predicting the dependent variable. Multivariable regression approaches provide us with models in which each variable makes its own independent contribution to the prediction.[12]

FIGURE 15.1-5

Distribution of Walk Test Results in Men and Women With High and Low FEV$_1$ (Sample of 219 Patients)

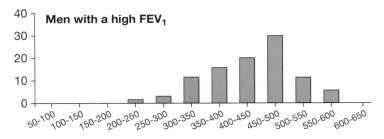

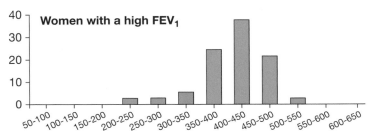

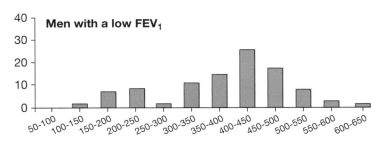

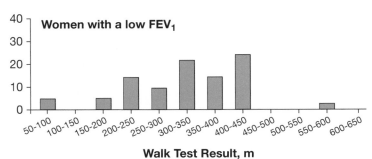

Walk Test Result, m

Abbreviation: FEV$_1$, forced expiratory volume in 1 second.

Reproduced from Guyatt et al,[1] by permission of the publisher. © 1995 Canadian Medical Association.

For example, FEV_1 and sex both make independent contributions to explaining walk test results ($P < .001$ for FEV_1 and $P = .03$ for sex in the multivariable regression analysis), but height (which was significant at the $P = .02$ level when considered in a bivariable regression) does not make a comparable contribution to the explanation.

If we had chosen both the FEV_1 and peak expiratory flow rates as independent variables, they would both reveal significant associations with walk test score. However, because FEV_1 and peak expiratory flow rates are associated strongly with one another, they are unlikely to provide independent contributions to explaining the variation in walk test scores. In other words, once we take FEV_1 into account, peak flow rates are not likely to be of any help in predicting walk test scores, and if we first took peak flow rate into account, FEV_1 would not provide further explanatory power to our predictive model. Similarly, height was a significant predictor of walk test score when considered alone but was no longer significant in the multivariable regression because of its correlation with sex and FEV_1.[1]

We have emphasized how the P value associated with a correlation provides little information about the strength of the relation between 2 values; the correlation coefficient itself is required. Similarly, knowing that a number of independent variables in a multivariable model explain some of the variation in the dependent variable tells us little about the power of our predictive model.

Regression equations can tell us much more: the proportion of the variation in the dependent variable that is explained by the model. If a model explains less than 10% of the variability, it is not very useful. If it explains more than 50% of the variability, it will be extremely useful. Intermediate proportions of variability explained are of intermediate value.

Returning to our example, Figure 15.1-5 gives us some sense of the model's predictive power. Although the distributions of walk test scores in the 4 subgroups differ appreciably, considerable overlap remains. In this case, FEV_1 explains 15% of the variation when it is the first variable entered into the model, sex explains an additional 2% of the variation, and the total model explains 17% of the variation. We therefore can conclude that there are many other factors that we have not measured—and, perhaps, that we cannot measure—that determine how far people with chronic lung disease can walk in 6 minutes. Other investigations that use regression techniques have found that patients' experience of the intensity of their exertion, as well as the perception of the severity of their illness, may be more powerful determinants of walk test distance than is their FEV_1.[13]

Regression Modeling With Dichotomous Target Variables

Frequently, we are interested in predicting a patient's status on a dichotomous dependent variable, such as death or myocardial infarction, in which the outcome is present or absent. We use the term *logistic regression* to refer to such models.

Some time ago, we addressed the question of whether we could predict which critically ill patients are at risk of clinically important upper gastrointestinal tract bleeding.[14] The dependent variable was whether patients had a clinically important bleeding episode. The independent variables included whether patients were breathing independently or required mechanical ventilation and the presence of coagulopathy, sepsis, hypotension, hepatic failure, or renal failure.

Table 15.1-1 gives some of the results from this study, in which we documented

TABLE 15.1-1

Odds Ratios and *P* Values According to Simple (Bivariable) and Multiple (Multivariable) Logistic Regression Analysis for Risk Factors for Clinically Important Gastrointestinal Bleeding in Critically Ill Patients

Risk Factor	Simple Regression		Multiple Regression	
	OR	*P* Value	OR	*P* Value
Mechanical ventilation	25.5	<.001	15.6	<.001
Coagulopathy	9.5	<.001	4.3	<.001
Hypotension	5.0	.03	2.1	.08
Sepsis	7.3	<.001	NS	
Hepatic failure	6.5	<.001	NS	
Renal failure	4.6	<.001	NS	
Enteral feeding	3.8	<.001	NS	
Corticosteroid administration	3.7	<.001	NS	
Organ transplant	3.6	.006	NS	
Anticoagulant therapy	3.3	.004	NS	

Abbreviations: OR, odds ratio; NS, not significant.
Reproduced from Guyatt et al,[1] by permission of the publisher. © 1995 Canadian Medical Association.

the frequency of major bleeding episodes in 2252 critically ill patients. The table indicates that in bivariable logistic regression equations, many independent variables (respiratory failure, coagulopathy, hypotension, sepsis, hepatic failure, renal failure, enteral feeding, corticosteroid administration, organ transplantation, and anticoagulant therapy) were significantly associated with clinically important bleeding. For a number of variables, the *odds ratio* (see Chapter 7, Therapy [Randomized Trials]), which indicates the strength of the association, is quite large.

When we constructed a multiple logistic regression equation, however, only 2 of the independent variables, mechanical ventilation and coagulopathy, were significantly and independently associated with risk of bleeding. All of the other variables that predicted bleeding in the bivariate analysis were correlated with mechanical ventilation or coagulopathy and, therefore, did not reach conventional levels of *statistical*

significance in the multiple regression model. Of those not requiring mechanical ventilation, 3 of 1597 (0.2%) experienced a bleeding episode; of those who received ventilatory support, 30 of 655 (4.6%) experienced a bleeding episode. Of those with no coagulopathy, 10 of 1792 (0.6%) bled; of those with coagulopathy, 23 of 455 (5.1%) experienced a bleeding episode.

Our primary clinical interest was to identify a subgroup with a sufficiently low bleeding risk that prophylaxis might be withheld. Separate from the regression analysis but suggested by its results, we divided the patients into 2 groups: those who were neither mechanically ventilated nor had a coagulopathy and in whom the incidence of bleeding was only 2 of 1405 (0.14%) and those who were either ventilated or had a coagulopathy and of whom 31 of 847 (3.7%) had a bleeding episode. We concluded that prophylaxis may reasonably be withheld in the former low-risk group.

CONCLUSION

Correlation is a statistical tool that permits researchers to examine the strength of the relationship between 2 variables when neither variable is necessarily considered the dependent variable. Regression, by contrast, examines the strength of the relationship between 1 or more predictor variable and a target variable. Regression can be very useful in formulating predictive models to assess risks; for example, the risk of subsequent death in patients presenting with acute coronary syndrome,[15] the risk of cardiac events in patients undergoing noncardiac surgery,[16]

or the risk of bleeding in critically ill patients.[14] Such predictive models can help us make better clinical decisions. Such models are also vital for examining causal associations, particularly with rare harmful events, in *observational studies* when *randomization* is not possible. Regardless of whether you are considering an issue of correlation or regression, you should note not only whether the relationship among variables is statistically significant but also the magnitude or strength of the relationship in terms of the proportion of variation explained, the extent to which groups with very different risks of the target event can be specified, or the odds ratio associated with a putative harmful *exposure*.

References

1. Guyatt G, Walter S, Shannon H, Cook D, Jaeschke R, Heddle N. Basic statistics for clinicians: 4. Correlation and regression. *CMAJ*. 1995;152(4):497-504.

2. McGavin CR, Gupta SP, McHardy GJ. Twelve-minute walking test for assessing disability in chronic bronchitis. *Br Med J*. 1976;1(6013):822-823.

3. Streiner DL. *A Guide for the Statistically Perplexed: Selected Readings for Clinical Researchers*. Toronto, Ontario: University of Toronto Press; 2013:187.

4. Guyatt GH, Berman LB, Townsend M. Long-term outcome after respiratory rehabilitation. *CMAJ*. 1987;137(12):1089-1095.

5. Guyatt G, Keller J, Singer J, Halcrow S, Newhouse M. Controlled trial of respiratory muscle training in chronic airflow limitation. *Thorax*. 1992;47(8):598-602.

6. Goldstein RS, Gort EH, Stubbing D, Avendano MA, Guyatt GH. Randomised controlled trial of respiratory rehabilitation. *Lancet*. 1994;344(8934):1394-1397.

7. Guyatt G, Jaeschke R, Heddle N, Cook D, Shannon H, Walter S. Basic statistics for clinicians: 2. Interpreting study results: confidence intervals. *CMAJ*. 1995;152(2):169-173.

8. Katz MH. Multivariable analysis: a primer for readers of medical research. *Ann Intern Med*. 2003;138(8):644-650.

9. Sedgwick P. Statistical question: correlation versus linear regression. *BMJ*. 2013;346:f2686.

10. Godfrey K. Simple linear regression in medical research. *N Engl J Med*. 1985;313(26):1629-1636.

11. Winker MA, Lurie SJ. Glossary of statistical terms. In: *AMA Manual of Style: A Guide for Authors and Editors*. 10th ed. New York, NY: Oxford University Press; 2007. http://www.amamanualofstyle.com/view/10.1093/jama/9780195176339.001.0001/med-9780195176339-div1-215. Accessed January 7, 2014.

12. Babyak MA. What you see may not be what you get: a brief, nontechnical introduction to overfitting in regression-type models. *Psychosom Med*. 2004;66(3):411-421.

13. Morgan AD, Peck DF, Buchanan DR, McHardy GJ. Effect of attitudes and beliefs on exercise tolerance in chronic bronchitis. *Br Med J (Clin Res Ed)*. 1983;286(6360):171-173.

14. Cook DJ, Fuller HD, Guyatt GH, et al; Canadian Critical Care Trials Group. Risk factors for gastrointestinal bleeding in critically ill patients. *N Engl J Med*. 1994;330(6):377-381.

15. Eagle KA, Lim MJ, Dabbous OH, et al; GRACE Investigators. A validated prediction model for all forms of acute coronary syndrome: estimating the risk of 6-month postdischarge death in an international registry. *JAMA*. 2004;291(22):2727-2733.

16. Detsky AS, Abrams HB, McLaughlin JR, et al. Predicting cardiac complications in patients undergoing non-cardiac surgery. *J Gen Intern Med*. 1986;1(4):211-219.

HARM (OBSERVATIONAL STUDIES)

JAMAevidence
Using Evidence to Improve Care

DIAGNOSIS

DIAGNOSIS

16

The Process of Diagnosis

W. Scott Richardson and Mark C. Wilson

IN THIS CHAPTER

DIAGNOSIS

Consider the following diagnostic situations:

1. A 43-year-old woman presents with a painful cluster of vesicles grouped in the T3 dermatome of her left thorax, which you recognize as shingles from reactivation of herpes zoster.

2. A 78-year-old man returns to your office for follow-up of hypertension. He has lost 10 kg since his last visit 6 months ago. He describes reduced appetite but otherwise has no localizing symptoms. You recall that his wife died a year ago and consider depression as a likely explanation, yet his age and exposure history (ie, smoking) suggest other possibilities.

TWO COMPLEMENTARY APPROACHES TO DIAGNOSIS

The first case in the opening scenarios illustrates the rapid, nonanalytic approach that expert diagnosticians use to recognize disorders they have seen many times before (ie, pattern recognition) and that is particularly relevant to the diagnostic properties of aspects of the physical examination.[1-6] The second case illustrates a more challenging circumstance in which simple pattern recognition fails, so expert diagnosticians slow down and toggle to a more analytic mode of diagnostic thinking.[7,8] This includes the probabilistic approach to clinical diagnosis that uses *evidence* from clinical research—the focus of this chapter (Figure 16-1). Using this probabilistic analytic approach, expert diagnosticians generate a list of potential diagnoses, estimate the *probability* associated with each, and conduct investigations, the results of which increase or decrease the probabilities, until they believe they have found the best answer to fit the patient's illness.[9-14]

Applying the probabilistic approach requires knowledge of human anatomy, pathophysiology, and the taxonomy of disease.[11,12,14] Evidence from clinical research represents another form of knowledge required for optimal diagnostic reasoning.[15-17] This chapter describes how evidence from clinical research can facilitate the probabilistic mode of diagnosis.

CLUSTERS OF FINDINGS DEFINE CLINICAL PROBLEMS

Using the probabilistic mode, clinicians begin with the medical interview and physical examination, which they use to identify individual findings

FIGURE 16-1

Pattern Recognition vs Probabilistic Diagnostic Reasoning

Pattern recognition	Probabilistic diagnostic reasoning
See it and recognize disorder	Clinical assessment generates pretest probability
↓	↓
Compare posttest probability with thresholds (usually pattern recognition implies probability near 100% and so above threshold)	New information generates posttest probability (may be iterative)
	↓
	Compare posttest probability with thresholds

as potential clues. For instance, in the second scenario, the clinician noted a 10-kg weight loss in 6 months that is associated with anorexia but without localizing symptoms. Experienced clinicians often group findings into meaningful clusters, summarized in brief phrases about the symptom, body location, or organ system involved, such as "involuntary weight loss with anorexia." These clusters, often termed "clinical problems," represent the starting point for the probabilistic approach to *differential diagnosis* (see Chapter 17, Differential Diagnosis).[11]

CLINICIANS SELECT A SMALL LIST OF DIAGNOSTIC POSSIBILITIES

When considering a patient's differential diagnosis, clinicians must decide which disorders to pursue. If they considered all known causes to be equally likely and tested for them all simultaneously (the "possibilistic" list), unnecessary testing would result. Instead, experienced clinicians are selective, considering those disorders that are more likely (a probabilistic list), more serious if left undiagnosed and untreated (a prognostic list), or more responsive to treatment (a pragmatic list). Wisely selecting an individual patient's prioritized differential diagnosis involves all 3 of these considerations (probabilistic, prognostic, and pragmatic).

One can label the best explanation for the patient's problem as the leading hypothesis or working diagnosis. In the second scenario, the clinician suspected depression as the most likely cause of the patient's anorexia and weight loss. A few (usually 1-5) other diagnoses may be worth considering at the initial evaluation because of their likelihood, seriousness if left undiagnosed and untreated, or responsiveness to treatment. In the case of unexplained weight loss, the man's age raises the specter of neoplasm, and in particular, his past smoking suggests the possibility of lung cancer.

Additional causes of the problem may be too unlikely to consider at the initial diagnostic evaluation but could arise subsequently if the initial hypotheses are later disproved. Most clinicians considering the 78-year-old man with weight loss would not select a disease that causes malabsorption as their initial differential diagnosis but might turn to this hypothesis if investigation ultimately excludes depression and cancer.

ESTIMATING THE PRETEST PROBABILITY FACILITATES THE DIAGNOSTIC PROCESS

Having assembled a short list of plausible target disorders to be investigated—the differential diagnosis for this patient—clinicians rank these conditions. The probabilistic approach to diagnosis encourages clinicians to estimate the probability of each target condition on the short list, the *pretest probability* (Figure 16-1) (see also Chapter 17, Differential Diagnosis).[18] The sum of the probabilities for all candidate diagnoses should equal 1.

How can the clinician estimate these pretest probabilities? One method is implicit, drawing on memories of previous cases with the same clinical problem(s) and using the frequency of disorders found in those previous patients to guide estimates of pretest probability for the current patient. Often, though, memory is imperfect, and we are excessively influenced by particularly vivid or recent experiences and by previous inferences, and we put insufficient weight on new evidence. Furthermore, our experience with a given clinical problem may be limited. All of these factors leave the probabilities arising from clinicians' intuition subject to *bias* and *random error*.[19-21]

A complementary approach uses evidence from research to guide pretest probability estimates. In one type of relevant research, patients with the same clinical problem undergo thorough diagnostic evaluation, yielding a set of frequencies of the underlying diagnoses made, which clinicians can use to estimate the initial pretest probability (see Chapter 17, Differential Diagnosis). Another category of relevant research generates *clinical decision rules* or *prediction rules*. Patients with a defined clinical problem undergo diagnostic evaluation, and investigators use statistical methods to identify clinical and diagnostic test features that segregate patients into subgroups with different probabilities

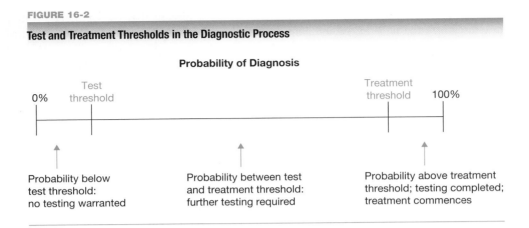

FIGURE 16-2

Test and Treatment Thresholds in the Diagnostic Process

Probability of Diagnosis

Test threshold

Treatment threshold

0%   100%

Probability below test threshold: no testing warranted

Probability between test and treatment threshold: further testing required

Probability above treatment threshold; testing completed; treatment commences

of a target condition (see Chapter 19.4, Clinical Prediction Rules).

NEW INFORMATION GENERATES POSTTEST PROBABILITIES

Clinical diagnosis is a dynamic process. As new information arrives, it may increase or decrease the probability of a target condition or diagnosis.[6] For instance, in the older man with involuntary weight loss, the presence of a recent major life event (his wife's death) raises the likelihood that depression is the cause, whereas the absence of localizing gut symptoms decreases the probability of an intestinal disorder. *Likelihood ratios* capture the extent to which new pieces of information revise probabilities (see Chapter 18, Diagnostic Tests, and Chapter 19.2, Examples of Likelihood Ratios).

Although intuitive estimates based on experience may, at times, serve clinicians well in interpreting test results, confidence in the extent to which a result increased or decreased probabilities requires systematic research. This research can take several forms, most notably individual *primary studies* of test accuracy (see Chapter 18, Diagnostic Tests) and *systematic reviews* of these test accuracy studies (see Chapter 22, The Process of a Systematic Review and Meta-analysis). Once these research results have been appraised for *risk of bias* and applicability, the discriminatory power of the clinical findings or test

results can be collected into reference resources useful for each clinical discipline.[22,23]

THE RELATION BETWEEN POSTTEST PROBABILITIES AND THRESHOLD PROBABILITIES DETERMINES CLINICAL ACTION

After the test result generates the *posttest probability*, one can compare this new probability to thresholds (Figure 16-2).[24-26] If the posttest probability is equal to 1, the diagnosis would be absolutely certain. Short of certainty, as the posttest probability approaches 1, the diagnosis becomes more and more likely and reaches a threshold of probability above which the clinician would recommend starting treatment for the disorder (the *treatment threshold*) (Figure 16-2). These thresholds apply to both pattern recognition and probabilistic or *Bayesian diagnostic reasoning* (Figure 16-1). For instance, consider the first scenario, the patient who presents with a painful eruption of grouped vesicles in the distribution of a single dermatome. In an instant, an experienced clinician would make a diagnosis of herpes zoster and consider whether to offer the patient therapy. In other words, the probability of herpes zoster is so high (near 1.0 or 100%) that it is above a threshold (the treatment threshold) that requires no further testing.

Alternatively, if the posttest probability equaled 0, the diagnosis would be disproved. Short

TABLE 16-1

Factors That Affect the Location of Test Thresholds

Factor	Lowers Test Threshold	Raises Test Threshold
Test safety	Low or zero-risk test	Higher risk (eg, invasive)
Test cost	Low-cost test	Higher cost
Test acceptability to patient	High acceptability	Lower acceptability
Prognosis of target disorder	Serious if left undiagnosed	Less serious if missed
Effectiveness of treatment	Treatment is effective	Treatment is less effective
Availability of treatment	Treatment is available	Treatment is not available

TABLE 16-2

Factors That Affect the Location of Treatment Thresholds

Factor	Lowers Treatment Threshold	Raises Treatment Threshold
Safety of next test	Higher risk from tests	Low or zero risk from tests
Costs of next test	More expensive tests	Lower costs of tests
Prognosis of target disorder	Serious if left untreated	Less serious if untreated
Effectiveness of treatment	Highly effective treatment	Less effective treatment
Safety of treatment	Low risk from treatment	Higher risk from treatment
Availability of treatment	Treatment readily available	Treatment is less available

of this certainty, as the posttest probability nears 0, the diagnosis becomes less and less likely, until a probability threshold is reached, below which the clinician would consider the diagnosis excluded (the *test threshold*).[24] Between the test and treatment thresholds are intermediate probabilities that mandate further testing.

For instance, consider a previously healthy athlete who presents with lateral rib cage pain after being unintentionally struck by an errant baseball pitch. Again, an experienced clinician would recognize the clinical problem (posttraumatic lateral chest pain), identify a leading hypothesis (rib contusion) and an active alternative (rib fracture), and plan a test (radiography) to investigate the latter. If asked, the clinician also could list disorders that are too unlikely to consider further (such as myocardial infarction). In other words, although not as likely as rib contusion, the probability of a rib fracture is above a threshold for testing, whereas the probability of myocardial infarction is below the threshold for testing.

What determines these test and treatment thresholds? They are a function of the properties of

the test, the disease prognosis, and the nature of the treatment (Tables 16-1 and 16-2). For the test threshold, the safer and less costly the testing strategy, the more serious the condition if left undiagnosed, and the more effective and safe the available treatment is, the lower we would place the test threshold. On the other hand, the less safe or more costly the test strategy, the less serious the condition if undiagnosed, and the less secure we are about the effectiveness and safety of treatment, the higher we would place the test threshold.

Consider, for instance, ordering a troponin test for suspected acute coronary syndrome. The condition, if present, can lead to serious consequences (such as fatal arrhythmias), and the test is inexpensive and noninvasive. This is the reason one sees emergency department physicians ordering the test for patients with even a very low probability of acute coronary syndrome: they have set a very low diagnostic threshold.

Contrast this with pulmonary angiography for suspected pulmonary embolism. Although the condition is serious, the test is invasive and may be complicated.

As a result, if after tests such as Doppler compression ultrasonography and ventilation-perfusion scanning or helical computed tomography they are left with a low probability of pulmonary embolism, clinicians may choose to monitor closely. The test threshold is higher because of the invasiveness and risks of the test.

For the treatment threshold, the safer and the less expensive our next test, the more benign the prognosis of the illness, and the higher the costs or greater the adverse effects of the treatment options, the higher we would place the threshold, requiring greater diagnostic certainty before exposing our patients to treatment. On the other hand, the more invasive and less safe the next test needed, the more ominous the prognosis, and the safer and less costly the proposed treatment, the lower we would place the treatment threshold because proceeding with treatment may be preferable to increasing diagnostic certainty. For instance, consider patients presenting with suspected malignant tumors. In general, before treating, clinicians will subject such patients to invasive diagnostic tests associated with possible serious complications. The

reason is that the treatment—surgery, radiation, or chemotherapy—is itself associated with morbidity or even mortality. Thus, clinicians set the treatment threshold very high.

Contrast this with a patient who presents with symptoms of heartburn and acid reflux. Even if symptoms are atypical, clinicians may be ready to prescribe a proton pump inhibitor for symptom relief rather than subject the patient to endoscopy. The lower treatment threshold is a function of the relatively benign nature of the treatment in relation to the invasiveness of the next test.

CONCLUSION

In this chapter, we outlined the probabilistic tradition of analytic diagnostic reasoning and identified how different types of clinical research evidence can inform our diagnostic decisions and actions. The next chapters highlight particular aspects of the diagnostic process.

References

1. Elstein AS, Shulman L, Sprafka S. *Medical Problem Solving: An Analysis of Clinical Reasoning.* Cambridge, MA: Harvard University Press; 1978.

2. Schmidt HG, Norman GR, Boshuizen HP. A cognitive perspective on medical expertise: theory and implication. *Acad Med.* 1990;65(10):611-621.

3. Eva KW. What every teacher needs to know about clinical reasoning. *Med Educ.* 2005;39(1):98-106.

4. Norman GR, Brooks LR. The non-analytical basis of clinical reasoning. *Adv Health Sci Educ Theory Pract.* 1997;2(2):173-184.

5. Norman GR. The epistemology of clinical reasoning: perspectives from philosophy, psychology, and neuroscience. *Acad Med.* 2000;75(10)(suppl):S127-S135.

6. Sackett DL. A primer on the precision and accuracy of the clinical examination. In: Simel DL, Rennie D, eds. *The Rational Clinical Examination: Evidence-Based Clinical Diagnosis.* New York, NY: McGraw-Hill; 2009. http://www.jamaevidence.com/content/3474001. Accessed January 7, 2014.

7. Moulton CA, Regehr G, Mylopoulos M, MacRae HM. Slowing down when you should: a new model of expert judgment. *Acad Med.* 2007;82(10)(suppl):S109-S116.

8. Croskerry P. A universal model of diagnostic reasoning. *Acad Med.* 2009;84(8):1022-1028.

9. Barrows HS, Pickell GC. *Developing Clinical Problem Solving Skills: A Guide to More Effective Diagnosis and Treatment.* New York, NY: WW Norton; 1991.

10. Kassirer JP, Wong JB, Kopelman RI. *Learning Clinical Reasoning.* 2nd ed. Baltimore, MD: Williams & Wilkins; 2009.

11. Barondess JA, Carpenter CCJ, eds. *Differential Diagnosis.* Philadelphia, PA: Lea & Febiger; 1994.

12. Bordage G. Elaborated knowledge: a key to successful diagnostic thinking. *Acad Med.* 1994;69(11):883-885.

13. Glass RD. *Diagnosis: A Brief Introduction.* Melbourne, Australia: Oxford University Press; 1996.

14. Cox K. *Doctor and Patient: Exploring Clinical Thinking.* Sydney, Australia: UNSW Press; 1999.

15. Kassirer JP. Diagnostic reasoning. *Ann Intern Med.* 1989; 110(11):893-900.

16. Richardson WS. Integrating evidence into clinical diagnosis. In: Montori VM, ed. *Evidence-Based Endocrinology.* Totowa, NJ: Humana Press; 2006:69-89.

17. Richardson WS. We should overcome the barriers to evidence-based clinical diagnosis! *J Clin Epidemiol.* 2007; 60(3):217-227.

18. Sox HC Jr, Higgins MC, Owens DK, eds. *Medical Decision Making.* Chichester, UK: Wiley-Blackwell; 2013.

19. Richardson WS. Where do pretest probabilities come from? [editorial, EBM Note]. *Evid Based Med.* 1999;4:68-69.

20. Richardson WS, Glasziou P, Polashenski WA, Wilson MC. A new arrival: evidence about differential diagnosis. *ACP J Club.* 2000;133(3):A11-A12.

21. Richardson WS. Five uneasy pieces about pre-test probability. *J Gen Intern Med*. 2002;17(11):882-883.

22. Fletcher RH, Fletcher SW, Fletcher GS. *Clinical Epidemiology: The Essentials*. 5th ed. Philadelphia, PA: Wolters-Kluwer/ Lippincott Williams & Wilkins; 2012.

23. Straus SE, Glasziou P, Richardson WS, Haynes RB, eds. *Evidence-Based Medicine: How to Practice and Teach It*. 4th ed. Edinburgh, UK: Elsevier/Churchill-Livingstone; 2011.

24. Pauker SG, Kassirer JP. The threshold approach to clinical decision making. *N Engl J Med*. 1980;302(20):1109-1117.

25. Gross R. *Making Medical Decisions: An Approach to Clinical Decision Making for Practicing Physicians*. Philadelphia, PA: ACP Publications; 1999.

26. Hunink M, Glasziou P, eds. *Decision Making in Health and Medicine: Integrating Evidence and Values*. Cambridge, England: Cambridge University Press; 2001.

17

Differential Diagnosis

W. Scott Richardson, Mark C. Wilson,
and Thomas McGinn

IN THIS CHAPTER

DIAGNOSIS

CLINICAL SCENARIO

Your patient is a 78-year-old man who, at today's routine visit for the follow-up of his longstanding hypertension, is surprised to be told that his weight has decreased 10 kg since his last visit 6 months ago. He reports eating less, with little appetite but no food-related symptoms. He takes a diuretic for his hypertension, with no change in dose for more than a year, and uses acetaminophen for occasional knee pain and stiffness. He stopped smoking 11 years ago, and he stopped drinking alcohol 4 decades ago. His examination reveals him to be extremely thin but provides no localizing clues. His initial blood and urine test results are normal.

You review the long list of the possible causes of involuntary weight loss, yet you realize that an immediate exhaustive search for all possibilities is not sensible. Instead, you will seek information about the causes of involuntary weight loss that are common and most plausible in this patient.

FINDING THE EVIDENCE

Using the Guide

You begin by framing your knowledge gap as a question: "In adults presenting with involuntary weight loss who undergo a diagnostic evaluation, how frequent are the important categories of underlying disease, such as neoplasms, gastrointestinal conditions, and psychiatric disorders?" As you sit at your computer to search for an answer, you notice your nearby files that store your article reprint collection. On a whim, you open the file for involuntary weight loss and find an article about the frequency of diseases in patients with involuntary weight loss that was published more than 30 years ago.[1] Hoping to find some newer evidence, you access PubMed and locate this older citation in the database. Clicking the "Related Articles" link yields 92 citations, of which the second listing, by Hernandez et al,[2] published in 2003, looks promising because it also explicitly addresses the frequency of underlying disorders in patients with weight loss.[2] Farther down the list, you find a similar, newer study that has fewer patients,[3] as well as 2 narrative review articles on unintentional weight loss,[4,5] which cites the article by Hernandez et al[2] as the largest of the recent studies of causes of weight loss. To double check, you scan the chapter on weight loss in an electronic text and find that no newer large study is mentioned. With some confidence that you have found recent evidence, you decide to start with the larger of the 2 studies and retrieve its full text to appraise critically.

Box 17-1 summarizes the guide for an article about disease probabilities for *differential diagnosis*.

HOW SERIOUS IS THE RISK OF BIAS?

Did the Study Patients Represent the Full Spectrum of Those With This Clinical Problem?

The patients in a study are identified or sampled from an underlying target population of people who seek care for the clinical problem being investigated. Ideally, this sample mirrors the target population in all important ways so that the frequency of underlying diseases found in the sample reflects the frequency in the population. A patient sample that mirrors the target population well is termed "representative." The more representative the sample, the more accurate the resulting disease *probabilities*. As shown in Box 17-2, we suggest 4 ways to examine how well the study patients represent the entire target population.

First, because this determines the target population from which the study patients should be drawn, find the investigators' definition of the presenting clinical problem. For instance, for a study of chest discomfort, you would want to find whether the investigators' definition included patients with chest discomfort who deny pain (like many patients with angina do), whether "chest" means discomfort only in the anterior thorax (vs also posterior), and whether patients with obvious recent trauma are excluded. In addition, investigators may specify the level of care or amount of previous evaluation (eg, "fatigue in primary care"[6] or "referred for persistent unexplained cough"[7]). Differing definitions would define differing target populations that would yield differing disease probabilities. A detailed, specific definition of the clinical problem makes it more likely you will be able to confidently judge whether the study population matches the patient before you.

Second, examine the settings from which patients are recruited. Patients with the same clinical problem could present to any of a number of different clinical settings, whether primary care offices, emergency departments, or referral clinics. The choice of where to seek care can involve several factors, including the duration and severity of illness, the availability of various settings, the referral habits of one's clinician, or patient preferences. Different clinical settings are likely to manage patient groups with different disease frequencies. Typically, the frequency of more serious or less common diseases will be greater in secondary or tertiary care settings than in primary care settings. For instance, in a study of patients presenting with chest pain, a higher proportion of referral practice patients had coronary artery disease than did primary care practice patients, even among patients with similar clinical histories.[8]

Investigators should avoid restricting recruitment to idiosyncratic settings that are likely to treat an unrepresentative patient sample. For instance, for the "fatigue in primary care" problem, although only primary care settings would be relevant, the investigators would ideally recruit from a broad spectrum of primary care settings (eg, those serving patients of varying socioeconomic status). In general, the fewer the relevant sites used for patient recruitment, the greater the risk that the setting will be idiosyncratic or unrepresentative.

Third, note the investigators' methods for identifying patients at each site and how carefully they avoided missing patients. Ideally, they would recruit a *consecutive sample* of all patients who seek care at the study sites for the clinical problem during a specified period. If patients are not included consecutively, selective inclusion could reduce the representativeness of the sample and reduce confidence in the resulting disease probabilities.

Fourth, examine the spectrum of severity and clinical features exhibited by the patients in the study sample. Are mild, moderate, and severely symptomatic patients included? Are all of the important variations of this presenting clinical problem found in the sample? For instance, for a study of chest discomfort,

DIAGNOSIS

you would want to determine whether patients with chest discomfort of any degree of severity were included and whether patients were included whether they did or did not have important associated symptoms, such as dyspnea, diaphoresis, or pain radiation. The fuller the clinical spectrum of patients in the sample is, the more representative the sample should be of the target population. Conversely, the narrower the clinical spectrum is, the less representative you would rate the sample. In particular, are patients similar to the one before you well represented?

USING THE GUIDE

Hernandez et al[2] defined the clinical problem for their study as "isolated involuntary weight loss," meaning a verified, unintentional loss of more than 5% of body weight during 6 months without localizing signs or symptoms and with no diagnosis made on initial testing. From January 1991 through December 1996, 1211 patients were referred consecutively from a defined geographic area to their general internal medicine outpatient and inpatient settings for involuntary weight loss, of whom 306 met their definition of "isolated." Men and women were included, and ages ranged from 15 to 97 years. The authors did not describe the patients' ethnic background or socioeconomic status. The investigators excluded patients if they lost less than 5 kg, if they had a previous diagnosis that could explain involuntary weight loss, if the initial evaluation identified the cause, or if weight loss was intentional. Thus, their study sample represents fairly well the target population of patients who are referred for the evaluation of involuntary weight loss. Your patient would have been included in their sample.

Was the Diagnostic Evaluation Definitive?

Articles about disease probability for differential diagnosis will provide valid evidence only if the investigators arrive at correct final diagnoses for the study patients. To judge the accuracy of the final diagnoses, you should examine the diagnostic evaluation undertaken. The more definitive this evaluation, the more likely that the frequencies of

the diagnoses made are accurate estimates of the disease frequencies in the target population. In Box 17-3, we suggest 6 ways to examine the question, "How definitive is the diagnostic evaluation?"

First, determine how comprehensive the investigators' diagnostic evaluation is. Ideally, the diagnostic evaluation would be able to detect all possible causes of the clinical problem, if any are present. For example, a retrospective study of stroke in 127 patients with mental status changes failed to include a comprehensive search for all causes of delirium, and 118 cases remained unexplained.[9] Because the investigators did not describe a complete and systematic search for causes of delirium, the disease probabilities appear less credible.

Second, examine how consistently the diagnostic evaluation was performed. This does not mean that every patient must undergo every test. Instead, for many clinical problems, the clinician takes a detailed yet focused medical history and performs a problem-oriented physical examination of the involved organ systems, along with a few initial tests. Then, depending on the diagnostic clues from this information, further inquiry proceeds down one of multiple branching pathways. Ideally, investigators would evaluate all patients with the same initial evaluation and then follow the resulting clues using prespecified multiple branching pathways of testing. Once a definitive test result confirms a final diagnosis, further testing is unnecessary.

BOX 17-3

Ensuring a Definitive Diagnostic Evaluation

Was the diagnostic evaluation sufficiently comprehensive?

Was the diagnostic evaluation consistently applied to all patients?

Were the criteria for all candidate diagnoses explicit and credible?

Were the diagnostic labels assigned reproducibly?

Were there few patients left with undiagnosed conditions?

For patients with undiagnosed conditions, was follow-up sufficiently long and complete?

You may find it easy to decide whether the patients' illnesses have been thoroughly and consistently investigated if they were evaluated prospectively with a predetermined diagnostic approach. When clinicians do not standardize their investigation, this becomes harder to judge. For example, in a study of precipitating factors in 101 patients with decompensated heart failure, although all patients underwent a medical history taking and physical examination, the lack of standardization of subsequent testing makes it difficult to judge the thoroughness of the investigations.[10]

Third, examine the criteria for each disorder used in assigning patients' final diagnoses. Ideally, investigators will develop or adapt a set of explicit criteria for each underlying candidate disorder that could be diagnosed and then apply these criteria consistently when assigning each patient a final diagnosis. When possible, these criteria should include not only the findings needed to confirm each diagnosis but also those findings useful for rejecting each diagnosis. For example, published diagnostic criteria for infective endocarditis include criteria for verifying the infection and criteria for rejecting it.[11,12] Investigators can then classify study patients into diagnostic groups that are mutually exclusive, with the exception of patients whose symptoms stem from more than 1 etiologic factor. Because a complete, explicit, referenced, and credible set of diagnostic criteria can be long, it may appear as an appendix or online-only supplement to the published article, such as in a study of patients with palpitations.[13]

While reviewing the diagnostic criteria, keep in mind that "lesion finding" is not necessarily the same thing as "illness explaining." In other words, when using credible diagnostic criteria, investigators may find that patients have 2 or more disorders that might explain the clinical problem, causing some doubt as to which disorder is the culprit. Better studies of disease probability will include some assurance that the disorders found actually accounted for the patients' illnesses. For example, in a sequence of studies of syncope, investigators required that the symptoms occur simultaneously with an arrhythmia before that arrhythmia was judged to be the cause.[14] In a study of chronic cough, investigators gave cause-specific therapy and used positive responses to this to strengthen the case for these disorders actually causing the chronic cough.[7]

Fourth, consider whether the assignments of the patients' final diagnoses were reproducible. Ensuring reproducibility begins with the use of explicit criteria and a comprehensive and consistent evaluation, as described above. Investigators can also use a formal test of reproducibility, such as *chance-corrected agreement* (κ statistic), as investigators did in a study of causes of dizziness.[15] The greater the investigators' agreement beyond chance on the final diagnoses assigned to their patients, the more confident you can be in the resulting disease probabilities.

Fifth, look at how many patients' conditions remain undiagnosed despite the study evaluation. Ideally, a comprehensive diagnostic evaluation would leave no patient's illness unexplained, yet even the best evaluation may fall short of this goal. The higher the proportion of undiagnosed patients, the greater the chance of error in the estimates of disease probability. For example, in a retrospective study of various causes of dizziness in 1194 patients in an otolaryngology clinic, approximately 27% had undiagnosed conditions.[16] With more than a quarter of patients' illnesses unexplained, the disease frequencies for the overall sample might be inaccurate.

Sixth, if the study evaluation leaves some patients' conditions undiagnosed, look at the length and completeness of their *follow-up* and whether additional diagnoses are made and the clinical outcomes are known. The longer and more complete the follow-up, the greater our confidence in the benign nature of the conditions in patients whose conditions remain undiagnosed and yet who are unharmed at the end of the study. How long is long enough? We suggest 1 to 6 months for symptoms that are acute and self-limited and 1 to 5 years for chronically recurring or progressive symptoms.

USING THE GUIDE

Hernandez et al[2] described the consistent use of a standardized initial evaluation of medical history, physical examination, blood tests (blood cell counts, sedimentation rate, blood chemical analyses, protein electrophoresis, and thyroid hormone levels), urinalysis, and radiography (chest and abdomen), after which further testing was performed at the discretion of the attending physician. The authors do not list the diagnostic criteria for each disorder. For the patients' final diagnoses, the investigators required finding not only a disorder recognized in the literature to cause weight loss but also a correlation of weight loss with the clinical outcome of the disorder (recovery or progression). Two investigators independently judged final diagnoses and resolved disagreements (<5%) by consensus. An underlying disorder explaining involuntary weight loss was diagnosed for 221 patients (72%); therefore, 85 patients (28%) initially had undiagnosed conditions. During follow-up and repeated evaluations at 3, 6, and 12 months, 55 of these 85 patients were seen, and diagnoses were made for 41, leaving 14 unexplained diagnoses at 1 year and 30 patients *lost to follow-up*. Thus, the reported diagnostic evaluation appears credible, although some uncertainty exists because of unspecified criteria and the 10% loss to follow-up.

WHAT ARE THE RESULTS?

What Were the Diagnoses and Their Probabilities?

In many studies of disease probability, the authors report the main results in a table that lists the diagnoses made, along with the numbers and percentages of patients found with those disorders. For some symptoms, patients may have more than 1 underlying disease coexisting with and presumably contributing to the clinical problem. In these situations, authors often identify the major diagnosis for such patients and separately tabulate contributing causes. Alternatively, authors could identify a separate multiple-cause group.

USING THE GUIDE

Hernandez et al[2] report in a table the diagnoses made by the end of the study follow-up in 276 of their 306 patients (90%). Neoplasms were found in 104 (34%) and psychiatric diseases in 63 (21%), whereas no known cause was identified in 14 (5%).

How Precise Are the Estimates of Disease Probability?

Even when valid, these disease frequencies found in the study sample are only estimates of the true disease probabilities in the target population. You can examine the precision of these estimates with the 95% *confidence intervals* (CIs).

Whether you will deem the CIs sufficiently precise depends on where the estimated proportion and CIs fall in relation to your *test threshold* or *treatment threshold*. If both the estimated proportion and the entire 95% CI are on the same side of your threshold, then the result is precise enough to permit firm conclusions about disease probability for use in planning tests or treatments. Conversely, if the confidence limit around the estimate crosses your threshold, the result may not be precise enough for definitive conclusions about disease probability. You may still use a valid but imprecise probability result, keeping in mind the uncertainty and what it might mean for testing or treatment.

USING THE GUIDE

Hernandez et al[2] do not provide the 95% CIs for the probabilities they found. If you were concerned about how close the probabilities were to your thresholds, you could calculate the 95% CIs. For instance, for psychiatric causes found in 23% of their patients, the 95% CI is 18.1% to 27.9%. In this situation, even the lower boundary of the 95% CI appears high enough for you to pursue an underlying psychiatric disease as the cause of involuntary weight loss.

HOW CAN I APPLY THE RESULTS TO PATIENT CARE?

Are the Study Patients and Clinical Setting Similar to Mine?

Earlier, we urged you to examine how the study patient sample was selected from the target population. In doing so, you should pay careful attention to its applicability to your patients—and, in particular, the patient before you. If, for instance, patients who present with this problem in your practice come from areas in which one of the underlying disorders is endemic, the probability of that condition would be much higher than its frequency found in a study performed in a nonendemic area, limiting the applicability of the study results to your practice.

USING THE GUIDE

For the 78-year-old man referred to you for evaluation of involuntary weight loss, the clinical setting described by Hernandez et al[2] appears to fit. The partial description of the sample patients sounds similar enough to this man in age and sex, so that despite some remaining uncertainty, you can use the results for your evaluation.

Is It Unlikely That the Disease Possibilities or Probabilities Have Changed Since This Evidence Was Gathered?

As time passes, evidence about disease frequency can become obsolete. Old diseases can be controlled or, as in the case of smallpox, eliminated.[17] New diseases or new epidemics of disease can arise. Such events can so alter the list of possible diseases or their likelihood that previously valid and applicable studies may lose their

relevance. For example, consider how markedly the arrival of human immunodeficiency virus transformed the possibilities and the probabilities for clinical problems, such as generalized lymphadenopathy, chronic diarrhea, and involuntary weight loss.

Similar changes can occur as the result of progress in medical science or public health. For instance, in studies of fever of unknown origin, new diagnostic technologies have substantially altered the proportions of patients who are found to have malignant tumors or whose fevers remain unexplained.[18-20] Treatment advances that improve survival, such as chemotherapy for childhood leukemia, can bring about shifts in disease likelihood because the treatment might cause complications, such as secondary malignant tumor, years after cure of the disease. Public health measures that control diseases such as cholera can alter the likelihood of occurrence of the remaining causes of the clinical problems that the prevented disease would have caused (in this example, acute diarrhea).

USING THE GUIDE

The study by Hernandez et al[2] was published in 2003, and the study period was 1991 to 1997. However, the PubMed search did not reveal any new developments likely to change the causes or probabilities of disease in patients with involuntary weight loss since this evidence was gathered.[4,5]

CLINICAL SCENARIO RESOLUTION

Let us return to the 78-year-old man being evaluated for involuntary weight loss. After an initial evaluation yielded no leads, a detailed interview turns up clues to a depressed mood with anorexia and reduced appetite after his wife died a year ago. Your leading hypothesis is that major depressive disorder is causing your patient's involuntary weight loss, yet this diagnosis is not sufficiently certain to stop testing to exclude other conditions. From the study by Hernandez et al,[2] you decide to include in your active alternatives selected neoplasms (common, serious, and treatable) and hyperthyroidism (less common yet serious and

treatable), and you arrange testing to exclude these disorders (ie, these alternatives are above your test threshold). Finally, given that few of the study patients had a malabsorption syndrome and because your patient has no other features of this disorder besides involuntary weight loss, you place it into your "other hypotheses" category (ie, below your test threshold) and decide to delay testing for this condition. You use the disease frequencies from the study as starting estimates for *pretest probability* and then raise the probability for depression, given the clues, which lowers the probabilities for the other conditions.

References

1. Marton KI, Sox HC Jr, Krupp JR. Involuntary weight loss: diagnostic and prognostic significance. *Ann Intern Med*. 1981;95(5):568-574.

2. Hernández JL, Riancho JA, Matorras P, González-Macías J. Clinical evaluation for cancer in patients with involuntary weight loss without specific symptoms. *Am J Med*. 2003;114(8):631-637.

3. Metalidis C, Knockaert DC, Bobbaers H, Vanderschueren S. Involuntary weight loss: does a negative baseline evaluation provide adequate reassurance? *Eur J Intern Med*. 2008;19(5):345-349.

4. McMinn J, Steel C, Bowman A. Investigation and management of unintentional weight loss in older adults. *BMJ*. 2011;342:d1732.

5. Stajkovic S, Aitken EM, Holroyd-Leduc J. Unintentional weight loss in older adults. *CMAJ*. 2011;183(4):443-449.

6. Elnicki DM, Shockcor WT, Brick JE, Beynon D. Evaluating the complaint of fatigue in primary care: diagnoses and outcomes. *Am J Med*. 1992;93(3):303-306.

7. Pratter MR, Bartter T, Akers S, DuBois J. An algorithmic approach to chronic cough. *Ann Intern Med*. 1993;119(10):977-983.

8. Sox HC Jr, Hickam DH, Marton KI, et al. Using the patient's history to estimate the probability of coronary artery disease: a comparison of primary care and referral practices. *Am J Med*. 1990;89(1):7-14.

9. Benbadis SR, Sila CA, Cristea RL. Mental status changes and stroke. *J Gen Intern Med*. 1994;9(9):485-487.

10. Ghali JK, Kadakia S, Cooper R, Ferlinz J. Precipitating factors leading to decompensation of heart failure: traits among urban blacks. *Arch Intern Med*. 1988;148(9):2013-2016.

11. Von Reyn CF, Levy BS, Arbeit RD, Friedland G, Crumpacker CS. Infective endocarditis: an analysis based on strict case definitions. *Ann Intern Med*. 1981;94(4 pt 1):505-518.

12. Durack DT, Lukes AS, Bright DK; Duke Endocarditis Service. New criteria for diagnosis of infective endocarditis: utilization of specific echocardiographic findings. *Am J Med*. 1994;96(3):200-209.

13. Weber BE, Kapoor WN. Evaluation and outcomes of patients with palpitations. *Am J Med*. 1996;100(2):138-148.

14. Kapoor WN. Evaluation and outcome of patients with syncope. *Medicine (Baltimore)*. 1990;69(3):160-175.

15. Kroenke K, Lucas CA, Rosenberg ML, et al. Causes of persistent dizziness: a prospective study of 100 patients in ambulatory care. *Ann Intern Med*. 1992;117(11):898-904.

16. Katsarkas A. Dizziness in aging: a retrospective study of 1194 cases. *Otolaryngol Head Neck Surg*. 1994;110(3):296-301.

17. Barquet N, Domingo P. Smallpox: the triumph over the most terrible of the ministers of death. *Ann Intern Med*. 1997;127 (8 pt 1):635-642.

18. Petersdorf RG, Beeson PB. Fever of unexplained origin: report on 100 cases. *Medicine (Baltimore)*. 1961;40:1-30.

19. Larson EB, Featherstone HJ, Petersdorf RG. Fever of undetermined origin: diagnosis and follow-up of 105 cases, 1970-1980. *Medicine (Baltimore)*. 1982;61(5):269-292.

20. Knockaert DC, Vanneste LJ, Vanneste SB, Bobbaers HJ. Fever of unknown origin in the 1980s: an update of the diagnostic spectrum. *Arch Intern Med*. 1992;152(1):51-55.

18

Diagnostic Tests

Toshi A. Furukawa, Sharon E. Straus, Heiner C. Bucher,
Thomas Agoritsas, and Gordon Guyatt

IN THIS CHAPTER

INTRODUCTION

In the previous 2 chapters (Chapter 16, The Process of Diagnosis, and Chapter 17, Differential Diagnosis), we explained the process of diagnosis, the way diagnostic test results move clinicians across the *test threshold* and the *therapeutic threshold*, and how to use studies to help obtain an accurate *pretest probability*. In this chapter, we explain how to use an article that addresses the ability of a diagnostic test to move clinicians toward the extremely high (ruling in) and extremely low (ruling out) *posttest probabilities* they seek. Later in this book, we explain how to use articles that integrate a number of test results into a *clinical prediction rule* (Chapter 19.4, Clinical Prediction Rules).

CLINICAL SCENARIO

How Can We Identify Dementia Quickly and Accurately?

You are a busy primary care practitioner with a large proportion of elderly patients in your practice. Earlier in the day, you saw a 70-year-old woman who lives alone and has been managing well. On this visit, she informed you of a long-standing problem, joint pain in her lower extremities. During the visit, you get the impression that, as you put it to yourself, "she isn't quite all there," although you find it hard to specify further. On specific questioning about memory and function, she acknowledges that her memory is not what it used to be but otherwise denies problems. Pressed for time, you deal with the osteoarthritis and move on to the next patient.

That evening, you ponder the problem of making a quick assessment of your elderly patients when the possibility of cognitive impairment occurs to you. The Mini-Mental State Examination (MMSE), with which you are familiar, takes too long. You wonder if there are any brief instruments that allow a reasonably accurate rapid diagnosis of cognitive impairment to help you identify patients who need more extensive investigation.

FINDING THE EVIDENCE

You formulate the clinical question, "In older patients with suspected cognitive impairment, what is the accuracy of a brief *screening* tool to identify patients who need more extensive investigation for possible dementia?" To conduct a rapid and specific search, you access the PubMed Clinical Queries page (see Chapter 5, Finding Current Best Evidence). Typing in the search terms "identify dementia brief MMSE," you select "diagnosis" as the clinical study category and "narrow" as the scope of the filter. This search strategy yields 8 citations.

You survey the abstracts, looking for articles that focus on patients with suspected dementia and report accuracy similar to your previous standard, the MMSE. An article that reports results for an instrument named Six-Item Screener (SIS) meets both criteria.[1] You retrieve the full-text article electronically and start to read it, hoping its methods and results will justify using the instrument in your office.

HOW SERIOUS IS THE RISK OF BIAS?

Box 18-1 summarizes our *Users' Guides* for assessing the *risk of bias*, examining the results, and determining the applicability of a study reporting on the accuracy of a diagnostic test.

Did Participating Patients Constitute a Representative Sample of Those Presenting With a Diagnostic Dilemma?

A diagnostic test is useful only if it distinguishes among conditions or disorders that might otherwise be confused. Although most tests can differentiate healthy persons from severely affected ones, this ability will not help us in clinical practice. Studies

The story of carcinoembryonic antigen (CEA) testing in patients with colorectal cancer reveals how choosing the wrong spectrum of patients can dash the hopes raised with the introduction of a diagnostic test. A study found that CEA was elevated in 35 of 36 people with known advanced cancer of the colon or rectum. The investigators found much lower levels in healthy people, pregnant women, or patients with a variety of other conditions.[5] The results suggested that CEA might be useful in diagnosing colorectal cancer or even in screening for the disease. In subsequent studies of patients with less advanced stages of colorectal cancer (and, therefore, lower disease severity) and patients with other cancers or other gastrointestinal disorders (and, therefore, different but potentially confused disorders), the accuracy of CEA testing as a diagnostic tool plummeted. Clinicians appropriately abandoned CEA measurement for new cancer diagnosis and screening.

Enrolling *target-positive* patients (those with the underlying condition of interest; in our scenario, people with dementia) and *target-negative* patients (those without the target condition) from separate populations results in overestimates of the diagnostic test's power. This *case-control design* (where cases are known to be target positive and controls are known to be target negative) of a diagnostic test may be likened to a phase 2 efficacy trial: if it fails (ie, the test fails to discriminate target-positive from target-negative patients), the test is hopeless; if it succeeds, it cannot guarantee real-world effectiveness.

Even if investigators enroll target-positive and target-negative patients from the same population, nonconsecutive patient sampling and retrospective data collection may inflate estimates of diagnostic test performances.

Did the Investigators Compare the Test to an Appropriate, Independent Reference Standard?

The accuracy of a diagnostic test is best determined by comparing it to the "truth." Readers must assure

that confine themselves to florid cases vs asymptomatic healthy volunteers are unhelpful because, when the diagnosis is obvious, we do not need a diagnostic test. Only a study that closely resembles clinical practice and includes patients with mild, early manifestations of the *target condition* can establish a test's true value.

We label studies with unrepresentative patient selection as suffering from *spectrum bias* (see Chapter 19.1, Spectrum Bias). There are 3 empirical studies that have systematically examined for various sources of *bias* in studies of diagnostic tests.[2-4] All 3 studies documented bias associated with unrepresentative patient selection.

themselves that investigators have applied an appropriate *reference, criterion,* or *gold standard* (such as biopsy, surgery, autopsy, or long-term *follow-up* without treatment) to every patient who undergoes the test under investigation.

One way a study can go wrong is if the test that is being evaluated is part of the reference standard. The incorporation of the test into the reference standard is likely to inflate the estimate of the test's diagnostic power. Thus, clinicians should insist on independence as one criterion for a satisfactory reference standard.

> For instance, consider a study that evaluated the utility of abdominojugular reflux for the diagnosis of congestive heart failure. Unfortunately, this study used clinical and radiographic criteria that included the abdominojugular reflex as the reference test.[6] Another example comes from a study evaluating screening instruments for depression in terminally ill people. The authors claimed perfect performance (*sensitivity* of 1.0 and *specificity* of 1.0) for a single question ("Are you depressed?") to detect depression. Their diagnostic criteria included 9 questions of which one was, "Are you depressed?"[7]

In reading articles about diagnostic tests, if you cannot accept the reference standard (within reason; after all, nothing is perfect), then the article is unlikely to provide trustworthy results.[3]

Were Those Interpreting the Test and Reference Standard Blind to the Other Result?

If you accept the reference standard, the next question is whether the interpreters of the test and reference standard were unaware of the results of the other investigation (*blind* assessment).

Consider how, once clinicians see a pulmonary nodule on a computed tomogram (CT), they can see the previously undetected lesion on the chest radiograph or, once they learn the results of an echocardiogram, they hear a previously inaudible cardiac murmur.

The more likely that knowledge of the reference standard result can influence the interpretation of a test, the greater the importance of independent interpretation. Similarly, the more susceptible the reference standard is to changes in interpretation as a result of knowledge of the test being evaluated, the more important the blinding of the reference standard interpreter. The empirical study of Lijmer et al[2] found bias associated with unblinded assessments, although the magnitude was small.

Did Investigators Perform the Same Reference Standard in All Patients Regardless of the Results of the Test Under Investigation?

The properties of a diagnostic test will be distorted if its results influence whether patients undergo confirmation by the reference standard (*verification*[8,9] or *work-up bias*).[10,11] This can occur in 2 ways.

First, only a selected sample of patients who underwent the index test may be verified by the reference standard. For example, patients with suspected coronary artery disease whose exercise test results are positive may be more likely to undergo coronary angiography (the reference standard) than those whose exercise test results are negative. This type of verification bias is known as *partial verification bias*.

Second, results of the index test may be verified by different reference standards. Use of different reference tests for positive and negative results is known as *differential verification bias*.

> Verification bias proved a problem for the Prospective Investigation of Pulmonary Embolism Diagnosis (PIOPED) study that evaluated the utility of ventilation perfusion scanning in the diagnosis of pulmonary embolism. Patients whose ventilation perfusion scan results were interpreted as "normal/near normal" and "low *probability*" were less likely to undergo pulmonary angiography (69%) than those with more positive ventilation perfusion scans (92%). This is not surprising because clinicians might be reluctant to subject patients with a low probability of pulmonary embolism to the *risks* of angiography.[12]

Most articles would stop here, and readers would have to conclude that the magnitude of the bias resulting from different proportions of patients with high-probability and low-probability ventilation perfusion scans undergoing adequate angiography is uncertain but perhaps large. The PIOPED investigators, however, applied a second reference standard to the 150 patients with low-probability or normal or near-normal scans who did not undergo angiography (136 patients) or in whom angiogram interpretation was uncertain (14 patients). They judged such patients to be free of pulmonary embolism if they did well without treatment. Accordingly, they followed up all such patients for 1 year without treating them with anticoagulant drugs. No patient developed clinically evident pulmonary embolism during follow-up, allowing us to conclude that patient-important pulmonary embolism (if we define patient-important pulmonary embolism as requiring anticoagulation therapy to prevent subsequent adverse events) was not present at the time they underwent ventilation perfusion scanning. Thus, the PIOPED study achieved the goal of applying a reference standard assessment to all patients but failed to apply the same standard to all.

USING THE GUIDE

The study of a brief diagnostic test for cognitive impairment included 2 *cohorts*. One was a random sample of black persons 65 years and older in the general population; the other, a *consecutive sample* of unscreened patients referred by family, caregivers, or health care professionals for cognitive evaluation at the Alzheimer Disease Center. In the former group, the authors included all patients with a high suspicion of dementia on a detailed screening test and a *random sample* of those with moderate and low suspicion. The investigators faced diagnostic uncertainty in both populations. The populations are not perfect: the former included individuals without any suspicion

of dementia, and the latter had already passed an initial screen at the primary care level (indeed, whether to refer for full geriatric assessment is one of the questions you are trying to resolve for the patient who triggered your search for evidence). Fortunately, test properties proved similar in the 2 populations, considerably lessening your concern.

All patients received the SIS, which asks the patient to remember 3 words (apple, table, penny), then to say the day of the week, month, and year, and finally to recall the 3 words without prompts. The number of errors provides a result with a range of 0 to 6.

For the reference standard diagnosis of dementia, patients had to satisfy both *Diagnostic and Statistical Manual of Mental Disorders* (Third Edition Revised) and *International Statistical Classification of Diseases, 10th Revision* (ICD-10) criteria, based on an assessment by a geriatric psychiatrist or a neurologist that included history, physical and neurologic examination, a complete neuropsychological test battery that included the MMSE and 5 other tests, and an interview with a relative of the participant.

Although you are satisfied with this reference standard, the published article leaves you unsure whether those making the SIS and the reference diagnosis were blind to the other result. To resolve the question, you email the first author and ask for clarification. A couple of emails later, you have learned that "research assistants who had been trained and tested" administered the neuropsychological battery. On the other hand, "a consensus team composed of a geriatric psychiatrist, and social psychologist, a geriatrician, and a neuropsychologist" made the reference standard diagnoses. The author reports, "There were open discussions of the case and they had access to the entire medical record including results of neuropsychological testing at their disposal." The 6 items included in the SIS are derived from the MMSE but "were not pulled out as a separate instrument in the consensus team conference."

Thus, although there was no blinding, you suspect that this did not create important bias and are therefore ready to consider its results.

DIAGNOSIS

WHAT ARE THE RESULTS?

What Likelihood Ratios Were Associated With the Range of Possible Test Results?

In deciding how to interpret diagnostic tests results, we will consider their ability to change our initial estimate of the likelihood the patient has the target condition (we call this the pretest probability) to a more accurate estimate (we call this the posttest probability of the target disorder). The *likelihood ratio* (LR) for a particular test result moves us from the pretest probability to a posttest probability.

Put yourself back in the shoes of the primary care physician in the scenario and consider 2 patients with suspected cognitive impairment with clear consciousness. The first is the 70-year-old woman in the clinical scenario who seems to be managing rather well but has a specific issue that her memory is not what it used to be.

The other is an 85-year-old woman, another long-standing patient, who arrives accompanied, for the first time, by her son. The concerned son tells you that she has, on one of her usual morning walks, lost her way. A neighbor happened to catch her a few miles away from home and notified him of the incident. On visiting his mother's house, he was surprised to find her room a mess. However, in your office she greets you politely and protests that

she was just having a bad day and does not think the incident warrants any fuss (at which point, the son looks to the ceiling in frustrated disbelief). Your clinical hunches about the probability of dementia for these 2 people (ie, their pretest probabilities) are quite different. In the first woman, the probability is relatively low, perhaps 20%; in the second, relatively high, perhaps 70%.

The results of a formal screening test (eg, the SIS) will not tell us definitively whether dementia is present. Rather the results modify the pretest probability of that condition, yielding a new posttest probability. The direction and magnitude of this change from pretest to posttest probability are determined by the test's properties, and the property of most value is the LR.

We will use the results of the study by Callahan et al[1] to illustrate the usefulness of LRs. Table 18-1 presents the distribution of the SIS scores in the cohort of patients from the study by Callahan et al.

How likely is a test result of 6 among people who have dementia? Table 18-1 indicates that 105 of 345 people (30.4%) with the condition made 6 errors. We can also see that of 306 people without dementia, 2 (0.65%) made 6 errors. How likely is this test result (ie, making 6 errors) in someone with dementia as opposed to someone without?

Determining this requires us to look at the ratio of the 2 likelihoods that we have just calculated (30.4/0.65) and equals 47. In other words, the test result of 6 is 47 times as likely to occur in a patient with as opposed to without dementia.

In a similar fashion, we can calculate the LR associated with a test result of each score. For example, the LR for the test score of 5 is (64/345)/(2/306) = 28. Table 18-1 provides the LR for each possible SIS score.

How can we interpret LRs? Likelihood ratios indicate the extent to which a given diagnostic test result will raise or lower the pretest probability of the target disorder. An LR of 1 tells us that the posttest probability is exactly the same as the pretest probability. Likelihood ratios greater than 1.0 increase the probability that the target disorder is present; the higher the LR, the greater the increase. Conversely, LRs less than 1.0 decrease the probability of the target disorder, and the smaller the LR, the greater the decrease in probability.

TABLE 18-1

Six-Item Screener (SIS) Scores in Patients With and Without Dementia and Corresponding Likelihood Ratios

SIS Score	Dementia	No Dementia	Likelihood Ratio
6	105	2	47
5	64	2	28
4	64	8	7.1
3	45	16	2.5
2	31	35	0.79
1	25	80	0.28
0	11	163	0.06
Total	345	306	

How big is a "big" LR, and how small is a "small" one? Use of LRs in your day-to-day practice will lead to your own sense of their interpretation, but consider the following a rough guide: LRs greater than 10 or less than 0.1 generate large and often conclusive changes from pretest to posttest probability, LRs of 5 to 10 and 0.1 to 0.2 generate moderate shifts in pretest to posttest probability, LRs of 2 to 5 and 0.5 to 0.2 generate small (but sometimes important) changes in probability, and LRs of 1 to 2 and 0.5 to 1 alter probability to a small (and rarely important) degree.

Having determined the magnitude and significance of LRs, how do we use them to go from pretest to posttest probability? One way is to convert pretest probability to odds, multiply the result by the LR, and convert the consequent posttest odds into a posttest probability. If you wonder why the conversion to odds is necessary, consider the fact that LRs compare the likelihood of a test result between patients with and without a target disease (corresponding to the odds of that disease). The calculation is complicated, but there are now several Internet pages and smartphone applications that do this for you (http://meta.cche.net/clint/templates/calculators/lr_nomogram.asp and http://www.cebm.net/nomogram.asp or http://medcalc3000.com and https://itunes.apple.com/app/twobytwo/id436532323?mt=8).

When you do not have access to them, one strategy is to use the *nomogram* proposed by Fagan[13] (Figure 18-1), which does all of the conversions and allows an easy transition from pretest to posttest probability. The left-hand column of this nomogram represents the pretest probability, the middle column represents the LR, and the right-hand column represents the posttest probability. You obtain the posttest probability by anchoring a ruler at the pretest probability and rotating it until it lines up with the LR for the observed test result.

Recall the elderly woman from the opening scenario with suspected dementia. We have decided that the probability of this patient having the condition is approximately 20%. Suppose that the patient made 5 errors on the SIS. Anchoring a ruler at her pretest probability of 20% and aligning it with the LR of 28 associated with the test result of 5, you can get a posttest probability of approximately 90%.

The pretest probability is an estimate. Although the literature dealing with differential diagnosis can

FIGURE 18-1

Likelihood Ratio Nomogram

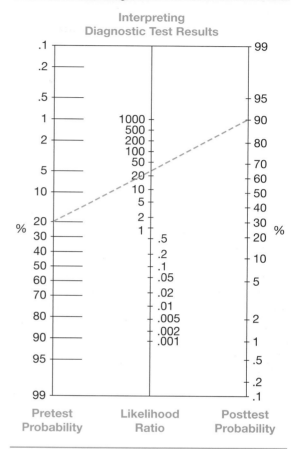

Interpreting
Diagnostic Test Results

sometimes help us in establishing the pretest probability (see Chapter 17, Differential Diagnosis), we know of no such study that will complement our intuition in arriving at a pretest probability when the suspicion of dementia arises. Although our intuition does not allow precise estimates of pretest probability, we can deal with residual uncertainty by examining the implications of a plausible range of pretest probabilities.

For example, if the pretest probability in this case is as low as 10% or as high as 30%, using the nomogram, we will get the posttest probability of approximately 80% and above 90%. Table 18-2 tabulates

TABLE 18-2

Pretest Probabilities, Likelihood Ratios of the Six-Item Screener, and Posttest Probabilities in the 70-Year-Old Woman With Moderate Suspicion of Dementia

Pretest Probability, % (Range)[a]	SIS Score (LR)	Posttest Probability, % (Range)[a]
20 (10-30)	6 (47)	92 (84-95)
	5 (28)	88 (76-92)
	4 (7.1)	64 (44-75)
	3 (2.5)	38 (22-52)
	2 (0.79)	16 (8-25)
	1 (0.28)	7 (3-11)
	0 (0.06)	1 (1-3)

Abbreviations: LR, likelihood ratio; SIS, Six-Item Screener.

[a]The values in parentheses represent a plausible range of pretest probabilities. That is, although the best guess as to the pretest probability is 20%, values of 10% to 30% would also be reasonable estimates.

TABLE 18-3

Pretest Probabilities, Likelihood Ratios of the Six-Item Screener, and Posttest Probabilities in the 85-Year-Old Woman With High Suspicion of Dementia

Pretest Probability, % (Range)[a]	SIS Score (LR)	Posttest Probability, % (Range)[a]
70 (60-80)	6 (47)	99 (99-99)
	5 (28)	98 (98-99)
	4 (7.1)	94 (91-97)
	3 (2.5)	85 (79-76)
	2 (0.79)	65 (54-76)
	1 (0.28)	40 (30-53)
	0 (0.06)	12 (8-19)

Abbreviations: LR, likelihood ratio; SIS, Six-Item Screener.

[a]The values in parentheses represent a plausible range of pretest probabilities. That is, although the best guess as to the pretest probability is 20%, values of 60% to 80% would also be reasonable estimates.

the posttest probabilities corresponding with each possible SIS score for the 65-year-old woman in the clinical scenario.

We can repeat this exercise for our second patient, the 85-year-old woman who had lost her way. You estimate that her history and presentation are compatible with a 70% probability of dementia. Using our nomogram (Figure 18-1), the posttest probability with an SIS score of 6 or 5 is almost 100%; with an SIS score of 4, it is 94%; with an SIS score of 3, it is 85%; and so on. The pretest probability (with a range of possible pretest probabilities of 60% to 80%), LRs, and posttest probabilities associated with each of these possible SIS scores are presented in Table 18-3.

Having learned to use LRs, you may be curious about where to find easy access to the LRs of the tests you use regularly in your own practice. The Rational Clinical Examination[14] is a series of systematic reviews of the diagnostic properties of the history and physical examination that have been published in *JAMA* (an updated database is available on the JAMAevidence homepage at http://jama evidence.com/resource/523). Chapter 19.2 lists a large number of examples of LRs. Further examples are accumulated on the JAMAevidence website (http://www.jamaevidence.com).

Dichotomizing Continuous Test Scores: Sensitivity, Specificity, and Likelihood Ratios

Readers who have followed the discussion to this point will understand the essentials of interpretation of diagnostic tests. In part because they remain in wide use, it is also helpful to understand 2 other terms in the lexicon of diagnostic testing: sensitivity and specificity. Many articles that address diagnostic tests report a 2 × 2 table and its associated sensitivity and specificity, as in Table 18-4, and to go along with it a figure that depicts the overall power of the diagnostic test (called a *receiver operating characteristic curve*).

Sensitivity is the proportion of people with a positive test result among those with the target condition. Specificity is the proportion of people with a negative test result among those without the target condition.

The study by Callahan et al recommends a cutoff of 3 or more errors for the diagnosis of dementia. Table 18-5 provides the breakdown of the cohort of referred patients according to this cutoff.

When we set the cutoff of 3 or more, the SIS has a sensitivity of 0.81 (278/345) and a specificity of 0.91 (278/306). We can also calculate the LRs, exactly as we did in Table 18-1. The LR for an SIS score of 3 or greater is therefore (278/345)/(28/306) = 8.8,

TABLE 18-4

Comparison of the Results of a Diagnostic Test With the Results of Reference Standard Using a 2 × 2 Table

Test Results	Reference Standard	
	Disease Present	**Disease Absent**
Test result positive	True positive (TP)	False positive (FP)
Test result negative	False negative (FN)	True negative (TN)

$$\text{Sensitivity} = \frac{TP}{TP + FN}$$

$$\text{Specificity} = \frac{TN}{FP + TN}$$

$$\text{Likelihood Ratio for Positive Test Result (LR+)} = \frac{\text{Sensitivity}}{1 - \text{Specificity}} = \frac{TP \text{ rate}}{FP \text{ rate}} = \frac{TP/(TP + FN)}{FP/(FP + TN)}$$

$$\text{Likelihood Ratio for Negative Test Result (LR−)} = \frac{1 - \text{Sensitivity}}{\text{Specificity}} = \frac{FN \text{ rate}}{TN \text{ rate}} = \frac{FN/(TP + FN)}{TN/(FP + TN)}$$

and the LR for an SIS score less than 3 is (67/345)/(278/306) = 0.21. The LR for a positive test result is often denoted as LR+ and that for a negative test result as LR−.

Let us now try to resolve our clinical scenario using this dichotomized 2 × 2 table. We had supposed that the pretest probability for the woman in the opening scenario was 20% and she had made 5 errors. Because the SIS score of 5 is associated here with an LR+ of 8.8, using Fagan's nomogram, we arrive at the posttest probability of approximately 70%, a figure considerably lower than the 90% that we had arrived at when we had a specific LR for 5 errors. This is because the dichotomized LR+ for SIS scores of 3 or more pooled strata for SIS scores of 3, 4, 5, and 6, and the resultant LR is thus diluted by the adjacent strata.

Although the difference between 70% and 90% may not dictate change in management strategies for the case in the clinical scenario, this will not always be the case. Consider a third patient, an elderly gentleman with a pretest probability of 50% of dementia who has surprised us by not making a single error on the SIS. With the dichotomous LR+/LR− approach (or, for that matter, with the sensitivity and specificity approach because these are mathematically equivalent and interchangeable), you combine the pretest probability of 50% with the

TABLE 18-5

Comparison of the Results of a Diagnostic Test (Six-Item Screener) With the Results of Reference Standard (Consensus *DSM-IV* and *ICD-10* Diagnosis) Using the Recommended Cutoff

SIS Score	Dementia	No Dementia
≥3	278	28
<3	67	278
Total	345	306

Abbreviations: *DSM-IV, Diagnostic and Statistical Manual of Mental Disorders* (Fourth Edition); *ICD-10, International Classification of Diseases, 10th Revision*; SIS, Six-Item Screener.

LR− of 0.21 and arrive at the posttest probability of approximately 20%, very likely necessitating further neuropsychological and other examinations. The true posttest probability for this man when we apply the LR associated with a score of 0 from Table 18-1 (0.06) is only approximately 5%. With this posttest probability, you (and the patient and his family) can feel relieved and, at least for the time being, be spared further testing.

In summary, use of multiple cuts or thresholds (sometimes referred to as multilevel LRs or stratum-specific LRs) has 2 key advantages over the sensitivity and specificity approach. First, for a test

DIAGNOSIS

that produces continuous scores or a number of categories (which many tests in medicine do, notably many laboratory tests), use of multiple thresholds retains as much information as possible. Second, knowing the LR of a particular test result, one can use a simple nomogram to move from the pretest to the posttest probability that is linked to your own patient.

USING THE GUIDE

Thus far, we have established that the results are likely true for the people who were included in the study, and we have calculated the multi-level LRs associated with each possible score of the test. We have indicated how the results could be applied to our patient (although we do not yet know the patient's score and have not decided how to proceed when we do).

HOW CAN I APPLY THE RESULTS TO PATIENT CARE?

Will the Reproducibility of the Test Result and Its Interpretation Be Satisfactory in My Clinical Setting?

The value of any test depends on its ability to yield the same result when reapplied to stable patients. Poor *reproducibility* can result from problems with the test itself (eg, variations in reagents in radioimmunoassay kits for determining hormone levels) or from its interpretation (eg, the extent of ST-segment elevation on an electrocardiogram). You can easily confirm this when you recall the clinical disagreements that arise when you and one or more colleagues examine the same electrocardiogram, ultrasonogram, or CT (even when all of you are experts).

Ideally, an article about a diagnostic test will address the reproducibility of the test results using a measure that corrects for agreement by chance (see Chapter 19.3, Measuring Agreement Beyond Chance), especially for issues that involve interpretation or judgment.

If the reported reproducibility of a test in the study setting is mediocre and disagreement between observers is common, and yet the test still discriminates well between those with and without the target condition, the test is likely to be very useful. Under these circumstances, there is a good chance that the test can be readily applied to your clinical setting.

If reproducibility of a diagnostic test is very high, either the test is simple and unambiguous or those interpreting the results are highly skilled. If the latter applies, less skilled interpreters in your own clinical setting may not do as well. You will either need to obtain appropriate training (or ensure that those interpreting the test in your setting have that training) or look for an easier and more robust test.

Are the Study Results Applicable to the Patients in My Practice?

Test properties may change with a different mix of disease severity or with a different distribution of competing conditions. When patients with the target disorder all have severe disease, LRs will move away from a value of 1.0 (ie, sensitivity increases). If patients are all mildly affected, LRs move toward a value of 1.0 (ie, sensitivity decreases). If patients without the target disorder have competing conditions that mimic the test results seen in patients who have the target disorder, the LRs will move closer to 1.0, and the test will appear less useful (ie, specificity decreases). In a different clinical setting in which fewer of the disease-free patients have these competing conditions, the LRs will move away from 1.0, and the test will appear more useful (ie, specificity increases). Differing prevalence in your setting may alert you to the possibility that the spectrum of target-positive and target-negative patients could differ in your practice.[15]

Investigators have reported the phenomenon of differing test properties in different subpopulations for exercise electrocardiography in the diagnosis of coronary artery disease. The more severe the coronary artery disease, the larger the LRs of abnormal exercise electrocardiograph results for angiographic narrowing of the coronary arteries.[16] Another example comes from the diagnosis of venous thromboembolism, where compression ultrasonography for proximal-vein thrombosis has proved more accurate in symptomatic outpatients than in asymptomatic postoperative patients.[17]

Sometimes, a test fails in just the patients one hopes it will best serve. The LR of a negative dipstick test result for the rapid diagnosis of urinary tract infection is approximately 0.2 in patients with clear symptoms and thus a high probability of urinary tract infection but is higher than 0.5 in those with low probability,[18] rendering it of little help in ruling out infection in the latter situation.

If you practice in a setting similar to that of the study and if the patient under consideration meets all of the study eligibility criteria, you can be confident that the results are applicable. If not, you must make a judgment. As with therapeutic interventions, you should ask whether here are compelling reasons why the results should not be applied to the patients in your practice, either because of the severity of disease in those patients or because the mix of competing conditions is so different that generalization is unwarranted. You may resolve the issue of *generalizability* if you can find a *systematic review* that summarizes the results of a number of studies.[19]

Will the Test Results Change My Management Strategy?

It is useful, when making and communicating management decisions, to link them explicitly to the probability of the target disorder. For any target disorder there are probabilities below which a clinician would dismiss a diagnosis and order no further tests: the test threshold. Similarly, there are probabilities above which a clinician would consider the diagnosis confirmed and would stop testing and initiate treatment (ie, the treatment threshold). When the probability of the target disorder lies between the test and treatment thresholds, further testing is mandated (see Chapter 16, The Process of Diagnosis).

If most patients have test results with LRs near 1.0, test results will seldom move us across the test or treatment threshold. Thus, the usefulness of a diagnostic test is strongly influenced by the proportion of patients suspected of having the target disorder whose test results have very high or very low LRs.

Among the patients suspected of having dementia, a review of Table 18-1 allows us to determine the proportion of patients with extreme results (LR >10 or <0.1). The proportion can be calculated as (105 + 2 + 64 + 2 + 11 + 163)/(345 + 306) or 347/651 = 53%. The SIS is likely to move the posttest probability in a decisive manner in half of the patients suspected of having dementia and examined—a very impressive proportion and better than for most of our diagnostic tests.

A final comment has to do with the use of sequential tests. The LR approach fits in particularly well in thinking about the diagnostic pathway. Each item of history—or each finding on physical examination—represents a diagnostic test in itself. We can use one test to get a certain posttest probability that can be further increased or decreased by using another, subsequent test. In general, we can also use laboratory tests or imaging procedures in the same way. If 2 tests are very closely related, however, application of the second test may provide little or no additional information, and the sequential application of LRs will yield misleading results. For example, once one has the results of the most powerful laboratory test for iron deficiency, serum ferritin, additional tests, such as serum iron or transferrin saturation, add no further useful information.[20] Once one has conducted an SIS, additional information from the MMSE is likely to be minimal.

Clinical prediction rules deal with the lack of independence of a series of tests and provide the clinician with a way of combining their results (see Chapter 19.4, Clinical Prediction Rules). For instance, in patients with suspected pulmonary embolism, one could use a rule that incorporates leg symptoms, heart rate, hemoptysis, and other aspects of the history and physical examination to accurately classify patients with suspected pulmonary embolism as being characterized by high, medium, and low probability.[21]

Will Patients Be Better Off as a Result of the Test?

The ultimate criterion for the usefulness of a diagnostic test is whether the benefits that accrue to patients are greater than the associated risks.[22] How can we establish the benefits and risks of applying a diagnostic test? The answer lies in thinking of a diagnostic test as a therapeutic maneuver (see Chapter 7, Therapy [Randomized Trials]). Establishing whether a test does more good than harm will involve (1) randomizing patients to a diagnostic strategy that includes the test under investigation and a management schedule linked to it, or to one in which the test is not available, and (2) following up patients in both groups forward in time to determine the frequency of *patient-important outcomes.*

When is demonstrating accuracy sufficient to mandate the use of a test and when does one require a *randomized clinical trial*? The value of an accurate test will be undisputed when the target disorder is dangerous if left undiagnosed, if the test has acceptable risks, and if effective treatment exists. This is the case for the CT-angiogram for suspected pulmonary embolism. A high probability or normal or near-normal results of the CT-angiogram may well eliminate the need for further investigation and may result in anticoagulant agents being appropriately given or appropriately withheld (with either course of action having a substantial positive influence on patient outcome).

Sometimes, a test may be completely benign, represent a low resource investment, be evidently accurate, and clearly lead to useful changes in management. Such is the case for use of the SIS in patients with suspected dementia, when test results may dictate reassurance or extensive investigation and ultimately planning for a tragic deteriorating course.

In other clinical situations, tests may be accurate and management may even change as a result of their application, but their effect on patient outcome may be far less certain. Consider one of the issues we raised in our discussion of framing clinical questions (see Chapter 4, What Is the Question?). There, we considered a patient with apparently resectable non–small cell carcinoma of the lung and wondered whether the clinician should order a positron emission tomogram (PET)–CT and base further management on the results or use alternative diagnostic strategies. For this question, knowledge of the accuracy of CT is insufficient. A randomized trial of PET-CT–directed management or an alternative strategy for all patients is warranted. Other examples include catheterization of the right side of the heart for critically ill patients with uncertain hemodynamic status and bronchoalveolar lavage for critically ill patients with possible pulmonary infection. For these tests, randomized trials have helped elucidate optimal management strategies.

CLINICAL SCENARIO RESOLUTION

Although the study itself does not report reproducibility, its scoring is simple and straightforward because you need only count the number of errors made to 6 questions. The SIS does not require any props or visual cues and is therefore unobtrusive, easy to administer, and takes only 1 to 2 minutes to complete (compared with 5 to 10 minutes for the MMSE). Although you note that trained research staff administered the SIS, the appendix of the article gives a detailed, word-by-word instruction on how to administer the SIS. You believe that you too can administer this scale reliably.

The patient in the clinical scenario is an older woman who was able to come to your clinic by herself but appeared no longer as lucid as she used to be. The Alzheimer Disease Center cohort in the study we had been examining in this chapter consists of people suspected of having dementia by their caregivers and brought to a tertiary care center directly. Their test characteristics were reported to be similar to those observed in the general population cohort, that is, in a sample with less severe presentations. You decide that there is no compelling reason that the study results would not apply to your patient.

You invite your patient back to the office for a follow-up visit and administer the SIS. The result is a score of 4, which, given your pretest probability of 20%, increases the probability to more than 60%. After hearing that you are concerned about her memory and possibly about her function, she agrees to a referral to a geriatrician for more extensive investigation.

References

1. Callahan CM, Unverzagt FW, Hui SL, Perkins AJ, Hendrie HC. Six-item screener to identify cognitive impairment among potential subjects for clinical research. *Med Care*. 2002;40(9):771-781.

2. Lijmer JG, Mol BW, Heisterkamp S, et al. Empirical evidence of design-related bias in studies of diagnostic tests. *JAMA*. 1999;282(11):1061-1066.

3. Rutjes AW, Reitsma JB, Di Nisio M, Smidt N, van Rijn JC, Bossuyt PM. Evidence of bias and variation in diagnostic accuracy studies. *CMAJ*. 2006;174(4):469-476.

4. Whiting P, Rutjes AW, Reitsma JB, Glas AS, Bossuyt PM, Kleijnen J. Sources of variation and bias in studies of diagnostic accuracy: a systematic review. *Ann Intern Med*. 2004; 140(3):189-202.

5. Thomson DM, Krupey J, Freedman SO, Gold P. The radioimmunoassay of circulating carcinoembryonic antigen of the human digestive system. *Proc Natl Acad Sci USA*. 1969;64(1): 161-167.

6. Marantz PR, Kaplan MC, Alderman MH. Clinical diagnosis of congestive heart failure in patients with acute dyspnea. *Chest*. 1990;97(4):776-781.

7. Chochinov HM, Wilson KG, Enns M, Lander S. "Are you depressed?" screening for depression in the terminally ill. *Am J Psychiatry*. 1997;154(5):674-676.

8. Begg CB, Greenes RA. Assessment of diagnostic tests when disease verification is subject to selection bias. *Biometrics*. 1983;39(1):207-215.

9. Gray R, Begg CB, Greenes RA. Construction of receiver operating characteristic curves when disease verification is subject to selection bias. *Med Decis Making*. 1984;4(2):151-164.

10. Ransohoff DF, Feinstein AR. Problems of spectrum and bias in evaluating the efficacy of diagnostic tests. *N Engl J Med*. 1978;299(17):926-930.

11. Choi BC. Sensitivity and specificity of a single diagnostic test in the presence of work-up bias. *J Clin Epidemiol*. 1992; 45(6):581-586.

12. PIOPED Investigators. Value of the ventilation/perfusion scan in acute pulmonary embolism: results of the Prospective Investigation of Pulmonary Embolism Diagnosis (PIOPED). *JAMA*. 1990;263(20):2753-2759.

13. Fagan TJ. Letter: Nomogram for Bayes theorem. *N Engl J Med*. 1975;293(5):257.

14. Sackett DL, Rennie D. The science of the art of the clinical examination. *JAMA*. 1992;267(19):2650-2652.

15. Leeflang MM, Rutjes AW, Reitsma JB, Hooft L, Bossuyt PM. Variation of a test's sensitivity and specificity with disease prevalence. *CMAJ*. 2013;185(11):E537-E544.

16. Hlatky MA, Pryor DB, Harrell FE Jr, Califf RM, Mark DB, Rosati RA. Factors affecting sensitivity and specificity of exercise electrocardiography. Multivariable analysis. *Am J Med*. 1984;77(1):64-71.

17. Ginsberg JS, Caco CC, Brill-Edwards PA, et al. Venous thrombosis in patients who have undergone major hip or knee surgery: detection with compression US and impedance plethysmography. *Radiology*. 1991;181(3):651-654.

18. Lachs MS, Nachamkin I, Edelstein PH, Goldman J, Feinstein AR, Schwartz JS. Spectrum bias in the evaluation of diagnostic tests: lessons from the rapid dipstick test for urinary tract infection. *Ann Intern Med*. 1992;117(2):135-140.

19. Leeflang MM, Deeks JJ, Gatsonis C, Bossuyt PM; Cochrane Diagnostic Test Accuracy Working Group. Systematic reviews of diagnostic test accuracy. *Ann Intern Med*. 2008; 149(12):889-897.

20. Guyatt GH, Oxman AD, Ali M, Willan A, McIlroy W, Patterson C. Laboratory diagnosis of iron-deficiency anemia: an overview. *J Gen Intern Med*. 1992;7(2):145-153.

21. van Belle A, Büller HR, Huisman MV, et al; Christopher Study Investigators. Effectiveness of managing suspected pulmonary embolism using an algorithm combining clinical probability, D-dimer testing, and computed tomography. *JAMA*. 2006;295(2):172-179.

22. Guyatt GH, Tugwell PX, Feeny DH, Haynes RB, Drummond M. A framework for clinical evaluation of diagnostic technologies. *CMAJ*. 1986;134(6):587-594.

19.1

ADVANCED TOPICS IN DIAGNOSIS

Spectrum Bias

Reem A. Mustafa, Victor M. Montori, Peter Wyer,
Thomas B. Newman, Sheri A. Keitz, and Gordon Guyatt

IN THIS CHAPTER

DIAGNOSIS

CHOOSING THE WRONG PATIENTS WILL BIAS ESTIMATES OF THE USEFULNESS OF A DIAGNOSTIC TEST

For clinicians to appropriately use diagnostic tests in clinical practice, they need to know how well the tests can distinguish between those who have the *target condition* and those who do not. If investigators choose clinically inappropriate populations for their study of a diagnostic test (introducing what is sometimes called *spectrum bias*), the results may seriously mislead clinicians (see Chapter 18, Diagnostic Tests).

In this chapter, we present a series of examples that expand on the points related to spectrum bias. Working through these examples, you will gain a deeper understanding of which characteristics of a study population are and are not likely to result in misleading results. Readers will find an elaborated version of this demonstration, intended to assist teachers in interactive sessions with small groups, in another publication.[1]

TARGET-POSITIVE PATIENTS WITH UNEQUIVOCALLY SEVERE DISEASE AND TARGET-NEGATIVE PATIENTS WITH NO REASON TO SUSPECT DISEASE ARE THE WRONG PATIENTS TO STUDY

Ideally, the ability of a test to correctly identify patients with a particular disease, condition, or outcome (*target-positive* patients) and those without (*target-negative* patients) would not vary from patient to patient. A test may, however, perform better when used to evaluate patients with more severe disease than it would in patients whose disease is less obvious and/or less advanced. Moreover, clinicians do not need diagnostic tests when the disease is clinically obvious or sufficiently unlikely that they need not seriously consider it.

A study of a diagnostic test involves performing the test of interest, together with a second test or investigation (which we will call the *reference standard*, *criterion standard*, or *gold standard*) in patients with and without the disease or condition of interest. We accept the results of the reference standard as the criterion by which the results of the test under investigation are assessed.

In designing such a study, investigators sometimes choose patients with unequivocally far-advanced disease together with unequivocally disease-free people, such as healthy asymptomatic volunteers. This approach ensures that the criterion standard will not misclassify any patients and may be appropriate in the early stages of developing a test. Any study performed on a population that lacks diagnostic uncertainty may, however, produce a biased estimate of a test's performance relative to a study restricted to patients for whom the test would be clinically indicated.

DISTRIBUTIONS OF TEST RESULTS ILLUSTRATE THE SPECTRUM PROBLEM

A crucial issue in the design of a diagnostic test study is the distribution of severity of illness or abnormality among the patients who were enrolled. We refer to this distribution as the spectrum of disease, illness, or abnormality.

For example, consider brain natriuretic peptide (BNP), which is a hormone that the ventricles of the heart secrete in response to expansion. Plasma levels of BNP increase in congestive heart failure (CHF). Consequently, investigators have suggested BNP as a test to distinguish between CHF and other causes of acute dyspnea among patients presenting to emergency departments.[2]

One study reported promising results using a BNP cutoff of 100 pg/mL.[3,4] In thinking about the use of BNP as a test for CHF among patients with acute dyspnea, consider Figure 19.1-1. The horizontal axis corresponds to increasing values of BNP. The 2 bell curves constitute hypothetical probability density plots of the distribution of BNP values among patients with and without CHF. The height of the vertical axis at any point in either curve reflects the proportion of emergency department patients having the corresponding BNP result. Aside from the choice of cutoff value, this figure is a hypothetical illustration that does not directly reflect the results of any actual study.

The bell curve on the left of Figure 19.1-1 represents a schematic of the distribution of BNP values in a group of young individuals with known asthma and no risk factors for CHF. They will tend to have very low levels of circulating BNP. The bell curve on the right represents the distribution of BNP values in older patients with unequivocal and severe acute

CHF. Such patients will have test results clustered on the high end of the scale.

If Figure 19.1-1 accurately represented the performance of BNP in distinguishing between patients with and without CHF as the cause of their symptoms, BNP would be a very good test: the 2 curves demonstrate very little overlap. For BNP values above

FIGURE 19.1-1

Distribution of Brain Natriuretic Peptide Values Among Patients With and Without Congestive Heart Failure: Patients With Asthma and Those With Severe Heart Failure

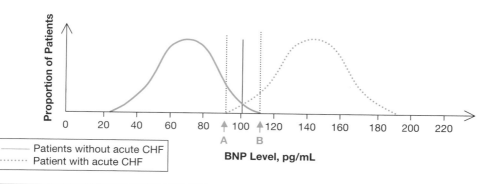

The height of the bell curve at each point reflects the proportion of the patient subgroup having the corresponding BNP value. Patients without CHF (left hand curve) are made up of younger patients with known asthma and no risk factors for CHF. The patients with CHF are older and are clinically severe and unequivocal. Treating clinicians in the emergency department have little uncertainty regarding the cause of dyspnea in any of these patients. Abbreviations: BNP, brain natriuretic peptide; CHF, congestive heart failure.

Reproduced from Montori et al,[1] by permission of the publisher. © 2005, Canadian Medical Association.

FIGURE 19.1-2

Distribution of Brain Natriuretic Peptide Values Among Patients With and Without Congestive Heart Failure

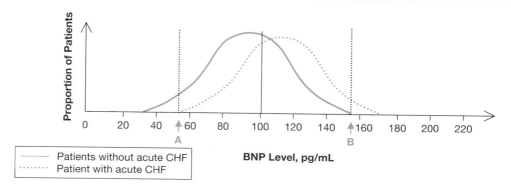

Individuals had a history of CHF and asthma with or without CHF. The probability density distributions now reflect a study population of middle-aged patients who all have recurrent asthma and chronic CHF. The patients whose dyspnea is due to asthma exacerbations manifest test results similar to those whose symptoms are being caused by acute CHF. Abbreviations: BNP, brain natriuretic peptide; CHF, congestive heart failure.

Reproduced from Montori et al,[1] by permission of the publisher. © 2005, Canadian Medical Association.

110 pg/mL (point B), all patients have CHF, and for BNP values below 85 pg/mL (point A), no patients have CHF. This means that you can be completely certain about the diagnosis for all individuals with BNP values above 110 pg/mL or below 85 pg/mL. Only for patients whose BNP values are within the narrow range of 85 to 110 pg/mL is there residual uncertainty after the test has been performed regarding their likelihood of CHF.

Before you embrace a test according to its performance in clinically unequivocal patients, however, you need to consider the likely distribution of test results in a population of patients for whom you would be less certain. In Figure 19.1-2, imagine that the entire population is made up of middle-aged patients, all of whom have a history of chronic CHF and also of asthma episodes. The distributions of BNP values among the subgroups with and without acute CHF are both closer to the middle. The extent of the overlap of the curves between points A and B is much greater. This means that even after the BNP test has been performed, residual uncertainty regarding the disease status of a large proportion of the tested patients remains.

In the cited study of performance of BNP, the *sensitivity* and *specificity* of the test, using the 100-pg/mL cutoff, were 90% and 76%, respectively, when all patients were included.[3] Only approximately 25% of the study population, however, comprised patients judged by the treating physicians to be in the intermediate range of probability of acute CHF.[3] When only patients in the latter range were considered in a number of studies, the specificity of BNP at a cutoff of 100 pg/mL decreased to 55%.[5]

As it turns out, BNP test performance appears adequate to aid clinicians in treating emergency department patients with suspected heart failure.[6-8] *Randomized clinical trials* in which patients with acute dyspnea and possible heart failure were randomized to BNP testing or no BNP testing have demonstrated that clinician access to BNP results decreases hospital admission rates and length of stay in those admitted to the hospital.[6-8]

THE RIGHT POPULATION INCLUDES ONLY PATIENTS WITH DIAGNOSTIC UNCERTAINTY

The message here is that clinicians seldom need new tests to differentiate normal from unequivocally severely diseased patients; rather, additional testing must differentiate between those who appear as if they might have the target condition and do from those who appear as if they might have the target condition and do not. Box 19.1-1 presents various ways of expressing the optimal population for a diagnostic test study.

DISTRIBUTIONS OF TEST RESULTS HELP THE UNDERSTANDING OF LIKELIHOOD RATIOS

As Chapter 18, Diagnostic Tests, describes at length, *likelihood ratios* are the best way of expressing and using diagnostic test results. As it turns out, the likelihood ratio for any given test value is represented by the ratio of respective heights of the curves at that point on the x-axis. As shown in Figure 19.1-3, the point on the x-axis below the intersection of the 2 curves is the test result with a likelihood ratio of 1. As the proportion of those in the target-positive and target-negative populations with particular test results diverges, likelihood ratios move farther and farther from 1.

FIGURE 19.1-3

Distribution of Brain Natriuretic Peptide Values Among Patients With and Without Congestive Heart Failure

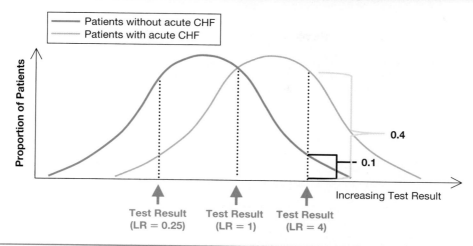

Note how the height of the curves relates to the LRs. The LR of a test result represented by a point on the horizontal line is the height of the right-hand distribution curve (patients with the disease of interest) divided by the height of the left-hand distribution curve (patients without the disease of interest) at that point. Abbreviations: CHF, congestive heart failure; LR, likelihood ratio.

Reproduced from Montori et al,[1] by permission of the publisher. © 2005, Canadian Medical Association.

SPECTRUM, NOT DISEASE PREVALENCE, DETERMINES TEST PROPERTIES

You may have learned that whereas *posttest probabilities* vary with disease prevalence, likelihood ratios do not. Is this true? The answer is yes, provided that the spectra of both diseased and not diseased remain the same in high-prevalence and low-prevalence populations. Recall that spectrum refers to the distribution of severity of illness or abnormality among patients. Therefore, likelihood ratios do not vary with disease prevalence provided that the spectrum of illness severity remains the same in high-prevalence and low-prevalence populations. This is, admittedly, a strong assumption, as we will note below.

Referring once again to Figure 19.1-1, let us consider 3 cases. In the first, we will assume that there were 2000 patients in whom CHF was unequivocally the cause of their dyspnea and 1000 in whom asthma was almost certainly the cause. The prevalence of CHF is 67%. Each bell curve corresponds to the distribution of BNP values within the respective subgroup.

Now consider a second case in which there are 1000 patients with severe CHF and 1000 patients with recurrent asthma and no risk factors for CHF. The prevalence of CHF is 50%.

Finally, consider a third case in which investigators study 1000 patients with CHF and 2000 with asthma. The prevalence of CHF is 33%.

In each case, regardless of the prevalence of CHF, the shapes of the 2 bell curves in Figure 19.1-1 do not change because the vertical axis represents the proportion, not the absolute number, of patients with that test value in that group. Changes in the total number of patients will therefore not alter the performance of the test, as measured by likelihood ratios. Hence, when the spectrum remains the same, the prevalence of CHF within the study population is irrelevant to the estimation of test characteristics. Having said that, we are not suggesting that an investigator should design a study with an arbitrary "prevalence" of disease because it will lead to a meaningless posttest probability.

TABLE 19.1-1A

Women Attending a Screening Clinic Located in a Community Center Serving a Moderately Growing Population Are Tested for Pregnancy

hCG Result	Pregnant	Not Pregnant	Total
Positive	A	B	A + B
	95	1	96
Negative	C	D	C + D
	5	99	104
Total	A + C	B + D	A + B + C + D
	100	100	200

Abbreviation: hCG, human chorionic gonadotrophin.

The urine pregnancy test has a sensitivity of 95% and a specificity of 99%. The sensitivity takes into account women who present fewer than 2 weeks after conception; 50% of the women are pregnant.

Reproduced from Montori et al,[1] by permission of the publisher. © 2005, Canadian Medical Association.

TABLE 19.1-1B

The Same Test Used in Table 19.1-1A Performed in a Similar Clinic Located in a Geographic Area Characterized by High Population Growth

hCG Result	Pregnant	Not Pregnant	Total
Positive	A × 4	B	4A + B
	380	1	381
Negative	C × 4	D	4C + D
	20	99	119
Total	4A + 4C	B + D	4A + B + 4C + D
	400	100	500

Abbreviation: hCG, human chorionic gonadotrophin.

The same proportion of women presents within 2 weeks of conception; 80% of the women are pregnant.

Reproduced from Montori et al,[1] by permission of the publisher. © 2005, Canadian Medical Association.

Let us take a different clinical example. A human chorionic gonadotrophin (hCG) urine test for pregnancy has a very high sensitivity and specificity when performed at least 2 weeks after conception.[9] It is an inherently dichotomized test (ie, yes/no, does not provide a range of values).

Let us assume that the hCG test result is positive in 95% of women who are pregnant and is negative in 99% of women who are not. Tables 19.1-1A, B, and C give the sensitivity and specificity of the test when it is administered in 3 geographic locations with high, moderate, and low population growth and where the proportion of women presenting at least 2 weeks after conception is constant. Again, for simplicity, we are considering only the prevalence of pregnancy in the population being studied, in other words, the percentage of women tested who are pregnant. A clinician might estimate the probability of pregnancy in an individual patient to be higher or lower than this on the basis of clinical features, such as use of birth control methods or history of recent sexual activity. As Tables 19.1-1A, B, and C indicate,

TABLE 19.1-1C

The Same Pregnancy Test Used in Tables 19.1-1A and B Is Now Used in a Similar Clinic Servicing a Population Characterized by Low Population Growth			
hCG Result	**Pregnant**	**Not Pregnant**	**Total**
Positive	A	B × 4	A + 4B
	95	4	99
Negative	C	D × 4	C + 4D
	5	396	401
Total	A + C	4B + 4D	A + 4B + C + 4D
	100	400	500

Abbreviation: hCG, human chorionic gonadotrophin.

The same proportion of women presents within 2 weeks of conception; only 20% of them are pregnant.

Reproduced from Montori et al,[1] by permission of the publisher. © 2005, Canadian Medical Association.

the prevalence of pregnancy in the population has no effect on the estimation of test characteristics.

There are many other examples of conditions that may present with equal severity in people with different demographics (age, sex, and ethnic origin) but that are much more prevalent in a certain group than in another. Mild osteoarthritis of the knee is rare in young patients but common in older patients. Asymptomatic thyroid abnormalities are rare in men but common in women. In both examples, as long as the spectrum of disease and of competing conditions is similar, an admittedly strong assumption, diagnostic tests will have the same likelihood ratios in young and old and in men and women.

PREVALENCE (OR PRETEST PROBABILITY) INFLUENCES POSTTEST PROBABILITY

Higher prevalence will, however, result in a higher proportion of those with either normal or abnormal results who are in fact target positive. Referring to Table 19.1-1B, in population B, of whom 80% are pregnant, 380 of 381 test-positive women (99.7%) are pregnant, as are 20 of 119 test-negative women (17%). In population C (Table 19.1-1C), of whom 20% are pregnant, 95 of 99 test-positive women (96%) are pregnant, but only 5 of 401 test-negative women (1.2%). The results indicate how test properties

can remain the same across populations of varying prevalence, but posttest probabilities may differ substantially.

LIKELIHOOD RATIOS SHOULD REFLECT APPROPRIATE SPECTRUMS OF TARGET-POSITIVE AND TARGET-NEGATIVE PATIENTS

Although differences in prevalence alone should not affect the sensitivity or specificity of a test, in many clinical settings, disease prevalence and disease spectrum may be related. For instance, rheumatoid arthritis observed in a family physician's office will be relatively uncommon, and most patients will have relatively mild disease. In contrast, rheumatoid arthritis will be common in a rheumatologist's office, and the patients will tend to have relatively severe disease. Tests to diagnose rheumatoid arthritis in the rheumatologist's waiting area (eg, hand inspection for joint deformity) are likely to be relatively more sensitive not because of the increased prevalence but because of the spectrum of disease present (ie, degree and extent of joint deformity) in this setting.

As long as both the family physician and the rheumatologist are facing diagnostic uncertainties, they both have their own setting-specific disease spectrums, which therefore yield different likelihood ratios. Family physicians and rheumatologists will both want to select the likelihood ratios obtained from study populations similar to those they see in practice.

CONCLUSION

In this chapter, we discussed spectrum bias and how it may affect the estimates of the usefulness of a diagnostic test. We described the importance of choosing only patients with diagnostic uncertainty to study to minimize this bias. We also highlighted that studying populations with different disease or condition prevalence will not affect test characteristics, such as the likelihood ratio, whereas studying populations with a different disease spectrum will affect test characteristics. Hence, the likelihood ratio should reflect the appropriate spectrum of target-positive and target-negative patients in clinicians' practice.

References

1. Montori VM, Wyer P, Newman TB, Keitz S, Guyatt G. Tips for learners of evidence-based medicine, 5: the effect of spectrum of disease on the performance of diagnostic tests. *CMAJ*. 2005;173(4):385-390 and online appendix.

2. Dao Q, Krishnaswamy P, Kazanegra R, et al. Utility of B-type natriuretic peptide in the diagnosis of congestive heart failure in an urgent-care setting. *J Am Coll Cardiol*. 2001;37(2):379-385.

3. Maisel AS, Krishnaswamy P, Nowak RM, et al; Breathing Not Properly Multinational Study Investigators. Rapid measurement of B-type natriuretic peptide in the emergency diagnosis of heart failure. *N Engl J Med*. 2002;347(3):161-167.

4. McCullough PA, Nowak RM, McCord J, et al. B-type natriuretic peptide and clinical judgment in emergency diagnosis of heart failure: analysis from Breathing Not Properly (BNP) Multinational Study. *Circulation*. 2002;106(4):416-422.

5. Schwam E. B-type natriuretic peptide for diagnosis of heart failure in emergency department patients: a critical appraisal. *Acad Emerg Med*. 2004;11(6):686-691.

6. Mueller C, Scholer A, Laule-Kilian K, et al. Use of B-type natriuretic peptide in the evaluation and management of acute dyspnea. *N Engl J Med*. 2004;350(7):647-654.

7. Mueller C, Laule-Kilian K, Scholer A, et al. Use of B-type natriuretic peptide for the management of women with dyspnea. *Am J Cardiol*. 2004;94(12):1510-1514.

8. Mueller C, Laule-Kilian K, Frana B, et al. The use of B-type natriuretic peptide in the management of elderly patients with acute dyspnoea. *J Intern Med*. 2005;258(1):77-85.

9. Cole LA. The hCG assay or pregnancy test. *Clin Chem Lab Med*. 2012;50(4):617-630.

19.2

ADVANCED TOPICS IN DIAGNOSIS

Examples of Likelihood Ratios

Luz Maria Letelier, Daniel Capurro, Jaime Cerda, Lorena Cifuentes Aguila, Juan Carlos Claro, Gabriel Rada, Solange Rivera Mercado, and Victor M. Montori

IN THIS CHAPTER

(continued on following page)

DIAGNOSIS

INTRODUCTION

Other chapters of this book have made the case for the usefulness of *likelihood ratios* (LRs) in the process of diagnosis (see Chapter 16, The Process of Diagnosis, and Chapter 18, Diagnostic Tests). In this chapter, we present some examples of LRs, along with their associated 95% *confidence intervals* (CIs), for many diagnostic tests. For each test, we describe the population to whom the test was applied and the range of *prevalence* (*pretest probability*) found for each *target condition* (disease). Our choice of conditions has been idiosyncratic and represents the interests of the authors. We restricted ourselves to tests in current use and so do not offer a technical description of the tests. The authors conducted all searches and summaries, without duplicate adjudication of eligibility or data extraction.

METHODS FOR SUMMARIZING THE INFORMATION ON LIKELIHOOD RATIOS

Eligibility Criteria

For each test and target condition under consideration, we included studies that met each of the following criteria:

- The study authors presented LRs or sufficient data to allow their calculation.
- The investigators compared the test with a *reference standard* (*criterion standard* or *gold standard*) that was defined in advance and that met the following criteria: (1) at the time of the study it was in wide use and no better standard was available; (2) when the decision to apply the criterion standard was unrelated to the results of the test, it was applied to at least 50% of eligible patients; and (3) when the decision to apply the criterion standard may have been influenced by test results, it was applied to 90% of eligible patients or it was blindly applied.
- The investigators enrolled patients similar to those treated in clinical practice for whom the test might be reasonably applied.
- Publications were in English or Spanish.

FIGURE 19.2-1

Search Strategy Template

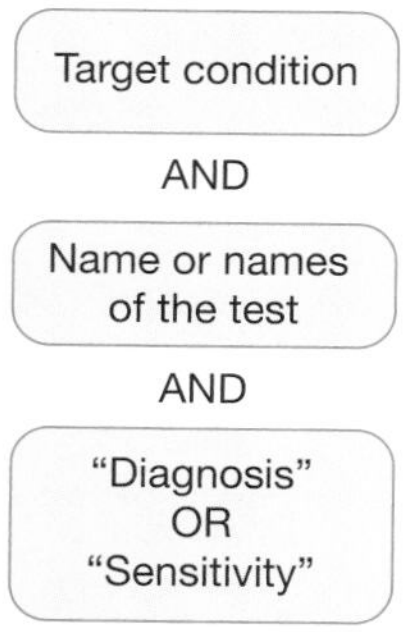

We excluded studies that met the following criteria:

- The study was concerned with predicting long-term outcomes.
- The study evaluated diagnostic models, including multiple tests such as decision trees, diagnostic algorithms, neural networks, or computer-based pattern recognition systems.

Literature Search

Our original search included Best Evidence (1991-2000) and MEDLINE (1966-2000). In addition, we hand-searched the *JAMA* series entitled The Rational Clinical Examination (1992-2000) and references from a diagnostic textbook.[1] We also reviewed the citations of articles we found for additional potentially eligible studies. Examples have been updated to 2013, and new examples have been added.

For every pair of target condition and test, we searched the databases with the following search strategy template, using both *Medical Subject Headings* (MeSH) and text words (Figure 19.2-1). An example of the typical search strategy is shown in Figure 19.2-2.

Selection Process

Whenever we found a good-quality *systematic review* with *meta-analysis*, we used it as our only data source, although we sometimes reviewed the original studies to obtain the data required for our own statistical analysis and searched for more recent studies on the topic.

DIAGNOSIS

FIGURE 19.2-2

Sample Search Strategy

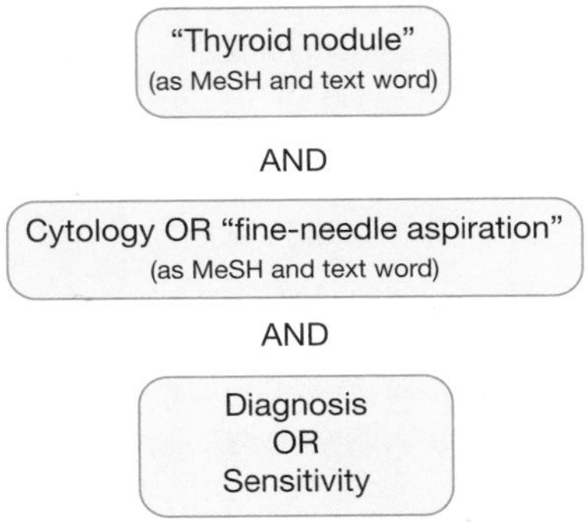

"Thyroid nodule"
(as MeSH and text word)

AND

Cytology OR "fine-needle aspiration"
(as MeSH and text word)

AND

Diagnosis
OR
Sensitivity

When we identified more than 1 systematic review, we either selected the better quality and more comprehensive one or presented the range of possible LRs.

Statistical Analysis

For topics without a systematic review and formal meta-analysis, LRs and 95% CIs for individual 2 × 2 and 2 × J (ie, 2 outcomes—*target positive* and *target negative*—but multiple levels of test result) tables were computed using methods described by Simel et al.[2] We computed *random-effect* pooled estimates of the LRs (with $\Delta = 0.25$ added to each

cell count) using the general meta-analytic method advanced by Fleiss.[3]

In calculating summary LRs, we did not take into account study quality, differences in calibration among centers, or differences in study populations beyond those of our eligibility criteria, so these results are not considered to qualify as a formal meta-analysis. For more thorough examples, see The Rational Clinical Examination chapters on the JAMAevidence website (http://www.jamaevidence.com).

EXAMPLES

Abdominal Aortic Aneurysm

We found 1 systematic review that included the following studies, in which investigators enrolled asymptomatic people with risk factors for abdominal aortic aneurysm. Their reference standard was abdominal ultrasonography (Table 19.2-1).[4]

Acute Appendicitis

Table 19.2-2 presents likelihood ratios for medical history, physical examination, ultrasonography, and computed tomography in patients older than 14 years with suspected acute appendicitis. The reference standard was surgical findings with pathologic

TABLE 19.2-1

Likelihood Ratios for Detection of AAA in Asymptomatic People With Risk Factors Compared With Abdominal Ultrasonography as Reference Standard

Prevalence (Pretest Probability, %)	Patients, No.	Test	Test Result	Likelihood Ratio (95% CI)	Reference
Target Condition: AAA ≥3 cm					
1-28	2955	Abdominal palpation directed toward AAA detection	Positive	12 (7.4-20)	4
			Negative	0.72 (0.65-0.81)	
Target Condition: AAA ≥4 cm					
1-28	2955	Abdominal palpation directed toward AAA detection	Positive	6 (8.6-29)	4
			Negative	0.51 (0.38-0.67)	

Abbreviations: AAA, abdominal aortic aneurysm; CI, confidence interval.

TABLE 19.2-2

Likelihood Ratios of Tests for the Diagnosis of Acute Appendicitis in Adults and Children

Prevalence (Pretest Probability, %)	Patients, No.	Test	Test Result	Likelihood Ratio (95% CI)	Reference
Adults					
12-60	6072	Medical history or physical examination			5-9
		Rigidity	Present	2.96 (2.43-3.59)	
			Absent	0.86 (0.72-1.02)	
		Psoas sign,[a] pain migration from periumbilical area or epigastrium to the RLQ, guarding, rebound sign,[b] or pain located in the RLQ	Present	1.52-2.48	
			Absent	0.36-0.67	
		Radiologic tests			
48-50	1516	US by radiologist or trained surgeon with or without graded compression technique	Positive	5.8-11.8	10-11
			Negative	0.19-0.18	
40-45	1172	High-resolution helical CT of abdominal and pelvic areas or focused on the appendix; with intravenous, oral, or colonic contrast media, or without intestinal contrast[c]	Positive	13.3-15.6	
			Negative	0.09-0.06	
38	1268	Surgeon-performed US	Positive	24 (16.8-34)	12
			Negative	0.09 (0.07-0.12)	
Children 18 Years or Younger					
10	246	Medical history or physical examination			13
		Fever	Present	3.4 (2.4-4.8)	
			Absent	0.32 (0.16-0.64)	
		Vomiting, diarrhea	Present	2.2-2.6	
			Absent	0.57-1.0	
37-89	1845	Pain migration from periumbilical area or epigastrium to the RLQ, pain located in the RLQ	Present	1.2-3.1	
			Absent	0.41-0.72	
		Rebound sign[a]	Present	3.0 (2.3-3-9)	
			Absent	0.28 (1.9-3.1)	
		Radiologic tests			

(Continued)

TABLE 19.2-2

Likelihood Ratios of Tests for the Diagnosis of Acute Appendicitis in Adults and Children *(Continued)*

Prevalence (Pretest Probability, %)	Patients, No.	Test	Test Result	Likelihood Ratio (95% CI)	Reference
31	6850	US by radiologist or trained surgeon with or without graded compression technique	Positive	15 (13-16)	11
			Negative	0.13 (0.11-0.14)	
31	598	High-resolution helical CT of abdominal and pelvic areas or focused on the appendix; with intravenous, oral, or colonic contrast media, or without intestinal contrast	Positive	19 (12-29)	11
			Negative	0.06 (0.04-0.11)	

Abbreviations: CI, confidence interval; CT, computed tomography; RLQ, right lower quadrant; US, ultrasonography.

aPsoas sign: A sign of irritation of the psoas muscle, which is elicited by having the patient extend the leg (ipsilateral to the location of abdominal pain) at the hip against resistance (by the examiner) while lying on the unaffected side. If abdominal pain appears or is exacerbated with this maneuver, the sign is considered positive. In acute appendicitis, this sign may be positive on the right side.

bRebound sign: A sign of peritoneal inflammation, which is elicited by first palpating deeply and slowly an area of the abdomen distant from the location of abdominal pain, followed by quick removal of the palpating hand. If abdominal pain appears or is exacerbated with removal of the palpating hand, the sign is considered positive.

cNo differences were found among different CT techniques.

analysis or clinical *follow-up* in patients who did not undergo surgery. For the likelihood ratios for surgeon-performed ultrasonography, investigators used pathologic analysis or radiologist-performed ultrasonography as the reference standard.[5-12] The study of children 18 years or younger in whom the diagnosis of appendicitis was considered used surgical pathologic findings or clinical follow-up in those who did not undergo surgery as the reference standard.[11,13]

Acute Cholecystitis

The reference standard was surgical findings with pathologic analysis or clinical follow-up in patients who did not undergo surgery (Table 19.2-3).[14,15]

Acute Myocardial Infarction

Likelihood ratios are based on 3 systematic reviews on the diagnostic value of symptoms, signs, and electrocardiographic (ECG) changes in patients with acute chest pain for the diagnosis of acute myocardial infarction (MI). The systematic reviews summarized 172 studies on clinical findings and

53 of ECG. The reference standard was the combination of clinical findings and ECG changes and cardiac biomarkers. Note that the tests are not independent from the reference standard, but this is the reference standard most widely used (Table 19.2-4).[16-18]

Airflow Limitation

The likelihood ratios in Table 19.2-5 are based on 2 systematic reviews, including 26 studies that used spirometry as the reference standard.[19,20]

Alcohol Abuse or Dependence

For the diagnosis of alcohol abuse or dependence with the CAGE (Cut down, Annoyed, Guilty, Eye opener) score, 1 systematic review[21] that involved the general population (excluding psychiatric facilities and emergency departments) is presented. The study, summarized in Table 19.2-6, used as a reference standard the *Diagnostic and Statistical Manual of Mental Disorders, Third Edition Revised* (DSM-III-R), or the *Diagnostic and Statistical Manual of Mental Disorders, Fourth Edition* (DSM-IV).

TABLE 19.2-3

Likelihood Ratios of Tests for Diagnosing Cholecystitis in Adult Patients With Abdominal Pain or Suspected Acute Cholecystitis

Prevalence (Pretest Probability, %)	Patients, No.	Test	Test Result	Likelihood Ratio (95% CI)	Reference
41-80		History			14
	1135	Anorexia	Present	1.1-1.7	
			Absent	0.5-0.9	
	669	Nausea	Present	1.0-1.2	
			Absent	0.6-1.0	
	1338	Emesis	Present	1.5 (1.1-2.1)	
			Absent	0.6 (0.3-0.9)	
41-80		Physical examination			14
	1292	Fever (temperature >38°C)	Present	1.5 (1.0-2.3)	
			Absent	0.9 (0.8-1.0)	
	1170	Guarding	Present	1.1-2.8	
			Absent	0.5-1.0	
	565	Murphy sign	Present	2.8 (0.8-8.6)	
			Absent	0.5 (0.2-1.0)	
	1381	Rebound	Present	1.0 (0.6-1.7)	
			Absent	1.0 (0.8-1.4)	
	1170	Rectal tenderness	Present	0.3-0.7	
			Absent	1.0-1.3	
	1140	Rigidity	Present	0.5-2.32	
			Absent	1.0-1.2	
	408	Right upper abdominal quadrant mass	Present	0.8 (0.5-1.2)	
			Absent	1.0 (0.9-1.1)	
	949	Right upper abdominal quadrant pain	Present	1.5 (0.9-1.1)	
			Absent	0.7 (0.3-1.6)	
	1001	Right upper abdominal quadrant tenderness	Present	1.6 (1.0-2.5)	
			Absent	0.4 (0.2-1.1)	
46	116	Bedside abdominal ultrasonography findings[a]	Present	2.7 (1.7-4.1)	15
			Absent	0.13 (0.04-0.39)	

(Continued)

DIAGNOSIS

TABLE 19.2-3

Likelihood Ratios of Tests for Diagnosing Cholecystitis in Adult Patients With Abdominal Pain or Suspected Acute Cholecystitis *(Continued)*

Prevalence (Pretest Probability, %)	Patients, No.	Test	Test Result	Likelihood Ratio (95% CI)	Reference
41-80		Laboratory			14
	556	Alkaline phosphatase >120 U/L	Present	0.8 (0.4-1.6)	
			Absent	1.1 (0.6-2.0)	
	592	Elevated ALT or AST[b]	Present	1.0 (0.5-2.0)	
			Absent	1.0 (0.8-1.4)	
	674	Total bilirubin >2 mg/dL	Present	1.3 (0.7-2.3)	
			Absent	0.9 (0.7-1.2)	
	270	Total bilirubin, AST, or alkaline phosphatase: all elevated	Present	1.6 (1.0-2.8)	
			Absent	0.8 (0.8-0.9)	
	270	Total bilirubin, AST, or alkaline phosphatase: any one elevated	Present	1.2 (1.0-1.5)	
			Absent	0.7 (0.6-0.9)	
	1197	Leukocytosis[c]	Present	1.5 (1.2-1.9)	
			Absent	0.6 (0.5-1.8)	

Abbreviations: ALT, alanine aminotransferase; AST, aspartate aminotransferase; CI, confidence interval.
[a]Bedside abdominal ultrasonography evidence of gallstones and a positive sonographic Murphy sign.
[b]Greater than upper limit of normal (ALT, 40 U/L; AST, 48 U/L).
[c]White blood cell count greater than 10 000/μL.

TABLE 19.2-4

Likelihood Ratios of Tests for the Diagnosis of Myocardial Infarction in Patients Admitted for Suspected Myocardial Infarction or Consulting Emergency Departments for Chest Pain

Prevalence (Pretest Probability, %)	Patients, No.	Test	Test Result	Likelihood Ratio (95% CI)	Reference
		Medical history			16
Not reported	5608	Left-sided radiation of pain	Present	0.85 (0.60-1.20)	
			Absent	1.06 (0.96-1.18)	
Not reported	1635	Right-sided radiation of pain	Present	1.39 (0.58-3.34)	
			Absent	0.96 (0.87-1.06)	
Not reported	10788	Central pain	Present	1.23 (1.10-1.38)	
			Absent	0.71 (0.50-0.99)	
Not reported	16316	Radiation to left arm/shoulder	Present	1.30 (1.12-1.52)	
			Absent	0.86 (0.78-0.95)	

(Continued)

TABLE 19.2-4

Likelihood Ratios of Tests for the Diagnosis of Myocardial Infarction in Patients Admitted for Suspected Myocardial Infarction or Consulting Emergency Departments for Chest Pain *(Continued)*

Prevalence (Pretest Probability, %)	Patients, No.	Test	Test Result	Likelihood Ratio (95% CI)	Reference
Not reported	2090	Radiation to right arm/shoulder	Present	4.43 (1.77-11.10)	
			Absent	0.87 (0.77-0.97)	
Not reported	11082	Stabbing pain	Present	0.69 (0.34-1.40)	
			Absent	1.04 (0.94-1.15)	
Not reported	2047	Burning pain	Present	1.35 (0.87-2.09)	
			Absent	0.97 (0.93-1.02)	
Not reported	12212	Time since onset of pain >6 h	Present	0.82 (0.59-1.14)	
			Absent	1.10 (0.93-1.29)	
Not reported	1673	Pain related to effort	Present	1.22 (0.50-2.96)	
			Absent	0.94 (0.69-1.28)	
Not reported	11939	Dyspnea	Present	0.89 (0.76-1.03)	
			Absent	1.06 (0.98-1.15)	
Not reported	2588	Palpitations	Present	0.47 (0.28-0.81)	
			Absent	1.12 (0.98-1.27)	
Not reported	16082	Nausea/vomiting	Present	1.54 (1.32-1.79)	
			Absent	0.83 (0.75-0.92)	
Not reported	16011	Sweating	Present	2.05 (1.73-2.42)	
			Absent	0.73 (0.61-0.87)	
9	38638	Physical examination			16-18
		Third heart sound	Present	3.21 (1.60-6.45)	
		SBP <80 mm Hg	Present	3.06 (1.80-5.22)	
Not reported	11516	Absence of chest wall tenderness	Present	1.47 (1.23-1.75)	
			Absent	0.23 (0.18-0.29)	
Not reported	19700	Rales	Present	1.81 (1.03-3.17)	
			Absent	0.88 (0.81-0.95)	
9	78515	Electrocardiogram			17
		Normal ECG	Present	0.14 (0.11-0.20)	
		ST-segment elevation	Present	13.1 (8.28-20.6)	
		ST-segment depression	Present	3.13 (2.50-3.92)	
		Abnormal T waves	Present	1.87 (1.41-2.48)	
		Q waves	Present	5.01 (3.56-7.06)	
		Left BBB	Present	0.49 (0.15-1.60)	
		Right BBB	Present	0.28 (0.04-2.12)	

Abbreviations: BBB, bundle branch block; CI, confidence interval; ECG, electrocardiograph; MI, myocardial infarction; SBP, systolic blood pressure.

DIAGNOSIS

TABLE 19.2-5

Likelihood Ratios of Clinical History and Signs for Diagnosis of Acute or Chronic Airflow Limitation in Symptomatic Patients

Prevalence (Pretest Probability, %)	Patients, No.	Test	Test Result	Likelihood Ratio (95% CI)[a]	Reference
Not reported	Not reported	History			19
		Smoking pack-year	>70	8.0	
			<70	0.63	
		Smoking	Ever	1.8	
			Never	0.16	
		Sputum production (>¼ cup)	Present	4.0	
			Absent	0.84	
		Wheezing	Present	3.8	
			Absent	0.66	
		Exertional dyspnea (grade 4)	Present	3.0	
			Absent	0.98	
		Exertional dyspnea (any grade)	Present	2.2	
			Absent	0.83	
		Physical examination			
		Wheezing	Present	36	
			Absent	0.85	
		Decreased heart dullness	Present	10	
			Absent	0.88	
Not reported	Not reported	Match test[b]	Positive	7.1	
			Negative	0.43	
		Chest hyperresonance on percussion	Present	4.8	
			Absent	0.73	
		Subxiphoid palpation of cardiac apex impulse	Present	4.6	
			Absent	0.94	
		Forced expiratory time, s	>9	4.8	
			9-6	2.7	
			<6	0.45	
Not reported	233	Maximal laryngeal height <4 cm	Present	4.2	20
Not reported	172	Reduced breath sounds	Present	3.38	
			Absent	0.49	
Not reported	172	Clinical impression on presence/absence of COPD	Present	4.26	
			Absent	0.21	

Abbreviations: CI, confidence interval; COPD, chronic obstructive pulmonary disease.
[a]Not enough data for 95% CI.
[b]Match test: inability to extinguish a lighted match held 10 cm from the mouth.

TABLE 19.2-6

Likelihood Ratios for CAGE Score on the Diagnosis of Alcohol Abuse or Dependence in the General Population[a]

Prevalence (Pretest Probability, %)	Patients, No.	Test	Test Result[b]	Likelihood Ratio (95% CI)	Reference
10-53	4562	CAGE questionnaire	4	25.18 (14.6-43.43)	21
			3	15.33 (8.22-28.6)	
			2	6.86 (4.17-11.31)	
			1	3.44 (2.31-5.11)	
			0	0.18 (0.11-0.29)	

Abbreviation: CI, confidence interval.

[a]Excluding psychiatric facilities and emergency departments, using as a reference standard *Diagnostic and Statistical Manual of Mental Disorders, Third Edition Revised* or *Fourth Edition*, criteria.

[b]The CAGE questionnaire score results from adding 1 point for each question answered affirmatively. CAGE: C, Have you ever felt you ought to *Cut* down on your drinking? A, Have people *Annoyed* you by criticizing your drinking? G, Have you ever felt bad or *Guilty* about your drinking? E, Have you ever had a drink first thing in the morning to steady your nerves or get rid of a hangover (*Eye* opener)?

Alcohol Abuse Among Inpatients, Ambulatory Medical Patients, and Primary Care Patients

For the diagnosis of hazardous drinking, a systematic review[22] that involved inpatients, ambulatory medical patients, and primary care patients assessed 2 other scores along with the CAGE score. The reference standard used for this systematic review was *DSM-III-R* or *DSM-IV* (Table 19.2-7).

Ascites

In the following study of the diagnosis of ascites, investigators enrolled patients suspected of having liver disease or ascites, using abdominal ultrasonography as their reference standard (Table 19.2-8).[23]

Carotid Artery Stenosis

Four studies of the diagnosis of carotid artery stenosis (defined as stenosis of more than 50% of the arterial lumen) enrolled patients undergoing angiography for transient ischemic attacks or other neurologic conditions. Investigators used the results of carotid angiography as the reference standard. One study enrolled asymptomatic patients using Doppler ultrasonography as the reference standard (Table 19.2-9).[24-28]

Celiac Disease

In the following study, investigators performed a systematic review to summarize evidence on the performance of different diagnostic tests to identify celiac disease in primary care patients and other populations with a similar prevalence or spectrum of disease. The systematic review included 16 studies (6085 patients), and all included studies had to use small-bowel biopsy and histologic analysis as the reference standard (Table 19.2-10).[29]

Community-Acquired Pneumonia

In the following studies of the diagnosis of community-acquired pneumonia, investigators enrolled patients with fever or acute respiratory symptoms or those suspected of having pneumonia, excluding patients with nosocomial infections, chronic pulmonary disease, and immunosuppression. Their reference standard was defined as the presence of definite or suspicious new infiltrates on chest radiograph. We found the results in 1 overview and 1 recent good-quality diagnostic study that described individual clinical findings. We also found a recent study that assessed the diagnostic accuracy of selected inflammatory markers combined to symptoms and signs (Table 19.2-11).[30-32]

DIAGNOSIS

Deep Venous Thrombosis

For deep venous thrombosis (DVT), we found 2 systematic reviews, one concerning ultrasonography and plethysmography–enrolled symptomatic hospitalized or ambulatory patients suspected of having a first episode of DVT. The reference standard was venography.

The systematic review that assessed D-dimer included 49 studies enrolling any patient with suspected DVT. The cutoff for most studies was 500. For

a reference standard, they used any "objective tests" (Table 19.2-12).[33,34]

Hypovolemia

For the diagnosis of hypovolemia, we found 1 systematic review that involved patients 60 years or older with acute conditions associated with vomiting, diarrhea, or decreased oral intake. The reference standard included chemical measures, such as serum sodium level, blood urea nitrogen level, the

TABLE 19.2-7

Likelihood Ratios for Scores on the Diagnosis of at Risk, Harmful, or Hazardous Drinking on Inpatients, Ambulatory Medical Patients, and Primary Care Patients

Prevalence (Pretest Probability, %)	Patients, No.	Test	Test Result[b]	Likelihood Ratio (95% CI)	Reference
2-29	Not reported	AUDIT-C >8[a]	Present	12 (5.0-30)	22
			Absent	0.62 (0.38-0.55)	
	Not reported	AUDIT >8[b]	Present	6.8 (4.7-10)	
			Absent	0.46 (0.38-0.55)	
	Not reported	CAGE[c] >2 (patients all >60 years)	Present	4.7 (3.7-6.0)	
			Absent	0.89 (0.86-0.91)	
	Not reported	CAGE >2	Present	3.4 (1.2-10)	
			Absent	0.66 (0.54-0.81)	

Abbreviations: AUDIT, Alcohol Use Disorders Identification Test; AUDIT-C, Alcohol Use Disorders Identification Test Consumption; CI, confidence interval.

[a]AUDIT-C questions. Circle the number that comes closest to your alcohol use in the PAST YEAR.

1. How often do you have a drink containing alcohol? Consider a "drink" to be 1 can or bottle of beer, 1 glass of wine, 1 wine cooler, 1 cocktail, or 1 shot of hard liquor (like scotch, gin, or vodka).
   (0) Never (1) Monthly or less (2) 2 to 4 times a month (3) 2 to 3 times a week (4) 4 or more times a week
2. How many drinks containing alcohol do you have on a typical day when you are drinking?
   (0) 1 or 2 (1) 3 or 4 (2) 5 or 6 (3) 7 to 9 (4) 10 or more
3. How often do you have 6 or more drinks on 1 occasion?
   (0) Never (1) Less than monthly (2) Monthly (3) Weekly (4) Daily or almost daily

[b]AUDIT: Circle the number that comes closest to your alcohol use in the PAST YEAR.

1. How often do you have a drink containing alcohol?
   (0) Never (1) Monthly or less (2) 2 to 4 times a month (3) 2 or 3 times a week, (4) 4 or more times a week
2. How many drinks containing alcohol do you have on a typical day when you are drinking?
   (0) 1 or 2 (1) 3 or 4 (2) 5 or 6 (3) 7 to 9 (4) 10 or more
3. How often do you have 6 or more drinks on 1 occasion?
4. How often during the last year have you found that you were not able to stop drinking once you had started?
5. How often during the last year have you failed to do what was expected from you because of drinking?

[c]The CAGE questionnaire score results from adding 1 point for each question answered affirmatively. CAGE: C, Have you ever felt you ought to Cut down on your drinking? A, Have people Annoyed you by criticizing your drinking? G, Have you ever felt bad or Guilty about your drinking? E, Have you ever had a drink first thing in the morning to steady your nerves or get rid of a hangover (Eye opener)?

TABLE 19.2-8

Likelihood Ratios of Tests for Diagnosing Ascites in Patients Suspected of Having Liver Disease or Ascites

Prevalence (Pretest Probability, %)	Patients, No.	Test	Test Result	Likelihood Ratio (95% CI)	Reference
29-33	Not reported	Increased girth	Present	4.16[a]	23
			Absent	0.17[a]	
		Recent weight gain	Present	3.2[a]	
			Absent	0.42[a]	
		Hepatitis	Present	3.2[a]	
			Absent	0.80[a]	
		Ankle swelling	Present	2.8[a]	
			Absent	0.10[a]	
		Fluid wave	Present	6.0 (3.3-11)	
			Absent	0.4 (0.3-0.6)	
		Shifting dullness	Present	2.7 (1.9-3.9)	
			Absent	0.3 (0.2-0.6)	
		Flank dullness	Present	2.0 (1.5-2.9)	
			Absent	0.3 (0.1-0.7)	
		Bulging flanks	Present	2.0 (1.5-2.6)	
			Absent	0.3 (0.2-0.6)	

Abbreviation: CI, confidence interval.
[a]Insufficient data to determine 95% CI.

TABLE 19.2-9

Likelihood Ratios for Carotid Bruit on Diagnosis of Carotid Artery Stenosis (>50% or >60%) in Symptomatic Patients Undergoing Cerebral Angiography for TIA or Other Neurologic Conditions

Prevalence (Pretest Probability, %)	Patients, No.	Test	Test Result	Likelihood Ratio (95% CI)	Reference
Carotid Artery Stenosis >50%					
8.2-38	2011	Carotid bruit	Present	4.4 (2.9-6.8)	24-27
			Absent	0.62 (0.45-0.86)	
Carotid Artery Stenosis >60%					
2.2	686	Carotid bruit	Present	28.25 (15.96-50.01)	28
			Absent	0.45 (0.26-0.78)	

Abbreviations: CI, confidence interval; TIA, transient ischemic attack.

DIAGNOSIS

TABLE 19.2-10

Likelihood Ratios for Tests on the Diagnosis of Celiac Disease in Primary Care and Other Populations With a Similar Prevalence or Spectrum of Disease

Prevalence (Pretest Probability, %)	Patients, No.	Test	Test Result	Likelihood Ratio (95% CI)	Reference
9	8 studies (3 primary care)	IgA antiendomysial antibodies	Positive	171 (56-522)	29
			Negative	0.11 (0.05-0.20)	
5.5	7 studies (1 primary care)	IgA antitissue transglutaminase antibodies	Positive	37.7 (18.7-76.0)	
			Negative	0.11 (0.06-0.19)	

Abbreviation: CI, confidence interval.

TABLE 19.2-11

Likelihood Ratios of Tests for the Diagnosis of Community-Acquired Pneumonia in Patients Suspected of Having Pneumonia or Patients With Acute Respiratory Symptoms but Without Chronic Pulmonary Disease or Immunosuppression

Prevalence (Pretest Probability, %)	Patients, No.	Test	Test Result	Likelihood Ratio (95% CI)	Reference
3-38		Medical history			30
	1118	Dementia[a]	Present	3.4 (1.6-6.5)	
			Absent	0.94 (0.90-0.99)	
3-38		Physical examination			30-31
	2234	Egophony	Present	4.0 (2.0-8.1)	
			Absent	0.93 (0.88-0.99)	
	1118	Bronchial breath sounds	Present	3.5 (2.0-5.6)	
			Absent	0.90 (0.83-0.96)	
	1751	Dullness to percussion	Present	3.0 (1.6-5.8)	
			Absent	0.86 (0.74-1.0)	
	633	Respiration rate >30/min	Present	2.6 (1.6-4.1)	
			Absent	0.80 (0.70-0.90)	
	2489	Decreased breath sounds, temperature >37.8°C (>100°F), crackles on chest auscultation, or any abnormal vital sign[b]	Present	1.3-2.4	
			Absent	0.18-0.78	
34	325	Cyanosis	Present	5.0 (2.07-12)	31
			Absent	0.88 (0.81-0.95)	
34	325	Chest retraction	Present	5.0 (1.68-15)	31
			Absent	0.92 (0.86-0.98)	

(Continued)

TABLE 19.2-11

Likelihood Ratios of Tests for the Diagnosis of Community-Acquired Pneumonia in Patients Suspected of Having Pneumonia or Patients With Acute Respiratory Symptoms but Without Chronic Pulmonary Disease or Immunosuppression *(Continued)*

Prevalence (Pretest Probability, %)	Patients, No.	Test	Test Result	Likelihood Ratio (95% CI)	Reference
34	325	Oxygen saturation <90%	Present	4.5 (2.44-8.3)	31
			Absent	0.78 (0.69-0.87)	
5	2820	Combination of clinical findings and serum C-reactive protein[c]			32
2	1556	Low risk[d]	Present	0.4 (0.29-0.54)	32
			Absent	1.8 (1.63-1.99)	
6	1132	Intermediate risk[d]	Present	1.2 (0.97-1.48)	32
			Absent	0.9 (0.78-1.03)	
31	132	High risk[d]	Present	9.7 (6.91-14)	32
			Absent	0.7 (0.66-0.81)	

Abbreviation: CI, confidence interval.

[a]Significant cognitive impairment with ineffective airway protection mechanisms.

[b]Individual clinical signs, not combined.

[c]Combination of clinical findings—absence of runny nose and presence of breathlessness, crackles and diminished breath sounds on auscultation, tachycardia (heart rate >100/min), and fever (temperature ≥37.8°C)—and serum C-reactive protein level greater than 30 mg/dL.

[d]Estimated probability for pneumonia: low risk, less than 2.5%; intermediate risk, 2.5% to 20%; and high risk, greater than 20%.

TABLE 19.2-12

Likelihood Ratios of Tests for Diagnosis of DVT in Symptomatic Hospitalized or Ambulatory Patients Suspected of Having a First Episode of DVT

Prevalence (Pretest Probability, %)	Patients, No.	Test	Test Result	Likelihood Ratio (95% CI)	Reference
Target Condition: All DVT, Including Distal (Isolated Calf DVT) and Proximal DVT					
Not reported	2658	Ultrasonography	Positive	15[a]	33
			Negative	0.12[a]	
	1156	Impedance plethysmography	Abnormal	10[a]	33
			Normal	0.18[a]	
3-78	Not reported	D-dimer (assay)			34
		ELISA microplate	Positive	2.00 (1.39-3.03)	
			Negative	0.11 (0.04-0.37)	

(Continued)

TABLE 19.2-12

Likelihood Ratios of Tests for Diagnosis of DVT in Symptomatic Hospitalized or Ambulatory Patients Suspected of Having a First Episode of DVT *(Continued)*

Prevalence (Pretest Probability, %)	Patients, No.	Test	Test Result	Likelihood Ratio (95% CI)	Reference
		ELISA membrane	Positive	1.89 (1.21-2.97)	
			Negative	0.21 (0.07-0.65)	
		ELFA	Positive	1.78 (1.28-2.51)	
			Negative	0.09 (0.03-0.35)	
		Latex quantitative	Positive	1.98 (1.65-2.44)	
			Negative	0.13 (0.08-0.24)	
		Latex semiquantitative	Positive	2.66 (1.45-4.89)	
			Negative	0.22 (0.09-0.60)	
		Latex qualitative	Positive	69.00 (4.50-∞)	
			Negative	0.31 (0.07-0.78)	
		Whole blood assay	Positive	2.86 (1.56-5.17)	
			Negative	0.24 (0.09-0.58)	
Target Condition: Proximal DVT (Popliteal or More Proximal Veins)					
2658		Ultrasonography	Positive	49[a]	33
			Negative	0.03[a]	
1156		Impedance plethysmography	Abnormal	8.4[a]	33
			Normal	0.09[a]	

Abbreviations: CI, confidence interval; DVT, deep venous thrombosis; ELFA, enzyme-linked immunofluorescence assay; ELISA, enzyme-linked immunosorbent assay.

[a]Insufficient data available to determine CI.

blood urea nitrogen–creatinine ratio, and osmolality (Table 19.2-13).[35]

Influenza

In the following study about the diagnostic accuracy of clinical findings for the diagnosis of influenza, the investigators enrolled patients who presented with acute respiratory symptoms during influenza seasons. The reference standards used were cultures, polymerase chain reaction for influenza A, enzyme-linked immunosorbent assay, immunofluorescence, or a 4-fold increase in influenza titers. One meta-analysis examined the accuracy of rapid influenza diagnostic tests (RIDTs) in adults and children with influenza-like illness, including 159 studies assessing 26 RIDTs (usually immunochromatographic assays that detect specific influenza viral antigens in respiratory specimens). The reference standard was either reverse transcriptase–polymerase chain reaction (first choice) or viral culture. Sensitivity estimates were highly heterogeneous, which was partially explained by lower sensitivity in adults than in children and a higher sensitivity for influenza A than for influenza B (Table 19.2-14).[36,37]

Iron Deficiency Anemia

For studies on the diagnosis of iron deficiency anemia, investigators enrolled patients with hemoglobin levels less than 11.7 g/dL and less than 13.0 g/dL for women and men, respectively. Their reference standard was a bone marrow aspirate stained for iron. We have added a systematic review that describes a new test (Table 19.2-15).[38-46]

TABLE 19.2-13

Likelihood Ratios for Diagnosis of Hypovolemia in Patients 60 Years or Older Experiencing Acute Conditions Associated With Volume Loss[31]

Prevalence (Pretest Probability, %)	Patients, No.	Test	Test Result	Likelihood Ratio (95% CI)	Reference
Not available	38	Sunken eyes	Present	3.4 (1.0-12)	35
			Absent	0.50 (0.3-0.7)	
	86	Dry axilla	Present	2.8 (1.4-5.4)	
			Absent	0.6 (0.4-1.0)	
	38	Dry tongue	Present	2.1 (0.8-5.8)	
			Absent	0.6 (0.3-1.0)	
	38	Dry mouth and nose mucosa	Present	2.0 (1.0-4.0)	
			Absent	0.3 (0.1-0.6)	
	38	Longitudinal furrows on tongue	Present	2.0 (1.0-4.0)	
			Absent	0.3 (0.1-0.6)	
	38	Unclear speech	Present	3.1 (0.9-11)	
			Absent	0.5 (0.4-0.8)	
	38	Weak upper or lower extremities	Present	2.3 (0.6-8.6)	
			Absent	0.7 (0.5-1.0)	
	38	Confusion	Present	2.1 (0.8-5.7)	
			Absent	0.6 (0.4-1.0)	

Abbreviation: CI, confidence interval.

TABLE 19.2-14

Likelihood Ratios of Clinical Tests for the Diagnosis of Influenza in Patients With Acute Respiratory Symptoms During Influenza Seasons

Prevalence (Pretest Probability, %)	Patients, No.	Test	Test Result	Likelihood Ratio (95% CI)	Reference
28-67	4712	Fever at any age	Present	1.8 (1.1-2.9)	36
			Absent	0.40 (0.25-0.66)	
7	1838	Fever at >60 years of age	Present	3.8 (2.8-5.0)	
			Absent	0.72 (0.64-0.82)	
66-67	3825	Feverishness at any age	Present	1.0 (0.86-1.2)	
			Absent	0.70 (0.27-2.5)	
8	614	Feverishness at >60 years of age	Present	2.1 (1.2-3.7)	
			Absent	0.68 (0.45-1.0)	

(Continued)

DIAGNOSIS

TABLE 19.2-14

Likelihood Ratios of Clinical Tests for the Diagnosis of Influenza in Patients With Acute Respiratory Symptoms During Influenza Seasons *(Continued)*

Prevalence (Pretest Probability, %)	Patients, No.	Test	Test Result	Likelihood Ratio (95% CI)	Reference
28-67	4793	Cough at any age	Present	1.1 (1.1-1.2)	36
			Absent	0.42 (0.31-0.57)	
7-8	2371	Cough at >60 years of age	Present	2.0 (1.1-3.5)	
			Absent	0.57 (0.37-0.87)	
50-67	4183	Myalgia at any age	Present	0.93 (0.83-1.0)	
			Absent	1.2 (0.90-1.16)	
7-8	2371	Myalgia at >60 years of age	Present	2.4 (1.9-2.9)	
			Absent	0.68 (0.58-0.79)	
67	81	Malaise at any age	Present	0.98 (0.75-1.3)	
			Absent	1.1 (0.51-2.2)	
50	1838	Malaise at >60 years of age	Present	2.6 (2.2-3.1)	
			Absent	0.55 (0.44-0.67)	
28-68	4793	Headache at any age	Present	1.0 (1.0-1.1)	
			Absent	0.75 (0.63-0.89)	
7-8	2371	Headache at >60 years of age	Present	1.9 (1.6-2.3)	
			Absent	0.70 (0.60-0.82)	
Not reported	159 studies	Rapid influenza diagnostic tests	Positive	34.5 (23.8-45.2)	37
			Negative	0.38 (0.34-0.43)	

Abbreviation: CI, confidence interval.

TABLE 19.2-15

Likelihood Ratios of Tests for Diagnosis of Iron Deficiency Anemia in Patients With Anemia

Prevalence (Pretest Probability, %)	Patients, No.	Test	Test Result	Likelihood Ratio (95% CI)	Reference
Patients With Anemia					
21-50	2798	Serum ferritin, µg/L	<15	55 (35-84)	38-39
			15-25	9.3 (6.3-14)	
			25-35	2.5 (2.1-3.0)	
			35-45	1.8 (1.5-2.2)	
			45-100	0.54 (0.48-0.60)	
			>100	0.08 (0.06-0.11)	
21-50	536	Mean cell volume, µm³	<70	13 (6.1-19)	38

(Continued)

TABLE 19.2-15

Likelihood Ratios of Tests for Diagnosis of Iron Deficiency Anemia in Patients With Anemia *(Continued)*

Prevalence (Pretest Probability, %)	Patients, No.	Test	Test Result	Likelihood Ratio (95% CI)	Reference
			70-75	3.3 (2.0-4.7)	
			75-85	1.0 (0.69-1.31)	
			85-90	0.76 (0.56-0.96)	
			>90	0.29 (0.21-0.37)	
21-50	764	Transferrin saturation, %	<5	11 (6.4-15)	38
			5-10	2.5 (2.0-3.1)	
			10-20	0.81 (0.70-0.92)	
			20-30	0.52 (0.41-0.63)	
			30-50	0.43 (0.31-0.55)	
			>50	0.15 (0.06-0.24)	
21-50	278	Red cell protoporphyrin, μg/dL	>350	8.3 (2.6-14)	38
			350-250	6.1 (2.8-9.3)	
			250-150	2.0 (1.4-2.6)	
			150-50	0.56 (0.48-0.64)	
			<50	0.12 (0.0-0.25)	
16-73	875	Serum soluble transferrin receptor[a]	Positive	3.85 (2.23-6.63)	40
			Negative	0.19 (0.11-0.33)	
Patients With Anemia and Chronic Renal Failure Receiving Hemodialysis or Peritoneal Dialysis					
9-50	190	Serum ferritin, μg/L	<50	12 (4.4-32)	41-45
			50-100	2.3 (0.70-7.3)	
			100-300	0.64 (0.32-1.2)	
			>300	0.27 (0.12-0.61)	
Patients With Anemia and Cirrhosis					
40	72	Serum ferritin, μg/L	<50	22[b]	46
			50-400	1.0-1.8[b]	
			400-1000	0.13[b]	
			1000-2200	0.19[b]	

Abbreviation: CI, confidence interval.

[a]Serum concentration cutoff: 1.55 to 3.3 mg/L.

[b]Insufficient data to determine CIs.

Irritable Bowel Syndrome

We identified 1 recent systematic review in which researchers assessed the diagnostic accuracy of individual symptoms and clinical scores to diagnose irritable bowel syndrome in adults with lower gastrointestinal symptoms. The study included adults with symptoms and a final diagnosis collected prospectively (Table 19.2-16).[47]

Melanoma

In the following study of the diagnosis of melanoma, investigators enrolled patients with pigmented skin lesions and used biopsy of the lesions as their reference standard (Table 19.2-17).[48]

Osteoporosis

A systematic review included patients older than 50 years (mostly women). The reference standard used was bone densitometry or documented vertebral fracture using either a semiquantitative technique or vertebral morphometry. Another study evaluated a screening strategy for selecting women for bone densitometry. It included 3 population-based samples of postmenopausal women of different ages. Selection was based on the presence of at

TABLE 19.2-16

Likelihood Ratios of Clinical Symptoms and Scores for the Diagnosis of Irritable Bowel Syndrome in Adults With Lower Gastrointestinal Tract Symptoms

Prevalence (Pretest Probability, %)	Patients, No.	Test	Test Result	Likelihood Ratio (95% CI)	Reference
21-78		Individual symptoms			47
		Lower abdominal pain	Present	1.3 (1.1-1.7)	
			Absent	0.29 (0.12-0.72)	
		Passage of mucus per rectum	Present	1.2 (0.93-1.6)	
			Absent	0.88 (0.72-1.1)	
		Feeling of incomplete evacuation	Present	1.3 (1.1-1.5)	
			Absent	0.62 (0.48-0.80)	
		Looser stools at onset of pain	Present	2.1 (1.4-3.0)	
			Absent	0.59 (0.45-0.79)	
		More frequent stools at onset of pain	Present	1.9 (1.2-2.9)	
			Absent	0.67 (0.54-0.84)	
		Pain relieved by defecation	Present	1.8 (1.4-2.2)	
			Absent	0.62 (0.52-0.75)	
		Patient-reported visible distension	Present	1.7 (0.90-3.2)	
			Absent	0.79 (0.56-1.1)	
		Scores and statistical models			
62	574	Manning criteria[a]	≥3 criteria	2.9 (1.3-6.4)	
			<3 criteria	0.29 (0.12-0.71)	
56	602	Rome I criteria[b]	Positive	4.8 (3.6-6.5)	
			Negative	0.34 (0.29-0.41)	
Not reported	Not reported	Kruis model[c]	≥44 points	8.6 (2.9-26.0)	
			<44 points	0.26 (0.17-0.41)	

Abbreviations: CI, confidence interval; ESR, erythrocyte sedimentation rate.

[a]Abdominal pain relieved by defecation, more frequent stools with pain onset, looser stools with pain onset, passage of mucus per rectum, feeling incomplete emptying, and patient-reported abdominal distension.

[b]Abdominal discomfort or pain relieved by defecation or associated with a change in stool frequency or consistency plus 2 of any of the following symptoms: altered stool frequency, form, or passage; passage of mucus per rectum; bloating; or distension.

[c]Statistical model that adds or subtracts points based on the presence of abdominal pain, flatulence or bowel irregularity, duration longer than 2 years, alternating constipation and diarrhea, description of the pain (burning, cutting, very strong, terrible, feeling of pressure, dull, boring, or "not so bad"), abnormal physical findings, ESR greater than 20 mm/h, leukocyte count greater than 10 000/μL, anemia, and history of blood in stool.

least 1 major risk factor for low bone mineral density: personal history of fracture, maternal history of hip fracture, low weight (<45 kg), and/or early menopause (before 40 years of age). The reference standard used was bone densitometry. Women were classified as osteoporotic if they had a bone mineral density value more than 2.5 SDs below the average (T score ≤−2.5) at either total hip or lumbar spine (60-80 years of age) or femoral neck (80 years or older) (Table 19.2-18).[49,50]

Peripheral Arterial Disease or Peripheral Vascular Insufficiency

For the diagnosis of peripheral arterial disease (PAD), we found 1 systematic review that determined the accuracy of the ankle-brachial index as a diagnostic tool to detect significant stenosis (>50%) in PAD using angiographic methods (arteriography, digital subtraction angiography, and computed tomography angiography) as the reference standard. For clinical tests, we used the results of a systematic review and its included studies in which investigators used the ankle-brachial systolic pressure index as the reference standard (Table 19.2-19).[51-56]

Pleural Effusion

In the following systematic review about the diagnostic accuracy of clinical findings for the diagnosis of pleural effusion, investigators included studies that enrolled patients with respiratory symptoms. The reference standard was a chest radiograph (Table 19.2-20).[57]

TABLE 19.2-17

Likelihood Ratios of Tests for Diagnosis of Melanoma in Patients With Pigmented Skin Lesions

Prevalence (Pretest Probability, %)	Patients, No.	Test	Test Result	Likelihood Ratio (95% CI)	Reference
3	192	ABCD(E) checklist	BCD positive	62 (19-170)	48
			BCD negative	0 (0-0.5)	

Abbreviations: CI, confidence interval; ABCD(E): A, asymmetry; B, border irregularity; C, color variegation; D, diameter greater than 6 mm; E, elevation.

TABLE 19.2-18

Likelihood Ratios of Tests for Diagnosis of Osteoporosis in Women

Prevalence (Pretest Probability, %)	Patients, No.	Test	Test Result	Likelihood Ratio (95% CI)	Reference
Patients With Clinical Signs and Symptoms of Osteoporosis					
50	4638	Height loss >3 cm	Present	1.1 (1.0-1.1)	49
			Absent	0.60 (0.4-0.9)	
50	4638	Weight <60 kg	Present	1.9 (1.8-2.0)	
			Absent	0.3 (0.3-0.4)	
50	4638	Grip strength <59 kPa	Present	1.2 (1.1-1.2)	
			Absent	0.6 (0.5-0.7)	
50	4638	Grip strength <44 kPa	Present	1.7 (1.5-1.9)	
			Absent	0.8 (0.7-0.9)	

(Continued)

TABLE 19.2-18

Likelihood Ratios of Tests for Diagnosis of Osteoporosis in Women *(Continued)*

Prevalence (Pretest Probability, %)	Patients, No.	Test	Test Result	Likelihood Ratio (95% CI)	Reference
8	1873	Weight <51 kg	Present	7.3 (5.0-10.8)	49
			Absent	0.8 (0.7-0.9)	
10	610	Kyphosis	Present	3.1 (1.8-5.3)	
			Absent	0.8 (0.7-1.0)	
63	225	Hand skinfold	Present	1.2 (1.0-1.3)	
			Absent	0.40 (0.2-0.8)	
11.5	190	Tooth count <20 teeth	Present	3.4 (1.4-8.0)	
			Absent	0.8 (0.6-1.0)	
Patients With Clinical Signs and Symptoms of Spinal Fracture					
3.4 (55-59 y) 21.9 (80-84 y)	449	Arm-span height difference >5 cm	Present	1.6 (1.1-2. 5)	
			Absent	0.8 (0.6-1.0)	
14	781	Rib-pelvis distance <2 fingerbreadths	Present	3.8 (2.9-5.1)	
			Absent	0.6 (0.5-0.7)	

Abbreviation: CI, confidence interval.

TABLE 19.2-19

Likelihood Ratios of Tests for Diagnosis of Varying Degrees of Peripheral Artery Disease in Different Populations

Prevalence (Pretest Probability, %)	Patient Legs, No.	Test	Test Result	Likelihood Ratio (95% CI)	Reference
12	569	Ankle brachial index (ABI <0.9)	Present	4.18 (2.14-8.14)	51
			Absent	0.29 (0.18-0.47)	
Patients: Asymptomatic or Symptomatic With Risk Factors for Atherosclerosis or Classical PAD History; Target Outcome: Severe PAD (AAI <0.5)					
Symptomatic or asymptomatic with risk factors[a]: 10-12	605	Venous filling time	>20 s	3.6 (1.9-6.8)	52-55
			<20 s	0.8 (0.7-1.0)	
With classic PAD history: 71	854	Tibial or dorsalis pedis pulse	Weak/absent	3.2 (2.7-3.9)	52-53
			Present	0.19 (0.03-1.15)	
	605	Absent lower limb hair; atrophic skin; cool skin; blue/purple skin; capillary refilling time >5 s	Any of them	0.5-2.0	56

(Continued)

Renovascular Hypertension

In the following studies of the diagnosis of renovascular hypertension, investigators enrolled patients with hypertension referred to arteriography and used renal arteriography as the reference standard (Table 19.2-21).[58-60]

Stroke

In the first systematic review[61] about the diagnostic accuracy of clinical findings for the diagnosis of stroke, the investigators enrolled patients who presented to the emergency department or were given prehospital attention for neurologic symptoms.

TABLE 19.2-19

Likelihood Ratios of Tests for Diagnosis of Varying Degrees of Peripheral Artery Disease in Different Populations *(Continued)*

Prevalence (Pretest Probability, %)	Patient Legs, No.	Test	Test Result	Likelihood Ratio (95% CI)	Reference
Patients: Asymptomatic or Symptomatic With Risk Factors for Atherosclerosis or With Any Leg Complaint on Walking With or Without Risk Factors; Target Outcome: Moderate PAD (AAI <0.9)					
10-12	4597	Tibial or dorsalis pedis pulse, or both	Weak/absent	8.9 (7.1-11)	53-55
			Present	0.33 (0.28-0.40)	
10-12	4910	Wound or sores on foot or toes	Present	6.9 (2.9-16)	55
			Absent	0.98 (0.97-1.0)	
10-12	5418	Femoral pulse	Weak/absent	6.7 (4.3-10)	54-55
			Present	0.94 (0.91-0.96)	
10-12	4910	Unilateral cooler skin	Present	5.8 (4.0-8.4)	55
			Absent	0.92 (0.89-0.95)	
10-12	5418	Femoral bruit	Present	5.4 (4.5-6.5)	54-55
			Absent	0.78 (0.70-0.86)	
10-12	4910	Abnormal color on feet or leg	Present	2.8 (2.4-3.2)	55
			Absent	0.74 (0.69-0.80)	
Patients: Classic PAD History; Target Outcome: Moderate PAD (AAI <0.9)					
71	4597	Tibial or dorsalis pedis pulse, or both	Weak/absent	8.9 (7.1-11)	53-55
			Present	0.33 (0.28-0.40)	

Abbreviations: AAI, ankle to arm (brachial) systolic pressure index; CI, confidence interval; PAD, peripheral artery disease.
[a]Risk factors include dyslipidemia, diabetes mellitus, smoking, hypertension, and cardiovascular disease.

TABLE 19.2-20

Likelihood Ratios of Clinical Tests for the Diagnosis of Pleural Effusion in Patients With Respiratory Symptoms

Prevalence (Pretest Probability, %)	Patients, No.	Test	Test Result	Likelihood Ratio (95% CI)	Reference
4-21	609	Dullness to conventional percussion	Present	8.7 (2.2-33.8)	57
			Absent	0.31 (0.03-3.3)	
21	278	Reduced tactile vocal fremitus	Present	5.7 (4.0-8.0)	57
			Absent	0.21 (0.12-0.37)	

Abbreviation: CI, confidence interval.

TABLE 19.2-21

Likelihood Ratios for Tests for Diagnosis of Renovascular Hypertension in Patients With Hypertension Referred to Arteriography

Prevalence (Pretest Probability, %)	Patients, No.	Test	Test Result	Likelihood Ratio (95% CI)	Reference
24	263	Systolic and diastolic abdominal bruit	Present	39 (9.4-160)	58
			Absent	0.62 (0.51-0.75)	
23-49	705	Epigastric or flank systolic bruit	Present	4.3 (2.3-8.0)	58-60
			Absent	0.52 (0.34-0.78)	
29	477	History of atherosclerotic disease	Present	2.2 (1.8-2.8)	60
			Absent	0.52 (0.40-0.66)	

Abbreviation: CI, confidence interval.

The prehospital patients had to be older than 45 years, have had symptoms for less than 24 hours, not be wheelchair bound or bedridden, and have a blood glucose level between 60 and 400 mg/dL. The reference standards used were neuroimaging studies. The second study[62] presents the diagnostic accuracy of stroke scores to detect hemorrhagic vs ischemic strokes (Table 19.2-22).[61,62]

Thromboembolism or Acute Pulmonary Embolism

In studies on the diagnosis of acute pulmonary embolism (PE), using clinical assessment or ECG or chest radiography or V/Q scan (scintigraphy), investigators used angiography or clinical follow-up for more than 1 year as their reference standard. Normal ventilation-perfusion scan was used to rule out PE on those trials using "clinical assessment," ECG, or chest radiography.

For D-dimer assessment, we used 1 recent systematic review that included 81 studies that enrolled patients with suspected PE. The D-dimer cutoff point was 500 for most studies. The criterion standard was any "objective test."

Another systematic review that included 48 studies (11 004 patients) assessed different images in patients suspected of having PE. The reference standard was angiography for individuals with positive results and angiography or follow-up for individuals with negative results. Another systematic review that included 24 studies focused specifically on the diagnostic accuracy of computed tomography pulmonary angiography (Table 19.2-23).[34,63-72]

Thyroid Cancer

For studies on the diagnosis of malignancy in thyroid nodules (primary or metastatic cancer or lymphoma), investigators enrolled patients with normal thyroid function and palpable thyroid nodules. The nodules could be solid or cystic and solitary or dominant if multiple nodules were present. Their reference standard was histopathologic examination after surgical excision or clinical follow-up. In a recent systematic review on studies of fine-needle aspiration that used The Bethesda System for Reporting Thyroid Cytopathology (TBSRTC), cytologic diagnoses were classified as negative (TBSRTC diagnostic category II: benign) or positive (TBSRTC

TABLE 19.2-22

Likelihood Ratios of Clinical Findings for the Diagnosis of Stroke

Prevalence (Pretest Probability, %)	Patient, No.	Test	Test Result	Likelihood Ratio (95% CI)	Reference
Assessment (Physical Examination) by Emergency Physicians					
24	161	Facial paresis or arm drift or abnormal speech	3 Findings (+)	14 (1.6-121)	61
			2 Findings (+)	4.2 (1.4-13)	
			1 Finding (+)	5.2 (2.6-11)	
			>1 Finding (+)	5.5 (3.3-9.1)	
			0 Findings (+)	0.39 (0.25-0.61)	
Assessment (Physical Examination) by Emergency Medical Personnel					
24	161	Facial paresis or arm drift or abnormal speech	3 Findings (+)	7.0 (3.3-14)	61
			2 Findings (+)	7.6 (3.7-16)	
			1 Finding (+)	4.4 (3.0-6.4)	
			≥1 Finding (+)	5.4 (4.1-7.0)	
			0 Findings (+)	0.46 (0.38-0.56)	
Prehospital Assessment (Physical Examination) by Paramedics					
16.5	206	One of 3 unilateral deficits (arm drift, altered handgrip strength, or facial paresis)	Present	31 (13-75)	61
			Absent	0.09 (0.03-0.027)	
Clinical Scores to Diagnose Hemorrhagic vs Ischemic Stroke					
24	1528	Siriraj Stroke Score[a]	<−1	0.29 (0.23-0.37)	62
			−1 to 1	0.94 (0.77-1.1)	
			>1	5.7 (4.4-7.4)	
		Besson Score[b]	<1	0.23 (0.01-5)	
			>1	1.4 (0.92-2.2)	

Abbreviation: CI, confidence interval.

[a](2.5 for semicoma or 5 for coma) + (2 for vomiting) + (2 for headache within 2 h) + (0.1 for diastolic blood pressure) − (3 for ≥ 1 of diabetes, angina, intermittent claudication) − 12.

[b](2 for alcohol consumption) + (1.5 for plantar response both extensor) + (3 for headache) + (3 for history of hypertension) − (5 for history of transient ischemic attack) − (2 for peripheral arterial disease) − (1.5 for history of hyperlipidemia) − (2.5 for atrial fibrillation on admission).

diagnostic category IV: follicular neoplasm/suspicion for a follicular neoplasm, V: suspicious for malignancy, and VI: malignant, all of the latter leading to recommend surgery). In a second scenario, only diagnostic categories V and VI were considered positive. Their reference standard was histopathologic examination after surgery (benign vs malignant histologic findings) (Table 19.2-24).[73-80]

TABLE 19.2-23

Likelihood Ratios of Tests for the Diagnosis of Pulmonary Embolism

Prevalence (Pretest Probability, %)	Patients, No.	Test	Test Result	Likelihood Ratio (95% CI)	Reference
Patients Suspected of Having Acute Pulmonary Embolism With Symptoms for the Past 24 Hours					
32-44		Medical history/physical examination			
	78	Blood pressure	<100/70	3.1[a]	63
			>100/70	0.8[a]	
	78	Ventricular diastolic gallop	Present	3.0[a]	63
			Absent	0.9[a]	
	78	Congestive heart failure	Present	0.3[a]	63
			Absent	1.2[a]	
	403	Risk factors[b]	Any	0.4-2.0[c]	63-66
			Symptoms[b]		
			Signs[b]		
		Chest pain	Present	1.07 (0.86-1.33)	66
			Absent	1.00 (0.84-1.19)	
		Dyspnea	Present	1.42 (1.14-1.78)	66
			Absent	0.52 (0.37-0.73)	
		Sudden dyspnea	Present	1.83 (1.07–3.13)	66
			Absent	0.43 (0.25-0.73)	
		Syncope	Present	2.38 (1.54–3.69)	66
			Absent	0.88 (0.790-0.978)	
		Current DVT	Present	2.05 (1.12–3.73)	66
			Absent	0.79 (0.65-0.95)	
		Shock	Present	4.07 (1.84-8.96)	66
			Absent	0.79 (0.65-0.97)	
41-44		Electrocardiogram			
	78	S-I/Q-III/T-III	Present	2.4[a]	63
			Absent	0.88[a]	
	78	Inverted T waves V→V3	Present	2.3[a]	63
			Absent	0.94[a]	
	78	Normal	Present	0.82[a]	63
			Absent	2.2[a]	
	78	Right bundle-branch block		0.5-2.0[c]	63
		Right ventricular hypertrophy			

(Continued)

TABLE 19.2-23

Likelihood Ratios of Tests for the Diagnosis of Pulmonary Embolism *(Continued)*

Prevalence (Pretest Probability, %)	Patients, No.	Test	Test Result	Likelihood Ratio (95% CI)	Reference
27-44	1203	Chest radiograph	Any sign	0.5-2.0[c]	67-68
		• Normal			
		• Pulmonary edema			
		• Enlarged hilum or mediastinum			
		• Prominent central artery			
		• Atelectasis			
		• Pleural effusion			
3-69	Not reported	D-dimer (assay)			34
		ELISA microplate	Positive	1.90 (1.18-3.41)	
			Negative	0.10 (0.01-0.55)	
		ELISA membrane	Positive	1.82 (0.73-0.98)	
			Negative	0.18 (0.03-0.93)	
		ELFA	Positive	1.70 (1.14-2.83)	
			Negative	0.07 (0.02-0.52)	
		Quantitative latex	Positive	1.90 (0.88-0.98)	
			Negative	0.23 (0.11-0.48)	
				0.10 (0.03-0.33)	
		Semiquantitative latex	Positive	2.59 (1.16-5.71)	
			Negative	0.18 (0.04-0.79)	
		Whole blood	Positive	2.81 (1.23-6.00)	
			Negative	0.19 (0.05-0.75)	
30	378	Leg vein ultrasonography	Positive	16.2 (5.6-46.7)	69
			Negative	0.67 (0.50-0.89)	
19-79	Not reported	CT pulmonary angiography	Positive	17.80 (9.22-47.50)	70
			Negative	0.11 (0.06-0.19)	
				0.12 (0.05-0.19)	
30		Ultrasonography and spiral tomography	Negative	0.04 (0.03-0.06)	69
29	881	Ventilation-perfusion scintigram (V/Q scan)	High probability	18 (11-31)	71
			Intermediate probability	1.2 (1.0-1.5)	
			Low probability	0.36 (0.26-0.49)	
			Normal	0.10 (0.04-0.25)	

(Continued)

TABLE 19.2-23

Likelihood Ratios of Tests for the Diagnosis of Pulmonary Embolism *(Continued)*

Prevalence (Pretest Probability, %)	Patients, No.	Test	Test Result	Likelihood Ratio (95% CI)	Reference
30	148	Echocardiography	Positive	5 (2.3-10.6)	69
			Negative	0.59 (0.41-0.86)	
30	221	Magnetic resonance angiography	Positive	11.7 (3.6-37.8)	69
			Negative	0.20 (0.12-0.34)	
Patients With Suspected PE and Normal Chest Radiograph Result					
15	133	V/Q scan	High probability	10[a]	72
			Intermediate probability	1.7[a]	
			Low probability	1.1[a]	
			Normal	0.2[a]	
15	110	Dyspnea and PaO_2	<70	2.8[a]	72
			>70	0.58[a]	
15	110	PaO_2	<70	2.2[a]	
			>70	0.62[a]	
Patients With Suspected PE and Normal Chest Radiograph Result and No Previous Cardiopulmonary Disease					
15	110	Dyspnea and PaO_2	<60	6[a]	72
			>60	0.84[a]	
			<70	3.6[a]	
			>70	0.77[a]	

Abbreviations: CI, confidence interval; CT, computed tomography; DVT, deep venous thrombosis; ELFA, enzyme-linked immunofluorescence assay; ELISA, enzyme-linked immunosorbent assay; PE, pulmonary embolism.
[a]Insufficient data to determine 95% CI.

[b]Risk factors: immobilization, surgery, trauma, malignancy, previous deep venous thrombosis, estrogen, postpartum, and stroke. Symptoms: dyspnea, hemoptysis, any type of chest pain, cough, leg pain, or swelling. Signs: fever, heart rate greater than 100/min, respiratory rate greater than 20/min, cyanosis, pulmonary rales, crackles, wheezes, third or fourth heart sounds, increased pulmonic component of second heart sound, Homan sign, actual deep venous thrombosis, edema, and varices.
[c]Range of possible LRs.

TABLE 19.2-24

Likelihood Ratios for the Diagnosis of Malignancy in Euthyroid Patients With a Single or Dominant Palpable Thyroid Nodule

Prevalence (Pretest Probability, %)	Patients, No.	Test	Test Result	Likelihood Ratio (95% CI)	Reference
20	132	Fine-needle aspiration cytology guided with ultrasonography	Malignant	226 (4.4-11 739)	73
			Suspicious	1.3 (0.52-3.2)	
			Insufficient	2.7 (0.52-15)	
			Benign	0.24 (0.11-0.52)	

(Continued)

TABLE 19.2-24

Likelihood Ratios for the Diagnosis of Malignancy in Euthyroid Patients With a Single or Dominant Palpable Thyroid Nodule *(Continued)*

Prevalence (Pretest Probability, %)	Patients, No.	Test	Test Result	Likelihood Ratio (95% CI)	Reference
7-22	868	Fine-needle aspiration cytology not guided	Malignant	34 (15-74)	74-79
			Suspicious	1.7 (0.94-3.0)	
			Insufficient	0.5 (0.27-0.76)	
			Benign	0.23 (0.13-0.42)	
39	4875	Fine-needle aspiration cytology using TBSRTC	Positive (DC IV, V, VI)	1.97 (1.90-2.04)	80
			Negative (DC II)	0.06 (0.05-0.08)	
47	3084	Fine-needle aspiration cytology using TBSRTC	Positive (DC V, VI)	11 (9.74-13)	80
			Negative (DC II)	0.04 (0.03-0.06)	

Abbreviations: CI, confidence interval; DC II, benign; DC IV, follicular neoplasm/suspicion for a follicular neoplasm; DC V, suspicious for malignancy; DC VI, malignant; TBSRTC, The Bethesda System for Reporting Thyroid Cytopathology.

TABLE 19.2-25

Likelihood Ratios of Tests for Diagnosis of Urinary Tract Infection in Symptomatic Adult Women Presenting to a Primary Care Setting

Patients, No.	Test	Test Result	Likelihood Ratio (95% CI)	Reference
	History			81
3407	Dysuria	Present Absent	1.30 (1.2-1.41) 0.51 (0.43-0.61)	
2807	Frequency	Present Absent	1.10 (1.04-1.16) 0.60 (0.49-0.74)	
635	Back pain	Present Absent	0.90 (0.71-1.14) 1.07 (0.90-1.28)	
1250	Fever	Present Absent	1.28 (0.64-2.58) 0.98 (0.91-1.05)	
1340	Flank pain	Present Absent	0.85 (0.67-1.08) 1.07 (0.98-1.17)	
1078	Hematuria	Present Absent	1.72 (1.30-2.27) 0.88 (0.83-0.93)	
1470	Lower abdominal pain	Present Absent	1.01 (0.89-1.15) 0.99 (0.87-1.13)	
1720	Nocturia	Present Absent	1.30 (1.08-1.56) 0.75 (0.60-0.94)	
2298	Urgency	Present Absent	1.22 (1.11-1.34) 0.73 (0.62-0.86)	
1261	Vaginal discharge	Present Absent	0.65 (0.51-0.83) 1.10 (1.01-1.20)	

Abbreviation: CI, confidence interval.

Urinary Tract Infection

This systematic review included 16 studies of adult women with suspected uncomplicated urinary tract infection who presented in a primary care setting. The reference standard used to confirm diagnosis was a urine culture from a clean-catch or catheterized urine specimen with a diagnostic threshold of 10^2 CFU/mL or higher (Table 19.2-25).[81]

CONCLUSION

This chapter describes a series of LRs supported by high-quality evidence for historical clues, physical examination signs, and laboratory or radiologic tests to aid in the diagnosis of common medical problems.

References

1. Black ER, Bordely DR, Tape TG, Panzer RJ, eds. *Diagnostic Strategies for Common Medical Problems.* 2nd ed. Philadelphia, PA: American College of Physicians; 1999.

2. Simel DL, Samsa GP, Matchar DB. Likelihood ratios with confidence: sample size estimation for diagnostic test studies. *J Clin Epidemiol.* 1991;44(8):763-770.

3. Fleiss JL. The statistical basis of meta-analysis. *Stat Methods Med Res.* 1993;2(2):121-145.

4. Lederle FA, Simel DL. The rational clinical examination: does this patient have abdominal aortic aneurysm? *JAMA.* 1999;281(1):77-82.

5. Nauta RJ, Magnant C. Observation versus operation for abdominal pain in the right lower quadrant. Roles of the clinical examination and the leukocyte count. *Am J Surg.* 1986;151(6):746-748.

6. Liddington MI, Thomson WH. Rebound tenderness test. *Br J Surg.* 1991;78(7):795-796.

7. Eskelinen M, Ikonen J, Lipponen P. The value of history-taking, physical examination, and computer assistance in the diagnosis of acute appendicitis in patients more than 50 years old. *Scand J Gastroenterol.* 1995;30(4):349-355.

8. Wagner JM, McKinney WP, Carpenter JL. Does this patient have appendicitis? *JAMA.* 1996;276(19):1589-1594.

9. Andersson RE. Meta-analysis of the clinical and laboratory diagnosis of appendicitis. *Br J Surg.* 2004;91(1):28-37.

10. Terasawa T, Blackmore CC, Bent S, Kohlwes RJ. Systematic review: computed tomography and ultrasonography to detect acute appendicitis in adults and adolescents. *Ann Intern Med.* 2004;141(7):537-546.

11. Doria AS, Moineddin R, Kellenberger CJ, et al. US or CT for diagnosis of appendicitis in children and adults? a meta-analysis. *Radiology.* 2006;241(1):83-94.

12. Carroll PJ, Gibson D, El-Faedy O, et al. Surgeon-performed ultrasound at the bedside for the detection of appendicitis and gallstones: systematic review and meta-analysis. *Am J Surg.* 2013;205(1):102-108.

13. Bundy DG, Byerley JS, Liles EA, Perrin EM, Katznelson J, Rice HE. Does this child have appendicitis? *JAMA.* 2007;298(4):438-451.

14. Trowbridge RL, Rutkowski NK, Shojania KG. Does this patient have acute cholecystitis? *JAMA.* 2003;289(1):80-86.

15. Rosen CL, Brown DF, Chang Y, et al. Ultrasonography by emergency physicians in patients with suspected cholecystitis. *Am J Emerg Med.* 2001;19(1):32-36.

16. Haasenritter J, Stanze D, Widera G, et al. Does the patient with chest pain have a coronary heart disease? diagnostic value of single symptoms and signs—a meta-analysis. *Croat Med J.* 2012;53(5):432-441.

17. Mant J, McManus RJ, Oakes RA, et al. Systematic review and modelling of the investigation of acute and chronic chest pain presenting in primary care. *Health Technol Assess.* 2004;8(2):iii, 1-158.

18. Bruyninckx R, Aertgeerts B, Bruyninckx P, Buntinx F. Signs and symptoms in diagnosing acute myocardial infarction and acute coronary syndrome: a diagnostic meta-analysis. *Br J Gen Pract.* 2008;58(547):105-111.

19. Holleman DR Jr, Simel DL. Does the clinical examination predict airflow limitation? *JAMA.* 1995;273(4):313-319.

20. Broekhuizen BD, Sachs AP, Oostvogels R, Hoes AW, Verheij TJ, Moons KG. The diagnostic value of history and physical examination for COPD in suspected or known cases: a systematic review. *Fam Pract.* 2009;26(4):260-268.

21. Aertgeerts B, Buntinx F, Kester A. The value of the CAGE in screening for alcohol abuse and alcohol dependence in general clinical populations: a diagnostic meta-analysis. *J Clin Epidemiol.* 2004;57(1):30-39.

22. Fiellin DA, Reid MC, O'Connor PG. Screening for alcohol problems in primary care: a systematic review. *Arch Intern Med.* 2000;160(13):1977-1989.

23. Williams JW Jr, Simel DL. The rational clinical examination: does this patient have ascites? how to divine fluid in the abdomen. *JAMA.* 1992;267(19):2645-2648.

24. Ziegler DK, Zileli T, Dick A, Sebaugh JL. Correlation of bruits over the carotid artery with angiographically demonstrated lesions. *Neurology.* 1971;21(8):860-865.

25. Ingall TJ, Homer D, Whisnant JP, Baker HL Jr, O'Fallon WM. Predictive value of carotid bruit for carotid atherosclerosis. *Arch Neurol.* 1989;46(4):418-422.

26. Hankey GJ, Warlow CP. Symptomatic carotid ischaemic events: safest and most cost effective way of selecting patients for angiography, before carotid endarterectomy. *BMJ.* 1990;300(6738):1485-1491.

27. Sauvé JS, Laupacis A, Ostbye T, Feagan B, Sackett DL. The rational clinical examination: does this patient have a clinically important carotid bruit? *JAMA.* 1993;270(23):2843-2845.

28. Ratchford EV, Jin Z, Di Tullio MR, et al. Carotid bruit for detection of hemodynamically significant carotid stenosis: the Northern Manhattan Study. *Neurol Res.* 2009;31(7):748-752.

29. van der Windt DA, Jellema P, Mulder CJ, Kneepkens CM, van der Horst HE. Diagnostic testing for celiac disease among patients with abdominal symptoms: a systematic review. *JAMA.* 2010;303(17):1738-1746.

30. Metlay JP, Kapoor WN, Fine MJ. Does this patient have community-acquired pneumonia? diagnosing pneumonia by history and physical examination. *JAMA.* 1997;278(17):1440-1445.

31. Saldías PF, Cabrera TD, de Solminihac LI, Hernández AP, Gederlini GA, Díaz FA. Predictive value of history and physical examination for the diagnosis of community-acquired pneumonia in adults [in Spanish]. *Rev Med Chil.* 2007;135(2):143-152.

32. van Vugt SF, Broekhuizen BD, Lammens C, et al; GRACE consortium. Use of serum C reactive protein and procalcitonin concentrations in addition to symptoms and signs to predict pneumonia in patients presenting to primary care with acute cough: diagnostic study. *BMJ.* 2013;346:f2450. doi:10.1136/bmj.f2450.

33. Kearon C, Julian JA, Newman TE, Ginsberg JS. Noninvasive diagnosis of deep venous thrombosis: McMaster Diagnostic Imaging Practice Guidelines Initiative. *Ann Intern Med.* 1998;128(8):663-677.

34. Di Nisio M, Squizzato A, Rutjes AWS, Büller HR, Zwinderman AH, Bossuyt PM. Diagnostic accuracy of D-dimer test for exclusion of venous thromboembolism: a systematic review. *J Thromb Haemost.* 2007;5(2):296-304.

35. McGee S, Abernethy WB III, Simel DL. The rational clinical examination: is this patient hypovolemic? *JAMA.* 1999;281(11):1022-1029.

36. Call SA, Vollenweider MA, Hornung CA, Simel DL, McKinney WP. Does this patient have influenza? *JAMA.* 2005;293(8):987-997.

37. Chartrand C, Leeflang MM, Minion J, Brewer T, Pai M. Accuracy of rapid influenza diagnostic tests: a meta-analysis. *Ann Intern Med.* 2012;156(7):500-511.

38. Guyatt GH, Oxman AD, Ali M, Willan A, McIlroy W, Patterson C. Laboratory diagnosis of iron-deficiency anemia: an overview. *J Gen Intern Med.* 1992;7(2):145-153.

39. Punnonen K, Irjala K, Rajamäki A. Serum transferrin receptor and its ratio to serum ferritin in the diagnosis of iron deficiency. *Blood.* 1997;89(3):1052-1057.

40. Infusino I, Braga F, Dolci A, Panteghini M. Soluble transferrin receptor (sTfR) and sTfR/log ferritin index for the diagnosis of iron-deficiency anemia: a meta-analysis. *Am J Clin Pathol.* 2012;138(5):642-649.

41. Hussein S, Prieto J, O'Shea M, Hoffbrand AV, Baillod RA, Moorhead JF. Serum ferritin assay and iron status in chronic renal failure and haemodialysis. *Br Med J.* 1975;1(5957):546-548.

42. Milman N, Christensen TE, Pedersen NS, Visfeldt J. Serum ferritin and bone marrow iron in non-dialysis, peritoneal dialysis and hemodialysis patients with chronic renal failure. *Acta Med Scand.* 1980;207(3):201-205.

43. Blumberg AB, Marti HR, Graber CG. Serum ferritin and bone marrow iron in patients undergoing continuous ambulatory peritoneal dialysis. *JAMA.* 1983;250(24):3317-3319.

44. Kalantar-Zadeh K, Höffken B, Wünsch H, Fink H, Kleiner M, Luft FC. Diagnosis of iron deficiency anemia in renal failure patients during the post-erythropoietin era. *Am J Kidney Dis.* 1995;26(2):292-299.

45. Fernández-Rodríguez AM, Guindeo-Casasús MC, Molero-Labarta T, et al. Diagnosis of iron deficiency in chronic renal failure. *Am J Kidney Dis.* 1999;34(3):508-513.

46. Intragumtornchai T, Rojnukkarin P, Swasdikul D, Israsena S. The role of serum ferritin in the diagnosis of iron deficiency anaemia in patients with liver cirrhosis. *J Intern Med.* 1998;243(3):233-241.

47. Ford AC, Talley NJ, Veldhuyzen van Zanten SJ, Vakil NB, Simel DL, Moayyedi P. Will the history and physical examination help establish that irritable bowel syndrome is causing this patient's lower gastrointestinal tract symptoms? *JAMA.* 2008;300(15):1793-1805.

48. Whited JD, Grichnik JM. The rational clinical examination: does this patient have a mole or a melanoma? *JAMA.* 1998;279(9):696-701.

49. Green AD, Colón-Emeric CS, Bastian L, Drake MT, Lyles KW. Does this woman have osteoporosis? *JAMA.* 2004;292(23):2890-2900.

50. Dargent-Molina P, Piault S, Bréart G. Identification of women at increased risk of osteoporosis: no need to use different screening tools at different ages. *Maturitas.* 2006;54(1):55-64.

51. Xu D, Zou L, Xing Y, et al. Diagnostic value of ankle-brachial index in peripheral arterial disease: a meta-analysis. *Can J Cardiol.* 2013;29(4):492-498.

52. Boyko EJ, Ahroni JH, Davignon D, Stensel V, Pigeon RL, Smith DG. Diagnostic utility of the history and physical examination for peripheral vascular disease among patients with diabetes mellitus. *J Clin Epidemiol.* 1997;50(6):659-668.

53. Christensen JH, Freundlich M, Jacobsen BA, Falstie-Jensen N. Clinical relevance of pedal pulse palpation in patients suspected of peripheral arterial insufficiency. *J Intern Med.* 1989;226(2):95-99.

54. Criqui MH, Fronek A, Klauber MR, Barrett-Connor E, Gabriel S. The sensitivity, specificity, and predictive value of traditional clinical evaluation of peripheral arterial disease: results from noninvasive testing in a defined population. *Circulation.* 1985;71(3):516-522.

55. Stoffers HE, Kester AD, Kaiser V, Rinkens PE, Knottnerus JA. Diagnostic value of signs and symptoms associated with peripheral arterial occlusive disease seen in general practice: a multivariable approach. *Med Decis Making.* 1997;17(1):61-70.

56. McGee SR, Boyko EJ. Physical examination and chronic lower-extremity ischemia: a critical review. *Arch Intern Med.* 1998;158(12):1357-1364.

57. Wong CL, Holroyd-Leduc J, Straus SE. Does this patient have a pleural effusion? *JAMA.* 2009;301(3):309-317.

58. Turnbull JM. The rational clinical examination. Is listening for abdominal bruits useful in the evaluation of hypertension? *JAMA.* 1995;274(16):1299-1301.

59. Perloff D, Sokolow M, Wylie EJ, Smith DR, Palubinskas AJ. Hypertension secondary to renal artery occlusive disease. *Circulation.* 1961;24:1286-1304.

60. Krijnen P, van Jaarsveld BC, Steyerberg EW, Man in 't Veld AJ, Schalekamp MA, Habbema JD. A clinical prediction rule for renal artery stenosis. *Ann Intern Med.* 1998;129(9):705-711.

61. Goldstein LB, Simel DL. Is this patient having a stroke? *JAMA.* 2005;293(19):2391-2402.

62. Runchey S, McGee S. Does this patient have a hemorrhagic stroke? clinical findings distinguishing hemorrhagic stroke from ischemic stroke. *JAMA.* 2010;303(22):2280-2286.

63. Hildner FJ, Ormond RS. Accuracy of the clinical diagnosis of pulmonary embolism. *JAMA.* 1967;202(7):567-570.

DIAGNOSIS

64. Stein PD, Terrin ML, Hales CA, et al. Clinical, laboratory, roentgenographic, and electrocardiographic findings in patients with acute pulmonary embolism and no pre-existing cardiac or pulmonary disease. *Chest*. 1991;100(3):598-603.

65. Nazeyrollas P, Metz D, Jolly D, et al. Use of transthoracic Doppler echocardiography combined with clinical and electrocardiographic data to predict acute pulmonary embolism. *Eur Heart J*. 1996;17(5):779-786.

66. West J, Goodacre S, Sampson F. The value of clinical features in the diagnosis of acute pulmonary embolism: systematic review and meta-analysis. *QJM*. 2007;100(12):763-769.

67. Worsley DF, Alavi A, Aronchick JM, Chen JT, Greenspan RH, Ravin CE. Chest radiographic findings in patients with acute pulmonary embolism: observations from the PIOPED Study. *Radiology*. 1993;189(1):133-136.

68. Moons KG, van Es GA, Michel BC, Büller HR, Habbema JD, Grobbee DE. Redundancy of single diagnostic test evaluation. *Epidemiology*. 1999;10(3):276-281.

69. Roy PM, Colombet I, Durieux P, Chatellier G, Sors H, Meyer G. Systematic review and meta-analysis of strategies for the diagnosis of suspected pulmonary embolism. *BMJ*. 2005;331(7511):259.

70. Hogg K, Brown G, Dunning J, et al. Diagnosis of pulmonary embolism with CT pulmonary angiography: a systematic review. *Emerg Med J*. 2006;23(3):172-178.

71. PIOPED Investigators. Value of the ventilation/perfusion scan in acute pulmonary embolism: results of the Prospective Investigation of Pulmonary Embolism Diagnosis (PIOPED). *JAMA*. 1990;263(20):2753-2759.

72. Stein PD, Alavi A, Gottschalk A, et al. Usefulness of noninvasive diagnostic tools for diagnosis of acute pulmonary embolism in patients with a normal chest radiograph. *Am J Cardiol*. 1991;67(13):1117-1120.

73. Cochand-Priollet B, Guillausseau PJ, Chagnon S, et al. The diagnostic value of fine-needle aspiration biopsy under ultrasonography in nonfunctional thyroid nodules: a prospective study comparing cytologic and histologic findings. *Am J Med*. 1994;97(2):152-157.

74. Walfish PG, Hazani E, Strawbridge HT, Miskin M, Rosen IB. A prospective study of combined ultrasonography and needle aspiration biopsy in the assessment of the hypofunctioning thyroid nodule. *Surgery*. 1977;82(4):474-482.

75. Prinz RA, O'Morchoe PJ, Barbato AL, et al. Fine needle aspiration biopsy of thyroid nodules. *Ann Surg*. 1983;198(1):70-73.

76. Jones AJ, Aitman TJ, Edmonds CJ, Burke M, Hudson E, Tellez M. Comparison of fine needle aspiration cytology, radioisotopic and ultrasound scanning in the management of thyroid nodules. *Postgrad Med J*. 1990;66(781):914-917.

77. Cusick EL, MacIntosh CA, Krukowski ZH, Williams VM, Ewen SW, Matheson NA. Management of isolated thyroid swellings: a prospective six year study of fine needle aspiration cytology in diagnosis. *BMJ*. 1990;301(6747):318-321.

78. Pérez JA, Pisano R, Kinast C, Valencia V, Araneda M, Mera ME. Needle aspiration cytology in euthyroid uninodular goiter [in Spanish]. *Rev Med Chil*. 1991;119(2):158-163.

79. Piromalli D, Martelli G, Del Prato I, Collini P, Pilotti S. The role of fine needle aspiration in the diagnosis of thyroid nodules: analysis of 795 consecutive cases. *J Surg Oncol*. 1992;50(4):247-250.

80. Bongiovanni M, Spitale A, Faquin WC, Mazzucchelli L, Baloch ZW. The Bethesda System for Reporting Thyroid Cytopathology: a meta-analysis. *Acta Cytol*. 2012;56(4):333-339.

81. Giesen LGM, Cousins G, Dimitrov BD, van de Laar FA, Fahey T. Predicting acute uncomplicated urinary tract infection in women: a systematic review of the diagnostic accuracy of symptoms and signs. *BMC Fam Pract*. 2010;11:78.

JAMAevidence

Using Evidence to Improve Care

19.3

ADVANCED TOPICS IN DIAGNOSIS

Measuring Agreement Beyond Chance

Thomas McGinn, Gordon Guyatt, Richard Cook,
Deborah Korenstein, and Maureen O. Meade

IN THIS CHAPTER

DIAGNOSIS

CLINICIANS OFTEN DISAGREE

Clinicians often disagree in their assessment of patients. When 2 clinicians reach different conclusions regarding the presence of a particular physical sign, either different approaches to the examination or different interpretations of the findings may be responsible for the disagreement. Similarly, disagreement between repeated applications of a diagnostic test may result from different application of the test or different interpretation of the results.

Researchers also may face difficulties in agreeing on issues such as whether patients meet the eligibility requirements for a *randomized trial*, whether patients in a trial have experienced the outcome of interest (eg, they may disagree about whether a patient has had a transient ischemic attack or a stroke or about whether a death should be classified as a cardiovascular death), or whether a study meets the eligibility criteria for a *systematic review*.

CHANCE WILL ALWAYS BE RESPONSIBLE FOR SOME OF THE APPARENT AGREEMENT BETWEEN OBSERVERS

Any 2 people judging the presence or absence of an attribute will agree some of the time simply by chance. Similarly, even inexperienced and uninformed clinicians may agree on a physical finding on occasion purely as a result of chance. This chance agreement is more likely to occur when the prevalence of a target finding (a physical finding, a disease, an eligibility criterion) is high—occurring, for instance, in more than 80% of a population. When investigators present agreement as raw agreement (or crude agreement)—that is, by simply counting the number of times agreement has occurred—this chance agreement gives a misleading impression.

ALTERNATIVES FOR DEALING WITH THE PROBLEM OF AGREEMENT BY CHANCE

This chapter describes approaches to addressing the problem of misleading results based on chance agreement. When we are dealing with categorical data (ie, placing patients in discrete categories, such as mild, moderate, or severe or stage 1, 2, 3, or 4), the most popular approach to dealing with chance agreement is with *chance-corrected agreement*. Chance-corrected agreement is statistically determined with *kappa* (κ) or *weighted* κ. Another option is the use of *chance-independent agreement* or *phi* (φ). One can use these 3 statistics to measure nonrandom agreement among observers, investigators, or measurements.

ONE SOLUTION TO AGREEMENT BY CHANCE: CHANCE-CORRECTED AGREEMENT OR κ

The application of κ removes most of the agreement by chance and informs clinicians of the extent of the possible agreement over and above chance. The total possible agreement on any judgment is always 100%. Figure 19.3-1 depicts a situation in which agreement by chance is 50%, leaving possible agreement above and beyond chance of 50%. As depicted in the figure, the raters have achieved an agreement of 75%. Of this 75%, 50% was achieved by chance alone. Of the remaining possible 50% agreement, the raters have achieved half, resulting in a κ value of 0.25/0.50, or 0.50.

CALCULATING κ

How is κ calculated? Assume that 2 observers are assessing the presence of Murphy sign, which may help clinicians detect an inflamed gallbladder.[2] Unfortunately, they have no skill at detecting the presence or absence of Murphy sign, and their

FIGURE 19.3-1

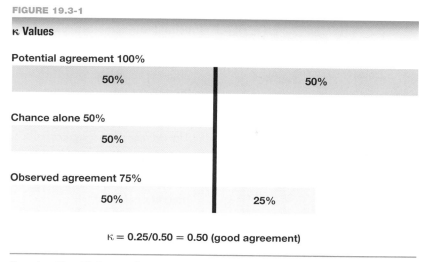

κ Values

Potential agreement 100%

| 50% | | 50% |

Chance alone 50%

| 50% |

Observed agreement 75%

| 50% | 25% |

κ = 0.25/0.50 = 0.50 (good agreement)

Reproduced from McGinn et al,[1] by permission of the publisher. © 2004 Canadian Medical Association.

evaluations are no better than blind guesses. Let us say they are both guessing in a ratio of 50:50; they guess that Murphy sign is present half the time and that it is absent half the time. On average, if both raters were evaluating the same 100 patients, they would achieve the results presented in Figure 19.3-2. Referring to that figure, you observe that these results demonstrate that the 2 cells that tally the raw agreement, A and D, include 50% of the observations. Thus, simply by guessing (and thus by chance), the raters have achieved 50% agreement.

What happens if the raters repeat the exercise of rating 100 patients, but this time, each rater guesses in a ratio of 80% positive and 20% negative? Figure 19.3-3 depicts what, on average, will occur. Now, the agreement (the sum of cells A and D) has increased to 68%.

What is the arithmetic involved in filling in the table to determine the level of agreement that occurs by chance? The procedure involves, for each cell, multiplying the total number of observations in the row of which that cell is a part by the number of observations in the column of which that cell is a part and dividing by the total number of patients. In the example in Figure 19.3-2, for instance, we can calculate how many observations we expect by

FIGURE 19.3-2

Agreement by Chance When Both Reviewers Are Guessing in a Ratio of 50% Target Positive and 50% Target Negative

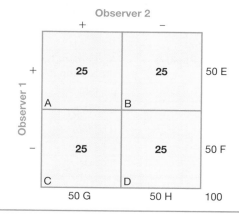

Plus sign refers to target positive and minus sign to target negative; in this case, the plus sign indicates that the Murphy sign is present and the minus sign that the Murphy sign is absent. A, Patients in which both observers find the sign present. B, Patients in which observer 1 finds the sign present and observer 2 finds the sign absent. C, Patients in which observer 1 finds the sign absent and observer 2 finds the sign present. D, Patients in which both observers find the sign absent.

Reproduced from McGinn et al,[1] by permission of the publisher. © 2004 Canadian Medical Association.

FIGURE 19.3-3

Agreement by Chance When Both Reviewers Are Guessing in a Ratio of 80% Target Positive and 20% Target Negative

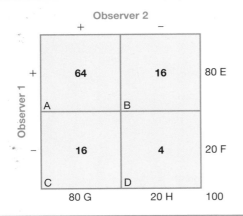

Plus sign refers to target positive and minus sign to target negative; in this case, the plus sign indicates that the Murphy sign is present and the minus sign that Murphy sign is absent.

Reproduced from McGinn et al,[1] by permission of the publisher. © 2004 Canadian Medical Association.

TABLE 19.3-1

Association Between the Proportion Positive and the Expected Agreement by Chance

Proportion Positive	Agreement by Chance, Proportion (%)
0.5	0.5 (50)
0.6	0.52 (52)
0.7	0.58 (58)
0.8	0.68 (68)
0.9	0.82 (82)

Reproduced from McGinn et al,[1] by permission of the publisher. © 2004 Canadian Medical Association.

chance to fall in cell A, which represents the number of positive results agreed on by both reviewers. First, we multiply the number of times observer 1 finds a Murphy sign (50) by the number of times observer 2 detects a Murphy sign (also 50), and we divide by 100, the total number of patients evaluated. Similarly, to calculate the number of observations we expect in cell D, we again multiply 50 by 50 (the 2 numbers of expected negatives) and divide by 100. Readers can

find a more detailed demonstration of the rationale behind this and other calculations presented here in the Evidence-Based Medicine Tips series.[1]

Were we to repeat this arithmetic exercise with different marginal totals, we would find that as the proportion of observations classified as positive becomes progressively more extreme (ie, as it moves away from 50%), the agreement by chance increases. The average chance agreement changes are shown in Table 19.3-1, with 2 observers classifying an increasingly higher proportion of patients in one category or the other (such as positive and negative or sign present or absent).

Figure 19.3-4 illustrates the calculation of κ with a hypothetical data set. First, we calculate the agreement observed: In 40 patients, the 2 observers agreed that Murphy sign was positive (cell A), and they further agreed that in another 40 patients, it was negative (cell D). Thus, the total agreement is 40 + 40, or 80.

Second, we calculate the agreement by chance by multiplying the proportions of test results read as positive by the 2 observers (0.5 × 0.5) and adding that to the product of the proportions of tests read as negative by the 2 observers (0.5 × 0.5). The total agreement by chance is 0.25 + 0.25, or 0.50, 50%.

We can then calculate κ using the principle illustrated in Figure 19.3-1.

$$\frac{\text{(agreement observed} - \text{agreement by chance)}}{\text{(agreement possible} - \text{agreement by chance)}}$$

or in this case:

$$\frac{80 - 50}{100 - 50} = \frac{30}{50} = 0.6$$

κ WITH 3 OR MORE RATERS OR 3 OR MORE CATEGORIES

Using similar principles, one can calculate chance-corrected agreement when there are more than 2 raters.[3] Furthermore, one can calculate κ when raters place patients into more than 2 categories (eg, patients with heart failure may be rated as New York Heart Association class I, II, III, or IV). In these situations, one may give partial credit for intermediate levels of agreement (for instance, one observer may classify a patient as having class II heart failure, whereas another may observe the same patient as having class III heart failure) by adopting a so-called weighted κ statistic. Weighting refers to calculations that give full credit to full agreement and partial credit to partial agreement (according to distance from the diagonal on an agreement table).[4]

There are a number of approaches to valuing the κ levels raters achieve. One option is the following: 0, poor agreement; 0 to 0.2, slight agreement; 0.21 to 0.4, fair agreement; 0.41 to 0.6, moderate agreement; 0.61 to 0.8, substantial agreement; and 0.81 to 1.0, almost perfect agreement.[5]

Examples of chance-corrected agreement that investigators have calculated in clinical studies are as follows: exercise stress test cardiac T-wave changes, κ = 0.25; jugular venous distention, κ = 0.50; arterial stenosis on cardiac catheterization, κ = 0.70; CAGE questionnaire score for alcoholism (Cut down, Annoyed, Guilty, Eye opener), κ = 0.82; tenderness on abdominal examination in the emergency department, κ = 0.42; and presence of retinopathy on examination, κ = 0.72-0.75.

A LIMITATION OF κ

Despite its intuitive appeal and widespread use, the κ statistic has an important disadvantage: As a result of the high level of chance agreement when distributions become more extreme, the possible agreement above chance becomes small, and even moderate values of κ are difficult to achieve. Thus, with the use of the same raters in a variety of settings, as the proportion of positive ratings becomes extreme, κ will decrease even if the raters' skill at interpretation does not.[6-8]

AN ALTERNATIVE TO κ: CHANCE-INDEPENDENT AGREEMENT OR φ

One solution to this problem is chance-independent agreement using the φ statistic.[9] Here, one begins by estimating the *odds ratio* (OR) from a 2 × 2 table indicating the agreement between 2 observers.

FIGURE 19.3-4

Observed and Expected Agreement

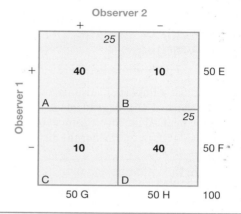

Plus sign refers to target positive and minus sign to target negative; in this case, the plus sign indicates that the Murphy sign is present and the minus sign that the Murphy sign is absent. Expected agreement by chance appears in italics in cells A and D.

Reproduced from McGinn et al,[1] by permission of the publisher. © 2004 Canadian Medical Association.

Figure 19.3-5 contrasts the formulas for raw agreement, κ, and φ.

The OR (*ad/bc*) in Figure 19.3-5 provides the basis for calculating φ. The OR is the odds of a positive classification by rater B when rater A gives a positive classification divided by the odds of a positive classification by rater B when rater A gives a negative classification (see Chapter 12.2, Understanding the Results: More About Odds Ratios). The OR would not change if we were to reverse the rows and columns. Thus, it does not matter which observer we identify as observer A and which we identify as observer B. The OR provides a natural measure of agreement. This agreement can be made more easily interpretable by converting it into a form that takes values from −1.0 (representing extreme disagreement) to 1.0 (representing extreme agreement). The φ statistic makes this conversion using the following formula:

$$\varphi = \frac{\sqrt{OR} - 1}{\sqrt{OR} + 1} = \frac{\sqrt{ad} - \sqrt{bc}}{\sqrt{ad} + \sqrt{bc}}$$

When both margins are 0.5 (ie, when both raters conclude that 50% of the patients are positive and 50% are negative for the trait of interest), φ is equal to κ.

ADVANTAGES OF φ OVER OTHER APPROACHES

The use of φ has 4 important advantages over other approaches. First, it is independent of the level of chance agreement. Thus, investigators could expect to find similar levels of φ whether the distribution of results is 50% positive and 50% negative or whether it is 90% positive and 10% negative. As we have pointed out, this is not true for κ.

Second, unlike κ, φ naturally accommodates statistical modeling. Such flexibility allows investigators to take advantage of all ratings when observers assess patients, radiographs, or other study outcomes on multiple occasions.[9] One also can examine which factors influence the degree of agreement through familiar OR-based regression modeling.

Third, φ allows testing of whether differences in agreement between pairings of raters are statistically significant, an option that is not available with κ.[9]

FIGURE 19.3-5

Calculations of Agreement

		Rater B	
		Observation present	Observation absent
Rater A	Observation present	A	B
	Observation absent	C	D

Raw agreement $= \dfrac{a+d}{a+b+c+d}$

$\kappa = \dfrac{\text{Observed agreement} - \text{Expected agreement}}{1 - \text{Expected agreement}}$

where observed agreement $= \dfrac{a+d}{a+b+c+d}$

and expected agreement $= \dfrac{(a+b)(a+c)}{a+b+c+d} + \dfrac{(c+d)(b+d)}{a+b+c+d}$

Odds ratio (OR) $= \dfrac{ad}{bc}$

$\Phi = \dfrac{\sqrt{OR}-1}{\sqrt{OR}+1} = \dfrac{\sqrt{ad}-\sqrt{bc}}{\sqrt{ad}+\sqrt{bc}}$

Fourth, because φ is based on the OR, one can perform so-called exact analyses. This feature is particularly attractive when the sample is small or if there is a 0 cell among the observations.[10]

Statisticians may disagree about the relative usefulness of κ and φ. Most important, from a clinician's point of view, is that either approach provides a major improvement over raw agreement.

References

1. McGinn T, Wyer PC, Newman TB, Keitz S, Leipzig R, For GG; Evidence-Based Medicine Teaching Tips Working Group. Tips for learners of evidence-based medicine, 3: measures of observer variability (kappa statistic). *CMAJ*. 2004;171(11):1369-1373.

2. Trowbridge RL, Rutkowski NK, Shojania KG. Does this patient have acute cholecystitis? In: Simel DL, Rennie D, eds. *The Rational Clinical Examination: Evidence-Based Clinical Diagnosis*. New York, NY: McGraw-Hill; 2009. http://www.jamaevidence.com/content/3477555. Accessed February 10, 2014.

3. Cohen J. Weighted kappa: nominal scale agreement with provision for scaled disagreement or partial credit. *Psychol Bull*. 1968;70(4):213-220.

4. Landis JR, Koch GG. The measurement of observer agreement for categorical data. *Biometrics*. 1977;33(1):159-174.

5. Sackett D, Hayes R, Guyatt G, Tugwell P. *Clinical Epidemiology: A Basic Science for Clinical Medicine*. 2nd ed. Boston, MA: Brown & Co; 1991:30.

6. Thompson WD, Walter SD. A reappraisal of the kappa coefficient. *J Clin Epidemiol*. 1988;41(10):949-958.

7. Feinstein AR, Cicchetti DV. High agreement but low kappa, I: the problems of two paradoxes. *J Clin Epidemiol*. 1990;43(6):543-549.

8. Cook R, Farewell V. Conditional inference for subject-specific and marginal agreement: two families of agreement measures. *Can J Stat*. 1995;23(4):333-344.

9. Meade MO, Cook RJ, Guyatt GH, et al. Interobserver variation in interpreting chest radiographs for the diagnosis of acute respiratory distress syndrome. *Am J Respir Crit Care Med*. 2000;161(1):85-90.

10. Armitage P, Colton T, eds. *Encyclopedia of Biostatistics*. Chichester, NY: John Wiley & Sons; 1998.

19.4

ADVANCED TOPICS IN DIAGNOSIS

Clinical Prediction Rules

Thomas McGinn, Peter Wyer, Lauren McCullagh,
Juan Wisnivesky, PJ Devereaux, Ian Stiell, W. Scott Richardson,
Thomas Agoritsas, and Gordon Guyatt

IN THIS CHAPTER

DIAGNOSIS

You are the medical director of a busy inner-city emergency department. Faced with a limited budget and pressure to improve efficiency, you have conducted an audit of radiologic procedures ordered for minor trauma and have found that the rate of radiographs ordered for ankle and knee trauma is high. You are aware of the Ottawa Ankle Rules, which help identify patients for whom it is safe to omit ankle radiographs without adverse consequences (Figure 19.4-1).[1,2] You are aware that only a small number of your institution's faculty and residents currently use the Ottawa Ankle Rules in the emergency department.

You are interested in knowing the accuracy of the Ottawa Ankle Rules, whether they are applicable to the population of patients in your hospital, and whether you should implement them in your own practice. Furthermore, you wonder whether implementing these rules can change clinical behavior and reduce costs without compromising *quality of care*. You decide to consult the original medical literature and assess the *evidence* for yourself.

FINDING THE EVIDENCE

To obtain a rapid overview of current best evidence that answers all of your questions, you start your search at the top of the pyramid of evidence-based medicine resources (see Chapter 5, Finding Current Best Evidence). You opt for the online summary in a preappraised-evidence resource, accessible through your institution. Using the term "ankle injury," you quickly find a relevant chapter on "Decision Rules for Imaging of Ankle and Foot Injuries." This chapter summarizes and provides detailed online references for the Ottawa *clinical prediction rule* for ankle fractures, its accuracy in ruling out ankle fractures, its validation in different populations and settings,

and its impact when implemented in various emergency centers.

However, you are also interested in the first derivation article, which does not seem to be cited in the summary chapter. To rapidly find it, you go to PubMed, then Clinical Queries (http://www.ncbi.nlm.nih.gov/pubmed/clinical), and type "ankle Ottawa decision rules." Under Clinical Study Categories, you choose the search filter "Clinical Prediction Guides" and choose as your scope "Broad" to find the derivation study. This retrieves 31 studies, of which the earliest one is the derivation study published in 1992.[1]

In reviewing the articles you have found, you require criteria for deciding on the strength of the inference you can make about the accuracy and impact of the Ottawa Ankle Rules. This chapter provides the tools to answer those questions.

WHAT IS A CLINICAL PREDICTION RULE?

Establishing a patient's diagnosis and *prognosis* is central to every physician's practice. The diagnoses we make—and our assessment of patients' prognoses—often determine our course of action and the recommendations we make to patients. Clinical experience provides us with an intuitive sense of which findings on history, physical examination, and laboratory or radiologic investigation are critical in making an accurate diagnosis or an accurate assessment of a patient's likely fate. Although intuition is sometimes extraordinarily accurate, it may be misleading. Clinical prediction rules attempt to increase the accuracy of clinicians' diagnostic and prognostic assessments.

We define a clinical prediction rule as a clinical tool that quantifies the individual contributions that various components of the medical history, physical examination, and basic laboratory results make toward the diagnosis, prognosis, or likely response to treatment in an individual patient.

FIGURE 19.4-1

Ottawa Ankle Rules

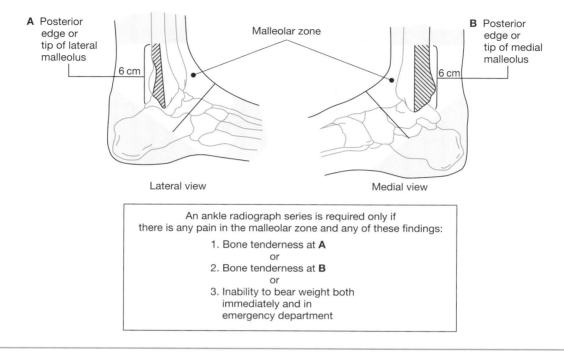

An ankle radiograph series is required only if there is any pain in the malleolar zone and any of these findings:

1. Bone tenderness at **A**
   or
2. Bone tenderness at **B**
   or
3. Inability to bear weight both immediately and in emergency department

Reproduced from Stiell et al,[3] with permission from *JAMA*.

Clinical prediction rules are potentially of great benefit because they are tailored to specific patients for real-time decision making.

"Prediction" implies helping the clinician to better appraise the likelihood of a future clinical event. "Decision" implies directing a clinician to a specific course of action. Application of clinical prediction rules sometimes results in a prediction and other times a decision but also may lead to a change between pretest and posttest likelihood of a specific diagnosis, often best summarized by a *likelihood ratio* (LR). The term "clinical prediction rule" is used in this chapter regardless of whether the output of the "rule" is a suggested clinical course of action, the probability of a future event, or an increase or decrease in the likelihood of a particular diagnosis.

Whatever the clinical prediction rule is generating—a decision, a prediction, or a change in diagnostic probability—clinicians are most likely to find it useful in common clinical situations in which decision making is complex, when the clinical stakes are high, or when opportunities exist to achieve cost savings without compromising patient care.

USERS' GUIDES TO CLINICAL PREDICTION RULES

Our usual approach to *Users' Guides—risk of bias,* results, and applicability—does not work well for clinical prediction rules because developing and testing a clinical prediction rule involves 3 steps: the creation or derivation of the rule, the testing or validation of the rule, and the assessment of the effect of the rule on clinical behavior—the impact analysis. The validation process may require several studies at different clinical sites to fully test the accuracy

FIGURE 19.4-2

Development and Testing of a Clinical Prediction Rule

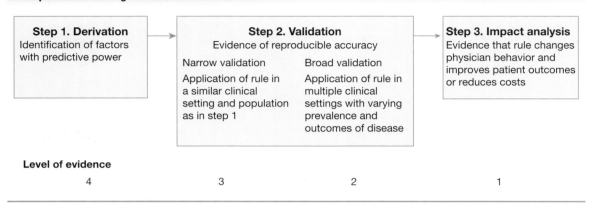

of the rule (Figure 19.4-2). Different authors may independently report the various steps in the evolution of a clinical prediction rule. Authors frequently label their report as a "derivation and validation" of a prediction rule, although the "validation" is limited to the use of statistical techniques on the same data set that was used for derivation. Under most circumstances, a statistical validation of this type would not qualify as an independent step beyond the derivation process. Box 19.4-1 presents a *hierarchy of evidence* that can guide clinicians in assessing the full range of evidence supporting the use of a clinical prediction rule in their practice. We now review the steps in the development and testing of a clinical prediction rule, relating each stage of the process to the *Users' Guides* presented in Box 19.4-1.

BOX 19.4-1

Users' Guide to Clinical Prediction Rules: Hierarchy of Evidence

Level 1: Has the rule undergone at least 1 prospective validation in a population separate from the derivation set plus 1 impact analysis that indicates a change in clinician behavior with beneficial consequences? If yes, clinicians can use the rule in a wide variety of settings with confidence that they can change clinician behavior, facilitate patient decision making, improve patient outcomes, or reduce costs.

Level 2: Has the rule shown accuracy either in 1 large prospective multicenter study, including a broad spectrum of patients and clinicians, or validation in several smaller settings that differ from one another? Has the rule been applied by clinicians rather than by research staff or by using results from a clinical database? If so, but if there is no impact analysis, clinicians can use it in various settings with confidence in their accuracy but with no certainty that patient outcomes will improve.

Level 3: Has the rule been validated in only 1 narrow prospective sample? If so, clinicians may consider using the clinical prediction rule with caution and only if patients in the study are similar to those in their clinical setting.

Level 4: Has the rule been derived but not validated or validated only in split samples, in large retrospective databases, or through statistical techniques? If so, this is a clinical prediction rule that needs further validation before it can be applied clinically.

DEVELOPING A CLINICAL PREDICTION RULE

Our search retrieved 3 relevant articles related to the Ottawa Ankle Rules[1,2,4]; the first described the rules' derivation.[1] Developers of clinical prediction rules begin by constructing a list of potential predictors of the outcome of interest—in this case, ankle fractures apparent on ankle radiograph. The list typically includes items from the medical history, physical examination, and basic laboratory tests. The investigators then examine a group of patients and determine (1) each patient's status regarding the clinical predictors and (2) each patient's status on the outcome of interest—in this case, the presence or absence of a fracture on an ankle radiograph.[5] Statistical analysis reveals which predictors are most powerful and which predictors can be omitted from the rule without loss of predictive power.

Typically, the statistical techniques used in this process are based on *logistic regression analysis* (see Chapter 15.1, Correlation and Regression). Other techniques that investigators sometimes use include *discriminant analysis,* which produces equations similar to regression analysis[6]; *recursive partitioning analysis*, which divides the patient population into smaller and smaller groups according to discriminating *risk factors*[7]; or *neural networks*.[8]

Clinical prediction rules that are not validated are usually not ready for clinical application (see Box 19.4-1). Nevertheless, clinicians can extract clinically relevant messages from an article that describes the development of a clinical prediction rule. They may wish to note the most important predictors and to consider them more carefully in their own practice. They also may consider giving less importance to variables that failed to show predictive power. Finally, if their instinct is that the unvalidated rule may nevertheless provide a more accurate prognosis than their clinical intuition, they may choose to use the rule in their practice. This is particularly true if the rule deals with prognostic models that aim to reduce uncertainty.

For instance, in developing a clinical prediction rule to predict mortality from pneumonia, investigators found that the white blood cell count had no bearing on subsequent mortality.[9,10] Hence, clinicians may wish to put less weight on the white blood cell count when making decisions about admitting pneumonia patients to the hospital.

DERIVATION—EVEN WHEN RIGOROUS—IS SELDOM SUFFICIENT

There are 3 reasons why even rigorously derived clinical prediction rules are generally not ready for application in clinical practice. First, the prediction rules derived from one set of patients may reflect associations between given predictors and outcomes that occur primarily because of the play of chance. If that is so, a different set of predictors will emerge in a different group of patients, even if they come from the same setting. This concern is influenced by the number of patients, the number of events or diagnoses, and the number of patients with the various risk factors evaluated. If the study is very large with many patients, many events, and many patients with the risk factor, this becomes less of a concern. In particular, if the study includes tens of thousands of patients with hundreds of events, the concern becomes minimal.

Second, predictors may be idiosyncratic to the population, to the clinicians using the rule, or to other aspects of the design of individual studies. If that is so, the rule may fail in a new setting. Again, a very large study conducted across dozens of settings reduces, or perhaps eliminates, this concern. Finally, because of problems in the feasibility of rule application in the clinical setting, clinicians may fail to implement a rule comprehensively or accurately, which would result in a rule that succeeds in theory but fails in practice. Large sample sizes cannot address this concern.

Statistical methods can deal with the problem of the play of chance resulting in misleading findings. For instance, investigators may split their population into 2 groups, using one to develop the rule and the other to test it. Alternatively, they may use statistical methods with interesting names (eg, *bootstrap* or *jackknife*) to estimate the performance of the clinical prediction rule in subsets of the derivation population.

Although statistical validations within the same setting or group of patients reduce the likelihood that the rule reflects the play of chance rather than true associations, they fail to address the other 2 threats to validity. Because of the risk that a clinical prediction rule will provide misleading information when applied in an actual clinical setting, a clinical prediction rule that has undergone development without validation is situated as level 4 in the hierarchy of evidence (Box 19.4-1). To ascend from level 4 in the hierarchy, studies must assess application of the rule by clinicians in clinical practice.

As an example, a study designed to develop a rule to identify a low-risk group of children presenting to emergency departments with signs and symptoms suggestive of acute appendicitis enrolled patients during a 16-month period.[11] Without altering any other aspect of the study protocol, the authors chose to define patients enrolled during the final 5 months of the study period as a "validation" group. The authors presented the resulting instrument as a prediction rule that had already undergone validation and therefore was ready for clinical application. This rule, although promising, is classified as level 4 within our hierarchy.

A clinical prediction rule developed to predict a serious outcome (including heart failure or ventricular arrhythmia) in patients with syncope further highlights the importance of clinical validation. Investigators derived the rule using data from 252 patients who presented to the emergency department; subsequently, they attempted to prospectively validate it in a sample of 374 patients.[12] The prediction rule gave individuals a score from 0 to 4, depending on the number of clinical predictors present.

Unfortunately, if one used results from the derivation patients, one would estimate that patients had almost twice the risk of a poor outcome than was the case for patients in the validation set. In the derivation set, the risk of a poor outcome among patients with a score of 3 was 52%; by contrast, patients with the same score in the validation set had a much lower probability of a poor outcome, 27%. This variation in results may have occurred as a result of differences in the severity of the syncope cases entered into the 2 studies, different criteria for generating a score of 3, or—given the small sample size in each study—chance. It is also possible that all 3 factors contributed.

As we have alluded to in referring to studies with very large sample sizes, there are instances in which one might question rigid application of this hierarchy. In one such example, Eagle et al[13] performed a multicenter study in more than 90 hospitals with 15 000 patients. The study evaluated predictors of mortality in patients who were discharged after an acute coronary syndrome. The prediction rule was developed with a prospective data set that included more than 15 000 patients and then validated in a second *cohort* of more than 7 000 patients.

Although this study was not a formal prospective validation, the sheer size of the validation would move the study into level 3 of the hierarchy of evidence (Figure 19.4-1, Box 19.4-1). Given, however, that the authors identified 9 variables predictive of 6-month mortality (older age, history of myocardial infarction, history of heart failure, increased pulse rate at presentation, lower systolic blood pressure at presentation, elevated initial serum creatinine level, elevated initial serum cardiac biomarker levels, ST-segment depression on presenting electrocardiogram, and not having a percutaneous coronary intervention performed in the hospital), clinicians are likely to have considerable difficulty applying the rule. Thus, the feasibility of application in clinical practice remains untested, and a compelling argument remains for further study to ensure feasibility and accuracy in actual clinical use. We would not consider this study for a designation of level 2 in the evidence hierarchy.

MOVING UP THE HIERARCHY— VALIDATION OF A CLINICAL PREDICTION RULE

To move up the evidence hierarchy, clinical prediction rules must provide additional evidence of validity. Another article in our search described the prospective validation of the Ottawa Ankle Rules. Validation of a clinical prediction rule involves demonstrating that its repeated application as part of the process of clinical care—that is, by clinicians actually taking care of patients—leads to the same results. Ideally, validation entails application of the rule prospectively in a new population (with dissimilar prevalence and spectrum of disease from the derivation population) and by a variety of clinicians in a variety of institutions. If the setting in which the prediction rule was originally developed was limited and its validation was confined to the same population, application by clinicians working in other settings is less secure. Validation in a similar setting can take a number of forms. Most simply, after developing the prediction rule, the investigators return to their population, draw a new sample of patients, and then test the rule's performance as actually implemented by physicians. Thus, we classify rules that have been validated in the same—or very similar—limited or narrow populations as the sample used in the development phase as level 3 on our hierarchy, and we recommend that clinicians be aware of the possible limitations of the clinical prediction rule (Box 19.4-1).

In the derivation phase, investigators draw patients from a sufficiently heterogeneous population across a variety of institutions; testing the rule in the same population provides strong validation. Validation in a new population by physicians in that setting provides the clinician with strong inferences about the usefulness of the rule, corresponding to level 2 in the evidence hierarchy (Box 19.4-1). The more numerous and diverse the settings in which the rule is tested and found accurate, the more likely it is that it will generalize to an untested setting, assuming that the testing is performed by clinicians actually using the rule in clinical practice.[14]

To demonstrate the importance of the progression from level 3 to level 2, consider a rule that was derived to predict preserved left ventricular (LV) function after myocardial infarction.[19] The initial derivation and validation were performed on 314 patients who were admitted to a tertiary care center. The prediction rule was first derived by using 162 patients and then was validated with 152 patients in the same setting. The prediction rule demonstrated that, of patients in whom the rule suggested LV function was preserved, this was, in fact, true in 99%.

At this stage of development, one would consider the rule as level 3, to be used only in settings similar to that of the validation study, that is, in similar cardiac care units. The rule was further validated in 2 larger trials, a trial using 213 patients from a single site and a larger trial using 1 891 patients from several institutions and in both cases applied by clinicians as part of patient care.[20,21] In both settings, 11% of patients in whom the rule suggested that LV function had been preserved had abnormal LV function. This decrease in accuracy, expected in validation studies, changes the potential use and implications of the rule in clinical practice. At this point in development, we would consider the rule to fall within the category of level 2, meaning that clinicians can use the rule in clinical settings with a high degree of confidence to identify patients with approximately a 90% probability of preserved LV function.

USING THE GUIDE

The Ottawa Ankle Rules were derived in 2 large, university-based emergency departments in Ottawa and then prospectively validated in a large sample of patients from the same emergency departments.[2] At this stage, the rule would be classified as level 2 in the hierarchy of evidence because of the large number and diversity of patients and physicians involved in the study and because the rule was actually applied by clinicians with their patients. Since then, other studies[15-18] have validated the rule in several clinical settings, with relatively consistent results. This evidence further strengthens our inference about its predictive power.

STRONG METHODS INCREASE CONFIDENCE IN VALIDATION STUDIES

Regardless of whether investigators have conducted their validation study in a similar, narrow (level 3) population or a broad, heterogeneous, and independent (level 2) population, their results allow stronger inferences if they have adhered to a number of methodologic standards (Box 19.4-2). Interested readers can find a complete discussion on the validation process and these criteria in an article by Laupacis et al.[5]

If those evaluating predictor status of study patients are aware (ie, unblinded) of the outcome or if those assessing the outcome are aware of patients' status with respect to the predictors, their assessments may be biased.

BOX 19.4-2

Methodologic Standards for Validation of a Clinical Prediction Rule

Were the patients chosen in an unbiased fashion and do they represent a wide spectrum of severity of disease?

Was there a blinded assessment of the criterion standard for all patients?

Was there an explicit and accurate interpretation of the predictor variables and the actual rule without knowledge of the outcome?

Was there 100% follow-up of those enrolled?

For instance, in a clinical prediction rule developed to predict the presence of pneumonia in patients who present with cough, the authors make no mention of blinding during either the derivation or validation process.[22] Knowledge of medical history or physical examination findings may have influenced the judgments of the unblinded radiologists.

USING THE GUIDE

The investigators testing the Ottawa Ankle Rules enrolled consecutive patients, obtained radiographs for all of them, and ensured not only that the clinicians were assessing the clinical predictors unaware of the radiologic results but also that the radiologists had no knowledge of the clinical data.

HOW TO DECIDE ON THE POWER OF THE RULE

Regardless of the level of evidence associated with a clinical prediction rule, its usefulness will depend on its ability to discriminate between patients who will experience an event and those who will not (or between patients who have a diagnosis and those without). Investigators may report their results in a variety of ways.

USING THE GUIDE

First, the results may dictate a specific course of action. For instance, the ankle component of the Ottawa Ankle Rules states that ankle radiographs are indicated only for patients with pain near the malleoli plus either inability to bear weight or localized bone tenderness at the posterior edge or tip of either malleolus (Figure 19.4-1).[2] Underlying this decision are the likelihood ratios associated with the rule as a diagnostic test (see Chapter 18, Diagnostic Tests). In the development process, all patients with fractures had a positive result (*sensitivity* of 100%), but only 40% of those without fractures had a negative result (*specificity* of 40%). These results suggest that if clinicians order radiographs only for those patients with a positive result, they will not miss any fractures and will avoid the test in 40% of those without a fracture.

The Ottawa Ankle Rules validation study confirmed these results.[2] The test maintained a sensitivity of 100%, with a 95% *confidence interval* (CI) around this estimate of 93% to 100%. Some clinicians might remain uncomfortable committing themselves to the use of the rule were the true sensitivity of the clinical prediction rule as low as 93%, the lower limit of this interval. Clinicians adopting the rule would nevertheless miss few, if any, fractures.

Another way of reporting results of a clinical prediction rule is in terms of probability of the target condition or outcome, given a particular result. When investigators report prediction rule results in this fashion, they are implicitly incorporating all clinical information. In doing so, they remove any need for clinicians to consider independent information in deciding about the likelihood of the diagnosis or about a patient's prognosis. For example, a prediction rule for pulmonary embolus derived and validated by Wells et al[23] accurately placed inpatients and outpatients presenting to tertiary care hospitals into low (3.4%; 95% CI, 2.2%-5.0%), intermediate (28%; 95% CI, 23.4%-32.2%), or high (78%; 95% CI, 69.2%-89.6%) probability categories.

Finally, investigators may report their findings about the accuracy of prediction rules as LRs, *absolute risks*, or *relative risks*. Using LRs, investigators are implicitly suggesting that clinicians should use other, independent information to generate a *pretest probability* (or prerule probability). Clinicians then can use the LRs generated from the rule to establish a *posttest probability*. (For approaches to using LRs, see Chapter 18, Diagnostic Tests.) For example, accuracy of the CAGE (Cut down, Annoyed, Guilty, Eye-opener) prediction rule for detecting alcoholism has been reported using LRs (eg, for CAGE scores of 0/4, LR = 0.14; for scores of 1/4, LR = 1.5; for scores of 2/4, LR = 4.5; for scores of 3/4, LR = 13; and for scores of 4/4, LR = 101).[24] In this example, the probability of disease (alcoholism) depends on the combination of the *prevalence* of disease in the community and/or other features of the presenting patient that may determine the pretest probability (eg, family history of alcoholism or knowing that the patient's partner is an alcoholic) and the score on the CAGE prediction rule.

TESTING THE CLINICAL IMPACT OF A CLINICAL PREDICTION RULE

Even an accurate prediction rule may fail to produce a change in behavior or an improvement in outcomes. First, clinicians' intuitive estimation of probabilities may be as good as, if not better than, the rule. Second, because use of clinical prediction rules involves remembering the relevant predictor variables and often entails making calculations to determine a patient's probability of having the target outcome, the calculations involved may be cumbersome, and as a result, clinicians may not use the rule or may use it incorrectly. Digital algorithms accessed on computers, tablets, and mobile devices can help clinicians perform the calculation and are likely to be mandatory in complex clinical prediction rules.

Third, there may be practical barriers to acting on the results of the clinical prediction rule. For instance, in the case of the Ottawa Ankle Rules, clinicians may be sufficiently concerned about protecting themselves against litigation that they may order radiographs despite a prediction rule result that suggests a negligible probability of fracture.

These are the considerations that lead us to classify a clinical prediction rule with evidence of accuracy in diverse populations as level 2 and insist on a positive result from a study of impact before a clinical prediction rule ascends to level 1.

Ideally, studies of the effect of clinical prediction rules would *randomize* patients—or health care practices—to either apply or not apply the clinical prediction rule and follow up patients for all relevant outcomes (including quality of life, morbidity, and resource use). Randomization of individual patients is unlikely to be appropriate because one would expect the participating clinicians to incorporate the rule into the care of all of their patients and not only the ones randomly allocated to the rule. A suitable alternative is to randomize institutions or practice settings and to conduct analyses appropriate to these larger units or to perform *cluster randomization* (this approach corresponds to cluster *randomized clinical trials* [RCTs]). Another potential design is to look at a single group before and after clinicians began to use the clinical prediction rule, but choice of a before-after study will substantially reduce the strength of inference.

USING THE GUIDE

Investigators examining the impact of the Ottawa Ankle Rules conducted 1 nonrandomized study in which they compared a hospital in which the rule was implemented with a *control* hospital in which it was not.[3] Results suggested a positive effect of implementation of the rule. Subsequently, they randomized 6 emergency departments to use or not use their prediction rule.[4] Just before initiating the study, 1 center dropped out, leaving a total of 5 emergency departments, 2 in the intervention group and 3 in the usual care group. The intervention consisted of introducing the prediction rule at a general meeting, distributing pocket cards that summarized the rule, posting the rule throughout the emergency department, and applying preprinted data collection forms to each patient's medical record. In the control group, the only intervention was the introduction of preprinted data collection forms without the Ottawa Ankle Rules attached to each medical record. A total of 1911 eligible patients were entered into the study: 1005 in the control group and 906 in the intervention group. There were 691 radiographs requested in the intervention group and 996 requested in the control group. In an analysis that focused on the ordering physician, the investigators found that the mean proportion of patients referred for radiography was 99.6% in the control group and 78.9% in the intervention group (*P* = .03). The investigators noted 3 missed fractures in the intervention group, none of which led to adverse outcomes. Thus, the investigators found a positive effect on resource use of the Ottawa Ankle Rules (decreased test ordering) without increase in adverse outcomes, moving the clinical prediction rule to level 1 in the hierarchy of evidence (Box 19.4-1).

Studies of the effect of clinical prediction rules on clinical practice have, by and large, thus far found little change in clinician behaviors. These results have often been a result of poor adoption (eg, if clinicians do not use the clinical prediction rule, it cannot improve outcomes). Increasing dissemination of electronic medical records and *clinical decision support systems* tools (see Chapter 11.6, Clinical Decision Support Systems) in outpatient and inpatient settings provides a means of implementing clinical prediction rules at the point of care and potentially increasing uptake. Doing so successfully, however, requires applying the science of usability testing to address workflow issues and other barriers to use.

An RCT conducted in several urban primary care settings examined the impact of integrating 2 clinical prediction rules for the management of patients with suspected pneumonia and strep throat into the clinics' electronic health records.[25] On the basis of very low rates of adoption of clinical decision support, before launching their trial, the team conducted iterative phases of usability testing (talk out loud, mock clinical scenarios, near live testing) and modification of the process, combined with user training and an information technology support group. These interventions resulted in high adoption rates and a significant impact on patient outcomes (fewer broad-spectrum antibiotic orders).[26,27]

Some prediction rules require, by their very nature, evidence of clinical effect as a condition of use. For example, the Pneumonia Outcomes Research Team's (PORT) rule for stratifying mortality risk in patients with community-acquired pneumonia does not itself prescribe a course of action for clinicians.[28] The authors of the original study included recommendations regarding appropriate assignment of patients in different risk classes to management as outpatients or inpatients or in intensive care units. It is, however, ultimately up to the treating physicians to make the site of care decision with each patient, and the PORT severity score is only 1 factor they must consider. A before-after study[29] incorporated the PORT score as part of an emergency department–based clinical pathway and found that clinicians were more inclined to manage low-risk patients outside the hospital when the scores were made available to them. More recently, Yealy et al[30] published a sound proposal for an RCT studying the clinical impact of the PORT rule, and preliminary results of their study confirm its clinical value.[31]

META-ANALYSIS OF CLINICAL PREDICTION RULES

As clinical prediction rules become more common, it is not unusual to encounter several rules to predict the same event or an individual rule that has been derived and validated in multiple populations and different settings. *Systematic reviews* and, if appropriate, *meta-analyses* are the preferred tools to assess the quality of prediction and the level of evidence. Researchers have used meta-analysis to generate best estimates of the predictive power of a clinical prediction rule the same way they use meta-analysis to generate best estimates of the properties of a diagnostic test.[32] Performing systematic reviews and meta-analyses of clinical prediction rules is very challenging because of the variable predictors that make up different clinical prediction rules.[32]

USING THE GUIDE

A systematic review and meta-analysis[33] summarized the results of 6 studies that involved 4249 adult patients addressing the Ottawa Ankle Rules. The authors calculated a pooled sensitivity of 98.5% (95% CI, 93.2%-100%) and a pooled specificity of 48.6% (95% CI, 43.4%-51.0%). Thus, combined evidence from these studies suggests that the Ottawa prediction rule accurately excludes knee fractures after acute knee injury.

CLINICAL SCENARIO RESOLUTION

You have found level 1 evidence supporting the use of the Ottawa decision rule in reducing unnecessary ankle radiographs in patients presenting to the emergency department with ankle injuries.[3,4] You therefore feel confident that you can use the rule in your own practice. Another study makes you aware that changing the behavior of your colleagues to realize the possible reductions in cost may be a challenge. Cameron and Naylor[34] reported on an initiative in which clinicians who were expert in the use of the Ottawa Ankle Rules trained 16 other individuals to teach the use of the rule. These individuals returned to their emergency departments armed with slides, overheads, a 13-minute instructional video, and a mandate to train their colleagues locally and regionally in the use of the rule. Unfortunately, this program led to no change in the use of ankle radiography.

Graham et al[35] conducted a structured survey of emergency practitioners in 5 countries to determine their awareness and use of the ankle and foot rules. Awareness of the rule by respondents in Canada,

the United Kingdom, and the United States ranged from 91% to 99%. However, only 32% of practitioners in the United States who were aware of the rule stated that they actually used it all or most of the time.

This contrasted with their counterparts in Canada and the United Kingdom, more than 80% of whom consistently used the instrument (the difference may be related to differing risk of malpractice lawsuits). In a similar survey of only Canadian emergency department staff, approximately 90% stated that they used the rule in practice and believed strongly that it was an important tool. More than 50% of respondents, however, stated that the Ottawa Ankle Rules were not the primary determinant in making decisions of whether to order an ankle radiograph.

The results indicate that even the availability of a level 1 clinical prediction rule may require local implementation strategies to change physician behavior. Finding ways of changing physician behavior is a principal agenda of the emerging field of knowledge translation.[36]

CONCLUSION

Clinical prediction rules inform our clinical judgment and have the potential to change clinical behavior and reduce unnecessary costs while maintaining quality of care and patient satisfaction. The challenge for

clinicians is to evaluate the strength of the rule and its likely effect and to find ways of efficiently incorporating level 1 rules into their daily practice. The importance of clinical prediction rules is likely to increase as they are built into systems providing probability estimates, LRs, and recommended actions.

DIAGNOSIS

References

1. Stiell IG, Greenberg GH, McKnight RD, Nair RC, McDowell I, Worthington JR. A study to develop clinical decision rules for the use of radiography in acute ankle injuries. *Ann Emerg Med*. 1992;21(4):384-390.

2. Stiell IG, Greenberg GH, McKnight RD, et al. Decision rules for the use of radiography in acute ankle injuries: refinement and prospective validation. *JAMA*. 1993;269(9):1127-1132.

3. Stiell IG, McKnight RD, Greenberg GH, et al. Implementation of the Ottawa ankle rules. *JAMA*. 1994;271(11):827-832.

4. Auleley GR, Ravaud P, Giraudeau B, et al. Implementation of the Ottawa ankle rules in France: a multicenter randomized controlled trial. *JAMA*. 1997;277(24):1935-1939.

5. Laupacis A, Sekar N, Stiell IG. Clinical prediction rules: a review and suggested modifications of methodological standards. *JAMA*. 1997;277(6):488-494.

6. Rudy TE, Kubinski JA, Boston JR. Multivariate analysis and repeated measurements: a primer. *J Crit Care*. 1992;7(5):30-41.

7. Cook EF, Goldman L. Empiric comparison of multivariate analytic techniques: advantages and disadvantages of recursive partitioning analysis. *J Chronic Dis*. 1984;37(9-10):721-731.

8. Baxt WG. Application of artificial neural networks to clinical medicine. *Lancet*. 1995;346(8983):1135-1138.

9. Fine MJ, Auble TE, Yealy DM, et al. A prediction rule to identify low-risk patients with community-acquired pneumonia. *N Engl J Med*. 1997;336(4):243-250.

10. Fine MJ, Hanusa BH, Lave JR, et al. Comparison of a disease-specific and a generic severity of illness measure for patients with community-acquired pneumonia. *J Gen Intern Med*. 1995;10(7):359-368.

11. Kharbanda AB, Taylor GA, Fishman SJ, Bachur RG. A clinical decision rule to identify children at low risk for appendicitis. *Pediatrics*. 2005;116(3):709-716.

12. Martin TP, Hanusa BH, Kapoor WN. Risk stratification of patients with syncope. *Ann Emerg Med*. 1997;29(4):459-466.

13. Eagle KA, Lim MJ, Dabbous OH, et al; GRACE Investigators. A validated prediction model for all forms of acute coronary syndrome: estimating the risk of 6-month postdischarge death in an international registry. *JAMA*. 2004;291(22):2727-2733.

14. Justice AC, Covinsky KE, Berlin JA. Assessing the generalizability of prognostic information. *Ann Intern Med*. 1999;130(6):515-524.

15. Lucchesi GM, Jackson RE, Peacock WF, Cerasani C, Swor RA. Sensitivity of the Ottawa rules. *Ann Emerg Med*. 1995;26(1):1-5.

16. Kelly AM, Richards D, Kerr L, et al. Failed validation of a clinical decision rule for the use of radiography in acute ankle injury. *N Z Med J*. 1994;107(982):294-295.

17. Stiell I, Wells G, Laupacis A, et al; Multicentre Ankle Rule Study Group. Multicentre trial to introduce the Ottawa ankle rules for use of radiography in acute ankle injuries. *BMJ*. 1995;311(7005):594-597.

18. Auleley GR, Kerboull L, Durieux P, Cosquer M, Courpied JP, Ravaud P. Validation of the Ottawa ankle rules in France: a study in the surgical emergency department of a teaching hospital. *Ann Emerg Med*. 1998;32(1):14-18.

19. Silver MT, Rose GA, Paul SD, O'Donnell CJ, O'Gara PT, Eagle KA. A clinical rule to predict preserved left ventricular ejection fraction in patients after myocardial infarction. *Ann Intern Med*. 1994;121(10):750-756.

20. Tobin K, Stomel R, Harber D, Karavite D, Sievers J, Eagle K. Validation in a community hospital setting of a clinical rule to predict preserved left ventricular ejection fraction in patients after myocardial infarction. *Arch Intern Med*. 1999;159(4):353-357.

21. Krumholz HM, Howes CJ, Murillo JE, Vaccarino LV, Radford MJ, Ellerbeck EF. Validation of a clinical prediction rule for left ventricular ejection fraction after myocardial infarction in patients > or = 65 years old. *Am J Cardiol*. 1997;80(1):11-15.

22. Heckerling PS, Tape TG, Wigton RS, et al. Clinical prediction rule for pulmonary infiltrates. *Ann Intern Med*. 1990;113(9):664-670.

23. Wells PS, Ginsberg JS, Anderson DR, et al. Use of a clinical model for safe management of patients with suspected pulmonary embolism. *Ann Intern Med*. 1998;129(12):997-1005.

24. Buchsbaum DG, Buchanan RG, Centor RM, Schnoll SH, Lawton MJ. Screening for alcohol abuse using CAGE scores and likelihood ratios. *Ann Intern Med*. 1991;115(10):774-777.

25. Mann DM, Kannry JL, Edonyabo D, et al. Rationale, design, and implementation protocol of an electronic health record integrated clinical prediction rule (iCPR) randomized trial in primary care. *Implement Sci*. 2011;6:109.

26. Li AC, Kannry JL, Kushniruk A, et al. Integrating usability testing and think-aloud protocol analysis with "near-live" clinical simulations in evaluating clinical decision support. *Int J Med Inform*. 2012;81(11):761-772.

27. McGinn TG, McCullagh L, Kannry J, et al. Efficacy of an evidence-based clinical decision support in primary care practices: a randomized clinical trial. *JAMA Intern Med*. 2013;173(17):1584-1591.

28. Atlas SJ, Benzer TI, Borowsky LH, et al. Safely increasing the proportion of patients with community-acquired pneumonia treated as outpatients: an interventional trial. *Arch Intern Med*. 1998;158(12):1350-1356.

29. Yealy DM, Fine MJ, Auble TE. Translating the pneumonia severity index into practice: a trial to influence the admission decision [abstract]. *Ann Emerg Med*. 2002;9:361.

30. Yealy DM, Auble TE, Stone RA, et al. The emergency department community-acquired pneumonia trial: methodology of a quality improvement intervention. *Ann Emerg Med*. 2004;43(6):770-782.

31. Yealy DM, Auble TE, Stone RA, et al. Effect of increasing the intensity of implementing pneumonia guidelines: a randomized, controlled trial. *Ann Intern Med*. 2005;143(12):881-894.

32. Irwig L, Macaskill P, Glasziou P, Fahey M. Meta-analytic methods for diagnostic test accuracy. *J Clin Epidemiol*. 1995;48(1):119-130, discussion 131-132.

33. Bachmann LM, Haberzeth S, Steurer J, ter Riet G. The accuracy of the Ottawa knee rule to rule out knee fractures: a systematic review. *Ann Intern Med*. 2004;140(2):121-124.

34. Cameron C, Naylor CD. No impact from active dissemination of the Ottawa Ankle Rules: further evidence of the need for local implementation of practice guidelines. *CMAJ*. 1999;160(8):1165-1168.

35. Graham ID, Stiell IG, Laupacis A, et al. Awareness and use of the Ottawa ankle and knee rules in 5 countries: can publication alone be enough to change practice? *Ann Emerg Med*. 2001;37(3):259-266.

36. Straus SE, Tetroe JM, Graham ID. Knowledge translation is the use of knowledge in health care decision making. *J Clin Epidemiol*. 2011;64(1):6-10.

PROGNOSIS

20

Prognosis

Adrienne G. Randolph, Deborah J. Cook, and Gordon Guyatt

IN THIS CHAPTER

CLINICAL SCENARIO

You are a pediatrician expecting to see an infant who was born at 26 weeks' gestation tomorrow for her first outpatient clinic visit at 4 months after birth. You know the family well because you care for their older child who was born at 35 weeks' gestation and is now a healthy 3-year-old girl. This infant had a prolonged stay in the neonatal intensive care unit but required relatively minimal respiratory support during her first 3 weeks of life. The neonatologist told you that the infant did extremely well, experiencing none of the complications that often occur in extremely preterm infants. He also informs you that he warned the family, "Your baby is at risk for long-term neurocognitive and motor complications related to being born so prematurely. Although some babies born this prematurely grow up to lead normal lives, many have minor disabilities, and there is a nontrivial chance that your baby could develop moderate to severe disabilities." You have 5 other children in your pediatric practice born at less than 27 weeks of gestation; all of them have major neurodevelopmental problems. On the basis of your professional experience, you wonder if the neonatologist has presented the family with an overly optimistic outlook. You decide to check out the *evidence* for yourself.

FINDING THE EVIDENCE

You use your clinic's free Internet connection to access MEDLINE at the National Library of Medicine website via PubMed. To find the appropriate search terms for your population of interest, you first type "premature" in the *Medical Subject Headings* database and find that there is a term called "Infant, Extremely Premature" defined as a human infant born before 28 weeks' gestation. You select it and click on the related link for Clinical Queries. Under Clinical Study Categories, you choose the search filter "Prognosis" and limit the scope to "Narrow." This retrieves 31 clinical studies and 5 potential reviews. You first look for a *systematic review* but do not find one that is relevant for evaluating outcomes across multiple extremely premature infant *cohorts*. However, the second *primary study* in the search results seems promising: Neurodevelopmental Outcome of Extremely Preterm Infants at 2.5 Years After Active Perinatal Care in Sweden.[1] This study reports the cognitive, language, and motor development of a prospective cohort of a *consecutive sample* of extremely preterm infants born before 27 weeks' gestation in Sweden between 2004 and 2007.[1]

WHY AND HOW WE MEASURE PROGNOSIS

Clinicians help patients in 3 broad ways: diagnosing or ruling out medical and health-related problems, administering treatment that does more good than *harm*, and giving them an indication of what the future is likely to hold. Clinicians require studies of *prognosis*—those examining the possible *outcomes* of a disease and the probability with which they can be expected to occur—to achieve the second and third goals.

Knowledge about prognosis can help clinicians make the right treatment decisions. If a patient is likely to improve without intervention, clinicians should not recommend treatments, particularly those that are expensive or potentially toxic. If a patient is at low *risk* of adverse outcomes, even beneficial treatments may not be worthwhile. On the other hand, some patients will experience poor outcomes regardless of which treatments are offered by the clinician. Whatever the treatment possibilities, by understanding prognosis and presenting the expected future course of a patient's illness, clinicians can offer reassurance and hope or preparation for long-term disability or death.

To estimate a patient's prognosis, we examine outcomes in groups of patients with a similar clinical presentation. We may then refine our prognosis by looking at subgroups defined by demographic variables, such as age, and by *comorbidity* and decide in which subgroup the patient belongs. When these variables or factors influence which patients do better or worse, we call them *prognostic factors*.

In this chapter, we focus on how to use articles that may contain trustworthy prognostic information that clinicians will find useful for counseling patients (Box 20-1).

HOW SERIOUS IS THE RISK OF BIAS?

Was the Sample of Patients in a Study Representative?

Bias has to do with systematic differences from the truth. A prognostic study is biased if it systematically overestimates or underestimates the likelihood of adverse outcomes in the group of patients under study. When a study sample is systematically different from the population of interest and is biased because patients will have a better or worse prognosis than those in the population of interest, we label the sample as unrepresentative.

How can you recognize an unrepresentative sample? First, determine whether patients pass through some sort of filter before entering the study. If they do, the result is likely a sample that is systematically different from the underlying population of interest. One such filter is the sequence of referrals that leads patients from primary to tertiary centers. Tertiary centers often care for patients with rare and unusual disorders or increased illness severity. Research describing the outcomes of patients in tertiary centers may not be applicable to the general patient with the disorder in the community (otherwise known as *referral bias*).

As an example, chronic hepatitis caused by infection with hepatitis C virus (HCV) can, after many years, lead to liver fibrosis, cirrhosis, and even hepatocellular carcinoma. Researchers have found that rates of progression to cirrhosis as diagnosed by liver biopsy can vary markedly, depending on how the patients are recruited.[2] For a group of

---

---

patients coming from the same demographic areas or health care settings, the mean estimated 20-year probability of progression to cirrhosis from their initial liver biopsy varied from 6% to 12% to 23%, depending, respectively, on whether the patients were recruited from a population-based posttransfusion HCV surveillance registry, referrals to general hospitals, or a tertiary referral center.[2] Those in a tertiary referral cohort may have other *risk factors* that predispose them to develop cirrhosis at higher rates than other patients.

Were the Patients Classified Into Prognostically Similar Groups?

Prognostic studies are most useful if individual members of the entire group of study participants are similar enough that the outcome of the group is applicable to each participant. This will be true only if patients are at a similar well-described point in their disease process. The point in the clinical course need not be early, but it does need to be consistent.

For instance, studies that evaluate the prognosis of patients with spinal cord injury could focus on in-hospital mortality right after the acute injury, patient outcomes after initial transfer to a rehabilitation center, or the ability of a group of patients to cope independently from the point of discharge to home.

After ensuring that patients were at the same disease stage, you must consider other factors that might influence patient outcome. If factors such as age or disease severity influence prognosis, then providing a single prognosis for young and old and those with mild and severe disease will be misleading for each of these subgroups. For instance, a study that evaluated the outcomes of 8 509 patients with traumatic brain injury[3] found that for each increase in age equal to the interquartile range of the patients (24 years), there was approximately double the risk of an unfavorable outcome (death or severe or moderate disability) at 6 months after injury. Patients with a more severe initial neurologic presentation as indicated by bilateral or unilateral absence of pupillary reactivity and those with no response or extensor response on the motor activity subcategory of the Glasgow Coma Scale also had markedly higher risk of having an unfavorable outcome. The percentage of patients having an unfavorable outcome at 6 months increased from 35% to 59% to 77% for patients in whom both pupils, 1 pupil, or neither pupil, respectively, was reactive on initial evaluation. Providing an overall intermediate prognosis across the entire study group (a 48% chance of an unfavorable outcome) to the family of a 20-year-old man who presented with reactive pupils could profoundly mislead them.

Not only must investigators consider all important prognostic factors, they must also consider prognostic factors in relation to one another. If sickness but not age truly determines outcome, and sicker patients tend to be older, investigators who fail to simultaneously consider age and severity of illness may mistakenly conclude that age is an important prognostic factor. For example, investigators in the Framingham study examined risk factors for stroke.[4] They reported that the rate of stroke in patients with atrial fibrillation and rheumatic heart disease was 41 per 1 000 person-years, which was similar to the rate for patients with atrial fibrillation but without rheumatic heart disease. Patients with rheumatic heart disease were, however, much younger than those who did not have rheumatic heart disease. To properly understand the influence of rheumatic heart disease, investigators in these circumstances must consider separately the relative risk of stroke in young people with and without rheumatic disease and the risk of stroke in elderly people with and without rheumatic disease. We call this separate consideration an *adjusted analysis*. Once adjustments were made for age, the investigators found that the rate of stroke was 6-fold greater in patients with rheumatic heart disease and atrial fibrillation than in patients with atrial fibrillation who did not have rheumatic heart disease.

If a large number of variables have a major effect on prognosis, investigators should use statistical techniques, such as *regression analysis*, to determine the most powerful predictors. Such an analysis may lead to a *clinical decision rule* that guides clinicians in simultaneously considering all of the important prognostic factors (see Chapter 19.4, Clinical Prediction Rules).

How can you decide whether the groups are sufficiently similar with respect to their risk? On the basis of your clinical experience and your understanding of the biology of the condition under study, can you think of factors that the investigators have neglected that are likely to define subgroups with very different prognoses? To the extent that the answer is yes, the risk of bias increases.

Was Study Follow-up Sufficiently Complete?

Investigators who lose track of a large number of patients increase the risk of bias associated with their prognostic study. The reason is that those who are followed up may have systematically higher or lower risk than those not followed up. As the number of patients who do not return for *follow-up* increases, the risk of bias also increases.

How many patients *lost to follow-up* is too many? The answer depends on the association between the proportion of patients who are lost and the proportion of patients who have had the adverse outcome of interest—the larger the number of patients whose fate is unknown relative to the number who have had the adverse event, the greater the risk of bias. For instance, let us assume that 30% of a particularly high-risk group (such as elderly patients with diabetes) have had an adverse outcome (such as cardiovascular death) during long-term follow-up in a study. If 10% of the patients have been lost to follow-up, the true rate of patients who had died may be as low as approximately 27% or as high as 37%. Across this range, the clinical implications would not change appreciably, and the loss to follow-up does not increase the risk of bias of the study. However, in a much lower-risk patient sample (otherwise healthy middle-aged patients, for instance), the observed event rate may be 1%. In this case, if we assumed that all 10% of the patients lost to follow-up had died, the event rate of 11% might have very different implications.

A large loss to follow-up constitutes a more serious risk of bias when the patients who are lost may be different from those who are easier to find. In one study, for example, investigators managed to follow up 180 of 186 patients treated for neurosis.[5] Of the 180 patients successfully followed up, 60% were easily traced. The death rate in these patients was 3%. The other 40% of the 180 were more difficult to find. The death rate in these patients was 27%.

Were Study Outcome Criteria Objective and Unbiased?

Outcome events may be objective and easily measured (eg, death), require some judgment (eg, myocardial infarction), or require considerable judgment and effort to measure (eg, disability, quality of life). Investigators should clearly specify and define their *target outcomes* and, whenever possible, base their criteria on objective measures.

The study of children with brain injury in a prolonged unconscious state provides a good example of the challenges involved in measuring outcome.[6] The study investigators found that children's family members frequently interpreted their interactions with the children with unfounded optimism. The investigators therefore required that family members' reports of development of a social response in the affected children be verified by study personnel.

USING THE GUIDE

Returning to our opening clinical scenario, the investigators who evaluated the outcome of extremely premature infants[1] captured the outcome of all infants born at less than 27 weeks' gestation in Sweden in a setting in which active perinatal care was available. This included easy and free access to care, a low threshold to provide life support at delivery, and transfer of extremely premature infants to specialized units in tertiary care centers. Because this is a population-based sample, it is likely to be representative and free of referral bias. The infants were classified into prognostic groups based on their gestational age at birth, which is known to be a strong prognostic factor. Of 707 extremely premature infants who were born alive, 497 (70%) were still alive at 1 year of age. Neurodevelopmental outcomes were assessed at 2.5 years of age in 456 (92%) of these infants. The most common nonmortality reason for loss to follow-up was an error in the identity number assigned at birth. Trained psychologists evaluated cognitive, language, and motor development using the Bayley Scales of Infant and Toddler Development (Bayley-III). Because the Bayley-III had not been standardized in Sweden, the investigators included a matched *control group* randomly selected from the Swedish Medical Birth Registry. Visual and hearing impairment and the development of cerebral palsy were evaluated by pediatric ophthalmologists and pediatric neurologists, respectively. Because the follow-up assessments were performed as part of clinical care, outcome assessors were not blinded to the fact that the patient was born extremely prematurely. Although knowledge of birth status could bias the assessment of future clinical outcomes, you are reassured that many of the assessments use standardized, objective criteria.

WHAT ARE THE RESULTS?

How Likely Are the Outcomes Over Time?

Results from studies of prognosis or risk are often reported as the proportion or percentage of patients with a certain outcome (eg, death, inability to walk, dependence on dialysis) after a certain period of time elapses (eg, 28 days, 3 months, 12 months, 5 years). A more informative way to depict these results is a *survival curve*, which is a graph of the number of events over time (or conversely, the chance of being free of these events over time) (see Chapter 9, Does Treatment Lower Risk? Understanding the Results). The events must be categorized as dichotomous variables, yes or no (eg, death, stroke, recurrence of cancer), and investigators must know the time at which the events occur. Figure 20-1 shows 2 survival curves: one of survival after a myocardial infarction[7] and the other of the need for revision surgery after hip replacement surgery.[8] The chance of dying after a myocardial infarction is highest shortly after the event (reflected by an initially steep downward slope of the curve, which then becomes flat), whereas few hip replacements require revision until much later (this curve, by contrast, starts out flat and then steepens).

How Precise Are the Estimates of Likelihood?

The more precise the estimate of prognosis a study provides, the more useful it is to us. Usually, authors report the risks of adverse outcomes with their associated 95% *confidence intervals* (CIs). If the study is unbiased, the 95% CI defines the range of risks within which it is highly likely that the true risk lies (see Chapter 10, Confidence Intervals: Was the Single Study or Meta-analysis Large Enough?). For example, a study of the prognosis of patients with dementia provided a 95% CI around the 49% estimate of survival at 5 years after presentation (ie, 39%-58%).[9] In most survival curves, the earlier follow-up periods usually include results from more patients than do the later periods (owing to losses to follow-up and because patients are not enrolled in the study at the same time), which means that the survival curves are usually more precise in the earlier periods, indicated by narrower confidence bands.

The number of patients evaluated and the number of events influence our confidence in the results. Table 20-1 reveals that in the case of extreme results (all or no patients have the outcome), confidence limits remain quite wide until the number of patients included is approximately 40 to 50, and they do not narrow until the numbers reach the hundreds.[10] When the numerator is 0 or 1 and there are at least

FIGURE 20-1

Survival Curves

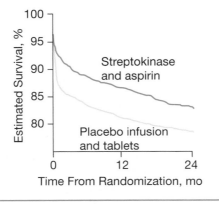 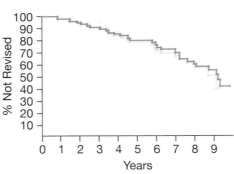

Left, Survival after myocardial infarction. Right, Results of hip replacement surgery: percentage of patients who survived without needing a new procedure (revision) after their initial hip replacement.

Reproduced from *The Lancet*,[7] Copyright ©1988, with permission from Elsevier (left). Reproduced from Dorey and Amstutz,[8] with permission from the *Journal of Bone and Joint Surgery* (right).

TABLE 20-1

95% Confidence Limits on Extreme Results[a]

If the denominator is:	And the % is 0%, the true % could be as high as:	And the % is 100%, the true % could be as low as:
1	95%	5%
2	78%	22%
3	63%	37%
4	53%	46%
5	45%	55%
10	26%	74%
25	11%	89%
50	6%	94%
100	3%	97%
150	2%	98%
300	1%	99%

[a]Adapted from Sackett et al.[10]

30 patients in the sample, a simple equation called "the rule of 3s" can be applied, where 100×3 divided by the number of patients estimates the upper limit of the 95% CI.[11]

USING THE GUIDE

Of the 456 children in the study who survived to 2.5 years of age whose neurodevelopment could be assessed, 42% were classified as healthy, 31% had mild disabilities, and 27% had moderate or severe disabilities.[1] However, the proportion of children with mild or no disabilities increased from 40% at 22 weeks to 83% at 26 weeks. Boys were at higher risk of moderate to severe disabilities (31%) than girls (23%). Figure 20-2 shows the mean Bayley-III composite cognitive, language, and motor scores at 2.5 years of corrected age according to gestational age at birth and compared with the control group. You are pleased to see in Figure 20-2 that the 99% confidence limits for the infants born at 26 completed weeks of pregnancy are fairly tight, in part because the number of patients in that group is the largest (n = 148), compared with the very wide CIs in the group of infants born at 23 weeks' gestation (n = 37).

HOW CAN I APPLY THE RESULTS TO PATIENT CARE?

Were the Study Patients and Their Management Similar to Those in My Practice?

Authors should describe the study patients explicitly and in sufficient detail that you can make a comparison with your patients. One factor sometimes neglected in prognostic studies that could strongly influence outcome is therapy. Therapeutic strategies often vary markedly among institutions and change over time as new treatments become available or old treatments regain popularity. In fact, investigators studying the cohort of extremely premature infants later reported major differences in 1-year mortality across health care regions in Sweden due to variation in perinatal practices.[12]

Was Follow-up Sufficiently Long?

Because the presence of illness often precedes the development of an outcome event by a long period, investigators must follow up patients for a period long enough to detect the outcomes of interest. For example, recurrence in some women with early breast cancer can occur many years after initial diagnosis and treatment.[13] A prognostic study may

FIGURE 20-2

Mean Bayley Scales of Infant and Toddler Development Composite Cognitive, Language, and Motor Scores at 2.5 Years of Corrected Age for Extremely Preterm Children by Gestational Age at Birth and for the Term Control Group[1]

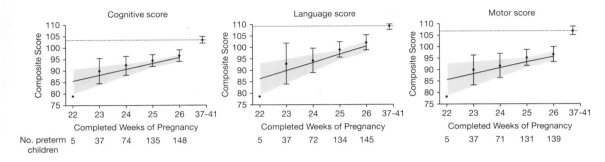

The diagonal line indicates the mean of the controls and the vertical bars represent the 99% confidence intervals (CIs) of the mean values. The regression lines with 99% CIs for respective scores of children in the preterm group are based on these equations in which GA indicates gestational age in completed weeks: cognitive score = 83.12 + (GA − 21) × 2.517, $P < .001$; language score = 82.78 + (GA − 21) × 3.551, $P < .001$; and motor score = 83.24 + (GA − 21) × 2.523, $P = .001$.

Reproduced from Serenius et al,[1] *JAMA* 2013.

provide an unbiased assessment of outcome during a short period if it meets the risk of bias criteria in Box 20-1, but it may be of little use if a patient is interested in prognosis during a long period.

Can I Use the Study Results in the Management of Patients in My Practice?

Prognostic data often provide the basis for sensible decisions about therapy. Even if the prognostic result does not help with selection of the appropriate therapy, it can help you in counseling a concerned patient or relative. Some conditions, such as asymptomatic hiatal hernia or asymptomatic colonic diverticulae, have such a good overall prognosis that they have been termed nondisease.[14] On the other hand, a result of uniformly bad prognosis could provide a clinician with a starting place for a discussion with a patient and family, leading to counseling about end-of-life care.

CLINICAL SCENARIO RESOLUTION

The active perinatal and follow-up care described in the study of extremely premature infants appears similar to the excellent prenatal care and neonatal intensive care that your patient received. Assuming that the same level of intensive follow-up care is provided, you conclude that the study is likely to provide a good estimate of the prognosis of the child under your care. As a pediatrician and parent, you know that many cognitive issues are not detected until a child begins elementary school, where learning issues sometimes reveal themselves. Although it would be ideal if the cohort were followed up to 6 years of age, you realize that more patients would

likely be lost to follow-up. One issue that bothered you is that many of the children died before reaching 2.5 years of age. With further investigation, you are reassured that approximately 84% of those born at 25 to 26 weeks' gestation survived to 2.5 years of age; most of the deaths occurred in those born at 22 to 23 weeks' gestation (approximately 38% survived to 2.5 years). You conclude that you agree with the neonatologist. At this point, this female infant has a nontrivial chance of having moderate to severe disabilities, a substantial chance of having minor disabilities, and even some chance of developing normally without neurocognitive disability.

References

1. Serenius F, Källén K, Blennow M, et al; EXPRESS Group. Neurodevelopmental outcome in extremely preterm infants at 2.5 years after active perinatal care in Sweden. *JAMA*. 2013;309(17):1810-1820.

2. Sweeting MJ, De Angelis D, Neal KR, et al; Trent HCV Study Group; HCV National Register Steering Group. Estimated progression rates in three United Kingdom hepatitis C cohorts differed according to method of recruitment. *J Clin Epidemiol*. 2006;59(2):144-152.

3. Steyerberg EW, Mushkudiani N, Perel P, et al. Predicting outcome after traumatic brain injury: development and international validation of prognostic scores based on admission characteristics. *PLoS Med*. 2008;5(8):e165, discussion e165.

4. Wolf PA, Dawber TR, Thomas HE Jr, Kannel WB. Epidemiologic assessment of chronic atrial fibrillation and risk of stroke: the Framingham study. *Neurology*. 1978;28(10):973-977.

5. Sims AC. Importance of a high tracing-rate in long-term medical follow-up studies. *Lancet*. 1973;2(7826):433-435.

6. Kriel RL, Krach LE, Jones-Saete C. Outcome of children with prolonged unconsciousness and vegetative states. *Pediatr Neurol*. 1993;9(5):362-368.

7. ISIS-2 (Second International Study of Infarct Survival) Collaborative Group. Randomised trial of intravenous streptokinase, oral aspirin, both, or neither among 17,187 cases of suspected acute myocardial infarction: ISIS-2. ISIS-2 (Second International Study of Infarct Survival) Collaborative Group. *Lancet*. 1988;2(8607):349-360.

8. Dorey F, Amstutz HC. The validity of survivorship analysis in total joint arthroplasty. *J Bone Joint Surg Am*. 1989;71(4):544-548.

9. Walsh JS, Welch HG, Larson EB. Survival of outpatients with Alzheimer-type dementia. *Ann Intern Med*. 1990;113(6):429-434.

10. Sackett DL, Haynes RB, Guyatt GH, Tugwell P. *Clinical Epidemiology: A Basic Science for Clinical Medicine*. 2nd ed. Toronto, Ontario: Little Brown & Company; 1991.

11. Hanley JA, Lippman-Hand A. If nothing goes wrong, is everything all right? interpreting zero numerators. *JAMA*. 1983;249(13):1743-1745.

12. Serenius F, Sjörs G, Blennow M, et al; EXPRESS study group. EXPRESS study shows significant regional differences in 1-year outcome of extremely preterm infants in Sweden. *Acta Paediatr*. 2014;103(1):27-37.

13. Early Breast Cancer Trialists' Collaborative Group. Systemic treatment of early breast cancer by hormonal, cytotoxic, or immune therapy. 133 randomised trials involving 31,000 recurrences and 24,000 deaths among 75,000 women. *Lancet*. 1992;339(8784):1-15.

14. Meador CK. The art and science of nondisease. *N Engl J Med*. 1965;272:92-95.

JAMAevidence
Using Evidence to Improve Care

21.1

ADVANCED TOPICS IN PROGNOSIS

How to Use an Article About Genetic Association

Elizabeth G. Holliday, John P. A. Ioannidis, Ammarin Thakkinstian, Mark McEvoy, Rodney J. Scott, Cosetta Minelli, John Thompson, Claire Infante-Rivard, Gordon Guyatt, and John Attia

IN THIS CHAPTER

(continued on following page)

INTRODUCTION

This chapter is a guide for clinicians using *genetic association studies* to inform their clinical practice. In this chapter, which is restricted to genetic association studies and does not deal with other types of designs, such as genetic *linkage* studies, we begin by summarizing the key concepts in genetics that are the necessary basis for understanding genetic association studies. We then introduce the idea of genetic association for both single-candidate gene and *genome-wide association studies* (GWASs). We use the *APOE* gene *polymorphism* and its association with Alzheimer disease as a case study to demonstrate the concepts and introduce the terms used in this field.

We then enumerate the major issues in judging the *validity* of these studies, including disease *phenotype* definition and potential differences between diseased and nondiseased groups, with a focus on ethnicity and the potential for population stratification. We discuss methods for evaluating the trustworthiness of genetic marker data, including assessment of Hardy-Weinberg equilibrium. We also discuss issues related to multiple comparisons.

Finally, we review issues related to applicability of the results to clinical practice. We provide guidance for evaluating the size and precision of genetic associations and whether the knowledge of genetic associations improves predictive power beyond easily measured clinical variables. We discuss absolute vs relative effects because even a strong genetic *risk* in relative terms may correspond with a very low *absolute risk*. We also discuss approaches to evaluating whether a particular genetic risk *allele* is likely to be present in a given patient. Finally, we provide guidelines for deciding whether a patient is likely better off in knowing the genetic information. Given that genes cannot be modified, one must weigh whether the genetic information is likely to be helpful in planning other health interventions or initiating behavior change.

The Human Genome Project has stimulated interest in genetic determinants of disease. The determinants of common mendelian diseases that involve a single gene (eg, cystic fibrosis, Huntington disease) are well established. More recent research addresses the role of genetics in major causes of human morbidity and mortality through chronic diseases that result from the concomitant effect of environmental, behavioral, and genetic factors. Since 2007, investigators have tested millions of genetic variations (polymorphisms) in GWASs, trying to establish the genetic determinants of chronic diseases, such as coronary artery disease,[1-3] type 2 diabetes,[4-6] stroke,[7-9] multiple sclerosis,[10-12] breast cancer,[13,14] schizophrenia,[15] bipolar disorder,[16,17] rheumatoid arthritis,[18,19] Crohn disease,[16,20] and Alzheimer disease.[21-26] Published GWASs are catalogued in the National Institutes of Health's Catalog of Published Genome-Wide Association Studies.[27] In March 2014, the catalog listed 1844 published GWASs, with 40 that addressed Alzheimer disease.

The basic construct of a gene-disease association study is relatively simple. In the same way that variation in an exposure (eg, cholesterol) is linked to a *health outcome* (eg, myocardial infarction) in a traditional epidemiologic study, variation in DNA sequence (eg, DNA variation in the cholesteryl ester transferase gene) is linked to an outcome (eg, myocardial infarction) in a genetic association study.

CLINICAL SCENARIO

A 55-year-old man consults you, worried about his risk of developing Alzheimer disease. His grandfather had Alzheimer disease in his 70s, and his father was diagnosed as having Alzheimer disease at 65 years of age. He has been a smoker since he was 20 years of age, works as an electrician, and has been taking antihypertensive medication (thiazide and a β-blocker) for the last 5 years. He has never had his cholesterol level checked. He recently read a news story about genetic tests and asks you whether he should have a genetic test for Alzheimer disease risk, in particular for a gene called *APOE*, and what this means for his risk of developing Alzheimer disease.

FINDING THE EVIDENCE

A colleague with an interest in genetics steers you toward a helpful website, the HuGE Navigator,[28] and you find that there are more than 2600 publications on the associations of Alzheimer disease with more than 1500 genes; the whole endeavor seems daunting. Consulting a preappraised-evidence resource, you find a chapter on the genetics of Alzheimer disease. You come across words such as allele, *single-nucleotide polymorphism* (SNP), and genetic association study. You realize that you need to review your basic genetics knowledge and discover more about how to read genetic association studies.

BACKGROUND CONCEPTS

The Genetic Blueprint

In 1953, James Watson and Francis Crick proposed a spiral staircase (double helix) structure of DNA (Figure 21.1-1). The sides of the staircase—which also resembles a winding ladder—are called strands, and they are formed by alternating sugar (deoxyribose) and phosphate molecules; the rungs of the ladder are formed by 4 nitrogen-containing ring compounds called bases: adenine (A), thymine (T), guanine (G), and cytosine (C). A pair of these bases forms each rung of the ladder; adenine always binds to thymine and cytosine always binds to guanine to form the full rung. Thus, each rung of the helix ladder is called a base pair. A single base plus its associated sugar and phosphate groups is called a nucleotide.

One long stretch of double-stranded DNA, forming the spiral staircase, constitutes 1 chromosome, on which there are many genes, a gene being a stretch of DNA that typically codes for 1 protein. Twenty-three chromosomes in the sperm and the corresponding 23 chromosomes in the egg come together at fertilization to form the entire DNA set of a human, called the *genome*. Each person therefore has 23 pairs of chromosomes, of which 1 pair are the sex chromosomes, which determine sex. The other 22 pairs are numbered 1 to 22, providing each person with 2 versions of each gene, 1 on the maternally inherited and 1 on the paternally inherited chromosome (Figure 21.1-2).

DNA is the blueprint for making the proteins that build cells and tissues, as well as the enzymes that catalyze biochemical reactions within a cell. The information encoded within DNA is used to produce proteins via a 2-step process of transcription and translation.

The first step involves transcribing DNA into messenger RNA (mRNA) within the cell nucleus (Figure 21.1-3). The mRNA molecule then migrates out of the nucleus to the cytoplasm to reach the protein-building machinery of the cell, known as the *ribosome*. Here, during the second step, the mRNA molecule is translated into protein, using the code to link amino acids one at a time. These processes of transcription and translation convert the genetic information contained within a gene into a protein that, in concert with other genes and their proteins, regulatory molecules, and environmental exposures, determines the final attribute: the phenotype (eg, hair color, height, thrombophilia).

Human Variation

Sequencing the human genome—identifying the entire sequence of base pairs in human DNA—has revealed that the genomic sequence is more than 99% identical across different people.[29] The human genome, however, includes 3.3 billion base pairs; thus, even with this high level of similarity, there are still tens of millions of potential variations between the genomes of any 2 people.[30-32] Differences in sequence that occur infrequently in populations (eg, <1%) are often called low-frequency variants, whereas differences that occur more frequently (eg, ≥1%) are called common variants. These variants, or polymorphisms, may take a number of different forms (Figure 21.1-4).

1. Variation in the identity of a single-base pair is called a SNP (pronounced snip). This is by far the most common type of polymorphism, and scientists have cataloged more than 35 million SNPs to date.[32] Because detecting SNPs is relatively easy and they are responsible for most of the genetic

FIGURE 21.1-1

Components and Structure of DNA

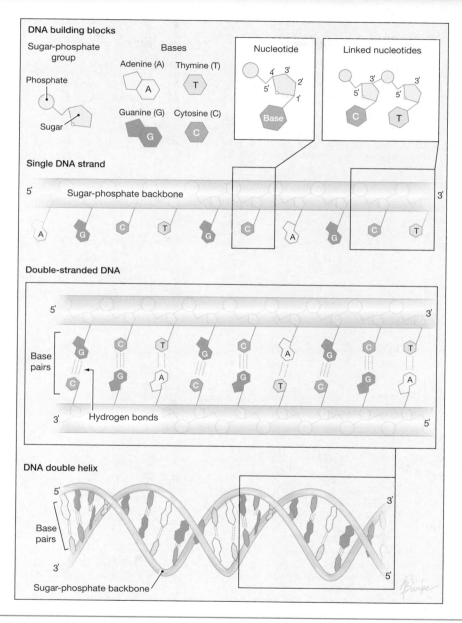

The building block of DNA is the nucleotide—a sugar (deoxyribose) with a phosphate group at the 5′ carbon and a base (adenine, thymine, guanine, or cytosine) at the 1′ carbon. Nucleotides link together by a bond between the phosphate group of one nucleotide and the 3′ carbon of the previous nucleotide to form a single DNA strand with a resulting directionality of 5′ to 3′. Two strands with opposite directionality combine to form a double helix that is held together by hydrogen bonds across the bases. Adenine always binds to thymine, and guanine always binds to cytosine. The sequence of base pairs encodes the genetic information.

FIGURE 21.1-2

Human Male Karyotype, Chromosome Structure and Mapping, and Location of *APOE*

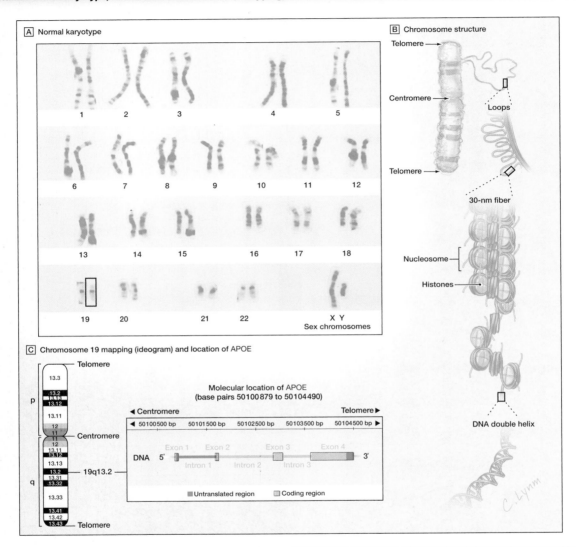

A, Typically, an individual has 23 pairs of chromosomes. One member of each pair is inherited from the mother and one from the father. Chromosomes shown in the karyotype were obtained when the cell was not dividing, stained using Giemsa, and ordered by size. B, The DNA double helix is wound around proteins called histones to form small packages called nucleosomes. The nucleosomes in turn are wound around themselves to form loops that make up the chromosome. The region of the chromosome near the center is called the centromere, and each end is called a telomere. C, The centromere is not exactly at the center of the chromosome, resulting in a shorter arm, named p for *petit* (French for small), and a longer arm, named q. Chromosome 19 is the site of the *APOE* gene, which is composed of sequences with regulatory functions (untranslated regions) and sequences with coding functions. Regions of the gene that are spliced out during transcription to messenger RNA are called introns. The remaining regions, exons, contain the sequences that code for the final protein product.

FIGURE 21.1-3

Transcription and Translation

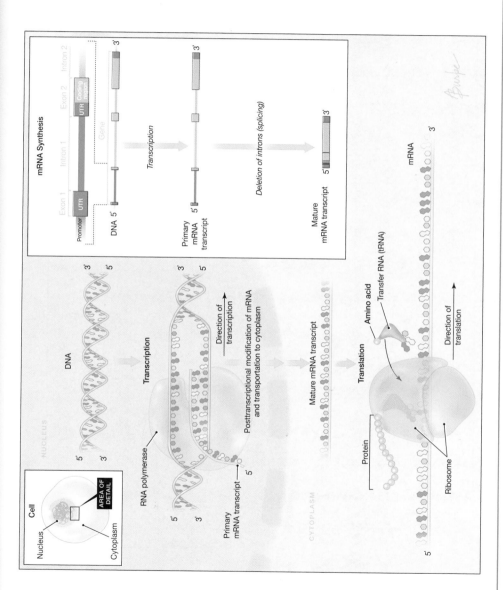

During transcription, the DNA double helix is split apart, and RNA polymerase synthesizes messenger RNA (mRNA) using one DNA strand as a template. Sections of the primary mRNA transcript, called introns, are spliced out to form the mature mRNA, which moves into the cytoplasm. The ribosome uses the mRNA sequence to build the protein. A specific sequence of 3 bases codes for each amino acid, which is delivered to the ribosome by transfer RNA. UTR indicates untranslated region.

FIGURE 21.1-4

Common (Wild-Type) Allele and 4 Types of Genetic Polymorphisms

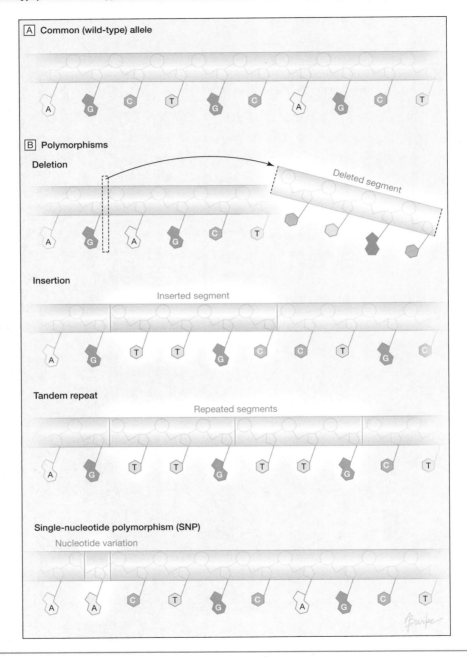

DNA polymorphisms include deletions, in which a DNA sequence is missing compared with the common allele, and insertions, in which a DNA sequence is added compared with the common allele. Repeats may also occur in which the same sequence repeats multiple times. Depending on the size of the repeating unit and the number of repeats, these variants may have different names, such as satellites, microsatellites, minisatellites, or copy number variants. Single-nucleotide polymorphisms (SNPs), variations at a single base-pair location, are the most common type of polymorphism in the human genome.

variation in humans, they have been the focus of most of the research exploring gene-disease associations. Some SNPs are in parts of the gene that are translated (ie, code for protein; among them, nonsynonymous SNPs lead to a change in amino acid sequence of the resultant protein, whereas synonymous SNPs do not result in amino acid change). Other SNPs are in areas of the chromosome that do not directly code for protein but may influence cellular functions through other means, such as controlling the amount of the protein that the cell builds. Given the very large number of SNPs, their nomenclature can be confusing, but the most common system uses a number with the prefix "rs" (for *reference SNP*) (eg, rs1228756).

2. Copy number variations can be divided into 3 main types. First, the insertion or deletion of short stretches of DNA sequence is called insertion or deletion polymorphisms or indels. More than 1 million short indels now have been cataloged.[32] Second, the deletion or duplication of relatively large stretches of DNA sequence results in variation in the number of repeated sequences, or copy number variants. Third, short stretches of DNA sequence (often 2 to 5 base pairs) can be repeated head-to-tail numerous times (from several up to 100 or more); such variants are known as short tandem repeats. Variant forms differ in the number of times the sequence is repeated.

3. Inversions in the order of the DNA sequence at a particular genomic location may involve a few base pairs to as many as 100 000 base pairs.

The different forms, or variants, that a particular polymorphism may take are called *alleles*. For example, the *APOE* gene in the clinical scenario has 3 alleles, named e2, e3, and e4 (e for epsilon; for historical reasons, there is no e1). According to this nomenclature, this polymorphism represents the combination of 2 different type 1 polymorphisms (SNPs), each of which is a nonsynonymous SNP that alters the amino acid sequence of the resultant protein. The location along the DNA strand at which a particular allele is present is called a *locus*. Geneticists decided to call the form of the gene that is most common in the population the *wild-type allele*; we use the less colorful term common allele, and we will call the less common alleles *variant*

alleles. Nonsynonymous SNPs, those in which different alleles result in the production of different forms of the protein, constitute only a small proportion of SNP alleles (most are synonymous). These different proteins are called *isoforms*.

The 3 alleles of the *APOE* gene lead to 3 protein isoforms. Of the *APOE* alleles, allele e3 is most common in white populations (78%) and thus represents the common allele; e2 and e4 are variant alleles (with a frequency of 6% and 16%, respectively, among white individuals). Physiologically, the apoE protein isoforms are plasma proteins that transport cholesterol. When these proteins bind apoE receptors on the surface of target cells, the cholesterol is taken into the cell and metabolized. Of the 3 protein isoforms corresponding to the 3 *APOE* alleles, the e2 isoform has less strength of binding, or affinity, to the apoE receptor relative to the e3 and e4 isoforms.

Because each person has 2 copies of each chromosome, 1 from the mother and 1 from the father, individuals have 2 *APOE* genes, 1 on each chromosome. The 2 chromosomes (in the case of *APOE*, chromosome 19) may both carry the e3 allele (denoted *e3/e3*) or 1 each of the e3 and e2 alleles (denoted *e2/e3*) or any other combination (eg, *e2/e4*, *e3/e3*). This shorthand denotes the genotype of the individual. Individuals with 2 copies of the same allele are said to be *homozygous* or a homozygote (ie, an individual with *e3/e3* is homozygous for e3 or an e3 homozygote). An individual with 2 different alleles (eg, *e2/e3*) is a heterozygote or *heterozygous*.

Individuals with *e2/e3* produce some e2 protein and some e3 protein. The question then follows: which protein function wins? If the variant allele is *dominant*, it need be present in only 1 of the 2 genes to carry all of its biological activity. In such cases, the allele on the other chromosome will remain biologically "silent." Conversely, an allele that is *recessive* will need to be present on both genes (homozygous) to affect function; it otherwise will remain silent. If neither of 2 differing protein isoforms resulting from 2 different alleles (eg, e2, e3) is dominant, the model of protein function is known as an *additive*, or per-allele, model. These dominant, recessive, and additive models are called models of inheritance or genetic models.

As it turns out, the *APOE* alleles act in an additive manner; thus, *e2/e3* individuals have overall apoE function that is partway between the reduced affinity of an e2 homozygote and the higher affinity of an e3 homozygote. With most genetic association studies for complex diseases, the underlying inheritance model remains unknown.

Examining Genes at the Population Level

In genetics, it is usual to describe the distribution of the alleles of interest in the population. In the same way that most continuous variables in medicine observe a normal distribution, most allele distributions observe what is called Hardy-Weinberg equilibrium (HWE). The Hardy-Weinberg law states that if there are 2 alleles at a particular locus, denoted A and a, with frequency p and q, respectively, then after 1 generation of random mating from the occurrence of the variation, the genotype frequencies of the *AA*, *Aa*, and *aa* combinations in the population will be p^2, $2pq$, and q^2, respectively, and that these genotype frequencies will remain constant in the population over time. Given that there are only 2 alleles possible, A or a, then $p + q = 1$. In turn, given the 3 possible genotypes—*AA*, *Aa*, and *aa*—then $p^2 + 2pq + q^2 = 1$. It is general practice in a genetic association study to check whether the allele frequencies observe HWE proportions.

Deviations from HWE in the population may be due to a number of population effects. (1) Inbreeding (ie, marrying close relatives) causes deviations because HWE depends on random mating. (2) Genetic drift refers to a process in which a population is isolated, with a limited number of possible matings (forced inbreeding). (3) Migration also can cause deviations in HWE. (4) Very new mutations can upset HWE, but equilibrium is usually reached within 1 generation in a sufficiently large population (the "equilibrium" in HWE). (5) Selection also can result in HWE deviation (eg, a selective disadvantage of a particular allele that leads to fetal death).

Deviations from HWE may signal methodologic problems within a genetic study, including issues with genotyping quality (eg, laboratory error) or population stratification, which could *bias* the results of a genetic association study. We will tell you what we mean by population stratification later in this chapter.

Candidate Gene vs Genome-wide Approaches

Investigators conducting genetic association studies may target genes for investigation according to the known or postulated biology and previous results, an approach known as candidate gene association, evaluated in *candidate gene studies*.

Alternatively, they may screen the entire genome for associations, an approach that has, in recent years, transformed the field of genetic association studies. These studies involve investigating hundreds of thousands (up to millions) of SNPs across the entire genome, without any previous hypotheses about potential candidates and their mechanism of action. This type of "agnostic" approach, termed a GWAS, has accelerated the pace of discovery of genetic associations, although some discoveries ultimately may prove to be false.[33-35]

As discussed in the next section in this chapter, testing so many potential genes carries the risk of finding many spurious associations. For this reason, SNPs with apparently strong signals in an initial GWAS are then tested for replication in independent studies. To ensure that the discoveries are not just statistical flukes, replication studies are often published along with the initial data.[16] The boundaries between candidate gene studies and agnostic GWASs can become blurred, and the 2 types of studies are not mutually exclusive: GWASs propose new candidates for replication but also may be used to confirm and estimate with higher precision the effects of prior apparent discoveries.

Whether hypothesis-driven or agnostic genetic association studies usually represent population-based investigations in which diseased and non-diseased individuals are unrelated. Genetic studies (either candidate or genome-wide) also may be performed within families in which multiple individuals are affected by a particular disease. The methods and interpretation of family studies differ radically from those of population-based studies,[36,37] and this article is restricted to discussion of the latter.

Linkage Disequilibrium

One goal of traditional epidemiology, elucidating causation, can be frustrated by noncausal associations. Traditional epidemiology tries to deal with this problem by *adjusted analyses* or *multivariable analysis*.

For example, an apparent association between obesity and stroke may not be due to obesity at all but rather to the higher incidence of smoking and diabetes in the obese. To deal with this problem, investigators will adjust for potential *confounding variables*, including age, sex, smoking, and obesity (see Chapter 6, Why Study Results Mislead: Bias and Random Error, and Chapter 14, Harm [Observational Studies]).

In genetic association studies, the goal may be to establish whether a SNP is causally associated with the outcome (eg, presence or absence of disease). This requires isolating the function of a particular SNP from the other SNPs that may be nearby in the gene. In practice, because stretches of the genome tend to be inherited together as a unit (a phenomenon known as *linkage disequilibrium*), this may be difficult. Thus, the association of a SNP with a disease, no matter how strong, cannot be considered a definitive causal link. It is possible, even likely, that some other SNP in linkage disequilibrium with the SNP under study is the true causal variable. Although this is an important distinction if the aim is to understand the underlying biology, it is not critical if the aim is to use the SNP simply as a marker of risk.

Stretches of DNA may be characterized by the presence of high linkage disequilibrium, or *correlation*, among the SNPs present. Two or more SNP alleles in linkage disequilibrium are called *haplotypes*, specific combinations of SNP alleles that tend to be inherited together.

As a hypothetical example, consider SNP A with a common allele frequency of 80% and SNP B with a common allele frequency of 60%. If there is no linkage disequilibrium (correlation) between SNP A and SNP B, allele A at SNP A and allele B at SNP B will be found together on a particular chromosome $0.80 \times 0.60 = 48\%$ of the time (ie, consistent with chance). With perfect linkage disequilibrium (eg, where the SNPs are very close together and always inherited together), it may happen that allele A is always found with allele B. The extent of this linkage disequilibrium may be expressed in different ways, commonly using metrics such as r^2 (a squared *correlation coefficient*), where 0 indicates that the alleles are found together no more often than chance and 1.0 means the alleles are always found together.

Armed with this background knowledge of genetic concepts and terms, you are now ready to evaluate the risk of bias, results, and applicability in genetic association studies. The remaining 2 sections in this chapter will address these issues.

USING THE GUIDE

You return to the chapter on the genetics of Alzheimer disease in the preappraised-evidence resource. Among the references cited, you choose a study based on its size (n = 6852), length of *follow-up* (up to 9 years), sample selection (a general, community-based population 55 years and older),[38] and choice of study design (*cohort* rather than *case-control;* see Chapter 14, Harm [Observational Studies]). The authors report a *relative risk* of 2.2 (95% *confidence interval* [CI], 1.6-2.9) for Alzheimer disease in *APOE e3/e4* heterozygotes and 7.0 (95% CI, 4.1-11.9) for *APOE e4* homozygotes compared with *e3/e3* individuals. They also report a cumulative, absolute risk of Alzheimer disease or vascular dementia by 80 years of age of approximately 15% to 20% for *APOE e4* heterozygotes and 40% to 50% for *APOE e4* homozygous individuals.

Initial Reports Tend to Overestimate Associations

Initial epidemiologic studies that addressed a novel association tend to overestimate the magnitude of association.[39] In candidate gene studies or studies in which only a few variants are examined, this commonly occurs as a result of *publication bias*: studies that address previously unreported associations are published only if they have significant results.[40] In GWASs, overestimation of genetic *effect sizes* is more likely to reflect the "winner's curse"—that is, an apparently exciting finding that, unfortunately, is due to chance.[41]

The investigators in a GWAS hope that by setting stringent threshold *P* values for declaring an association, they protect themselves from chance associations. Unfortunately, this is not so. Picture a situation in which a particular genetic variant has a weak association with an outcome of interest (such as Alzheimer disease) in a population. The association between this variant and disease will appear strongest in those individual studies that, simply by chance, reveal the largest differences in the frequency of this genetic variant between disease cases and unaffected controls. Thus, the population of studies with "positive" results will yield an upwardly biased estimate of genetic effects, and we should be conservative in interpreting genetic associations for newly discovered variants.[42] The result is that publication of all of the relevant studies, and their simultaneous consideration, is required for an accurate picture of the magnitude of the association.

STRUCTURE OF THIS GUIDE

We adopt the 3-step process used in other chapters of this book: (1) How serious is the risk of bias? (2) What are the results? (3) Will the results help me in caring for my patients? (Box 21.1-1)

HOW SERIOUS IS THE RISK OF BIAS?

Similar to traditional prognostic or etiologic studies, genetic association studies may use cohort or case-control designs (see Chapter 14, Harm [Observational Studies], and Chapter 20, Prognosis). Cohort studies sample a group of people (eg, older individuals) who vary in their genetic characteristics (eg, *APOE e2/e2, e2/e3, e2/e4*) and follow them forward in time to determine who has the outcome of interest (eg, Alzheimer disease). In case-control studies, investigators choose affected individuals (case patients or those with Alzheimer disease) and a sample of unaffected individuals from the same underlying population and determine the genetic characteristics of the individuals in the 2 groups.

Case-control studies in traditional epidemiology are subject to a number of potential biases, many of which are less of a concern in genetic studies. In contrast to most environmental exposures, the genetic "exposure" does not vary with age or calendar year, there is no *recall bias* and no choice of exposure made by the participant, and the exposure is not influenced by disease (or treatment). The case-control design also facilitates larger case sample sizes and therefore power, which is particularly important for

---

BOX 21.1-1
Critical Appraisal Guide to Genetic Association Studies

How serious is the risk of bias?

Was the disease phenotype properly defined and accurately recorded by someone blind to the genetic information? Have any potential differences between diseased and nondiseased groups, particularly ethnicity, been properly addressed?

Was measurement of the genetic variants unbiased and accurate? Do the genotype proportions observe Hardy-Weinberg equilibrium?

Have the investigators adjusted their inferences for multiple comparisons?

Are the results consistent with those of other studies?

What are the results of the study?

How large and precise are the associations?

How can I apply the results to patient care?

Does the genetic association improve predictive power beyond easily measured clinical variables?

What are the absolute and relative effects? Is the risk-associated allele likely to be present in my patient?

Is the patient likely better off knowing the genetic information?

---

detecting potentially small genetic effects. In comparison, cohort designs typically result in smaller case numbers but can offer other advantages, including the assessment of outcome incidence, cumulative risks, and the investigation of multiple outcomes. Our discussion focuses on the biases of particular relevance for genetic studies.

Was the Disease Phenotype Properly Defined and Accurately Recorded by Someone Blind to the Genetic Information?

In the absence of a standardized definition of the disease or trait of interest, investigators may run association analyses with varying definitions and report only the most significant findings, resulting in spurious associations.[43] On the other hand, what appears at first glance to be a single disease entity may in fact consist of many genetically different but clinically similar diseases, which may introduce genetic heterogeneity. In this situation, inclusion of diseases with different genetic causes may dilute or obscure a true association.

Even if the disease definition is well standardized, it is important to ask whether the disease phenotype has been appropriately measured during the study. Misclassification (here, categorizing people as having Alzheimer disease when they do not or vice versa) may affect the strength of the genetic association. If the misclassification is a result of *random error*, the association will be diluted. If misclassification errors are influenced by previous knowledge of the genotype of each individual (eg, if the *APOE* genotype influences the diagnosis of Alzheimer disease, then the genetic effect may be overestimated). Thus, individuals conducting the phenotyping should be *blind* to the genotyping result (and vice versa).

USING THE GUIDE

In our clinical scenario, because different causes of late dementia are likely to have different genetic determinants, researchers who do not separate individuals with Alzheimer disease from those with vascular dementia (common) and Lewy body dementia (rare) may fail to establish genetic links. Slooter et al[38] separated Alzheimer disease from vascular dementia and used widely accepted definitions. Moreover, the investigators made meticulous efforts to minimize misclassification caused by measurement error by using a panel of several tests and by blinding appropriately.

Have Any Potential Differences Between Diseased and Nondiseased Groups, Particularly Ancestry, Been Properly Addressed?

As we have pointed out, some common variables that, in traditional epidemiologic studies, can cause bias as

a result of an association with the condition of interest and maldistribution in exposed and unexposed populations (we call such variables *confounders*) are less likely to introduce bias in genetic epidemiology. Genetic studies, however, may yield misleading results if their diseased and nondiseased populations include a different ethnic/racial mix; this particular form of confounding is referred to as population stratification. The problem occurs if the likelihood of developing the condition of interest, or the proportion of cases and controls, varies with ancestry. If ancestry groups also happen to differ in allele frequency of genetic polymorphisms unrelated to the condition of interest, the result will be misleading associations—the association, rather than being with the disease of interest, will really be with an ancestral group.

Most association studies of unrelated individuals try to avoid this problem by using populations that are homogeneous in terms of ancestry. Self-reporting may suffice for homogeneous European populations[16,44,45] but is unlikely to work well in the presence of ancestrally mixed populations, such as the US population. To address this issue, a number of techniques are available to check and correct for ancestral differences; these corrections use self-reported ethnicity, family-based controls, or statistical techniques, such as *principal components analysis* or genomic control to test for patterns in unlinked markers.[46,47] For example, a spurious association between the *CYP3A4-V* polymorphism and prostate cancer in blacks disappeared when results were adjusted for additional genetic markers associated with ancestry in the population studied.[48]

Ancestry is not the only potential factor that may influence the interpretation of an identified genetic association. For example, 2 GWASs found an association between type 2 diabetes and a SNP in the *FTO* gene (associated with fat mass and obesity).[4,49] These studies selected patients with diabetes and controls irrespective of their body mass index (BMI); another study that matched patients with diabetes and controls on BMI found no association. Thus, although the study accurately identified the association between diabetes and the particular SNP, the causal association is probably between the candidate allele and BMI regulation/obesity rather than type 2 diabetes. In other words, the causal path is that the allele predisposes to obesity and obesity predisposes to diabetes. There is no direct causal connection between the allele and diabetes. In this case, the association is real, but the causal inference is spurious.

When considering issues of causation, clinicians should consider whether diseased and nondiseased groups were similar with respect to other important characteristics that are likely to be genetically determined and associated with the outcome of interest. Alternatively, they may determine whether the investigators adjusted for such characteristics in their statistical analysis.

USING THE GUIDE

Returning to the clinical scenario, one might imagine that ancestry and alcoholism are characteristics that are both genetically influenced and that would be associated with Alzheimer disease. Slooter et al[38] recruited their entire cohort from among the white population of the Netherlands, which is likely a homogeneous group with little genetic variability; this is verified by results from a recent GWAS from the same cohort.[50] They did not, however, consider alcohol history, which could potentially confound the *APOE*-Alzheimer association if the *APOE* polymorphisms, or variants correlated with these polymorphisms, were also associated with alcoholism.

Was Measurement of the Genetic Variants Unbiased and Accurate?

Genotyping error threatens the validity of genetic association studies. Genotyping may go wrong if there is a problem with the biological material (eg, the samples) or with the application of the molecular technique that is used to determine the alleles.

The biological material used for genotyping may differ between diseased and nondiseased participants in ways that lead to genotyping inaccuracies. For example, in a GWAS of type 2 diabetes, blood stored in 1958 provided the basis for genotyping nondiseased individuals, whereas blood drawn more recently was used for genotyping diseased individuals. The older blood resulted in genotyping errors[51] that led to some *false-positive* SNP associations.

Genotyping error may occur even when disease and nondisease samples are drawn and stored in identical ways. Although laboratory-based methods and DNA information may have the cachet of being absolute, these data are subject to error in the same way as traditional epidemiologic information. Genotyping error rates in candidate gene studies vary widely, from negligible to 30%,[52] and rates of up to a few percent were not uncommon in even the best studies.[53-55] Typically, GWASs have lower error rates, but they should still aim to minimize genotyping error and identify and remove any markers with high rates of error. Another useful piece of information is the proportion of samples in which the genotyping provides an unambiguous reading. If this proportion is not high, then information is lost. In GWASs, investigators should exclude SNPs with readings for less than a prespecified proportion of the sample, typically in the range of 95% to 98%. Even high rates can, however, fail to prevent bias if specific genotypes have lower rates than others (eg, if heterozygotes are more likely to produce ambiguous readings or false readings than homozygotes).

These sources of error are most easily detected by the researchers handling the raw data. A reader may, however, seek a description of how samples were handled, what genotyping method was used, whether any quality checks were implemented, whether any rules were established to say when the genotyping results would be considered valid, and the extent of missing data.

USING THE GUIDE

Returning to our clinical scenario, Slooter et al[38] refer to an earlier article from their team for genotyping details.[56] In this article, they state that genotyping was performed independently and in triplicate and without knowledge of the outcome status. They also state that their original cohort had 7983 persons, and they had to exclude 14% of the participants (n = 1131) because *APOE* genotype could not be determined. There is no mention about whether this loss may have been related to underlying genotype (eg, heterozygous vs homozygous) or to Alzheimer disease, but at face value, it seems unlikely. Although the method was not specified, given the prospective cohort design, one may assume that samples were stored in similar conditions regardless of the subsequent development of Alzheimer disease. We also may deduce that, given the blinding, allele identification could not be influenced by knowledge of the disease status.

Do the Genotype Proportions Observe Hardy-Weinberg Equilibrium?

Failure to observe HWE is one way of detecting possible genotyping error, although it is nonspecific and may be insensitive.[57-59] Investigators conduct statistical tests to check whether the observed genotype frequencies are consistent with HWE. In candidate gene studies, $P < .05$ is a typical threshold for declaring Hardy-Weinberg "disequilibrium." However, with simultaneous testing of a large number of possible associations, as in GWASs, it is expected that 5% of SNPs will violate HWE simply because of multiple testing. In this setting, investigators use more stringent P value thresholds, typically in the range of 10^{-4} to 10^{-6}. Empirical studies suggest that disequilibrium is common and many articles do not explicitly acknowledge this[60,61]; as discussed in the first section, there are many sources of disequilibrium aside from genotyping error.

Readers should look for evidence that the investigators have tested for HWE and raise their level of skepticism about the results if they have not. Given that erroneous reports of HWE occur, they may even check for HWE themselves by using a simple, freely available statistical program (Box 21.1-2).[62] For a cohort study, investigators should test for HWE in the whole study population; for a case-control study, they should test in the controls if they are intended to be representative of the general population.

USING THE GUIDE

In our scenario, Slooter et al[38] found that their study population did observe HWE ($P = .45$ in a well-powered study of n = 6852). Given that this is a 3-allele system, we are not able to use the online program to check HWE.

BOX 21.1-2

Checking Hardy-Weinberg Equilibrium

Readers can check whether the data at a biallelic single-nucleotide polymorphism (SNP) are consistent with Hardy-Weinberg equilibrium (HWE) by inserting the numbers in each genotype group into an online program.[62] For example, an article may report that among 100 controls, there are 80 homozygote wild types, 12 heterozygotes, and 2 homozygous variants. The program calculates the expected distribution among the 3 genotype groups, the χ^2 value, and the corresponding P value.

Genotypes	Observed, No.	Expected, No.
Homozygote reference	80	79.2
Heterozygote	18	19.6
Homozygote variant	2	1.2
SNP minor allele frequency	0.11	

$$x^2 = 0.65$$
x^2 test P value = .42 with 1 df
(if <.05 then not consistent with HWE)

There are limitations to the hypothesis testing, whether performed by the authors or the online program. Most HWE tests are weak because most sample sizes are small, and thus the likelihood of a *false-negative* result because of inadequate power is high. On the other hand, with very large sample sizes, the tests can detect very small deviations from HWE that are of no importance. In the setting of genome-wide association studies, a large number of SNPs are expected to have nominally significant deviations from HWE. For example, with 500 000 tested SNPs, 25 000 of them may have $P < .05$ on HWE testing by chance alone. Therefore, in GWASs, far more strict thresholds are appropriate to identify worrisome HWE deviation.

Have the Investigators Adjusted for Multiple Comparisons?

One of the main reasons for false-positive results is inadequate attention to the problem of multiple comparisons. The scenario of a candidate gene experiment testing 100 SNPs for association with a disease outcome in which no real association exists illustrates the magnitude of the problem. If the threshold P value of .05 is left unchanged, then the chance of finding at least 1 apparent but spurious positive association in this scenario can be calculated as $((1 - (1 - .05)^{100}) \times 100)$, or 99.4%. The simplest method to correct for this problem of multiple comparisons is the Bonferroni method, in which the threshold P value is divided by the number of independent tests. In this example, the P value would be set at .05/100 or .0005. This may, however, be overly conservative and stringent, and authors have suggested many other methods[45,63-66] (Box 21.1-3).[67,68]

BOX 21.1-3

Some Options for Adjustment for Multiple Comparisons

The *Bonferroni correction* is overly conservative and stringent, and there have been many suggestions for other methods. Two of the more popular ones include the following.

False-discovery rate calculations estimate the proportion of associations that are seemingly "discovered" (pass some required threshold of evidence) but are nevertheless expected to be false-positive results. The Benjamini-Hochberg method is used when loci (or single-nucleotide polymorphisms) are independent,[67] whereas the Benjamini-Lui method is applied when there is correlation or linkage disequilibrium among loci.[68] Both methods work on ranking the P values of the associations within a study and adjusting that P value by its position in the ranking list.

The false-report probability rate similarly states how likely an association is to be false if it emerges with a given level of statistical significance, given the power of the study and the perceived prior odds of an association being true.[45] The developers of this method have constructed a user-friendly spreadsheet to allow easy calculations.[45]

The potential for false-positive results also makes candidate gene association studies particularly susceptible to publication bias, in which initially strongly positive results find their way into publication more easily, and studies with negative results take longer to get published.[69] This bias is not corrected by simply accounting for multiple comparisons.

In GWASs, in which millions of SNPs are tested simultaneously, the multiple comparison problem takes on a magnitude never imagined in traditional epidemiology. To avoid false-positive results in such large-scale studies, $P < 5 \times 10^{-8}$ (as opposed to the usual 5×10^{-2}) is the accepted threshold for claiming what is called genome-wide significance.[33,70] This is equivalent to a Bonferroni correction for 1 million independent tests. This stringent threshold, combined with common journal requirements for independent replication of GWAS findings, provides appropriate insurance against spurious findings.

USING THE GUIDE

In our scenario, Slooter et al[38] have not adjusted their results for multiple comparisons since they test only the *APOE* polymorphism (although they address 3 outcomes: myocardial infarction, stroke, and Alzheimer disease). Given the extensive prior work raising the hypothesis, they reasonably consider theirs a hypothesis-testing study rather than a hypothesis-generating study.

Are the Results Consistent With Those of Other Studies?

Any *Users' Guide*—whether for diagnosis, therapy, *prognosis*, or *harm*—could include a validity criterion demanding replication. Although we have not included this criterion in considering other sorts of individual studies, the multiple-comparison problem and the forces that lead to differential publication of positive results suggest that, here, it is particularly important. Until putative genetic associations are replicated in similar but independent populations, one should interpret them with caution.[71,72]

Most of the genetic associations between SNPs and complex diseases are small (much smaller than the *odds ratios* [ORs] >2.0 observed for apoE e2/e3/e4),[73] and therefore even sizeable studies may fail to detect underlying associations.[74] Therefore, given that most individual studies are not large enough to detect these small effect sizes, typically, GWASs select SNPs with the lowest *P* values and test them in additional replication samples (either other GWASs or focused studies that target only the specific SNPs) to increase sample size and power, until the cumulative results pass genome-wide significance or similar thresholds. Even more teams may then continue to try to replicate these associations, and all of these data become essential in judging the *credibility* of these associations.

Therefore, we suggest—just as we do for issues of therapy, diagnosis, prognosis, and harm—that clinicians interested in genetic associations first seek a *systematic review*.[75,76] The Human Genome Epidemiology Network (HuGE Net) group has emerged as the Cochrane equivalent for genetic association studies. The HuGE Net website lists many of the *meta-analyses* performed to date[77,78] and also hosts the HuGE Navigator, where one can determine what single studies, GWASs, meta-analyses, and *synopses* are available.[28,79] Another useful aid in searching for GWASs is the Catalog of Published Genome-Wide Association Studies maintained by the National Institutes of Health.[27]

A MEDLINE search using "apoE" and "dementia" as search terms and restricted to English and meta-analysis, or a search on the HuGE Navigator, leads to 61 meta-analyses in the general population and a website collating all of the Alzheimer disease genetic association studies as an all-encompassing synopsis.[80] The Catalog of Published Genome-Wide Association Studies also lists 38 published GWASs of Alzheimer disease.[27] Taken together, the results for the *APOE e2/e3/e4* polymorphism are largely consistent across studies. This probably reflects the fact that the *apoE*–Alzheimer disease association is among the strongest genetic associations recorded to date.

USING THE GUIDE

Slooter et al[38] seem to have minimized bias:

The authors defined a homogeneous group of patients with dementia, separating Alzheimer disease from vascular dementia and using proper definitions and meticulous measurement schemes to determine outcomes.

They chose a homogeneous ethnic group and provided a table reporting similar characteristics in diseased and nondiseased groups, although alcohol is a possible confounder that was not included.

They did not report sufficient information to ensure that genotyping error had been eliminated, but the population observes HWE and the association is too strong to be accounted for by genotyping error.

They did not adjust for multiple comparisons in their study, but they studied only 1 polymorphism chosen according to previous work suggesting an association.

Most importantly, the specific *APOE* association with Alzheimer disease has been reproduced many times. Meta-analyses of the results also had consistent results across studies.

Given that we are satisfied with the validity of the study, we continue our critical appraisal. In the next section, we discuss how to interpret results of genetic association studies and how to apply this information in the context of patient care.

WHAT ARE THE RESULTS OF THE STUDY?

How Large and Precise Are the Associations?

Sometimes, investigators will tell you only whether an association is *statistically significant,* which will be of little use to you. Application depends on knowing the magnitude of the association (ie, it makes a difference whether the increase in risk is 1.4-fold or 8-fold).

Fortunately, investigators usually report the magnitude of a genetic association by using traditional measures of association: *relative risks* (RRs) in cohort studies, ORs in case-control studies, and *hazard ratios* (HRs) in *survival analyses* that consider the timing of events (see Chapter 9, Does Treatment

Lower Risk? Understanding the Results). If the variant allele is dominant—that is, it produces a protein isoform that dominates function—its presence in even 1 copy will result in maximal increase in risk. If the variant allele is recessive and present in only 1 gene, it produces a protein isoform that will fail to exert its biological effect; both variant alleles must be present to result in an increase in risk. In both cases, a single RR, OR, or HR describes the magnitude of the association.

If the effect of a variant allele is additive, its presence in a single gene will lead to an increase in risk; its presence in both genes will lead to a further increase. Investigators may present the RR, OR, or HR associated with heterozygous (variant allele present in only 1 gene) and homozygous (variant allele present in both genes) individuals. Alternatively, they may present the RR, OR, or HR associated with the presence of only a single variant allele, in which case you must calculate what the expected risk is for the homozygous individual. There are 2 ways to do this: the most common approach is to take the square of the risk (called log-additive or per-allele or multiplicative risk model); the other approach is to take 2 times the risk (called the linear additive model). Ideally, the choice of which calculation to use should be guided by the relevant biology, although this is often unknown.

USING THE GUIDE

Slooter et al[38] found that *APOE e2* may decrease the risk of Alzheimer disease, with an RR of 0.5 (95% CI, 0.3-0.9) for *e2/e3* heterozygous individuals compared with *e3/e3*; the e2 allele is sufficiently rare that the *e2/e2* group is small. The risk of Alzheimer disease increases with e4 (OR for the *e3/e4* heterozygous individual, 2.2; 95% CI, 1.6-2.9) and the presence of 2 e4 alleles increases the risk to 7.0 (95% CI, 4.1-11.9), even more than one would expect under either the log-additive model (2.2^2 or 4.8) or linear model (2.2×2 or 4.4). Given that this is a late-stage replication with many thousands of participants and that the results are consistent with prior literature likely free of publication bias, the winner's curse is probably not an issue here.

Our confidence in estimates is also influenced by precision, reflected in the CI. Small genetic association studies lack power and thus may fail to detect an association that is actually present.[69] If a CI around the RR has a lower boundary less than 1.0 and a higher boundary greater than 1.0, then the results are consistent with chance but do not exclude the possibility that the gene may either reduce or increase risk. That is, the possibilities of no association or an association remain (and if the CI is wide, the unestablished association may be important) as a result of small sample size. Although earlier candidate gene studies were often small, GWASs now routinely involve samples that include many thousands of cases and controls.

A new approach to the sample-size problem is the statistical synthesis of results from multiple, individual studies via meta-analysis. Indeed, hundreds of GWAS meta-analyses have been published since 2007, with most genetic disease associations published in recent years being discovered via meta-analysis.[81] By increasing the available sample size, meta-analysis provides greater power to detect the small genetic effects underlying many complex human diseases. Larger samples also result in narrow CIs and hence more precise estimates of effect.

Large sample sizes are necessary to detect small effects, and the effect of any single gene variant is likely to be small. In fact, *APOE* is a major exception: most genetic effects in the recent GWAS literature for other complex disorders have ORs or RRs in the range of 1.1 to 1.4. These small, seemingly unimportant ORs have generated interest in combining the effect of many genes in polygenic models or panels (ie, creating a genetic risk "profile" that assigns points for the presence of various risk alleles and calculates an overall risk of disease).[82] For example, in a study of 5 SNPs associated with prostate cancer, the investigators expressed the risk of disease associated with the increasing presence of risk alleles.[83] They found an OR of 1.6 for individuals who were homozygous or heterozygous for the risk allele at 1 SNP and up to 4.5 for those who were homozygous or heterozygous for the risk allele at 4 SNPs. However, there are potential problems in creating these polygenic models; in particular, the independence of each genetic effect—a fundamental assumption—may not hold.

We are not aware that any such polygenic score has yet been generated and rigorously tested for association with Alzheimer disease. The synopsis of the association studies in AlzGene[80] and the National Institutes of Health catalog[27] suggests that dozens of SNPs have nominal statistically significant associations and could potentially be considered for generating a risk profile. All but *APOE* confer small risk increases, on average per-allele ORs of less than 1.3.

Given the small effect sizes of most variants underlying the risk of Alzheimer disease (and other complex diseases), there are certainly numerous additional variants that evade detection in available sample sizes because of their very small ORs. Given this, there is increasing interest in considering the combined effects of large panels of common genetic variants. In fact, a recent GWAS that included 3290 Alzheimer disease cases and 3849 controls revealed that 24% of case-control differences in Alzheimer disease risk could be attributed to the additive effects of approximately 500 000 common SNPs distributed across the entire genome, regardless of their individual association with disease.[84] This finding suggests that Alzheimer disease results from known clinical risk factors acting in concert with potentially thousands of unidentified, common genetic variants, each with individually very small effects. The number of SNPs reported as associated with Alzheimer disease is thus likely to increase as larger samples are included in GWASs. The ongoing identification of additional genetic associations for Alzheimer disease may assist with the future selection of SNPs for predicting individual risk.

HOW CAN I APPLY THE RESULTS TO PATIENT CARE?

Does the Genetic Association Improve Predictive Power Beyond Easily Measured Clinical Variables?

The immediate clinical utility of a genetic association is to provide prognostic information to patients and clinicians. To do this, the genetic marker must provide independent predictive power above and beyond traditional clinical predictive variables (age; sex; family history; exposures to other causal agents, such

as cigarettes; simple laboratory tests, such as serum lipid levels; and other risk factors, such as hypertension). This independent contribution may well not be the case, particularly if the genetic polymorphism exerts its effect through some of these variables (eg, a gene that controls lipids exerts its effect on outcomes such as cardiovascular risk through increases in low-density lipoprotein).

Typically, a useful gene predictor will exert a biological influence that we cannot measure at some other level. The exception is if the biological factor measurement has large measurement error and day-to-day variability, whereas the gene is measured with high accuracy. In the previous example, if there is large lifetime variability and measurement error in lipid levels for a single individual, assessing the patient's gene variants that control lipid levels may provide more decisive information.[85]

To determine whether the genetic information adds substantial predictive power beyond easily measured clinical and laboratory variables, the clinician must look for the appropriate analysis. Does the association persist after adjusting for other clinical variables?

For *dichotomous outcomes*, there are a number of statistical tools to decide how much, if any, additional predictive power the genetic information adds. One is to calculate the area under the *receiver operating characteristic curve* (ROC curve), an approach often used for diagnostic tests.[86] As shown in Figure 21.1-5, the ROC curve plots the *true-positive* rate (y-axis) against the false-positive rate (x-axis). The ROC curve with no greater predictive ability than chance would approximate a straight diagonal line from the origin (0, 0) to the upper right-hand corner (1.0, 1.0) (Figure 21.1-5A). The area under the curve would be 0.5. The visual representation of a perfectly predictive test would be a line that goes straight up the y-axis to 1.0 and then straight across the x-axis to 1.0, and it would have an area under the curve of 1 (Figure 21.1-5B).[87]

The 2002 Prospective Cardiovascular Munster study, which developed a risk prediction score for cardiovascular disease, provides an example of the use of the ROC curve (Figure 21.1-5C).[88] Fitting this model to the Northwick Park Heart Study II by using normal clinical variables gave an area under the curve of 0.65. Adding genetic information based on candidate gene associations did not significantly

FIGURE 21.1-5

Example of a Receiver Operating Characteristic (ROC) Curve for Cardiovascular Risk Related to *APOE*

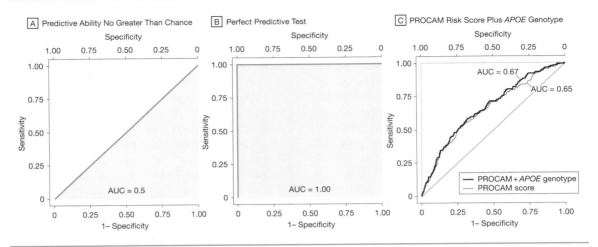

Abbreviation: AUC, area under the curve.

A, Example of a ROC curve for a test that performs no better than chance. B, Example of a ROC curve for a test with perfect predictive ability (100% sensitivity and specificity). C, ROC curves for cardiovascular disease calculated using PROCAM (Prospective Cardiovascular Munster study) risk score plus *APOE* genotype. On the basis of 2451 men (of 3012 eligible) who had complete data for PROCAM and *APOE* genotyping, the *APOE* genotype was fitted as a class variable with 3 categories: 33, 22/23, and 34/44. Factors included age, body mass index, total cholesterol, triglycerides, systolic blood pressure, and family history. Other factors in PROCAM were not measured in all men. For the PROCAM score, the ROC value was 0.65 (95% confidence interval [CI], 0.61-0.70), with a detection rate of 11.7% for a false-positive rate of 5.0%. In univariate analysis, *APOE* genotype was significant at $P = .01$. In multivariate analysis, the area under the curve increased to 0.67 (95% CI, 0.63-0.71) (detection rate, 14%), but this improvement was not significant ($P = .11$). Panel C data based on Humphries et al.[87]

increase this area, thus demonstrating that genotyping could not add important predictive information at that time (2004).[87]

Another study reports the advances facilitated by GWASs.[89] This 2013 study focused on risk prediction for coronary heart disease in the Edinburgh Artery Study. Clinical risk factors included age, sex, blood pressure, smoking status, diabetes/glucose intolerance, and total and high-density lipoprotein cholesterol. Models that included these clinical variables produced an area under the curve of 0.67, which increased by a significant increment to 0.74 ($P = .001$) when the model additionally included 36 SNPs associated with coronary heart disease in large-scale GWAS meta-analyses.

Perhaps the most striking example of risk prediction facilitated by genetic data is in type 1 diabetes. Candidate gene and genome-wide studies of type 1 diabetes have now identified more than 50 associated genetic variants, which together produce an

area under the curve of nearly 0.9,[90,91] the highest of any studied disease.

With regard to Alzheimer risk prediction using *APOE* genotype, Seshadri et al[92] found that adding *APOE* genotype to a model that included only age and sex in the Rotterdam Study increased the area under the curve from 0.83 to 0.85, but the increment was not statistically significant. The addition of 2 additional associated SNPs to the model produced a miniscule increase (0.002), consistent with the relatively larger genetic effect of *APOE* compared with other Alzheimer-associated variants.

USING THE GUIDE

Slooter et al[38] added age, sex, and education to regression models that included *APOE* genotype. The RRs they presented considered (ie, adjusted for) these clinical variables. However, their study would be stronger if they had considered other clinical variables that are also associated with Alzheimer risk, such as total cholesterol level and family history of Alzheimer disease. In general, it is important that investigators include family history in statistical models because it is easily measured and can help to predict an individual's risk of disorders with a known genetic component. To evaluate the predictive utility of risk genotypes, one then can assess whether including the *APOE* genotype can improve prediction over and above what can be predicted simply by family history. The failure of Slooter et al[38] to take family history into consideration results in some doubt about the utility of the genetic information and limits our use of the information in helping our patient. Other investigators have found that *APOE* information provides additional predictive ability beyond family history[93] but not necessarily beyond expert clinical diagnosis with standardized criteria. Mayeux et al[94] found that adding *APOE* genotype to expert diagnosis by using standardized criteria increased the area under the curve from 0.84 to 0.87, an increment that was not statistically significant.

What Are the Absolute vs Relative Genetic Effects?

If the patient's risk of disease in the absence of a variant risk allele is low, even a 5-fold or 10-fold increase in risk in the presence of the allele may represent a small absolute increase in risk. Conversely, if the baseline risk is high, even a modest increase in RR could affect clinical decision making. We also note that RRs are additive; thus, an individual's risk increase due to a risk genotype may add to the risk due to positive family history. In this example, an analysis of case-control studies[95] reports that having a first-degree relative with dementia is associated with a 3.5-fold increased risk of Alzheimer disease. Aggregation of *APOE* genotype within affected families may contribute partly to this increase in risk.

USING THE GUIDE

Slooter et al[38] estimated the RR of Alzheimer disease in *APOE e4* heterozygous individuals at 2.2 and the RR associated with *APOE e4* homozygous individuals at 7.0. Results were similar for Alzheimer disease and vascular dementia. They took baseline risk into account to estimate a cumulative, absolute risk of Alzheimer disease or vascular dementia by 80 years of age of approximately 15% to 20% for *APOE e4* heterozygous individuals and 40% to 50% for *APOE e4* homozygous individuals. Other studies confirm these high absolute risk estimates.[96]

Is the Risk-Associated Allele Likely to Be Present in My Patient?

In applying the results, clinicians must consider the likelihood that the culprit allele is present in a particular patient, given the patient's ancestral population and the respective allele frequencies in that population group. Allele frequencies for various genes and populations of interest are available in the Allele Frequency Database[97] or at the HapMap website.[98]

Similarly, some gene-disease associations may be restricted to a selected subgroup. For example, BRCA1 was identified in patients with early-onset breast cancer who had a strong family history.[99] This group of individuals, however, accounts for only approximately 5% of all breast cancers. Hence, although this genetic association is valid, individuals who present with late-onset breast cancer without a strong family history have no need to be tested for it. However, for certain ancestry groups, such as Ashkenazi Jews, who have a high prevalence of BRCA1 mutations, testing may be appropriate in women with breast or ovarian cancer.[100] Knowledge of BRCA1 genotype status could help these women assess their own future risk of further breast and other gynecologic cancer and also may be relevant for family members.

USING THE GUIDE

In our clinical scenario, the Allele Frequency Database[97] reveals that the *APOE4* allele frequencies are similar across a broad range of ancestries.

Is the Patient Likely Better Off Knowing the Genetic Information?

Knowing that one's genes increase the risk of a serious health problem years in the future may have substantial adverse consequences, including worry, anxiety, and potentially increased payments for life or disability insurance. These adverse consequences become particularly compelling if there is no productive action that follows knowledge of increased risk.

On the other hand, genetic information may prompt specific beneficial action or avoidance of harmful actions. In particular, some associations pertain to outcomes that are also related to the likelihood of satisfactory and unsatisfactory responses to specific treatments. For example, a SNP in the TPMT gene identifies children with acute leukemia who are at increased risk of a life-threatening adverse event with the chemotherapeutic agent mercaptopurine.[101] Genotyping this SNP can avoid substantial morbidity and mortality by substitution of an alternative chemotherapeutic agent in individuals with the high-risk genotype.

When associations pertain to risk related not to treatment but to development of disease, genetic information may facilitate behavior change to reduce nongenetically mediated risk.[102] For example, early evidence suggests that providing information about glutathione-S-transferase genotypes (which affect nicotine metabolism) may influence smoking cessation rates.[103]

Understanding genetic risk may be problematic for lay people,[104] and there is still uncertainty about how to use and convey genetic information and how to optimize genetic services. A systematic review on the influence of genetic services[105] found that behavioral outcomes have found mixed results and clinical outcomes were less well studied, genetics knowledge tends to be poor, and the most consistently identified barrier has been the self-assessed inadequacy of the primary care workforce to deliver genetic services. Additional barriers have included lack of oversight of genetic testing and concerns about privacy and discrimination because accessibility to genetic risk profiles may jeopardize an individual's ability to obtain employment or health insurance.

These deficiencies need to be addressed quickly, particularly given the direct-to-consumer availability of genetic testing.[106] Several companies are marketing genetic tests for common variants, including intense direct-to-consumer advertisement campaigns, often for indications without proven validity or usefulness,[107] and for at least one test the US Food and Drug Administration has ordered a genomics company to cease marketing.[108]

CLINICAL SCENARIO RESOLUTION

Recapping our critical appraisal, Slooter et al[38] used an optimal study design for the question (a longitudinal cohort), characterized dementia well (separating Alzheimer disease from vascular dementia), ensured similar ethnicity in diseased and nondiseased populations, and demonstrated HWE in the genotype results. Their results are consistent with a large number of other studies that addressed the association. The RRs associated with 1 or 2 copies of *APOE e4*, 2.2 and 7.0, respectively, are substantial, the culprit allele is common (25% of the white population has at least 1 *APOE e4* allele), and the absolute risks of Alzheimer disease by the age of 80 years of 15% and 40% to 50% in heterozygous and homozygous variant populations, respectively,

are impressive. Perhaps the most important limitation is that the incremental increase in risk with *APOE e4* beyond family history was not considered. Other studies suggest that the *APOE e4* genotype can provide additional information beyond family history[87] but not necessarily beyond expert clinical diagnosis.[94] Nevertheless, there may be a role for *APOE* genotyping in helping nonexperts arrive at a diagnosis.

You can therefore inform the patient that results of genetic testing may reveal an increased risk of Alzheimer disease. This may increase his estimated risk beyond the 3.5-fold increase due to family history but perhaps not considerably so. More extensive testing using a genome-wide platform, as offered by several companies, may reveal information for further gene variants with small contributions to Alzheimer risk, but the interpretation of this extra information is uncertain.

Discussion with the patient about why he is seeking the genetic information would be worthwhile. If knowledge of increased risk would increase his resolve to modify other factors that would affect his risk of Alzheimer disease (eg, quitting smoking and ensuring adherence with antihypertensive medication), the genetic information may offer a useful stimulus. Such actions might decrease not only his risk of Alzheimer disease but also his risk of stroke and other diseases. On the other hand, if a negative result would give him a false sense of security and even increase risky behaviors, the outcome of genetic testing may be less desirable. Ultimately, understanding the article by Slooter et al[38] and its implications will help you to work with the patient to arrive at the optimal course of action.

After discussing with the patient his increased risk due to family history, smoking, and high blood pressure, he decides to focus on modifiable risk factors, that is, to stop smoking, exercise to improve his blood pressure, and have his cholesterol level checked. Given the uncertain amount of additional risk attributable to *APOE* genotype, he decides to forgo the genetic test.

References

1. Samani NJ, Erdmann J, Hall AS, et al; WTCCC and the Cardiogenics Consortium. Genomewide association analysis of coronary artery disease. *N Engl J Med*. 2007;357(5):443-453.

2. Deloukas P, Kanoni S, Willenborg C, et al; CARDIoGRAMplusC4D Consortium; DIAGRAM Consortium; CARDIOGENICS Consortium; MuTHER Consortium; Wellcome Trust Case Control Consortium. Large-scale association analysis identifies new risk loci for coronary artery disease. *Nat Genet*. 2013;45(1):25-33.

3. Coronary Artery Disease (C4D) Genetics Consortium. A genome-wide association study in Europeans and South Asians identifies five new loci for coronary artery disease. *Nat Genet*. 2011;43(4):339-344.

4. Zeggini E, Weedon MN, Lindgren CM, et al; Wellcome Trust Case Control Consortium (WTCCC). Replication of genomewide association signals in UK samples reveals risk loci for type 2 diabetes. *Science*. 2007;316(5829):1336-1341.

5. Morris AP, Voight BF, Teslovich TM, et al; Wellcome Trust Case Control Consortium; Meta-Analyses of Glucose and Insulin-related traits Consortium (MAGIC) Investigators; Genetic Investigation of ANthropometric Traits (GIANT) Consortium; Asian Genetic Epidemiology Network–Type 2 Diabetes (AGEN-T2D) Consortium; South Asian Type 2 Diabetes (SAT2D) Consortium; DIAbetes Genetics Replication And Meta-analysis (DIAGRAM) Consortium. Large-scale association analysis provides insights into the genetic architecture and pathophysiology of type 2 diabetes. *Nat Genet*. 2012;44(9):981-990.

6. Scott RA, Lagou V, Welch RP, et al; DIAbetes Genetics Replication and Meta-analysis (DIAGRAM) Consortium. Large-scale association analyses identify new loci influencing glycemic traits and provide insight into the underlying biological pathways. *Nat Genet*. 2012;44(9):991-1005.

7. Traylor M, Farrall M, Holliday EG, et al; Australian Stroke Genetics Collaborative, Wellcome Trust Case Control Consortium 2 (WTCCC2); International Stroke Genetics Consortium. Genetic risk factors for ischaemic stroke and its subtypes (the METASTROKE collaboration): a meta-analysis of genome-wide association studies. *Lancet Neurol*. 2012;11(11):951-962.

8. Holliday EG, Maguire JM, Evans TJ, et al; Australian Stroke Genetics Collaborative; International Stroke Genetics Consortium; Wellcome Trust Case Control Consortium 2. Common variants at 6p21.1 are associated with large artery atherosclerotic stroke. *Nat Genet*. 2012;44(10):1147-1151.

9. Bellenguez C, Bevan S, Gschwendtner A, et al; International Stroke Genetics Consortium (ISGC); Wellcome Trust Case Control Consortium 2 (WTCCC2). Genome-wide association study identifies a variant in HDAC9 associated with large vessel ischemic stroke. *Nat Genet*. 2012;44(3):328-333.

10. Hafler DA, Compston A, Sawcer S, et al; International Multiple Sclerosis Genetics Consortium. Risk alleles for multiple sclerosis identified by a genomewide study. *N Engl J Med*. 2007;357(9):851-862.

11. Patsopoulos NA, Esposito F, Reischl J, et al; Bayer Pharma MS Genetics Working Group; Steering Committees of Studies Evaluating IFNβ-1b and a CCR1-Antagonist; ANZgene Consortium; GeneMSA; International Multiple Sclerosis Genetics Consortium. Genome-wide meta-analysis identifies novel multiple sclerosis susceptibility loci. *Ann Neurol*. 2011;70(6):897-912.

12. Sawcer S, Hellenthal G, Pirinen M, et al; International Multiple Sclerosis Genetics Consortium; Wellcome Trust Case Control Consortium 2. Genetic risk and a primary role for cell-mediated immune mechanisms in multiple sclerosis. *Nature*. 2011; 476(7359):214-219.

13. Easton DF, Pooley KA, Dunning AM, et al; SEARCH collaborators; kConFab; AOCS Management Group. Genome-wide association study identifies novel breast cancer susceptibility loci. *Nature*. 2007;447(7148):1087-1093.

14. Garcia-Closas M, Couch FJ, Lindstrom S, et al. Genomewide association studies identify four ER negative–specific

breast cancer risk loci. *Nat Genet*. Apr 2013;45(4):392-398, 398e391-392.

15. Ripke S, O'Dushlaine C, Chambert K, et al; Multicenter Genetic Studies of Schizophrenia Consortium; Psychosis Endophenotypes International Consortium; Wellcome Trust Case Control Consortium 2. Genome-wide association analysis identifies 13 new risk loci for schizophrenia. *Nat Genet*. 2013;45(10):1150-1159.

16. Wellcome Trust Case Control Consortium. Genome-wide association study of 14,000 cases of seven common diseases and 3,000 shared controls. *Nature*. 2007;447(7145):661-678.

17. Chen DT, Jiang X, Akula N, et al. Genome-wide association study meta-analysis of European and Asian-ancestry samples identifies three novel loci associated with bipolar disorder. *Mol Psychiatry*. 2013;18(2):195-205.

18. Plenge RM, Seielstad M, Padyukov L, et al. TRAF1-C5 as a risk locus for rheumatoid arthritis—a genomewide study. *N Engl J Med*. 2007;357(12):1199-1209.

19. Eyre S, Bowes J, Diogo D, et al; Biologics in Rheumatoid Arthritis Genetics and Genomics Study Syndicate; Wellcome Trust Case Control Consortium. High-density genetic mapping identifies new susceptibility loci for rheumatoid arthritis. *Nat Genet*. 2012;44(12):1336-1340.

20. Jostins L, Ripke S, Weersma RK, et al; International IBD Genetics Consortium (IIBDGC). Host-microbe interactions have shaped the genetic architecture of inflammatory bowel disease. *Nature*. 2012;491(7422):119-124.

21. Coon KD, Myers AJ, Craig DW, et al. A high-density whole-genome association study reveals that APOE is the major susceptibility gene for sporadic late-onset Alzheimer's disease. *J Clin Psychiatry*. 2007;68(4):613-618.

22. Li H, Wetten S, Li L, et al. Candidate single-nucleotide polymorphisms from a genomewide association study of Alzheimer disease. *Arch Neurol*. 2008;65(1):45-53.

23. Reiman EM, Webster JA, Myers AJ, et al. GAB2 alleles modify Alzheimer's risk in APOE epsilon4 carriers. *Neuron*. 2007;54(5):713-720.

24. Kamboh MI, Demirci FY, Wang X, et al; Alzheimer's Disease Neuroimaging Initiative. Genome-wide association study of Alzheimer's disease. *Transl Psychiatry*. 2012;2:e117.

25. Naj AC, Jun G, Beecham GW, et al. Common variants at MS4A4/MS4A6E, CD2AP, CD33 and EPHA1 are associated with late-onset Alzheimer's disease. *Nat Genet*. 2011;43(5):436-441.

26. Hollingworth P, Harold D, Sims R, et al; Alzheimer's Disease Neuroimaging Initiative; CHARGE consortium; EADI1 consortium. Common variants at ABCA7, MS4A6A/MS4A4E, EPHA1, CD33 and CD2AP are associated with Alzheimer's disease. *Nat Genet*. 2011;43(5):429-435.

27. National Human Genome Research Institute. A Catalog of Published Genome-Wide Association Studies. http://www.genome.gov/gwastudies/. Accessed February 28, 2014.

28. Yu W, Gwinn M, Clyne M, Yesupriya A, Khoury MJ. A navigator for human genome epidemiology. *Nat Genet*. 2008;40(2):124-125.

29. Lander ES, Linton LM, Birren B, et al; International Human Genome Sequencing Consortium. Initial sequencing and analysis of the human genome. *Nature*. 2001;409(6822):860-921.

30. International HapMap Consortium. A haplotype map of the human genome. *Nature*. 2005;437(7063):1299-1320.

31. Frazer KA, Ballinger DG, Cox DR, et al; International HapMap Consortium. A second generation human haplotype map of over 3.1 million SNPs. *Nature*. 2007;449(7164):851-861.

32. Abecasis GR, Auton A, Brooks LD, et al; 1000 Genomes Project Consortium. An integrated map of genetic variation from 1,092 human genomes. *Nature*. 2012;491(7422):56-65.

33. McCarthy MI, Abecasis GR, Cardon LR, et al. Genome-wide association studies for complex traits: consensus, uncertainty and challenges. *Nat Rev Genet*. 2008;9(5):356-369.

34. Pearson TA, Manolio TA. How to interpret a genome-wide association study. *JAMA*. 2008;299(11):1335-1344.

35. Visscher PM, Brown MA, McCarthy MI, Yang J. Five years of GWAS discovery. *Am J Hum Genet*. 2012;90(1):7-24.

36. Dawn Teare M, Barrett JH. Genetic linkage studies. *Lancet*. 2005;366(9490):1036-1044.

37. Risch N. Evolving methods in genetic epidemiology. II. Genetic linkage from an epidemiologic perspective. *Epidemiol Rev*. 1997;19(1):24-32.

38. Slooter AJ, Cruts M, Hofman A, et al. The impact of APOE on myocardial infarction, stroke, and dementia: the Rotterdam Study. *Neurology*. 2004;62(7):1196-1198.

39. Ioannidis JP. Contradicted and initially stronger effects in highly cited clinical research. *JAMA*. 2005;294(2):218-228.

40. Ioannidis JP, Trikalinos TA. Early extreme contradictory estimates may appear in published research: the Proteus phenomenon in molecular genetics research and randomized trials. *J Clin Epidemiol*. 2005;58(6):543-549.

41. Ioannidis JP. Why most discovered true associations are inflated. *Epidemiology*. 2008;19(5):640-648.

42. Zollner S, Pritchard JK. Overcoming the winner's curse: estimating penetrance parameters from case-control data. *Am J Hum Genet*. 2007;80(4):605-615.

43. Contopoulos-Ioannidis DG, Alexiou GA, Gouvias TC, Ioannidis JP. An empirical evaluation of multifarious outcomes in pharmacogenetics: beta-2 adrenoceptor gene polymorphisms in asthma treatment. *Pharmacogenet Genomics*. 2006;16(10):705-711.

44. Evangelou E, Trikalinos TA, Salanti G, Ioannidis JP. Family-based versus unrelated case-control designs for genetic associations. *PLoS Genet*. 2006;2(8):e123.

45. Wacholder S, Chanock S, Garcia-Closas M, El Ghormli L, Rothman N. Assessing the probability that a positive report is false: an approach for molecular epidemiology studies. *J Natl Cancer Inst*. 2004;96(6):434-442.

46. Barnholtz-Sloan JS, McEvoy B, Shriver MD, Rebbeck TR. Ancestry estimation and correction for population stratification in molecular epidemiologic association studies. *Cancer Epidemiol Biomarkers Prev*. 2008;17(3):471-477.

47. Pritchard JK, Rosenberg NA. Use of unlinked genetic markers to detect population stratification in association studies. *Am J Hum Genet*. 1999;65(1):220-228.

48. Kittles RA, Chen W, Panguluri RK, et al. CYP3A4-V and prostate cancer in African Americans: causal or confounding association because of population stratification? *Hum Genet*. 2002;110(6):553-560.

49. Frayling TM, Timpson NJ, Weedon MN, et al. A common variant in the FTO gene is associated with body mass index and predisposes to childhood and adult obesity. *Science*. 2007;316(5826):889-894.

50. Richards JB, Rivadeneira F, Inouye M, et al. Bone mineral density, osteoporosis, and osteoporotic fractures: a genome-wide association study. *Lancet.* 2008;371(9623):1505-1512.

51. Clayton DG, Walker NM, Smyth DJ, et al. Population structure, differential bias and genomic control in a large-scale, case-control association study. *Nat Genet.* 2005;37(11):1243-1246.

52. Akey JM, Zhang K, Xiong M, Doris P, Jin L. The effect that genotyping errors have on the robustness of common linkage-disequilibrium measures. *Am J Hum Genet.* 2001;68(6):1447-1456.

53. Bogardus ST Jr, Concato J, Feinstein AR. Clinical epidemiological quality in molecular genetic research: the need for methodological standards. *JAMA.* 1999;281(20):1919-1926.

54. Mein CA, Barratt BJ, Dunn MG, et al. Evaluation of single nucleotide polymorphism typing with invader on PCR amplicons and its automation. *Genome Res.* 2000;10(3):330-343.

55. Pompanon F, Bonin A, Bellemain E, Taberlet P. Genotyping errors: causes, consequences and solutions. *Nat Rev Genet.* 2005;6(11):847-859.

56. Slooter AJ, Cruts M, Kalmijn S, et al. Risk estimates of dementia by apolipoprotein E genotypes from a population-based incidence study: the Rotterdam Study. *Arch Neurol.* 1998;55(7):964-968.

57. Cox DG, Kraft P. Quantification of the power of Hardy-Weinberg equilibrium testing to detect genotyping error. *Hum Hered.* 2006;61(1):10-14.

58. Hosking L, Lumsden S, Lewis K, et al. Detection of genotyping errors by Hardy-Weinberg equilibrium testing. *Eur J Hum Genet.* 2004;12(5):395-399.

59. Leal SM. Detection of genotyping errors and pseudo-SNPs via deviations from Hardy-Weinberg equilibrium. *Genet Epidemiol.* 2005;29(3):204-214.

60. Salanti G, Amountza G, Ntzani EE, Ioannidis JP. Hardy-Weinberg equilibrium in genetic association studies: an empirical evaluation of reporting, deviations, and power. *Eur J Hum Genet.* 2005;13(7):840-848.

61. Xu J, Turner A, Little J, Bleecker ER, Meyers DA. Positive results in association studies are associated with departure from Hardy-Weinberg equilibrium: hint for genotyping error? *Hum Genet.* 2002;111(6):573-574.

62. Tufts University Comparative and Molecular Pharmacogenomics Laboratory. A simple calculator to determine whether observed genotype frequencies are consistent with Hardy-Weinberg equilibrium. http://www.tufts.edu/~mcourt01/Documents/Court%20lab%20-%20HW%20calculator.xls. Accessed September 3, 2013.

63. Freimer N, Sabatti C. The use of pedigree, sib-pair and association studies of common diseases for genetic mapping and epidemiology. *Nat Genet.* 2004;36(10):1045-1051.

64. Ioannidis JP. Calibration of credibility of agnostic genome-wide associations. *Am J Med Genet B Neuropsychiatr Genet.* 2008;147B(6):964-972.

65. Province MA. Sequential methods of analysis for genome scans. *Adv Genet.* 2001;42:499-514.

66. Sabatti C. Avoiding false discoveries in association studies. *Methods Mol Biol.* 2007;376:195-211.

67. Benjamini Y, Hochberg Y. Controlling the false discovery rate: a practical and powerful approach to multiple testing. *J Royal Stat Soc Series B.* 1995;57(1):289-300.

68. Benjamini Y, Yekutieli D. The control of the false discovery rate in multiple testing under dependency. *Ann Stat.* 2001;29(4):1165-1188.

69. Ioannidis JP, Ntzani EE, Trikalinos TA, Contopoulos-Ioannidis DG. Replication validity of genetic association studies. *Nat Genet.* 2001;29(3):306-309.

70. Hoggart CJ, Clark TG, De Iorio M, Whittaker JC, Balding DJ. Genome-wide significance for dense SNP and resequencing data. *Genet Epidemiol.* 2008;32(2):179-185.

71. Chanock SJ, Manolio T, Boehnke M, et al; NCI-NHGRI Working Group on Replication in Association Studies. Replicating genotype-phenotype associations. *Nature.* 2007;447(7145):655-660.

72. Ioannidis JP, Boffetta P, Little J, et al. Assessment of cumulative evidence on genetic associations: interim guidelines. *Int J Epidemiol.* 2008;37(1):120-132.

73. Ioannidis JP, Trikalinos TA, Khoury MJ. Implications of small effect sizes of individual genetic variants on the design and interpretation of genetic association studies of complex diseases. *Am J Epidemiol.* 2006;164(7):609-614.

74. Moonesinghe R, Khoury MJ, Liu T, Ioannidis JP. Required sample size and nonreplicability thresholds for heterogeneous genetic associations. *Proc Natl Acad Sci U S A.* 2008;105(2):617-622.

75. Munafò MR, Flint J. Meta-analysis of genetic association studies. *Trends Genet.* 2004;20(9):439-444.

76. Salanti G, Sanderson S, Higgins JP. Obstacles and opportunities in meta-analysis of genetic association studies. *Genet Med.* 2005;7(1):13-20.

77. Khoury MJ, Dorman JS. The Human Genome Epidemiology Network. *Am J Epidemiol.* 1998;148(1):1-3.

78. Little J, Higgins J. *The HuGENet HuGE Review Handbook.* 2008; http://www.hugenet.ca. Accessed September 3, 2013.

79. Human Genome Epidemiology Network. A navigator for human genome epidemiology. http://www.hugenavigator.net/. Accessed September 3, 2013.

80. Bertram L, McQueen MB, Mullin K, Blacker D, Tanzi RE. Systematic meta-analyses of Alzheimer disease genetic association studies: the AlzGene database. *Nat Genet.* 2007; 39(1):17-23.

81. Evangelou E, Ioannidis JP. Meta-analysis methods for genome-wide association studies and beyond. *Nat Rev Genet.* 2013;14(6):379-389.

82. Yang Q, Khoury MJ, Friedman J, Little J, Flanders WD. How many genes underlie the occurrence of common complex diseases in the population? *Int J Epidemiol.* 2005;34(5): 1129-1137.

83. Zheng SL, Sun J, Wiklund F, et al. Cumulative association of five genetic variants with prostate cancer. *N Engl J Med.* 2008;358(9):910-919.

84. Lee SH, Harold D, Nyholt DR, et al; ANZGene Consortium; International Endogene Consortium; Genetic and Environmental Risk for Alzheimer's Disease Consortium. Estimation and partitioning of polygenic variation captured by common SNPs for Alzheimer's disease, multiple sclerosis and endometriosis. *Hum Mol Genet.* 2013;22(4):832-841.

85. Kathiresan S, Melander O, Anevski D, et al. Polymorphisms associated with cholesterol and risk of cardiovascular events. *N Engl J Med.* 2008;358(12):1240-1249.

86. Irwig L, Bossuyt P, Glasziou P, Gatsonis C, Lijmer J. Designing studies to ensure that estimates of test accuracy are transferable. *BMJ*. 2002;324(7338):669-671.

87. Humphries SE, Ridker PM, Talmud PJ. Genetic testing for cardiovascular disease susceptibility: a useful clinical management tool or possible misinformation? *Arterioscler Thromb Vasc Biol*. 2004;24(4):628-636.

88. Assmann G, Cullen P, Schulte H. Simple scoring scheme for calculating the risk of acute coronary events based on the 10-year follow-up of the prospective cardiovascular Münster (PROCAM) study. *Circulation*. 2002;105(3):310-315.

89. Bolton JL, Stewart MC, Wilson JF, Anderson N, Price JF. Improvement in prediction of coronary heart disease risk over conventional risk factors using SNPs identified in genome-wide association studies. *PLoS One*. 2013;8(2):e57310.

90. Jostins L, Barrett JC. Genetic risk prediction in complex disease. *Hum Mol Genet*. 2011;20(R2):R182-R188.

91. Clayton DG. Prediction and interaction in complex disease genetics: experience in type 1 diabetes. *PLoS Genet*. 2009; 5(7):e1000540.

92. Seshadri S, Fitzpatrick AL, Ikram MA, et al; CHARGE Consortium; GERAD1 Consortium; EADI1 Consortium. Genome-wide analysis of genetic loci associated with Alzheimer disease. *JAMA*. 2010;303(18):1832-1840.

93. Cupples LA, Farrer LA, Sadovnick AD, Relkin N, Whitehouse P, Green RC. Estimating risk curves for first-degree relatives of patients with Alzheimer's disease: the REVEAL study. *Genet Med*. 2004;6(4):192-196.

94. Mayeux R, Saunders AM, Shea S, et al; Alzheimer's Disease Centers Consortium on Apolipoprotein E and Alzheimer's Disease. Utility of the apolipoprotein E genotype in the diagnosis of Alzheimer's disease. *N Engl J Med*. 1998;338(8):506-511.

95. van Duijn CM, Clayton D, Chandra V, et al; EURODEM Risk Factors Research Group. Familial aggregation of Alzheimer's disease and related disorders: a collaborative re-analysis of case-control studies. *Int J Epidemiol*. 1991;20(suppl 2):S13-S20.

96. Myers RH, Schaefer EJ, Wilson PW, et al. Apolipoprotein E epsilon4 association with dementia in a population-based study: The Framingham study. *Neurology*. 1996;46(3):673-677.

97. The ALlele FREquency Database. http://alfred.med.yale.edu. Accessed February 28, 2014.

98. International HapMap Project. HapMap. http://hapmap.ncbi. nlm.nih.gov/. Accessed February 28, 2014.

99. Miki Y, Swensen J, Shattuck-Eidens D, et al. A strong candidate for the breast and ovarian cancer susceptibility gene BRCA1. *Science*. 1994;266(5182):66-71.

100. National Comprehensive Cancer Network. Testing of women with breast or ovarian cancer. http://www.nccn.org/index.asp. Accessed September 3, 2013.

101. McLeod HL, Krynetski EY, Relling MV, Evans WE. Genetic polymorphism of thiopurine methyltransferase and its clinical relevance for childhood acute lymphoblastic leukemia. *Leukemia*. 2000;14(4):567-572.

102. Marteau TM, Lerman C. Genetic risk and behavioural change. *BMJ*. 2001;322(7293):1056-1059.

103. Hamajima N, Suzuki K, Ito Y, Kondo T. Genotype announcement to Japanese smokers who attended a health checkup examination. *J Epidemiol*. 2006;16(1):45-47.

104. Lipkus IM, McBride CM, Pollak KI, Lyna P, Bepler G. Interpretation of genetic risk feedback among African American smokers with low socioeconomic status. *Health Psychol*. 2004;23(2):178-188.

105. Scheuner MT, Sieverding P, Shekelle PG. Delivery of genomic medicine for common chronic adult diseases: a systematic review. *JAMA*. 2008;299(11):1320-1334.

106. Hunter DJ, Khoury MJ, Drazen JM. Letting the genome out of the bottle—will we get our wish? *N Engl J Med*. 2008;358(2):105-107.

107. Janssens AC, Gwinn M, Bradley LA, Oostra BA, van Duijn CM, Khoury MJ. A critical appraisal of the scientific basis of commercial genomic profiles used to assess health risks and personalize health interventions. *Am J Hum Genet*. 2008; 82(3):593-599.

108. Downing NS, Ross JS. Innovation, risk, and patient empowerment: the FDA-mandated withdrawal of 23 and Me's Personal Genome Service. *JAMA*. 2014;311(8):793-794.

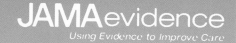
JAMAevidence
Using Evidence to Improve Care

SUMMARIZING THE EVIDENCE

SUMMARIZING THE EVIDENCE

22 The Process of a Systematic Review and Meta-analysis

M. Hassan Murad, Roman Jaeschke, PJ Devereaux, Kameshwar Prasad, Alonso Carrasco-Labra, Thomas Agoritsas, Deborah J. Cook, and Gordon Guyatt

IN THIS CHAPTER

CLINICAL SCENARIO

Should Patients Undergoing Noncardiac Surgery Receive β-Blockers?

You receive a request for consultation from a general surgeon regarding the perioperative management of a 66-year-old man undergoing hip replacement surgery in 2 days. The patient has a history of type 2 diabetes and hypertension and is a smoker. He has no history of heart disease. The patient's blood pressure is 135/80 mm Hg. Because the patient has multiple *risk factors* for heart disease, you are considering whether he should be treated perioperatively with β-blockers to reduce the risk of death, nonfatal myocardial infarction, and other vascular complications.

FINDING THE EVIDENCE

Being aware that a large amount of literature exists on this controversial topic, you decide to conduct a search that will provide you with an accurate and rapid overview of current best *evidence*. Because the question is about therapy, you are particularly interested in finding a recent *systematic review* and *meta-analysis* of *randomized clinical trials* (RCTs) that deal with this topic. Using the free *federated search engine* ACCESSSS (http://plus.mcmaster.ca/accessss; see Chapter 5, Finding Current Best Evidence), you enter these search terms: beta blockers, perioperative, and mortality.

Starting with the summaries at the top of your search output, you locate 2 relevant preappraised summaries on the "management of cardiac risk for noncardiac surgery." Both summaries cite the results of a large systematic review and meta-analysis published in 2008,[1] along with references to current US and European *clinical practice guidelines*. However, you notice that the last updates of these chapters date back 4 to 6 months ago. You therefore look further down

in your search output to check preappraised research (see Chapter 5, Finding Current Best Evidence) and rapidly identify a more recently published systematic review and meta-analysis addressing your question and that was highly rated for relevance and newsworthiness by clinicians from 4 specialties.[2] You download the full text of the article reporting this meta-analysis.

SYSTEMATIC REVIEWS AND META-ANALYSIS: AN INTRODUCTION

Definitions

A systematic review is a summary of research that addresses a focused clinical question in a systematic, reproducible manner. Systematic reviews can provide estimates of therapeutic efficacy, *prognosis*, and diagnostic test accuracy and can summarize the evidence for questions of "how" and "why" addressed by *qualitative research* studies. Although we will refer to other sorts of questions, this chapter focuses on systematic reviews that address the effect of therapeutic interventions or harmful *exposures* on *patient-important outcomes*.

A systematic review is often accompanied by a meta-analysis (a statistical pooling or aggregation of results from different studies) to provide a single best estimate of effect. The pooling of studies increases precision (ie, narrows the *confidence intervals* [CIs]), and the single best effect estimate generated facilitates clinical decision making. Therefore, you may see a published systematic review in which the authors chose not to do a meta-analysis, and you may see a meta-analysis conducted without a systematic review (ie, studies were combined statistically but were not selected following a comprehensive, explicit, and reproducible approach) (Figure 22-1). Most useful clinically will be a well-performed systematic review—the methods for which we describe in this chapter—with an accompanying meta-analysis.

In contrast to systematic reviews, traditional *narrative reviews* typically address multiple aspects of the disease (eg, etiology, diagnosis, prognosis, or management), have no explicit criteria for selecting the included studies, do not include systematic assessments of the *risk of bias* associated with *primary studies,* and do not provide quantitative best estimates or rate the confidence in these estimates. The traditional narrative review articles are useful for obtaining a broad overview of a clinical condition but may not provide a reliable and unbiased answer to a focused clinical question.

Why Seek Systematic Reviews?

When searching for evidence to answer a clinical question, it is preferable to seek a systematic review, especially one that includes a meta-analysis, rather than looking for the best individual study or studies. The reasons include the following:

1. Single studies are liable to be unrepresentative of the total body of evidence, and their results may therefore be misleading.
2. Collecting and appraising a number of studies take time you probably do not have.
3. A systematic review is often accompanied by a meta-analysis to provide the best estimate of effect that increases precision and facilitates clinical decision making.
4. If the systematic review is performed well, it will likely provide all of the relevant evidence with an assessment of the best estimates of effect and the confidence they warrant.
5. Systematic reviews include a greater range of patients than any single study, potentially enhancing your confidence in applying the results to the patient before you.

A Synopsis of the Process of a Systematic Review and Meta-analysis

In applying the *Users' Guides,* you will find it useful to have a clear understanding of the process of conducting a systematic review and meta-analysis. Figure 22-2 shows how the process begins with the definition of the question, which is synonymous with specifying eligibility criteria for deciding which studies to include in a review. These criteria define the population, the exposures or interventions, and the outcomes of interest. A systematic review also

may restrict studies to those that minimize the risk of bias. For example, systematic reviews that address a question of therapy often will include only RCTs.

FIGURE 22-1

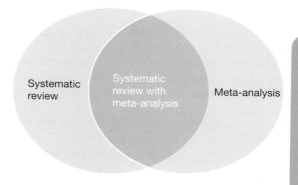

The Overlap of Study Designs: Systematic Review and Meta-analysis

Systematic review — Systematic review with meta-analysis — Meta-analysis

FIGURE 22-2

The Process of Conducting a Systematic Review and Meta-analysis

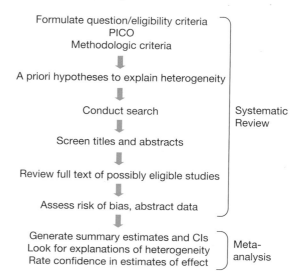

Formulate question/eligibility criteria PICO Methodologic criteria

A priori hypotheses to explain heterogeneity

Conduct search

Screen titles and abstracts

Review full text of possibly eligible studies

Assess risk of bias, abstract data

Systematic Review

Generate summary estimates and CIs Look for explanations of heterogeneity Rate confidence in estimates of effect

Meta-analysis

In a systematic review without meta-analysis, the step of generating summary estimates and confidence intervals is not applicable. If the systematic review includes a meta-analysis and presents estimates of effect from individual studies, seeking explanation for heterogeneity and rating confidence in estimates is possible.

Abbreviations: CI, confidence interval; PICO, Patient, Intervention, Comparison, Outcome.

Having specified their selection criteria, reviewers will conduct a comprehensive search of the literature in all relevant medical databases, which typically yields a large number of potentially relevant titles and abstracts. They then apply the selection criteria to the titles and abstracts, arriving at a smaller number of articles that they retrieve. Once again, the reviewers apply the selection criteria, this time to the complete reports.

Having completed the culling process, the reviewers assess the risk of bias of the individual studies and abstract data from each study. Finally, they summarize the results, including, if appropriate, a quantitative synthesis or meta-analysis. The meta-analysis provides *pooled estimates* (ie, combined estimates) of the effect on each of the outcomes of interest, along with the associated CIs. Meta-analyses frequently include an examination of the differences in effect estimates across included studies in an attempt to explain differences in results (exploring *heterogeneity*). If based on previously specified hypotheses about possible differences in patients, interventions, or outcomes that may explain differences in results, such explorations become more credible (see Chapter 25.2, How to Use a Subgroup Analysis).

BOX 22-1

Users' Guides for Credibility of the Systematic Review Process

Did the review explicitly address a sensible clinical question?

Was the search for relevant studies exhaustive?

Was the risk of bias of the primary studies assessed?

Did the review address possible explanations of between-study differences in results?

Did the review present results that are ready for clinical application?

Were selection and assessments of studies reproducible?

Did the review address confidence in effect estimates?

Judging the Credibility of the Effect Estimates

When applying the results of a systematic review to patient care, you can look for estimates of effect. A systematic review without a meta-analysis typically presents results from individual studies; the meta-analysis adds a single pooled (combined) estimate of effect, with an associated CI, for each relevant outcome. Pooled estimates could be for therapy outcomes (eg, death, myocardial infarction, quality of life, late catastrophic adverse effects), estimates of the properties of diagnostic tests (eg, *likelihood ratios*), or estimates of patients' likely outcomes (eg, prognosis). Clinicians need to know the extent to which they can trust these estimates.

Two fundamental problems can undermine this trust. One is the extent to which systematic review authors have applied rigorous methods in conducting their review. We refer to this as the *credibility* of the review.[3] By credibility, we mean the extent to which the design and conduct of the review are likely to have protected against misleading results.[4] As you will see, credibility may be undermined by eligibility criteria that are inappropriate or not specified, the conduct of an inadequate search, and the omission of risk of bias assessments of individual studies (see Box 22-1 for issues to be considered in the credibility of the review process; these issues are applicable to any systematic review, with or without a meta-analysis).

A highly credible review—one that has adhered to methodologic standards—may nevertheless leave us with only very low confidence in estimates of effect. Common reasons for this include the following: the individual studies may be plagued by high risk of bias and inconsistent results, even the pooled (combined) sample sizes may be small and the results may be imprecise, and the patients enrolled in the studies may differ in important ways from those in whom we are interested. This chapter deals with credibility assessment of the review process; the next chapter (Chapter 23, Understanding and Applying the Results of a Systematic Review and Meta-analysis) will guide you in deciding how much confidence we can place on estimates of effect in the presence of a credible review process.

WAS THE PROCESS CREDIBLE?

Did the Review Explicitly Address a Sensible Clinical Question?

A systematic review has, relative to a traditional narrative review, a narrow focus and addresses a specific question that—for questions of therapy or harm—is defined by particular patients, interventions, comparisons, and outcomes. When review authors conduct a meta-analysis, the issue of how narrow or wide is the scope of the question becomes particularly important. Let us look at these hypothetical examples of 4 meta-analyses with varying scope:

1. A meta-analysis that pooled results from all modalities of cancer therapy for all types of cancer to generate a single estimate of the effect on mortality.

2. A meta-analysis that pooled the results of the effect of all doses of all antiplatelet agents (including aspirin, sulfinpyrazone, dipyridamole, ticlopidine, and clopidogrel) on major thrombotic events (including myocardial infarctions, strokes, and acute arterial insufficiency in the lower extremities).

3. A meta-analysis that pooled the results of the effect of all doses of all antiplatelet agents on mortality in patients with clinically manifest atherosclerosis (whether in the heart, brain, or lower extremities).

4. A meta-analysis that pooled the results of the effect of a wide range of aspirin doses to *prevent* thrombotic stroke in patients presenting with a transient ischemic attack (TIA) due to carotid artery disease.

Clinicians will clearly be uncomfortable with the first meta-analysis, which addresses all treatments for all cancers. Clinicians are unlikely to find the second and third meta-analyses on antiplatelet agents in major thrombotic events and mortality useful because they remain too broad. In contrast, most clinicians may be comfortable with the fourth, more focused meta-analysis of aspirin and thrombotic stroke, although they may express concerns about pooling across a wide range of aspirin doses.

What makes a meta-analysis too broad or too narrow? When deciding whether the question posed in the meta-analysis is sensible, clinicians need to ask themselves whether the underlying biology is such that they would anticipate more or less the same *treatment effect* across the range of patients included (Box 22-2). They should ask a parallel question about the other components of the study question: Is the underlying biology such that, across the range of interventions and outcomes studied, they expect more or less the same treatment effect? Clinicians also can construct a similar set of questions for other areas of clinical inquiry. For example, across the range of patients, ways of testing, and *reference* or *gold standard* for diagnosis, does one expect more or less the same likelihood ratios associated with studies that examine a diagnostic test[5] (see Chapter 18, Diagnostic Tests)?

Clinicians reject a meta-analysis that pools data across all modes of cancer therapy for all types of cancer because they know that some cancer treatments are effective in certain cancers, whereas others are not effective. Combining the results of these studies would yield an estimate of effect that would make little sense or be misleading for most of the interventions. Clinicians who reject the meta-analysis on all antiplatelet agents and mortality in patients with atherosclerosis would argue that the biologic variation in

---

BOX 22-2

Were Eligibility Criteria for Inclusion in the Systematic Review Appropriate?

Are results likely to be similar across the range of included patients (eg, older and younger, sicker and less sick)?

Are results likely to be similar across the range of studied interventions or exposures (eg, for therapy, higher dose or lower dose; for diagnosis, test results interpreted by experts or nonexperts)?

Are results likely to be similar across the range of ways the outcome was measured (eg, shorter or longer follow-up)?

SUMMARIZING THE EVIDENCE

BOX 22-3

Guides for Selecting Articles That Are Most Likely to Provide Results at Lower Risk of Bias

Therapy	Were patients randomized?
	Was follow-up complete?
Diagnosis	Was the patient sample representative of those with the disorder?
	Was the diagnosis verified using credible criteria that were independent of the items of medical history, physical examination, laboratory tests, or imaging procedures under study?
Harm	Did the investigators find similarity in all known determinants of outcome or adjust for differences in the analysis?
	Was follow-up sufficiently complete?
Prognosis	Was there a representative sample of patients?
	Was follow-up sufficiently complete?

---

antiplatelet agents is likely to lead to important differences in treatment effect. Furthermore, they may contend that there are important differences in the biology of atherosclerosis in the vessels of the heart, brain and neck, and legs. Those who would endorse this meta-analysis would argue for the similar underlying biology of antiplatelet agents—and atherosclerosis in different parts of the body—and thus anticipate a similar magnitude of treatment effects.

For the last, more focused review, most clinicians would accept that the biology of aspirin action is likely to be similar in patients whose TIA reflected right-sided or left-sided brain ischemia, in patients older than 75 years and in younger patients, in men and women, across different aspirin doses, during periods of *follow-up* ranging from 1 to 5 years, and in patients with stroke who have been identified by the attending physician and those identified by a team of experts. The similar biology is likely to result in a similar magnitude of treatment effect, which explains the comfort of the meta-analysis authors with combining studies of aspirin in patients who have had a TIA.

The clinician's task is to decide whether, across the range of patients, interventions or exposures, and outcomes, it is plausible that the intervention will have a similar effect. This judgment is possible only if the review authors have provided a precise statement of what range of patients, exposures, and outcomes they decided to include; in other words, the explicit eligibility criteria for their review.

In addition, systematic review authors must specify the criteria for study inclusion related to the risk of bias. Generally, these should be similar to the most important criteria used to evaluate the risk of bias in primary studies[6] (Box 22-3). Explicit eligibility criteria not only facilitate the decision regarding whether the question was sensible but also make it less likely that the authors will preferentially include or exclude studies that support their own previous conclusions or beliefs.

Clinicians may legitimately ask, even within a relatively narrowly defined question, whether they can be confident that results will be similar across patients, interventions, and outcome measurement. Referring to the question of aspirin use by patients with a TIA, the effect could conceivably differ in those with more or less severe underlying atherosclerosis, across aspirin doses, or during short-term and long-term follow-up. Thus, at the time of examining the results, we need to ask whether the assumption with which we started proved accurate: was the effect the same across patients, interventions, and outcomes? We return to this issue in the next chapter (see Chapter 23, Understanding and Applying the Results of a Systematic Review and Meta-analysis).

Was the Search for Relevant Studies Detailed and Exhaustive?

Systematic reviews are at risk of presenting misleading results if they fail to secure a complete, or at least representative, sample of the available eligible studies. To achieve this objective, reviewers search bibliographic databases. For most clinical questions, searching a single database is insufficient and can lead to missing important studies. Therefore, searching MEDLINE, EMBASE, and the Cochrane Central Register of Controlled Trials is recommended for most clinical questions.[7] Searching other databases may be required, depending on the nature of the review question. The systematic review authors check the reference lists of the articles they retrieve and seek personal contact with experts in the area. It also may be important to examine recently published abstracts presented at scientific meetings and to look at less frequently used databases, including those that summarize doctoral theses and databases of ongoing trials held by pharmaceutical companies or databases of ongoing registered trials.

Another important source of unpublished studies is the US Food and Drug Administration (FDA) reviews of new drug applications. A study that evaluated the risk of dyspepsia associated with the use of nonsteroidal anti-inflammatory drugs found that searching FDA records yielded 11 trials, of which only 1 was published.[8] Another study of FDA reports found that they included numerous unpublished studies, and the findings of these studies can appreciably alter the estimates of effect.[9] Unless the authors of systematic reviews tell us what they did to locate the studies, it is difficult to know how likely it is that relevant studies were missed.

Reporting bias occurs in a number of forms, the most familiar of which is the failure to report or publish studies with negative results. This *publication bias* may result in misleading results of systematic reviews that fail to include unpublished studies.[10,11]

If authors include unpublished studies in a review, they should try to obtain full reports, and they should use the same criteria to appraise the risk of bias of both published and unpublished studies. There is a variety of techniques available to explore the possibility of publication bias, but none of them are fully satisfactory. Systematic reviews based on a small number of studies with limited total sample sizes are particularly susceptible to publication bias, especially if most or all of the studies have been sponsored by a commercial entity with a vested interest in the results.

Another increasingly recognized form of reporting bias occurs when investigators measure a number of outcomes but report only those that favor the *experimental intervention* or those that favor the intervention most strongly (*selective outcome reporting bias*). If reviewers report that they have successfully contacted authors of primary studies and were assured of the full disclosure of results, concern about reporting bias decreases.

Reviewers may go even farther than simply contacting the authors of primary studies. They may recruit these investigators as collaborators in their review, and in the process, they may obtain individual patient records. Such *individual patient data meta-analysis* can facilitate powerful analyses (addressing issues such as true *intention-to-treat* analyses and informed *subgroup analyses*), which may strengthen the inferences from a systematic review.

Was the Risk of Bias of the Primary Studies Assessed?

Even if a systematic review includes only RCTs, knowing the extent to which each individual trial used safeguards against bias is important. Differences in study methods might explain important differences among the results.[12] For example, less rigorous studies sometimes overestimate the effectiveness of therapeutic and preventive interventions.[13] Even if the results of different studies are consistent, determining their risk of bias is still important. Consistent results are less compelling if they come from studies with a high risk of bias than if they come from studies with a low risk of bias.

Consistent results from *observational studies* putatively addressing treatment issues also should raise concern. Clinicians may systematically select patients with a good prognosis to receive therapy, and this pattern of practice may be consistent over time and geographic setting. There are many examples of observational studies that found misleading results subsequently contradicted by large RCTs. For example, considerable preclinical and epidemiologic evidence suggested that antioxidant vitamins reduced the risk of prostate cancer. However, a trial of 35 533 healthy men found that dietary supplementation with vitamin E significantly increased the risk of prostate cancer.[14] Similarly, laboratory experiments suggested that antioxidants may slow or prevent atherosclerotic plaque formation, but a trial of 14 641 male physicians found that neither vitamin E nor vitamin C supplementation reduced the risk of major cardiovascular events.[15] Many other examples and a discussion of misleading results of observational studies and RCTs can be found in Chapter 11.2, Surprising Results of Randomized Trials.

There is no one correct way to assess the risk of bias.[16] Some reviewers use long checklists to evaluate risk of bias, whereas others focus on 3 or 4 key aspects of the study. When considering whether to trust the results of a review, check to see whether the authors examined criteria similar to those we have presented in other chapters of this book (see Chapter 7, Therapy [Randomized Trials]; Chapter 14, Harm [Observational Studies]; Chapter 18, Diagnostic Tests; and Chapter 20, Prognosis). Reviewers should apply these criteria with a relatively low threshold (such as restricting eligibility to RCTs) in selecting studies (Box 22-3) and more comprehensively (such as considering *concealment*, *blinding*, and *stopping early* for benefit) in assessing the risk of bias of the included studies. The authors of systematic reviews should explicitly report the extent of the risk of bias of each included study in their review.

Did the Review Address Possible Explanations of Between-Study Differences in Results?

Studies included in a systematic review are unlikely to show identical results. Whether or not their review includes a meta-analysis, systematic review authors should attempt to explain the reasons for variability in results. When the studies are combined in a meta-analysis, the difference in results becomes easily quantifiable. Chance always represents a possible explanation. Alternatively, differences in the

characteristics of the patients enrolled, in the way the intervention was administered, in the way the outcome was assessed, or in the risk of bias may be responsible. For example, the intervention may be more effective in older patients than in younger patients or in those with diabetes than in those without diabetes. We often refer to inconsistency in results among studies as heterogeneity.

Systematic review authors should hypothesize possible explanations for heterogeneity (a priori, when they plan the review) and test their hypotheses in a subgroup analysis. Subgroup analyses may provide important insights, but they also may be misleading (see Chapter 25.2, How to Use a Subgroup Analysis). In Chapter 23, Understanding and Applying the Results of a Systematic Review and Meta-analysis, we discuss how to evaluate heterogeneity and how it affects the confidence in estimates.

Did the Review Present Results That Are Ready for Clinical Application?

If you and your patients are told that treatment lowers the risk of myocardial infarction by 50%, it sounds impressive, but that could mean a reduction from 1% to 0.5% or from 40% to 20%. In the former situation, when the *risk difference* (also referred to as *absolute risk reduction*) is 0.5%, your patient may decide to decline a treatment with appreciable adverse effect, *burden*, or cost. In the latter situation, that is much less likely to be the case. Therefore, you and your patients need to know the absolute effect of the intervention. The absolute benefit (or harm) that patients will achieve with therapy depends on their *baseline risk* (the likelihood of the outcome when receiving no or standard therapy).

For example, statins reduce fatal and nonfatal cardiovascular events[17] by approximately 25% (*relative risk* [RR], 0.75); the absolute benefit, however, may be greater for a patient with an elevated Framingham risk score (or other risk stratification method) than for a patient with a low score (Box 22-4).

Although we are primarily interested in absolute effects, relative effects tend to be much more consistent across studies (see Chapter 9, Does Treatment Lower Risk? Understanding the Results). That is the reason that meta-analyses of binary outcomes

BOX 22-4

The Impact of Baseline Risk on the Magnitude of Absolute Risk Reduction

Patient 1

65-year-old male smoker with cholesterol level of 250 mg/dL, high-density lipoprotein (HDL) of 30 mg/dL, and systolic blood pressure of 140 mm Hg

Absolute risk of having a cardiac event during the next 10 years: 28%

Risk after treatment with statin: 28% × 0.75 = 21%

Absolute risk reduction: 28% − 21% = 7%

Patient 2

50-year-old female smoker with cholesterol of 170 mg/dL, HDL of 55 mg/dL, and systolic blood pressure of 130 mm Hg

Absolute risk of having a cardiac event during the next 10 years: 2%

Risk after treatment with statin: 2% × 0.75 = 1.5%

Absolute risk reduction: 2% − 1.5% = 0.5%

---

usually should and do combine and present relative effects, such as the relative risk, *odds ratio*, or occasionally *hazard ratio*. So how, then, do we determine the absolute effects in which we are really interested? The best way is to obtain an estimate of the patients' baseline risk (ideally from an observational study of a representative population, from a risk-stratification instrument, or, if neither is available, from the randomized trials in the meta-analysis)[18] and then use the relative risk[19] to estimate that patient's risk difference.

Review authors also can present outcomes that are *continuous variables* in ways that are more or less useful and applicable. For instance, the weighted mean difference and standardized mean difference represent common statistical approaches for pooling across studies. Clinicians, however, may have difficulty grasping the significance of the effect of a respiratory rehabilitation program presented as a weighted mean difference of 0.71 units on the Chronic Respiratory Questionnaire (CRQ) scale. They may have less difficulty if told that the *minimal important difference* on the CRQ is 0.5 units. Clinicians are likely to have at least equal difficulty if told that the treatment effect on disease-specific *health-related quality of life* is a standardized mean difference of 0.71. Again, they may have less difficulty if told that 0.2, 0.5, and 0.8 may represent small, moderate, and large effects. Clinicians are likely to have the least amount of difficulty if told that 30% of patients have an important improvement in function as a result of

the program (a *number needed to treat* of approximately 3).[20]

Were Selection and Assessments of Studies Reproducible?

As we have seen, authors of systematic reviews must decide which studies to include, the extent of risk of bias, and what data to abstract. These decisions always require judgment by the reviewers and are subject to both mistakes (ie, *random errors*) and bias (ie, *systematic errors*). Having 2 or more people participate in each decision guards against errors, and if there is good agreement beyond chance among the reviewers, the clinician can have more confidence in the results of the systematic review. Systematic reviewers often report a measure of agreement (eg, a measure of *chance-corrected agreement* such as the κ *statistic*) (see Chapter 19.3, Measuring Agreement Beyond Chance) to quantify their level of agreement on study selection and appraisal of the risk of bias.

Did the Review Address Confidence in Effect Estimates?

As we have pointed out, a review can follow optimal systematic review and meta-analytic methods, and the evidence may still warrant low confidence in estimates of effect. Ideally, systematic review authors will explicitly address the risk of bias that can diminish confidence in estimates as well as imprecision (ie, wide CIs) and inconsistency (ie, large variability in results from study to study). If systematic review authors do not make explicit assessments themselves, they should at least provide the information you need to make your own assessment. The next chapter

(Chapter 23, Understanding and Applying the Results of a Systematic Review and Meta-analysis) describes in detail how the systematic review authors—or you, in the absence of the authors doing so explicitly—can address these issues to make an appropriate rating of confidence in estimates of effect.

CLINICAL SCENARIO RESOLUTION

Returning to our opening scenario, the systematic review and meta-analysis you located included 11 trials that enrolled more than 10 000 patients who were having noncardiac surgery and were randomized to either β-blockers or a *control group*.[2] The trials addressed the main outcomes of interest (death, nonfatal myocardial infarction, and nonfatal stroke). The β-blocker, dose, timing, and duration of administration all varied across the trials.

The systematic review authors had searched MEDLINE, EMBASE, CINAHL, the Cochrane Library Central Register of Randomised Controlled Trials, and other trial databases and registries. They also checked the reference lists of identified articles and previous systematic reviews for additional references. They did not restrict the search to a particular language or location. They had 2 independent reviewers assess trial eligibility and select studies, and disagreements were resolved by a third review author. They did not quantitatively report the

agreement level among reviewers, a feature you would have preferred to know.

The systematic review authors used the *Cochrane Collaboration* risk of bias assessment methods. They explicitly described the risk of bias of each trial by reporting on the adequacy of generation of the allocation sequence, allocation concealment, and blinding of participants, personnel, and outcome assessors. As part of the meta-analysis, the authors conducted a separate *sensitivity analysis* that excluded the studies with a higher risk of bias. They tested for publication bias. They did not report that they had contacted authors of primary studies, which you would have preferred they did.

Overall, you conclude that the credibility of the methods of this systematic review and meta-analysis is moderate to high, and you decide to examine the estimates of effect and the associated confidence in these estimates.

References

1. Bangalore S, Wetterslev J, Pranesh S, Sawhney S, Gluud C, Messerli FH. Perioperative beta blockers in patients having non-cardiac surgery: a meta-analysis. *Lancet*. 2008;372(9654):1962-1976.

2. Bouri S, Shun-Shin MJ, Cole GD, Mayet J, Francis DP. Meta-analysis of secure randomised controlled trials of β-blockade to prevent perioperative death in non-cardiac surgery. *Heart*. 2014;100(6):456-464.

3. Alkin M. *Evaluation Roots: Tracing Theorists' Views and Influences*. Thousand Oaks, CA: Sage Publications Inc; 2004.

4. Oxman AD. Checklists for review articles. *BMJ*. 1994;309(6955): 648-651.

5. Irwig L, Tosteson AN, Gatsonis C, et al. Guidelines for meta-analyses evaluating diagnostic tests. *Ann Intern Med*. 1994;120(8):667-676.

6. Oxman AD, Guyatt GH. The science of reviewing research. *Ann N Y Acad Sci*. 1993;703:125-134.

7. The Cochrane Collaboration. *Cochrane Handbook for Systematic Reviews of Interventions*. Version 5.1.0. http://handbook.cochrane.org/. Accessed July 26, 2014.

8. MacLean CH, Morton SC, Ofman JJ, Roth EA, Shekelle PG. How useful are unpublished data from the Food and Drug Administration in meta-analysis? *J Clin Epidemiol*. 2003;56(1):44-51.

9. McDonagh MS, Peterson K, Balshem H, Helfand M. US Food and Drug Administration documents can provide unpublished evidence relevant to systematic reviews. *J Clin Epidemiol*. 2013;66(10):1071-1081.

10. Stern JM, Simes RJ. Publication bias: evidence of delayed publication in a cohort study of clinical research projects. *BMJ*. 1997;315(7109):640-645.

11. Ioannidis JP. Effect of the statistical significance of results on the time to completion and publication of randomized efficacy trials. *JAMA*. 1998;279(4):281-286.

12. Moher D, Pham B, Jones A, et al. Does quality of reports of randomised trials affect estimates of intervention efficacy reported in meta-analyses? *Lancet*. 1998;352(9128):609-613.

13. Odgaard-Jensen J, Vist GE, Timmer A, et al. Randomisation to protect against selection bias in healthcare trials. *Cochrane Database Syst Rev*. 2011;(4):MR000012.

14. Klein EA, Thompson IM Jr, Tangen CM, et al. Vitamin E and the risk of prostate cancer: the Selenium and Vitamin E Cancer Prevention Trial (SELECT). *JAMA*. 2011;306(14):1549-1556.

15. Sesso HD, Buring JE, Christen WG, et al. Vitamins E and C in the prevention of cardiovascular disease in men: the Physicians' Health Study II randomized controlled trial. *JAMA*. 2008;300(18):2123-2133.

16. Jüni P, Witschi A, Bloch R, Egger M. The hazards of scoring the quality of clinical trials for meta-analysis. *JAMA*. 1999;282(11):1054-1060.

17. Taylor F, Huffman MD, Macedo AF, et al. Statins for the primary prevention of cardiovascular disease. *Cochrane Database Syst Rev*. 2013;1:CD004816.

18. Guyatt GH, Eikelboom JW, Gould MK, et al; American College of Chest Physicians. Approach to outcome measurement in the prevention of thrombosis in surgical and medical patients: *Antithrombotic Therapy and Prevention of Thrombosis*, 9th ed: American College of Chest Physicians Evidence-Based Clinical Practice Guidelines. *Chest*. 2012;141(2)(suppl):e185S-e194S.

19. Murad MH, Montori VM, Walter SD, Guyatt GH. Estimating risk difference from relative association measures in meta-analysis can infrequently pose interpretational challenges. *J Clin Epidemiol*. 2009;62(8):865-867.

20. Thorlund K, Walter SD, Johnston BC, Furukawa TA, Guyatt GH. Pooling health-related quality of life outcomes in meta-analysis—a tutorial and review of methods for enhancing interpretability. *Res Synth Methods*. 2012;2(3):188-203.

SUMMARIZING THE EVIDENCE

23

Understanding and Applying the Results of a Systematic Review and Meta-analysis

M. Hassan Murad, Victor M. Montori, John P. A. Ioannidis,
Ignacio Neumann, Rose Hatala, Maureen O. Meade,
PJ Devereaux, Peter Wyer, and Gordon Guyatt

IN THIS CHAPTER

In the previous chapter (Chapter 22, The Process of a Systematic Review and Meta-analysis), we provided guidance on how to evaluate the *credibility* of the process of a *systematic review* with or without a *meta-analysis*. In this chapter, we address how—if the systematic review is sufficiently credible—to decide on the degree of confidence in the estimates that the *evidence* warrants. As you will see, systematic review authors may have conducted a credible review and analysis and one may still have little confidence in the estimates of effect. We will return to the clinical scenario discussed in the previous chapter and obtain the relative and absolute effects of the intervention from a credible systematic review and meta-analysis[1] and determine the confidence in these estimates (quality of evidence). The general framework for judging confidence in estimates is based on the approach offered by the *GRADE (Grading of Recommendations Assessment, Development and Evaluation)* Working Group.[2] This chapter focuses on questions of therapy or harm. This framework can, however, be adapted for other types of questions, such as issues of prognosis[3] or diagnosis.[4]

CLINICAL SCENARIO

We continue with the scenario of a 66-year-old male smoker with type 2 diabetes and hypertension undergoing noncardiac surgery for whom we are considering prescribing perioperative β-blockers to prevent the cardiovascular complications of nonfatal infarction, death, and nonfatal stroke.

UNDERSTANDING THE SUMMARY ESTIMATE OF A META-ANALYSIS

If the systematic review authors decide that combining results to generate a single estimate of effect is inappropriate, a systematic review will likely end with a table or tables describing results of individual *primary studies*. Often, however, systematic reviews include a meta-analysis with a best estimate of effect (often called a *summary* or *pooled estimate*) from the weighted averages of the results of the individual

studies. The weighting process depends on sample size or number of events (see Chapter 12.3, What Determines the Width of the Confidence Interval?) or, more specifically, study precision. Studies that are more precise have narrower *confidence intervals* (CIs) and larger weight in meta-analysis.

In a meta-analysis of a therapeutic question looking at *dichotomous outcomes* (yes/no) for estimates of the magnitude of the benefits or *risks*, you should look for the *relative risk* (RR) and *relative risk reduction* (RRR) or the *odds ratio* (OR) and *relative odds* reduction (see Chapter 9, Does Treatment Lower Risk? Understanding the Results). When the outcome is analyzed using time-to-event methods (eg, *survival analysis*), the results could be presented as a *hazard ratio*. In a meta-analysis addressing diagnosis, you should look for summary estimates of *likelihood ratios* or diagnostic ORs (see Chapter 18, Diagnostic Tests).

In the setting of *continuous variables* rather than dichotomous outcomes, meta-analysts typically use 1 of 2 options to aggregate data across studies. If the outcome is measured the same way in each study (eg, duration of hospitalization), the results from each study are combined, taking into account each study's precision to calculate what is called a *weighted mean difference*. This measure has the same units as the outcomes reported in the individual studies (eg, pooled estimate of reduction in hospital stay with treatment, 1.1 days).

Sometimes the outcome measures used in the primary studies are similar but not identical. For example, one trial might measure *health-related quality of life* using a validated questionnaire (the Chronic Respiratory Questionnaire), and another trial might use a different validated questionnaire (the St. George's Questionnaire). Another example of this situation is a meta-analysis of studies using different measures of severity of depression.

If the patients and the interventions are similar, generating a pooled estimate of the effect of the intervention on quality of life or depression, even when investigators have used different measurement instruments, is likely to be worthwhile. One way of generating the pooled estimate in this instance is to standardize the measures by looking at the mean difference between treatment and control and dividing this by the SD.[5] The *effect size* that results from this calculation provides a summary estimate of the treatment effect expressed in

SD units (eg, an effect size of 0.5 means that the mean effect of treatment across studies is half of an SD unit). A rule of thumb for understanding effect sizes suggests that 0.2 SD represents small effects; 0.5 SD, moderate effects; and 0.8 SD, large effects.[6]

Clinicians may be unfamiliar with how to interpret effect size, and systematic review authors may help you interpret the results by using one of a number of alternative presentations. One is to translate the summary effect size back into natural units.[7] For instance, clinicians may have become familiar with the significance of differences in walk test scores in patients with chronic lung disease. Investigators can then convert the effect size of a

treatment on a number of measures of functional status (eg, the walk test and stair climbing) back into differences in walk test scores.[8]

Even better may be the translation of continuous outcomes into dichotomies: the proportion of patients who, for instance, have experienced an important reduction in pain, fatigue, or dyspnea. Methods of making such translations are increasingly well developed.[9,10] For examples on how systematic review authors can present results that are ready for clinical applications, see Chapter 22, The Process of a Systematic Review and Meta-analysis.

The results of a traditional meta-analysis are usually depicted in what is called a *forest plot* (Figures 23-1,

SUMMARIZING THE EVIDENCE

FIGURE 23-1

Results of a Meta-analysis of the Outcomes of Nonfatal Infarction in Patients Receiving Perioperative β-Blockers

Study	β-Blockers Events	β-Blockers Total	Control Events	Control Total	RR (95% CI)
Low Risk of Bias					
DIPOM	3	462	2	459	1.49 (0.25-8.88)
MaVS	19	246	21	250	0.92 (0.51-1.67)
POISE	152	4174	215	4177	0.71 (0.58-0.87)
POBBLE	3	55	5	48	0.52 (0.13-2.08)
BBSA	1	110	0	109	2.97 (0.12-72.19)
Subtotal (I^2 = 0%, P = .70)					0.73 (0.61-0.88)
High Risk of Bias					
Poldermans	0	59	9	53	0.05 (0.00-0.79)
Dunkelgrun	11	533	27	533	0.41 (0.20-0.81)
Subtotal (I^2 = 57%, P = .13)					0.21 (0.03-1.61)

I^2 = 29%, P = .21
Interaction test between groups, P = .22

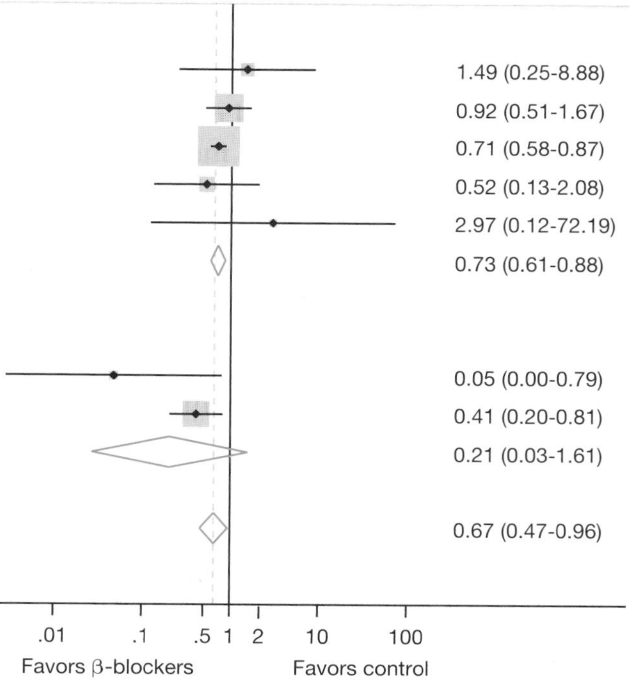

0.67 (0.47-0.96)

.01 .1 .5 1 2 10 100
Favors β-blockers   Favors control

Abbreviations: BBSA, Beta Blocker in Spinal Anesthesia study; CI, confidence interval; DIPOM, Diabetic Postoperative Mortality and Morbidity trial; MaVS, Metoprolol after Vascular Surgery study; POBBLE, Perioperative β-blockade trial; POISE, PeriOperative ISchemic Evaluation trial.
Solid line indicates no effect. Dashed line is centered on meta-analysis pooled estimate.
Data are from Bouri et al.[1]

FIGURE 23-2

Results of a Meta-analysis of the Outcomes of Death in Patients Receiving Perioperative β-Blockers

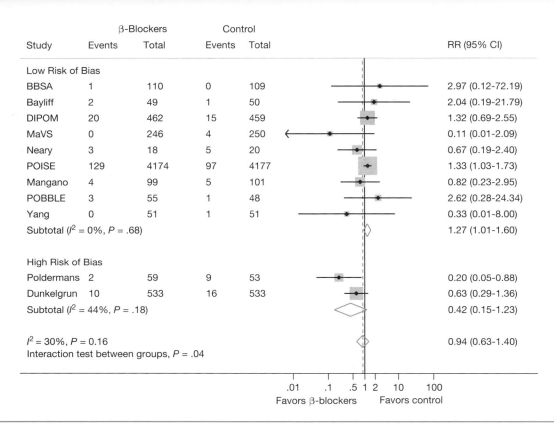

Abbreviations: BBSA, Beta Blocker in Spinal Anesthesia study; CI, confidence interval; DIPOM, Diabetic Postoperative Mortality and Morbidity trial; MaVS, Metoprolol after Vascular Surgery study; POBBLE, Perioperative β-blockade trial; POISE, PeriOperative ISchemic Evaluation trial. Solid line indicates no effect. Dashed line is centered on meta-analysis pooled estimate.

Data from Bouri et al.[1]

23-2, and 23-3). This forest plot shows the effect (ie, result) from every study; the *point estimate* is presented as a square with a size that is proportional to the weight of the study, and the CI is presented as a horizontal line. The solid line at 1.0 indicates no effect, and the dashed line is centered on the meta-analysis combined summary effect. The combined summary effect is usually presented as a diamond, with its width representing the CI for the combined effect. As the CI widens, uncertainty about the magnitude of effect increases; when the CI crosses no effect (RR or OR of 1.0), there is uncertainty about whether the intervention has any effect at all (see Chapter 10, Confidence Intervals: Was the Single Study or Meta-analysis Large Enough?).

USING THE GUIDE

Returning to the perioperative β-blockers scenario, you found a systematic review that you considered as having a credible process that included a meta-analysis for the outcomes of nonfatal infarction, mortality, and nonfatal stroke.[1] The forest plots reveal the estimates of effect for these outcomes from the relevant *randomized trials* (Figures 23-1, 23-2, and 23-3).

Perioperative administration of β-blockers decreases the risk of 1 adverse outcome—nonfatal myocardial infarction (RR, 0.67; 95% CI, 0.47-0.96).

FIGURE 23-3

Results of a Meta-analysis of the Outcomes of Nonfatal Stroke in Patients Receiving Perioperative β-Blockers

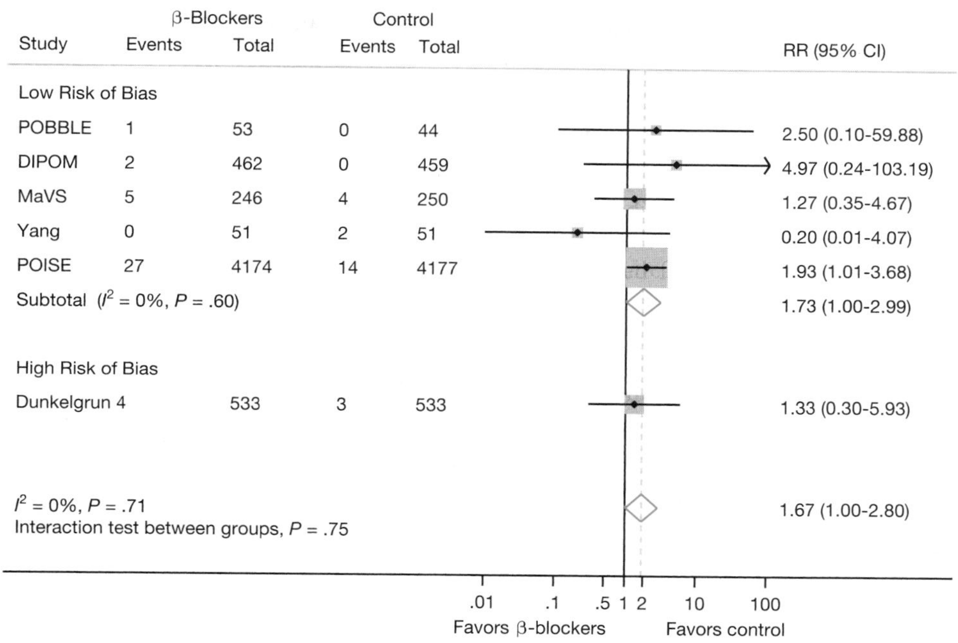

Study	β-Blockers		Control			RR (95% CI)
	Events	Total	Events	Total		
Low Risk of Bias						
POBBLE	1	53	0	44		2.50 (0.10-59.88)
DIPOM	2	462	0	459		4.97 (0.24-103.19)
MaVS	5	246	4	250		1.27 (0.35-4.67)
Yang	0	51	2	51		0.20 (0.01-4.07)
POISE	27	4174	14	4177		1.93 (1.01-3.68)
Subtotal (I^2 = 0%, P = .60)						1.73 (1.00-2.99)
High Risk of Bias						
Dunkelgrun 4		533	3	533		1.33 (0.30-5.93)
I^2 = 0%, P = .71						1.67 (1.00-2.80)
Interaction test between groups, P = .75						

.01　.1　.5 1 2　10　100

Favors β-blockers　　Favors control

Abbreviations: CI, confidence interval; DIPOM, Diabetic Postoperative Mortality and Morbidity trial; MaVS, Metoprolol after Vascular Surgery study; POBBLE, Perioperative β-blockade trial; POISE, PeriOperative ISchemic Evaluation trial.

Solid line indicates no effect. Dashed line is centered on meta-analysis pooled estimate.

Data from Bouri et al.[1]

SUMMARIZING THE EVIDENCE

The summary effect reached the threshold for *statistical significance* because the CI does not cross 1.0 (no effect) (Figure 23-1). However, β-blockers likely increased the risk of nonfatal stroke, the lower boundary of the CI just touching no effect (RR, 1.67; 95% CI, 1.00-2.80) (Figure 23-3). You are not sure about the effect of β-blockers on the outcome of death because the CI crosses 1.0 and is wide, including a large reduction (37%) and a large increase (40%) in death (RR, 0.94; 95% CI, 0.63-1.40) (Figure 23-2).

You note, however, that there is appreciable *inconsistency* in the results for the *end points* of death and myocardial infarction and that, in particular, the studies with low or high *risk of*

bias studies yield different results. This raises the question of which results are more credible, an issue to which we return later in this chapter.

Understanding the Estimate of Absolute Effect

The goal of a systematic review and meta-analysis is often to present evidence users (clinicians, patients, and policymakers) with best estimates of the effect of an intervention on each *patient-important outcome*. When interpreting and applying the results, you and your patients must balance the desirable and undesirable consequences to decide on the best course of action.

As we pointed out in the previous chapter (Chapter 22, The Process of a Systematic Review and Meta-analysis), knowledge of the RRs associated with the intervention is insufficient for making a decision about the trade-off between desirable and undesirable consequences; rather, it requires knowledge of the *absolute risk* associated with the intervention. For instance, the relative estimates we have presented so far suggest an RRR of myocardial infarction of 33% with use of β-blockers in noncardiac surgery but an increase in nonfatal strokes of 67%. The decision about whether to use β-blockers will be different, depending on whether the reduction in myocardial infarction is from 10% to 7% or from 1% to 0.7% and whether the increase in nonfatal strokes is from 0.5% to 0.8% or from 5% to 8%.

However, before we arrive at the best estimates of absolute effect we need to resolve a pending question: does the most trustworthy estimate of relative effect come from all of the studies or does it come from the studies with low risk of bias? We resolve this issue and present the best estimates of absolute effect later in this chapter.

RATING CONFIDENCE IN THE ESTIMATES (THE QUALITY OF EVIDENCE)

Consistent with the second principle of *evidence-based practice*—some evidence is more trustworthy and some less so—application of evidence requires a rating of how confident we are in our estimates of the magnitude of intervention effects on the outcomes of interest. This confidence rating is important for *clinical practice guideline* developers when they make their recommendations and for clinicians and patients when they decide on their course of action (see Chapter 26, How to Use a Patient Management Recommendation: Clinical Practice Guidelines and Decision Analyses, and Chapter 28.1, Assessing the Strength of Recommendations: The GRADE Approach).

The judgment about our confidence in the effect estimates applies not to a single study but rather a body of evidence. For any management decision, confidence in estimates can differ across outcomes. Historically, the word "quality" has been used synonymously with both risk of bias and confidence in estimates. Because of the ambiguity, we avoid the use of the word "quality" (although when we do use it, it is synonymous with confidence). Instead, we use the other 2 terms (risk of

bias and confidence in estimates). In this chapter, the focus is on confidence in effect estimates.

The GRADE Approach

The GRADE approach is one of several systems to rate the quality of evidence. The GRADE Working Group is a group of health care professionals, researchers, and guideline developers who, in 2000, began to work together to develop an optimal system of rating confidence in estimates for systematic reviews and health technology assessments of questions of the impact of interventions and to determine the strength of recommendations for clinical practice guidelines.[2] The GRADE approach has been disseminated widely and endorsed by more than 70 organizations worldwide,[11,12] including the Cochrane Collaboration, the UK National Institutes of Clinical Excellence, the World Health Organization, and the American College of Physicians. Several hundred publications have since described, demonstrated the feasibility and usefulness, evaluated the use of, and provided guidance on the GRADE approach.

GRADE suggests rating confidence in estimates of effect in 4 categories: high, moderate, low, or very low. Some organizations, including UpToDate, combine the low and very low. The lower the confidence, the more likely the underlying true effect is substantially different from the observed estimate of effect, and thus, it is more likely that further research would reveal a change in the estimates.[13]

Confidence ratings begin by considering study design. Randomized trials are initially assigned high confidence and *observational studies* are given low confidence, but a number of factors may modify these initial ratings (Figure 23-4). Confidence ratings may decrease when there is increased risk of bias, inconsistency, *imprecision*, *indirectness*, or concern about *publication bias*. An increase in confidence rating is uncommon and mainly occurs when the effect size is large (Figure 23-4).

These factors defined by GRADE should affect our confidence in estimates whether or not systematic review authors formally use GRADE. In one way or another, therefore, your consideration of evidence from a systematic review of alternative management strategies must include consideration of these issues. We now provide a description of how authors of systematic reviews and meta-analyses apply these criteria.

FIGURE 23-4

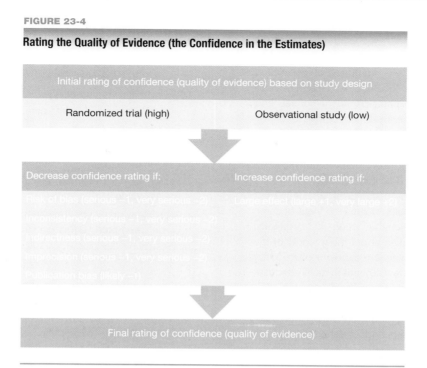

Rating the Quality of Evidence (the Confidence in the Estimates)

Initial rating of confidence (quality of evidence) based on study design

Randomized trial (high)   Observational study (low)

Decrease confidence rating if: Increase confidence rating if:

Risk of bias (serious −1, very serious −2)   Large effect (large +1, very large +2)

Inconsistency (serious −1, very serious −2)

Indirectness (serious −1, very serious −2)

Imprecision (serious −1, very serious −2)

Publication bias (likely −1)

Final rating of confidence (quality of evidence)

How Serious Is the Risk of Bias in the Body of Evidence?

Authors of systematic reviews evaluate the risk of bias for each of the outcomes measured in each individual study. *Bias* represents systematic rather than random error (see Chapter 6, Why Study Results Mislead: Bias and Random Error).

For randomized trials, risk of bias increases if there are problems with the *randomization* (defects in generation of the randomization sequence or lack of appropriate *allocation concealment*); if patients, caregivers, and study personnel are not *blinded;* or if a large number of patients are *lost to follow-up* (see Chapter 7, Therapy [Randomized Trials]). The effect of these problems can differ across outcomes. For example, lack of blinding and inadequate allocation concealment lead to greater bias for subjective outcomes than for objective hard clinical outcomes, such as death.[14] Stopping trials early because of a large apparent effect also can exaggerate the treatment effects (see Chapter 11.3, Randomized Trials Stopped Early for Benefit).[15] In observational studies, the main concerns associated with increased risk of bias include inappropriate measurement of

exposure and outcome, inadequate statistical adjustment for prognostic imbalance, and loss to follow-up (see Chapter 14, Harm [Observational Studies]).

Ideally, the authors of systematic reviews will present a risk of bias evaluation for every individual study and provide a statement about the overall risk of bias for all of the included studies. The reproducibility of this judgment affects the credibility of the process of the systematic review (see Chapter 22, The Process of a Systematic Review and Meta-analysis). Following the GRADE approach, the risk of bias can be expressed as "not serious," "serious," or "very serious." The assessment of the level of risk of bias can then result in no decrease in the confidence rating in estimates of effect or a decrease by 1 or 2 levels (eg, from high to moderate or low confidence) (Figure 23-4).[13]

USING THE GUIDE

The authors of the systematic review and meta-analysis addressing perioperative β-blockers[1] used the Cochrane Collaboration risk of bias assessment methods (see Chapter 22, The Process of a Systematic Review and Meta-analysis). They explicitly described the risk of bias of each trial and reported on the adequacy of generation of the allocation sequence; allocation concealment; blinding of participants, personnel, and outcome assessors; the extent of loss to follow-up; and the use of the *intention-to-treat principle*.

Of the 11 trials included in the analysis, 2 were considered to have high risk of bias[16,17]; limitations included lack of blinding and, in one trial, *stopping early* because of large apparent benefit.[17] The results of these 2 trials became even more questionable when, subsequently, concerns were raised about the integrity of the data.[1] The remaining 9 trials were deemed by the systematic review authors to have adequate bias protection measures and represented a body of evidence that was overall at low risk of bias for the 3 key outcomes—nonfatal myocardial infarction, death, and nonfatal stroke.

BOX 23-1

Evaluating Variability in Study Results

Visual evaluation of variability

    How similar are the point estimates?

    To what extent do the confidence intervals overlap?

Statistical tests evaluating variability

    Yes-or-no tests for heterogeneity that generate a P value

    I^2 test that quantifies the variability explained by between-study differences in results

---

Are the Results Consistent Across Studies?

The starting assumption of a meta-analysis that provides a summary estimate of treatment effect is that across the range of study patients, interventions, and outcomes included in the analysis, the effect of interest is more or less the same (see Chapter 22, The Process of a Systematic Review and Meta-analysis). On the one hand, a meta-analysis question framed to include a broad range of patients, interventions, and ways of measuring outcome helps avoid spurious effects from *subgroup analyses* (see Chapter 25.2, How to Use a Subgroup Analysis), leads to narrower CIs, and increases applicability across a broad range of patients. On the other hand, combining the results of diverse studies may violate the starting assumption of the analysis and lead to spurious conclusions (for instance, that the same estimate of effect applies to different patient groups or different ways of administering an intervention, when it in fact does not).

The solution to this dilemma is to evaluate the extent to which results differ from study to study, that is, the variability or *heterogeneity* of study results. Box 23-1 summarizes 4 approaches to evaluating

variability in study results, and the subsequent discussion expands on these principles.[18]

Visual Assessment of Variability

Studies combined in a meta-analysis and depicted in a forest plot will inevitably have some inconsistency (heterogeneity) of their point estimates. The question is whether that heterogeneity is sufficiently great to make us uncomfortable with combining results from a group of related studies to generate a single summary effect.[19]

Consider the results of the 2 meta-analyses shown in Figures 23-5A and B (meta-analysis A and meta-analysis B, respectively). When reviewing the results of these studies, would clinicians be comfortable with a single summary result in either or both meta-analyses? Although the results of meta-analysis A seem extremely unlikely to meet the assumption of a single underlying treatment effect across studies, the results of meta-analysis B are completely consistent with the assumption. Therefore, we would be uncomfortable applying the pooled estimate to all studies in A but comfortable doing so in B.

Constructing a rule to capture these inferences, one might suggest that "we are comfortable with a single summary effect when all studies suggest benefit or all studies suggest harm" (the case for B but not A). Figure 23-5C, however, highlights the limitation of such a rule: this hypothetical meta-analysis C also shows point estimates on both sides of the line of no effect, but here we would be comfortable combining the results.

FIGURE 23-5

Results of Hypothetical Meta-analyses

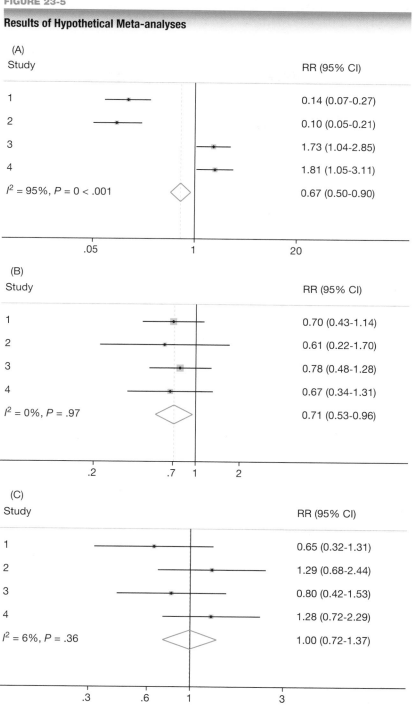

Abbreviations: CI, confidence interval; RR, relative risk.

A better approach to assessing heterogeneity focuses on the magnitude of the differences in the point estimates of the studies. Large differences in point estimates make clinicians less confident in the pooled estimate (as in meta-analysis A). Small differences in the magnitude of point estimates (as in meta-analyses B and C) support the underlying assumption that, across the range of study patients, interventions, and outcomes included in the meta-analysis, the effect of interest is more or less the same.

There is a second, equally important criterion that clinicians should apply when judging whether combining the studies is appropriate. If CIs overlap widely (as in meta-analyses B and C), *random error*, or chance, remains a plausible explanation for the differences in the point estimates. When CIs do not overlap (as in meta-analysis A), random error becomes an unlikely explanation for differences in apparent treatment effect across studies. Visual assessment of heterogeneity is useful; formal statistical testing can provide complementary information.

Yes-or-No Statistical Tests of Heterogeneity

The *null hypothesis* (see Chapter 12.1, Hypothesis Testing) of the *test for heterogeneity* is that the underlying effect is the same in each of the studies[20] (eg, the RR derived from study 1 is the same as that from studies 2, 3, and 4). Therefore, the null hypothesis assumes that all of the apparent variability among individual study results is due to chance. *Cochran Q*, the most commonly used test for heterogeneity, generates a *probability* based on a χ^2 distribution that between-study differences in results equal to or greater than those observed are likely to occur simply by chance.

Meta-analysts may consider different thresholds for the significance of the test of heterogeneity (eg, a conventional threshold of $P < .05$ or a more conservative threshold of $P < .10$). As a general principle, however, a low P value of the test for heterogeneity means that random error is an unlikely explanation for the differences in results from study to study. Thus, a low P value decreases confidence in a single summary estimate that represents the treatment effect for all patients and all variations in the administration of a treatment. A high P value of the test of heterogeneity, on the other hand, increases our confidence that the assumption underlying combining studies holds true.

In Figure 23-5A, the P value associated with the test for heterogeneity is small ($P < .001$), indicating that it is unlikely that we would observe results this disparate if all studies had the same underlying effect. On the other hand, the corresponding P values in Figure 23-3B and C are fairly large (.97 and .36, respectively). Therefore, in these 2 meta-analyses, chance is a likely explanation for the observed differences in effect.

When a meta-analysis includes studies with small sample sizes and a correspondingly small number of events, the test of heterogeneity may not have sufficient power to detect existing heterogeneity. Conversely, in a meta-analysis that includes studies with large sample sizes and a large number of events, the test for heterogeneity may provide potentially misleading results that reveal statistically significant but unimportant differences in point estimates. This is another reason why clinicians need to use their own visual assessments of heterogeneity (similarity of point estimates, overlap of CIs) and consider the results of formal statistical tests in that context.

Magnitude of Heterogeneity Statistical Tests

The I^2 *statistic* is a preferred alternative approach for evaluating heterogeneity that focuses on the magnitude of variability rather than the statistical significance of variability.[21]

When the I^2 is 0%, chance provides a satisfactory explanation for the variability in the individual study point estimates, and clinicians can be comfortable with a single summary estimate of treatment effect. As the I^2 increases, we become progressively less comfortable with a single summary estimate, and the need to look for explanations of variability other than chance becomes more compelling. Figure 23-6 provides a guide for interpreting the I^2.

If provided by the meta-analysis authors, a 95% CI associated with the I^2 can provide further insight regarding assessment of inconsistency. In most meta-analyses with a limited number of relatively small studies, this CI is quite large, suggesting the need for caution in making strong inferences regarding inconsistency.[22]

The results in Figure 23-5A generate an I^2 of more than 75% (suggesting high heterogeneity), whereas the results in Figure 23-5B and C

FIGURE 23-6

Interpretation of the I^2 Statistic

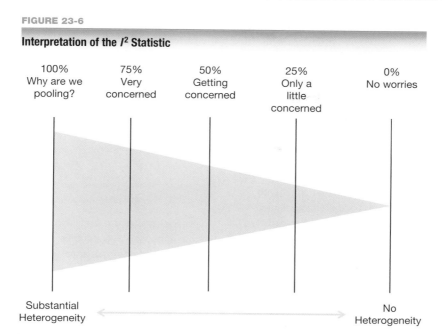

yield low I^2 percentages of 0% and 6%, respectively (suggesting low heterogeneity).

What to Do When Between-Study Variability in Results Is Large?

One of the credibility criteria introduced in Chapter 22 is whether the authors have addressed possible explanations of heterogeneity. When between-study variability is large, such an exploration becomes crucial.

Differences between study results can arise from differences in the population enrolled (eg, large effects in the more ill, smaller in the less ill), differences in the interventions (eg, if large doses are more effective than small doses), differences in the comparators (eg, smaller effects when standard care is optimal than when it is not), and study methods (eg, larger effect in studies with high risk of bias vs those with low risk of bias). Meta-analysis authors should conduct a test of interaction to determine whether the difference in effect estimates among subgroups is attributable to chance. Apparent subgroup effects are more likely to be true when they are based on within-trial rather than between-trial comparisons, are very unlikely to be due to chance, and are based on a small

number of hypotheses specified a priori, including a specified direction. If these criteria are not met, any subgroup hypothesis warrants a high level of skepticism (see Chapter 25.2, How to Use a Subgroup Analysis). For a discussion of additional issues in statistical analysis related to heterogeneity of study results, see Chapter 25.1, Fixed-Effects and Random-Effects Models.

What if, in the end, we are left with a large degree of unexplained between-study heterogeneity for which chance does not provide an adequate explanation? This is not an uncommon situation. Some argue that, in this situation, meta-analysis authors should not combine the results. Clinicians and patients, however, still need a best estimate of the treatment effect to inform their decisions. Pending further research that may explain the differences between results of different studies that address the same question, the summary estimate remains the best estimate of the treatment effect. Although clinicians and patients must use the best estimate to make their decisions, substantial unexplained inconsistency between studies appreciably reduces confidence in the summary estimate.[23]

In Figures 23-1 and 23-2, for both nonfatal myocardial infarction and death, we note substantial differences in point estimates across studies. In the case of death, there is minimal CI overlap. Although the heterogeneity P values of .21 and .16 are not statistically significant, the I^2 of 29% for nonfatal myocardial infarction and 30% for death suggest the presence of variability for which seeking a possible explanation is worthwhile.

Examining the data, we find that trials with a high risk of bias reveal a substantially larger reduction in the risk of nonfatal myocardial infarction. A test of interaction between the 2 groups of studies (those with high risk of bias and those with low risk of bias) yields a nonsignificant P value of .22, which indicates that the difference in the reduction in nonfatal myocardial infarction risk between these 2 subgroups of studies could be due to chance.

However, for the outcome of death, a test of interaction between the 2 groups of studies yields a significant P value of .04, which suggests that the risk of bias explains the observed heterogeneity (Figure 23-2). As we have mentioned previously, our inclination to use only the studies with low risk of bias is reinforced by our awareness of the doubts that have been raised regarding the integrity of the data from the 2 studies with high risk of bias. Results of the studies with low risk of bias are consistent (I^2 of 0% and P value for heterogeneity test of .68).

Meta-analysis of the outcome of nonfatal stroke reveals consistent results across trials with an I^2 value of 0% and P value for the heterogeneity test of .71 (Figure 23-3).

How Precise Are the Results?

Meta-analysis generates an estimate of the mean effect across studies and a CI around that estimate, that is, a range of values with a specified probability (typically 95%) of including the true effect (see Chapter 10, Confidence Intervals: Was the Single Study or Meta-analysis Large Enough?). When applying research evidence to a clinical question, one should determine whether clinical action would differ if the upper or the lower boundaries of the CI represented the truth. If the clinical decision is the same whether the upper or lower boundary of the CI represents the true effect, then the evidence is sufficiently precise. If across the range of the CI values our decision making would change, then we should have less confidence in the evidence and lower the confidence rating (eg, from high to moderate confidence).[24]

To determine the precision of the estimate of the effect of perioperative β-blockers on the risk of nonfatal myocardial infarction, you need to calculate the absolute effect, which requires knowledge of the RR and the *control event rate* (ie, the event rate in patients who did not receive β-blockers). Having decided that the best estimate of RR comes from focusing on the trials with low risk of bias rather than all trials included in the meta-analysis, we note that the RR is 0.73 (95% CI, 0.61-0.88) (Figure 23-1). We obtain the control event rate from the trial that is by far the largest—and the one that likely enrolled the most representative population[25]—which was 215/4177 or approximately 52 per 1000. You can then calculate the decreased risk of nonfatal myocardial infarction in those using β-blockers as follows:

Risk with intervention = risk with control × relative risk = 52/1000 × 0.73 = approximately 38 per 1000

Risk difference = risk with control − risk with intervention = 52/1,000 − 38/1000 = −14 (approximately 14 fewer myocardial infarctions per 1000)

You can use the same process to calculate the CIs around the *risk difference*, substituting the boundaries of the CI (in this case, 0.61 and 0.88) for the point estimate (in this case, 0.73). For instance, for the upper boundary of the CI:

Risk with intervention = 52/1000 × 0.88 = approximately 46 per 1000

Risk with intervention − risk with control = 46 − 52 = −6 (approximately 6 fewer per 1000)

The estimate of absolute difference in nonfatal myocardial infarction when using β-blockers is therefore approximately 14 fewer per 1000, with a CI of approximately 6 to 20 fewer per 1000.

The corresponding absolute difference for nonfatal stroke is 2 more nonfatal strokes per 1000, with a CI of approximately 0 to 6 more per 1000; for death, the absolute difference is 6 deaths more per 1000 with a CI of approximately 0 to 13 more per 1000 (Table 23-1).

Lowering a confidence rating because of imprecision is always a judgment call. There seems to be no doubt about the need to lower confidence for nonfatal stroke (the effect ranges from no difference to an appreciable increase in nonfatal stroke) and likely for death (some may consider 1 additional death in 1000 acceptable given the reduction in myocardial infarction; most would not consider 6 in 1000 trivial). Regarding nonfatal myocardial infarction, our judgment was not to lower confidence for imprecision (Table 23-1).

Do the Results Directly Apply to My Patient?

The optimal evidence for decision making comes from research that directly compared the interventions in which we are interested, evaluated in the populations in which we are interested, and measured outcomes important to patients. If populations, interventions, and outcomes in studies differ from those of interest (ie, the patient before us), we lose confidence in estimates of effect. In GRADE, the term "indirectness" is used as a label for these issues.[26]

So, for instance, the patient at hand may be very elderly and the trials may have included few, if any, such patients. The dose of a drug tested in the trials may be greater than the dose your patient can tolerate.

Decisions regarding indirectness of patients and interventions depend on an understanding of whether biologic or social factors are sufficiently different that one might expect substantial differences in the magnitude of effect (see Chapter 13.1, Applying Results to Individual Patients). Do elderly patients metabolize a drug differently from younger patients? Are there competing risks that will be responsible for the demise of elderly patients long

SUMMARIZING THE EVIDENCE

TABLE 23-1

Evidence Profile: Explicit Presentation of the Best Estimates of the Effect of Perioperative β-Blockers and the Confidence in Estimates

Confidence Assessment			
Outcome	Myocardial infarction	Stroke	Death
No. of Participants (No. of Studies)	10 189 (5)	10 186 (5)	10 529 (9)
Risk of Bias	No serious limitations	No serious limitations	No serious limitations
Consistency	No serious limitations	No serious limitations	No serious limitations
Directness	No serious limitations	No serious limitations	No serious limitations
Precision	No serious limitations	Imprecise	Imprecise
Reporting Bias	Not detected	Not detected	Not detected
Summary of Findings			
Confidence	High	Moderate	Moderate
Relative Effect (95% CI)	0.73 (0.61-0.88)	1.73 (1.00-2.99)	1.27 (1.01-1.60)
Risk Difference per 1000 Patients	14 fewer (6 fewer to 20 fewer)	2 more (0 more to 6 more)	6 more (0 more to 13 more)

Abbreviation: CI, confidence interval.

USING THE GUIDE

Assessing directness regarding the evidence bearing on the use of β-blockers in noncardiac surgery,[1] we note that the age of most patients enrolled across the trials ranged from 50 to 70 years, similar to your patient, who is 66 years old. Almost all of the trials enrolled patients undergoing surgical procedures classified as intermediate surgical risk, similar to the hip surgery of your patient. Most of the trials enrolled many patients who, like yours, had risk factors for heart disease. Although the drug used and the dose varied across trials, the consistent results suggest you can use a modest dose of the β-blocker with which you are most familiar. The outcomes of death, nonfatal stroke, and nonfatal infarction are the key outcomes of importance to your patients. Overall, the available evidence presented in the systematic review is direct and applicable to your patient and addresses the key outcomes (benefits and harms) needed for decision making.

before they experience the benefits of the intervention? Is there evidence that the tissue effect of a medication is highly dose dependent?

Another issue of indirectness arises when outcomes assessed in the studies differ from those of interest to patients. Trials often measure laboratory or *surrogate outcomes* that are not themselves important but are measured in the presumption that changes in the surrogate reflect changes in an outcome important to patients (see Chapter 13.4, Surrogate Outcomes). For instance, we have excellent information about the effect of medications used in type 2 diabetes on hemoglobin A_{1C} but limited information on their effect on macrovascular and microvascular disease. In almost every instance, we should reduce our confidence in estimates of effect on patient-important outcomes when all we have available is the effect on surrogates.

Lastly, a different type of indirectness occurs when clinicians must choose among interventions that have not been tested in head-to-head comparisons.

For instance, we may want to choose among alternative bisphosphonates for managing osteoporosis. We will find many trials that compare each agent to placebo, but few, if any, that have compared them directly against one another.[27] Making comparisons among treatments under these circumstances requires extrapolating results for the existing comparisons and requires multiple assumptions (see Chapter 24, Network Meta-analysis).[26]

Is There Concern About Reporting Bias?

The most difficult types of bias for systematic review authors to address stem from the inclination of authors of original studies to publish material, either entire studies or specific outcomes, based on the magnitude, direction, or statistical significance of the results. We call the systematic error in the body of evidence that results from this inclination *reporting bias*. When an entire study remains unreported, the standard term is publication bias. The reason for publication bias is that studies without statistically significant results (*negative studies*) are less likely to be published than studies that reveal apparent differences (*positive studies*). The magnitude and direction of a study's results may be more important determinants of publication than study design, relevance, or quality,[28] and positive studies may be as much as 3 times more likely to be published than negative studies.[29] When authors or study sponsors selectively manipulate and report specific outcomes and analyses, we use the term *selective outcome reporting bias*.[30] Selective reporting bias can be a serious problem. Empirical evidence suggests that half of the analysis plans of randomized trials are different in protocols than in published reports.[31] When the publication is delayed because of the lack of significance of results, authors have used the term *time lag bias*.[32]

Selective outcome reporting can also create misleading estimates of effect. A study of US Food and Drug Administration (FDA) reports found that they often included numerous unpublished studies and the findings of these studies can appreciably alter the estimates of effect.[33]

Reporting bias can intrude at virtually all stages of the planning, implementation, and dissemination of research. Even if studies with negative results succeed and get published, they may still suffer from *dissemination bias*: they may be published in less prominent journals, may not receive adequate attention from policymakers, may be omitted (whether identified or not) in narrative reviews, may be omitted (if unidentified) from systematic reviews, and may have minimal or no effect on formulation of policy guidelines. On the other hand, studies with positive results may receive disproportionate attention. For instance, they are more likely to appear in subsequent evidence summaries and in an evidence *synopsis*.[34]

The consequences of publication and reporting bias can corrupt the body of evidence, usually exaggerating estimates of magnitude of *treatment effect*. Systematic reviews that fail to identify and include unpublished studies face a risk of presenting overly sanguine estimates of treatment effectiveness.

The risk of publication bias is probably higher for systematic reviews and meta-analyses that are based on small studies. Small studies are more likely to produce nonsignificant results due to lack of statistical power and are easier to hide. Larger studies are not, however, immune. Sponsors and authors who are not pleased with the results of a study may delay publication or chose to publish their study in a journal with limited readership or a lower impact factor.[32]

An example of reporting bias is the Salmeterol Multicenter Asthma Research Trial, which was a randomized trial designed to examine the effect of salmeterol or placebo on a *composite end point* of respiratory-related deaths and life-threatening experiences. In September 2002, after a data safety and monitoring board review of 25 858 randomized patients that found a nearly significant increase in the primary outcome in salmeterol-treated patients, the sponsor terminated the study. In a significant deviation from the original protocol, the sponsor submitted to the FDA an analysis, including events in the 6 months after the termination of the trial, which produced an apparent diminution of the dangers associated with salmeterol. The FDA, through specific inquiry, eventually obtained the data and the results were finally published in January 2006, revealing the increased likelihood of respiratory-related deaths with salmeterol.[35,36]

Strategies to Address Reporting Bias

Several tests have been developed to detect publication bias (Box 23-2); unfortunately, all have serious limitations. The tests require a large number of

---

BOX 23-2

Four Strategies to Address Reporting Bias

1. Examine whether the smaller studies show bigger effects
   a. Funnel plots, visually assessed
   b. Funnel plots, statistical analysis
2. Reconstruct evidence by restoring the picture after accounting for postulated publication bias
   a. Trim and fill
3. Estimate the chances of publication according to the statistical significance level
4. Examine the evolution of effect size over time as more data appear

---

studies (ideally 30 or more), although many meta-analysis authors use them in analyses including few studies. Moreover, none of these tests has been validated against a *criterion standard* (or *gold standard*) of real data in which we know whether publication bias or other biases existed or not.[37]

The first category of tests examines whether small studies differ from larger ones in their results. In a figure that relates the precision (as measured by sample size, inverse of *standard error* or *variance*) of studies included in a meta-analysis to the magnitude of treatment effect, the resulting display should resemble an inverted funnel (Figure 23-7A). Such *funnel plots* should be symmetric, around the point estimate (dominated by the largest trials) or the results of the largest trials themselves. A gap or empty area in the funnel suggests that studies have been conducted and not published (Figure 23-7B). Because visual determination of symmetry can be subjective, meta-analysts sometimes apply statistical tests for the symmetry of the funnel.[37]

Even when the funnel shape or the tests suggest publication bias, other explanations for asymmetry are possible. The small studies may have a higher risk of bias, which may explain their larger effects. On the other hand, the small studies may have chosen a more responsive patient group or administered the intervention more meticulously. Finally, there is always the possibility of a chance finding.

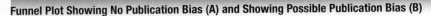

FIGURE 23-7

Funnel Plot Showing No Publication Bias (A) and Showing Possible Publication Bias (B)

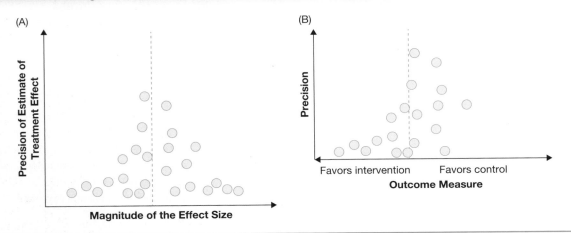

A, The circles represent the point estimates of the trials. The pattern of distribution resembles an inverted funnel. Larger studies tend to be closer to the summary estimate (the dashed line). In this case, the effect sizes of the smaller studies are more or less symmetrically distributed around the summary estimate. B, This funnel plot shows that the smaller studies are not symmetrically distributed around either the point estimate (dominated by the larger trials) or the results of the larger trials themselves. The trials expected in the bottom right quadrant are missing. This suggests publication bias and an overestimate of the treatment effect relative to the underlying truth.

A second set of tests imputes and corrects for missing information and address its effect (*trim-and-fill method*). Again, the availability of few studies and the presence of heterogeneity make this second strategy inappropriate for most meta-analyses.

A third set of tests estimates whether there are differential chances of publication according to the level of statistical significance.[38-40] The excess significance test can be used in single meta-analyses and collections of multiple meta-analyses in the same field where similar biases may be operating.

Finally, a set of tests aims to examine whether evidence changes over time as more data accumulate. Continuously diminishing effects are characteristic of time lag bias.[41]

More compelling than any of these theoretical exercises is the success of systematic review authors in obtaining the results of unpublished studies that appear to be a complete collection of all of the studies that have been undertaken.

Prospective study registration with accessible results represents the best solution to reporting bias.[42,43] Prospective registration makes publication bias potentially identifiable; however, more detailed information is necessary to identify potential selective outcome and analysis reporting bias. Until complete reporting becomes a reality,[44] clinicians using research reports to guide their practice must remain cognizant of the dangers of reporting biases.

USING THE GUIDE

The authors of the systematic review and meta-analysis[1] addressing perioperative β-blockers constructed funnel plots that appear to be symmetrical, and the statistical tests for the symmetry of the plot were nonsignificant. The total number of patients included (>10 000) further reduces concern about publication bias, leaving no reason for lowering our confidence rating due to publication or reporting bias.

Are There Reasons to Increase the Confidence Rating?

Some uncommon situations warrant an increase in the confidence rating of effect estimates from observational studies. Consider our confidence in the effect of hip replacement on reducing pain and functional limitations in severe osteoarthritis, epinephrine to prevent mortality in anaphylaxis, insulin to prevent mortality in diabetic ketoacidosis, or dialysis to prolong life in patients with end-stage renal failure.[45] In each of these situations, we are confident of a substantial treatment effect despite the absence of randomized trials. Why is that? The reason is a very large treatment effect that was achieved during a short period among patients with a condition that would have inevitably worsened in the absence of an intervention.

The GRADE approach provides specific guidance regarding large effect sizes: consider increasing the confidence rating by 1 level when there is a 2-fold reduction or increase in risk and consider increasing the confidence rating by 2 levels in the presence of a 5-fold reduction or increase in risk. For example, a systematic review and meta-analysis of observational studies examining the relationship between infant sleeping position and sudden infant death syndrome (SIDS) found an OR of 4.9 (95% CI, 3.6-6.6) of SIDS occurring with front vs back sleeping positions.[46] The "back to sleep" campaigns that were started in the 1980s were associated with a relative decrease in the incidence of SIDS by 50% to 70% in numerous countries.[46] This large effect increases our confidence in a true association.[45]

AN EVIDENCE-BASED SUMMARY OF THE FINDINGS: THE EVIDENCE PROFILE

To optimally apply evidence summarized in a systematic review, practitioners need succinct, easily digestible presentations of confidence in effect estimates (quality of evidence) and magnitude of effects. They need this information to trade benefits and harms and communicate risks to their patients. They need to know the confidence we have in a body of evidence to convey the uncertainty to their patients.

Systematic reviews may provide this summary in different ways. The GRADE Working Group recommends what are called *evidence profiles* (or a shortened version called *summary of findings tables*). Such tables present the relative and absolute effects of an intervention on each of the critical outcomes most important to patients, including a confidence rating. If stratifying patients' baseline risk for the outcome is possible, the absolute effect is presented for each risk strata separately.

CLINICAL SCENARIO RESOLUTION

Table 23-1 presents the evidence profile summarizing the results of the systematic review addressing perioperative β-blockers. We see that evidence warranting high confidence suggests that individuals with underlying cardiovascular disease or risk factors for disease can expect a reduction in their risk of a perioperative nonfatal infarction of 14 in 1000 (from approximately 20 per 1000 to 6 per 1000). Unfortunately, they can also expect an increase in their risk of dying or experiencing a nonfatal stroke. Because most people are highly averse to the disability associated with stroke and at least equally averse to death, it is likely that most patients faced with this evidence would decline β-blockers as part of their perioperative regimen. Indeed, that is what our 66-year-old man with diabetes decides when you discuss the evidence with him.

References

1. Bouri S, Shun-Shin MJ, Cole GD, Mayet J, Francis DP. Meta-analysis of secure randomised controlled trials of β-blockade to prevent perioperative death in non-cardiac. *Heart.* 2014:100(6):456-464.

2. Guyatt GH, Oxman AD, Vist GE, et al; GRADE Working Group. GRADE: an emerging consensus on rating quality of evidence and strength of recommendations. *BMJ.* 2008;336(7650):924-926.

3. Spencer FA, Iorio A, You J, et al. Uncertainties in baseline risk estimates and confidence in treatment effects. *BMJ*. 2012;345:e7401.

4. Schünemann HJ, Oxman AD, Brozek J, et al; GRADE Working Group. Grading quality of evidence and strength of recommendations for diagnostic tests and strategies. *BMJ*. 2008;336(7653):1106-1110.

5. Rosenthal R. *Meta-analytic Procedures for Social Research*. 2nd ed. Newbury Park, CA: Sage Publications; 1991.

6. Cohen J. *Statistical Power Analysis for the Behavioral Sciences*. 2nd ed. Hillsdale, NJ: Lawrence Earlbaum Associates; 1988.

7. Smith K, Cook D, Guyatt GH, Madhavan J, Oxman AD. Respiratory muscle training in chronic airflow limitation: a meta-analysis. *Am Rev Respir Dis*. 1992;145(3):533-539.

8. Lacasse Y, Martin S, Lasserson TJ, Goldstein RS. Meta-analysis of respiratory rehabilitation in chronic obstructive pulmonary disease. A Cochrane systematic review. *Eura Medicophys*. 2007;43(4):475-485.

9. Thorlund K, Walter S, Johnston B, Furukawa T, Guyatt G. Pooling health-related quality of life outcomes in meta-analysis—a tutorial and review of methods for enhancing interpretability. *Res Synth Methods*. 2011;2(3):188-203.

10. Guyatt GH, Thorlund K, Oxman AD, et al. GRADE guidelines: 13. Preparing summary of findings tables and evidence profiles-continuous outcomes. *J Clin Epidemiol*. 2013;66(2):173-183.

11. Guyatt GH, Oxman AD, Schünemann HJ, Tugwell P, Knottnerus A. GRADE guidelines: a new series of articles in the Journal of Clinical Epidemiology. *J Clin Epidemiol*. 2011;64(4):380-382.

12. Organizations. *The GRADE Working Group*. http://www.grade-workinggroup.org/society/index.htm. Accessed April 9, 2014.

13. Balshem H, Helfand M, Schünemann HJ, et al. GRADE guidelines: 3. Rating the quality of evidence. *J Clin Epidemiol*. 2011;64(4):401-406.

14. Wood L, Egger M, Gluud LL, et al. Empirical evidence of bias in treatment effect estimates in controlled trials with different interventions and outcomes: meta-epidemiological study. *BMJ*. 2008;336(7644):601-605.

15. Bassler D, Briel M, Montori VM, et al; STOPIT-2 Study Group. Stopping randomized trials early for benefit and estimation of treatment effects: systematic review and meta-regression analysis. *JAMA*. 2010;303(12):1180-1187.

16. Dunkelgrun M, Boersma E, Schouten O, et al; Dutch Echocardiographic Cardiac Risk Evaluation Applying Stress Echocardiography Study Group. Bisoprolol and fluvastatin for the reduction of perioperative cardiac mortality and myocardial infarction in intermediate-risk patients undergoing noncardiovascular surgery: a randomized controlled trial (DECREASE-IV). *Ann Surg*. 2009;249(6):921-926.

17. Poldermans D, Boersma E, Bax JJ, et al; Dutch Echocardiographic Cardiac Risk Evaluation Applying Stress Echocardiography Study Group. The effect of bisoprolol on perioperative mortality and myocardial infarction in high-risk patients undergoing vascular surgery. *N Engl J Med*. 1999;341(24):1789-1794.

18. Hatala R, Keitz S, Wyer P, Guyatt G; Evidence-Based Medicine Teaching Tips Working Group. Tips for learners of evidence-based medicine: 4. Assessing heterogeneity of primary studies in systematic reviews and whether to combine their results. *CMAJ*. 2005;172(5):661-665.

19. Lau J, Ioannidis JP, Schmid CH. Summing up evidence: one answer is not always enough. *Lancet*. 1998;351(9096):123-127.

20. Lau J, Ioannidis JP, Schmid CH. Quantitative synthesis in systematic reviews. *Ann Intern Med*. 1997;127(9):820-826.

21. Higgins JP, Thompson SG, Deeks JJ, Altman DG. Measuring inconsistency in meta-analyses. *BMJ*. 2003;327(7414):557-560.

22. Ioannidis JP, Patsopoulos NA, Evangelou E. Uncertainty in heterogeneity estimates in meta-analyses. *BMJ*. 2007;335(7626):914-916.

23. Guyatt GH, Oxman AD, Kunz R, et al; GRADE Working Group. GRADE guidelines: 7. Rating the quality of evidence—inconsistency. *J Clin Epidemiol*. 2011;64(12):1294-1302.

24. Guyatt GH, Oxman AD, Kunz R, et al. GRADE guidelines 6. Rating the quality of evidence--imprecision. *J Clin Epidemiol*. 2011;64(12):1283-1293.

25. Devereaux PJ, Yang H, Yusuf S, et al; POISE Study Group. Effects of extended-release metoprolol succinate in patients undergoing non-cardiac surgery (POISE trial): a randomised controlled trial. *Lancet*. 2008;371(9627):1839-1847.

26. Guyatt GH, Oxman AD, Kunz R, et al; GRADE Working Group. GRADE guidelines: 8. Rating the quality of evidence—indirectness. *J Clin Epidemiol*. 2011;64(12):1303-1310.

27. Murad MH, Drake MT, Mullan RJ, et al. Clinical review. Comparative effectiveness of drug treatments to prevent fragility fractures: a systematic review and network meta-analysis. *J Clin Endocrinol Metab*. 2012;97(6):1871-1880.

28. Easterbrook PJ, Berlin JA, Gopalan R, Matthews DR. Publication bias in clinical research. *Lancet*. 1991;337(8746):867-872.

29. Stern JM, Simes RJ. Publication bias: evidence of delayed publication in a cohort study of clinical research projects. *BMJ*. 1997;315(7109):640-645.

30. Chan AW, Hróbjartsson A, Haahr MT, Gøtzsche PC, Altman DG. Empirical evidence for selective reporting of outcomes in randomized trials: comparison of protocols to published articles. *JAMA*. 2004;291(20):2457-2465.

31. Saquib N, Saquib J, Ioannidis JP. Practices and impact of primary outcome adjustment in randomized controlled trials: meta-epidemiologic study. *BMJ*. 2013;347:f4313.

32. Ioannidis JP. Effect of the statistical significance of results on the time to completion and publication of randomized efficacy trials. *JAMA*. 1998;279(4):281-286.

33. McDonagh MS, Peterson K, Balshem H, Helfand M. US Food and Drug Administration documents can provide unpublished evidence relevant to systematic reviews. *J Clin Epidemiol*. 2013;66(10):1071-1081.

34. Carter AO, Griffin GH, Carter TP. A survey identified publication bias in the secondary literature. *J Clin Epidemiol*. 2006;59(3):241-245.

35. Lurie P, Wolfe SM. Misleading data analyses in salmeterol (SMART) study. *Lancet*. 2005;366(9493):1261-1262, discussion 1262.

36. Nelson HS, Weiss ST, Bleecker ER, Yancey SW, Dorinsky PM; SMART Study Group. The Salmeterol Multicenter Asthma Research Trial: a comparison of usual pharmacotherapy for asthma or usual pharmacotherapy plus salmeterol. *Chest*. 2006;129(1):15-26.

37. Lau J, Ioannidis JP, Terrin N, Schmid CH, Olkin I. The case of the misleading funnel plot. *BMJ*. 2006;333(7568):597-600.

38. Hedges L, Vevea J. Estimating effect size under publication bias: small sample properties and robustness of a random effects selection model. *J Educ Behav Stat*. 1996;21(4):299-333.

39. Vevea J, Hedges L. A general linear model for estimating effect size in the presence of publication bias. *Psychometrika*. 1995;60(3):419-435.

40. Ioannidis JP, Trikalinos TA. An exploratory test for an excess of significant findings. *Clin Trials*. 2007;4(3):245-253.

41. Ioannidis JP, Contopoulos-Ioannidis DG, Lau J. Recursive cumulative meta-analysis: a diagnostic for the evolution of total randomized evidence from group and individual patient data. *J Clin Epidemiol*. 1999;52(4):281-291.

42. Boissel JP, Haugh MC. Clinical trial registries and ethics review boards: the results of a survey by the FICHTRE project. *Fundam Clin Pharmacol*. 1997;11(3):281-284.

43. Horton R, Smith R. Time to register randomised trials. The case is now unanswerable. *BMJ*. 1999;319(7214):865-866.

44. Dickersin K, Rennie D. The evolution of trial registries and their use to assess the clinical trial enterprise. *JAMA*. 2012;307(17):1861-1864.

45. Guyatt GH, Oxman AD, Sultan S, et al; GRADE Working Group. GRADE guidelines: 9. Rating up the quality of evidence. *J Clin Epidemiol*. 2011;64(12):1311-1316.

46. Gilbert R, Salanti G, Harden M, See S. Infant sleeping position and the sudden infant death syndrome: systematic review of observational studies and historical review of recommendations from 1940 to 2002. *Int J Epidemiol*. 2005;34(4):874-887.

SUMMARIZING THE EVIDENCE

24

Network Meta-analysis

Edward J. Mills, John P. A. Ioannidis, Kristian Thorlund,
Holger J. Schünemann, Milo A. Puhan, and Gordon Guyatt

SUMMARIZING THE EVIDENCE

IN THIS CHAPTER

CLINICAL SCENARIO

Your patient is a 45-year-old woman who experiences frequent migraine headaches that last from 4 to 24 hours and prevent her from attending work or looking after her children. She has exhausted efforts to manage the symptoms with nonsteroidal anti-inflammatory drugs and seeks additional treatment. You decide to recommend a triptan for the patient's migraine headaches but are wondering how to choose from the 7 available triptans. You retrieve a *network meta-analysis* (NMA) that evaluates the different triptans among this patient population.[1] You are not familiar with this type of study, and you wonder if there are special issues to which you should attend in evaluating its methods and results.

FINDING THE EVIDENCE

You start by typing "migraine triptans" in the search box of an evidence-based summary website with which you are familiar. You find several chapters related to the management of migraine and drug information on the different drugs that are available. However, despite the profusion of *evidence* comparing single regimens, you wonder if all triptans have been compared, ideally in a in a single *systematic review*. To search for such a review, you type "migraine triptans comparison" in PubMed's Clinical Queries (http://www.ncbi.nlm.nih.gov/pubmed/clinical; see Chapter 5, Finding Current Best Evidence). In the results page, the middle column, which applies a broad filter for potential systematic reviews, retrieves 21 citations. The first strikes you as the most relevant to your question. It is a network meta-analysis that evaluates the different triptans among your patient population.[1] You are not familiar with this type of study, and you wonder if there are special issues to which you should attend in evaluating its methods and results.

INTRODUCTION

Traditionally, a meta-analysis addresses the merits of one intervention vs another (eg, *placebo* or another active intervention). Data are combined from all studies—often *randomized clinical trials* (RCTs)—that meet eligibility criteria in what we will term a pairwise meta-analysis. Compared with a single RCT, a *meta-analysis* improves the power to detect differences and also facilitates examination of the extent to which there are important differences in *treatment effects* across eligible RCTs—variability that is frequently called *heterogeneity*.[2,3] Large unexplained heterogeneity may reduce a reader's confidence in estimates of treatment effect (see Chapter 23, Understanding and Applying the Results of a Systematic Review and Meta-analysis).

A drawback of traditional pairwise meta-analysis is that it evaluates the effects of only 1 intervention vs 1 comparator and does not permit inferences about the relative effectiveness of several interventions. For many medical conditions, however, there are a selection of interventions that have most frequently been compared with placebo and occasionally with one another.[4,5] For example, despite 91 completed and ongoing RCTs that address the effectiveness of the 9 biologic drugs for the treatment of rheumatoid arthritis, only 5 compare biologics directly against each other.[4]

Recently, another form of meta-analysis, called an NMA (also known as a multiple or mixed treatment comparison meta-analysis) has emerged.[6,7] The NMA approach provides estimates of effect sizes for all possible pairwise comparisons whether or not they have actually been compared head to head in RCTs. Figure 24-1 displays examples of common networks of treatments.

Our ability to provide estimates of relative effect when 2 interventions, A and B, have not been tested head to head against one another comes from what are called indirect comparisons. We can make an indirect comparison if the 2 interventions (eg, paroxetine and lorazepam in Figure 24-2A) have each been compared directly against another intervention, C (eg, placebo).

For instance, assume that A (eg, paroxetine) substantially reduces the odds of an adverse outcome relative to C (placebo) (*odds ratio* [OR], 0.5).

FIGURE 24-1

Examples of Possible Network Geometry

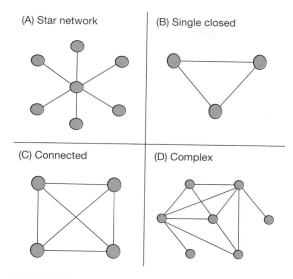

The figure shows 4 network graphs. In each graph, the lines show where direct comparisons exist from 1 or more trials. Figure 24-1A shows a star network, where all interventions have just 1 mutual comparator. Figure 24-1B shows a single closed loop that involves 3 interventions and can provide data to calculate both direct comparisons and indirect comparisons. Figure 24-1C shows a well-connected network, where all interventions have been compared against each other in multiple randomized clinical trials. Figure 24-1D is an example of a complex network with multiple loops and also arms that have sparse connections.

FIGURE 24-2

A Simple Indirect Comparison and Simple Closed Loop

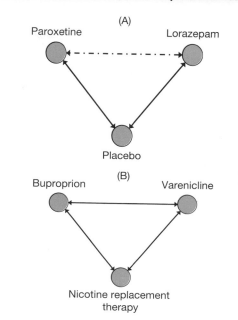

In the first example (A), there is direct evidence from paroxetine compared with placebo and direct evidence of lorazepam compared with placebo. Therefore, the indirect comparison can be applied to determine the effect of paroxetine compared with lorazepam, even if no direct head-to-head comparison exists on these 2 agents. In the second example (B), there is direct evidence that compares nicotine replacement therapy with both varenicline and bupropion. There is also direct evidence that compares bupropion with varenicline. Therefore, one has enough information to evaluate whether the results are coherent between direct and indirect evidence.

Intervention B (eg, lorazepam), on the other hand, has no impact relative to C on that outcome (OR, 1.0). One might then reasonably deduce that A is substantially superior to C—indeed, our best estimate of the OR of A vs B would be 0.5/1.0 or 0.5. The ratio of the OR in such a situation is our way of estimating the effect of A vs B on the outcome of interest.[8]

Network meta-analyses, which simultaneously include both direct and *indirect evidence* (see Figure 24-2B for an example in which both direct and indirect evidence is available, sometimes called a closed loop), are subject to 3 chief considerations. The first is an assumption that is also necessary for a conventional meta-analysis (see Chapter 23, Understanding and Applying the Results of a Systematic Review and Meta-analysis). Among trials available for pairwise comparisons, are the studies sufficiently *homogenous* to combine for each intervention?

Second, are the trials in the network sufficiently similar, with the exception of the intervention (eg, in important features, such as populations, design, or outcomes)?[9] For instance, if trials of drug A vs placebo differ substantially in the characteristics of the population studied from the population in drug B vs placebo, inferences about the relative effect of A and B on the basis of how each did against placebo become questionable. Third, where direct and indirect evidence exists, are the findings sufficiently consistent to allow confident pooling of direct and indirect evidence together?

By including evidence from both direct and indirect comparisons, an NMA may increase precision of estimates of the relative effects of treatments and facilitate simultaneous comparisons, or even ranking, of these treatments.[7] However, because NMAs are methodologically sophisticated, they are often challenging to interpret.[10]

One challenge clinicians will face with NMAs is that they usually use *Bayesian analysis* approaches rather than the *frequentist analysis* approaches with which most of us are more familiar. Clinicians need not worry further about this, and the main reason for pointing it out is as an alert to a difference in terms. Clinicians are used to considering *confidence intervals* (CIs) around estimates of treatment effect. The Bayesian equivalent are called *credible intervals* and can be interpreted in conceptually the same way as CIs.

Here, we demystify NMAs by using the 3 questions of *risk of bias*, results, and applicability of results. Box 24-1 includes all of the issues relevant to evaluating systematic reviews. Our discussion in this chapter does not include all of the issues but rather highlights those that are most important, or differ, in NMAs.

HOW SERIOUS IS THE RISK OF BIAS?

Did the Meta-analysis Include Explicit and Appropriate Eligibility Criteria?

One can formulate questions of optimal patient management in terms of the *PICO* framework of patients (P), interventions (I), comparisons (C), and outcomes (O).

Broader eligibility criteria may enhance *generalizability* of the results but may be misleading if participants are too dissimilar and as a consequence heterogeneity is large. Diversity of interventions may also be excessive if authors pool results from different doses or even different agents in the same class (eg, all statins), based on the assumption that effects are similar. You should ask whether investigators have been too broad in their inclusion of different populations, different doses or different agents in the same class, or different outcomes to make comparisons across studies credible.

Was Biased Selection and Reporting of Studies Unlikely?

Some NMAs apply the search strategies from other systematic reviews as the basis for identifying potentially eligible trials. Readers can be confident in such approaches only if authors have updated the search to include recently published trials.[11]

The eligible interventions can be unrestricted. Sometimes, however, the authors may choose to include only a specific set of interventions, eg, those available in their country. Some industry-initiated NMAs may choose to consider only a sponsored agent and its direct competitors.[12] This may omit the optimal agent for some situations and tends to give a fragmented picture of the evidence. It is typically best to include all interventions[13] because data on clearly suboptimal or abandoned interventions may still offer indirect evidence for other comparisons.[14]

In an NMA of 12 treatments for major depression, the authors chose to exclude placebo-controlled RCTs and included only head-to-head active treatment RCTs.[15] However, *publication bias* in the antidepressant literature is well acknowledged,[16,17] and by excluding placebo-controlled trials, the analysis loses the opportunity to benefit from additional available evidence.[18] Exclusion of eligible interventions, in this case placebo, may not just decrease statistical power but may also change the overall results.[14] Placebo-controlled trials may be different than head-to-head comparison trials in their conduct or in the degree of bias (eg, they may have more or less publication bias or *selective outcome reporting* and selective analysis reporting). Thus, their exclusion may also have an impact on the *point estimates* of the effects of pairwise comparisons and may affect the relative ranking of regimens.[14] When an NMA of second-generation antidepressants was later conducted and included placebo-controlled trials, relying only on the relative differences among treatments using the same depression scale, the authors reached a different interpretation than the earlier NMA.[15,19,20]

Finally, original trials often address multiple outcomes. Selection of NMA outcomes should not be data driven but based on importance for patients and consider both outcomes of benefit and *harm*.

Did the Meta-analysis Address Possible Explanations of Between-Study Differences in Results?

When substantial clinical variability is present (this is usually, and appropriately, the case), authors may conduct *subgroup analyses* or *meta-regression* to explain heterogeneity. If such analyses are successful in explaining heterogeneity, the NMA may provide results that more optimally fit the clinical setting and characteristics of the patient you are treating.[21] For example, in an NMA evaluating different statins for cardiovascular disease protection, the authors used meta-regression to address whether it was appropriate to combine results across primary and secondary prevention populations, different statins, and different doses of statins.[22] Meta-regression suggested heightened efficacy in those with prior cardiac events and those with a history of hypertension, possibly suggesting a more compelling case for statin use in such populations.

Inclusion of multiple control interventions (eg, placebo, no intervention, older standard of care) may enhance the robustness and connectedness of the treatment network. It is, however, important to gauge and account for potential differences between control groups. For example, because of potential placebo effects, patients receiving placebo in a *blinded* RCT may have differing responses than patients receiving no intervention in a nonblinded RCT. Thus, if an active treatment, A, has been compared with placebo and another active treatment, B, has been compared with no intervention, the different choice of control groups may produce misleading results (B may appear superior, but the use of placebo as the comparator in the A trials may be responsible for the difference). As with active interventions, meta-regression may address this problem.

For example, in an NMA evaluating the effectiveness of smoking cessation therapies, the authors combined placebo-controlled arms with standard-of-care control arms and then used meta-regression to examine whether the choice of control changed the *effect size*.[23] The authors found that trials that used placebo controls had smaller effect sizes than those that used standard of care, which explained the heterogeneity.

Did the Authors Rate the Confidence in Effect Estimates for Each Paired Comparison?

The treatment effects in an NMA are typically reported with common effect sizes along with 95%

credible intervals. Credible intervals are the Bayesian equivalent to the more commonly understood CIs. When there are K interventions included in the treatment network, there are $K*(K-1)/2$ possible pairwise comparisons. For example, if there are 7 interventions, then there are $7*(7-1)/2$, or 21, possible pairwise comparisons. Like authors of conventional meta-analyses, authors of NMAs need to address confidence in estimates of effect for each paired comparison (A vs B, A vs C, B vs C, etc—15 comparisons in the NMA example with 7 interventions). The necessity for these confidence ratings is that evidence may warrant strong inferences (ie, high confidence in estimates) for the superiority of one treatment over another (A vs B, for instance) and only weak inferences (ie, very low confidence in estimates) for the judgment of superiority of another pairing (A vs C).

The GRADE Working Group has provided a framework that is well suited to addressing confidence in estimates (see Chapter 23, Understanding and Applying the Results of a Systematic Review and Meta-analysis). We lose confidence in direct comparisons of alternative treatments if the relevant randomized trials have failed to protect against risk of bias by *allocation concealment*, blinding, and preventing loss to *follow-up* (see Chapter 7, Therapy [Randomized Trials]). We also lose confidence when CIs (or in the case of a Bayesian NMA, credible intervals) on pooled estimates are wide (imprecision); results vary from study to study and we cannot explain the differences (*inconsistency*); the population, intervention, or outcome differ from that of primary interest (*indirectness*); or we are concerned about publication bias.

Ideally, for each paired comparison, authors will present the pooled estimate for the direct comparison (if there is one) and its associated rating of confidence, the indirect comparison(s) that contributed to the pooled estimate from the NMA and its associated rating of confidence, and the NMA estimate and the associated rating of confidence. Criteria for judging confidence in estimates for direct comparisons are well established. Although these criteria provide considerable guidance in assessing confidence in indirect estimates, judgments regarding confidence in estimates from indirect comparisons present additional challenges. Criteria for addressing these challenges are still evolving, reflecting that NMA is still a very new method.

USING THE GUIDE

Returning to our opening scenario, the NMA we identified compared the efficacy of different triptans for the abortive treatment of migraine headaches.[1] Patients of interest included adults 18 to 65 years old who experience migraines, with or without aura. Experimental and control interventions included available oral triptans, placebos, and no-treatment controls. The outcomes of interest were pain-free response at 2 hours and 24 hours after the onset of headache. Patients in the included RCTs met similarly broad diagnostic criteria based on criteria from the International Headache Society and had to experience at least 1 migraine headache every 6 weeks. The outcomes assessed are important to patients, and their definitions were consistent across trials. Moreover, the authors planned to assess dose as a potential effect modifier.

The authors conducted a comprehensive search for published literature and sought unpublished RCTs via contact with industry trialists. Two reviewers conducted the search and extracted data independently, in duplicate. The authors did not rate the confidence in estimates from paired comparisons but provided information that allows conclusions about confidence. The authors reported events as proportions with ORs for treatment effects.

WHAT ARE THE RESULTS?

What Was the Amount of Evidence in the Treatment Network?

One can gauge the amount of evidence in the treatment network from the number of trials, total sample size, and number of events for each treatment and comparison. Furthermore, the extent to which the treatments are connected in the network is an important determinant of the confidence we can have in the estimates that emerge from the NMA. Understanding the *geometry of the network* (nodes and links) will permit clinicians to examine the larger picture and see what is compared to what.[24] Authors will generally present the structure of the network (as in the examples in Figure 24-1).

When alternative interventions have been compared with a single common comparator (eg, placebo), we call this a star network (Figure 24-1A). A star network only allows for indirect comparisons among active treatments, which reduces confidence in effects, particularly if there are a limited number of trials, patients, and events.[25] When there are data available that use both direct and indirect evidence of the same interventions, we refer to this as a closed loop (Figure 24-1B). The presence of direct evidence increases our confidence in the estimates of interest.

Often, a treatment network will include a mixture of exclusively indirect links and closed loops (Figures 24-1C and D). Most networks have unbalanced shapes with many trials of some comparisons, but few or none of others.[24] In this situation (and indeed, in many situations, as we have pointed out in our discussion of the need for a confidence rating of each paired comparison), evidence may warrant high confidence for some treatments and comparisons but low confidence for others. The credible intervals around direct, indirect, and NMA estimates provide a helpful index of the amount of information available for each paired comparison.

Were the Results Similar From Study to Study?

In a traditional meta-analysis of paired treatment comparisons, results often vary from study to study. Investigators can address possible explanations of differences in treatment effects using a subgroup analysis and meta-regression. However, these analyses are limited in the presence of small numbers of trials, and apparent subgroup effects often prove spurious, an issue to which we return in our discussion of applicability.[26-28]

Network meta-analyses, with larger numbers of patients and studies, present opportunities for more powerful exploration of explanations of between-study differences. Indeed, as we have pointed out in a prior section of this chapter—Did the Review Address Possible Explanations of Between-Study Differences in Results?—the search conducted by NMA authors for explanations for heterogeneity may be informative.

Nevertheless, as is true for conventional meta-analyses, NMA is vulnerable to unexplained differences in results from study to study. Ideally, NMA authors will, in summarizing the results of each paired comparison, alert you to the extent of inconsistency in results in both the direct and indirect comparisons

and the extent to which confidence in estimates decreases accordingly (see Chapter 23, Understanding and Applying the Results of a Systematic Review and Meta-analysis).

Were the Results Consistent in Direct and Indirect Comparisons?

Direct comparisons of treatments are generally more trustworthy than indirect comparisons. However, these head-to-head trials can also yield misleading estimates (eg, when conflicts of interest influence the choice of comparators used or result in selective reporting). Therefore, indirect comparisons may on occasion provide more trustworthy estimates.[29]

Deciding what estimates are most trustworthy (direct, indirect, or network) requires assessing whether the direct and indirect estimates are consistent or discrepant. One can assess whether direct and indirect estimates yield similar effects whenever there is a closed loop in the network (as in Figure 24-2B). Statistical methods exist for checking this type of inconsistency, typically called a test for *incoherence*.[30,31]

A group of investigators applied a test of incoherence to 112 interventions in which direct and indirect evidence was available. They found that the results were statistically inconsistent 14% of the time.[9] This same evaluation found that comparisons with smaller number of trials and measuring subjective outcomes had a greater risk of incoherence.

Authors' presentation of direct and indirect estimates for each paired comparison will allow you to easily examine the extent of incoherence between direct and indirect estimates. Authors can perform statistical tests to determine whether chance can explain the difference between direct and indirect estimates. Often, however, the amount of data are limited and not sufficient, and important differences may still exist in the absence of a statistically significant difference.

When incoherence is present, there are many explanations for the authors—and for you—to consider (Box 24-2). Just as unexplained heterogeneity in any direct paired comparison decreases confidence in the pooled estimate, unexplained incoherence reduces confidence in the estimate that arises from the network. Indeed, when large incoherence is present, the more credible estimate may come from either the direct (usually) or indirect (seldom) comparison rather than from the network.

BOX 24-2

Potential Reasons for Incoherence Between the Results of Direct and Indirect Comparisons

Chance

Genuine differences in results

Differences in enrolled participants (eg, entry criteria, clinical setting, disease spectrum, baseline risk, selection based on prior response)

Differences in the interventions (eg, dose, duration of administration, prior administration [second-line treatment])

Differences in background treatment and management (eg, evolving treatment and management in more recent years)

Differences in definition or measurement of outcomes

Bias in head-to-head (direct) comparisons

Optimism bias with unconcealed analysis

Publication bias

Selective reporting of outcomes and of analyses

Inflated effect size in *stopped early trials* and in early evidence

Limitations in allocation concealment, blinding, loss to follow-up, analysis as randomized

Bias in indirect comparisons

Each of the biasing issues above can affect the results of the direct comparisons on which the indirect comparisons are based

---

For example, a meta-analysis examining the analgesic efficacy of paracetamol plus codeine in surgical pain found a direct comparison that indicated the intervention was more efficacious than paracetamol alone (mean difference in pain intensity change, 6.97; 95% CI, 3.56-10.37). The *adjusted indirect comparison* did not find a significant difference between paracetamol plus codeine and paracetamol alone (−1.16; 95% CI, −6.95 to 4.64).[32] In this example, the direct and indirect evidence was statistically significantly incoherent ($P = .02$). The explanation for incoherence may be that the direct trials included patients with lower pain intensity at baseline, and such patients may be more responsive to the addition of codeine.

How Did Treatments Rank and How Confident Are We in the Ranking?

Besides presenting treatment effects, authors may also present the probability that each treatment is superior to all other treatments, allowing ranking of treatments.[33,34] Although this approach is appealing, it may be misleading because of fragility in the rankings, because differences among the ranks may be too small to be important, or because of other limitations in the studies (eg, risk of bias, inconsistency, indirectness).

We have already provided one example of such a misleading ranking: in an NMA of drug treatments to prevent fragility hip fractures, the authors' conclusion that teriparatide had the highest probability of being ranked first across 10 treatments[24] was misleading because comparison of teriparatide with all other agents, including placebo, warranted only low or very low confidence.

In another example, an NMA that examined direct-acting agents for hepatitis C found no statistical difference for sustained virologic response between telaprevir and boceprevir (OR, 1.42; 95% credible interval, 0.89-2.25); on the basis of these results, the probability of being the best favors teleprevir by far (93%) over boceprevir (7%).[35,36] However, this 93% probability provides a misleadingly strong endorsement for teleprevir. The lower boundary of the credible interval tells us that our confidence in substantial superiority of teleprevir is very low.

Examination of the confidence in estimates from each paired comparisons provides insight into the trustworthiness of any rankings, and reveals the importance of providing such ratings.

Were the Results Robust to Sensitivity Assumptions and Potential Biases?

Given the complexity of some NMAs, authors may assess the robustness of their study findings by applying sensitivity analyses that reveal how the results change if some criteria or assumptions change. Sensitivity analyses may include restricting the analyses to trials with low risk of bias only or examining different but related outcomes. The Cochrane Handbook provides a discussion of sensitivity analyses.[37]

For example, in an NMA on prevention of chronic obstructive pulmonary disease (COPD) exacerbations, the authors used the incidence rate as the primary outcome. However, there is some debate on whether incidence rates should be used in COPD trials,[38] and so the authors conducted sensitivity analyses with the binary outcome of ever having an exacerbation. The results were sufficiently similar to consider the analyses robust.[39]

USING THE GUIDE

Returning to our clinical scenario, Figure 24-3 displays the network of considered treatments for pain-free response at 2 hours. The authors included 74 RCTs that examined triptans for the treatment and prevention of migraine attacks. Placebo was compared with eletriptan, sumatriptan, rizatriptan, zolmitriptan, almotriptan, naratriptan, and frovatriptan in 15, 30, 16, 5, 9, 5, and 4 trials, respectively. The amount of evidence varied across these comparisons. For example, naratriptan had only been compared with placebo in 2 trials; therefore, confidence in these estimates is likely to be low. Evidence for sumatriptan and rizatriptan was based on a larger amount of evidence from both direct and indirect comparisons. Sumatriptan (n = 30), rizatriptan (n = 20), and eletriptan (n = 16) had the most links, whereas placebo was the most connected node (n = 68). The most common direct comparisons (n = 4 trials) were between sumatriptan and rizatriptan

(the 2 most commonly tested treatments). Of these, 15 comparisons were informed direct evidence, but 7 of the direct connections had only 1 trial, and several of the comparisons were informed only by indirect evidence. Frovatriptan was poorly connected to other treatments, and all comparisons that involved this agent warranted, therefore, only moderate confidence at best.

Sixty-three trials reported the outcome of pain-free response at 2 hours, and 25 reported 24 hours of sustained pain-free response. The authors used the I^2 value to assess heterogeneity in pairwise meta-analysis before conducting their NMA; however, they did not report the specific values. They checked the coherence between direct and indirect comparisons from closed loops and provided this information as a supplemental appendix online. Direct and indirect evidence were consistently similar, with no statistical evidence of incoherence (Table 24-1). The authors also conducted several sensitivity analyses to assess the role of dose.

Figure 24-4 displays the results of the NMA of triptans vs placebo. For pain-free response at 2 hours, the authors found that eletriptan, sumatriptan, and rizatriptan exhibited the largest treatment effects against placebo. The results were largely similar for pain-free response at 24 hours.

When the authors examined the comparative effectiveness of each triptan vs the other triptans, evidence warranted at least moderate confidence for some differences among triptans. For example, eletriptan was superior in pain-free response at 2 hours compared with sumatriptan (OR, 1.53;

95% CI, 1.16-2.01), almotriptan (OR, 2.03; 95% CI, 1.38-2.96), zolmitriptan (OR, 1.46; 95% CI, 1.02-2.09), and naratriptan (OR, 2.95; 95% CI, 1.78-4.90).

For all but naratriptan, we have at least moderate confidence in treatment effects vs placebo at 2 and 24 hours. Eletriptan was associated with the largest probability (68%) of being the best treatment for pain-free response at 2 and 24 hours (54.1%). The only other drug that ranked favorably was rizatriptan (22.6% at 2 hours and 9.2% at 24 hours). Given that comparisons between eletriptan and a number of other agents warrant at least moderate confidence, the first rank of elitriptan carried considerable weight.

FIGURE 24-3

Treatment Network for the Drugs Considered in the Example Network Meta-analysis on Triptans for the Abortive Treatment of Migraine for Pain-Free Response at 2 Hours

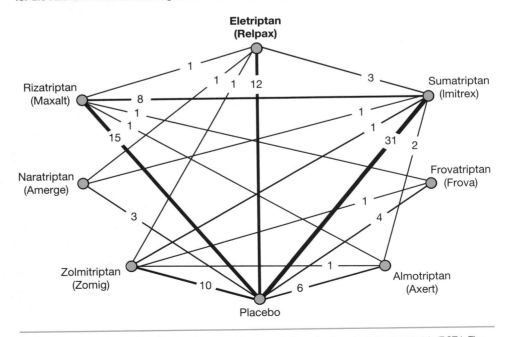

The lines between treatment nodes indicate the comparisons made throughout randomized clinical trials (RCTs). The numbers on the lines indicate the number of RCTs informing a particular comparison.

TABLE 24-1

Consistency Check for a Pain-free Response at 2 Hours With Triptan in Usual Doses

Comparison	No. of Trials	Direct Estimate[a]	Indirect Estimate[a]
Three-treatment loops where inconsistency can be checked			
Eletriptan (40 mg) vs sumatriptan (50 mg)	2	1.48 (1.14-2.79)	1.58 (0.60-5.87)
Eletriptan (40 mg) vs zolmitriptan (12.5 mg)	2	1.52 (0.96-1.81)	1.21 (0.35-3.55)
Eletriptan (40 mg) vs naratriptan (2.5 mg)	1	2.46 (1.53-3.98)	2.75 (0.37-19.8)
Sumatriptan (50 mg) vs almotriptan (2.5 mg)	1	1.49 (1.12-1.98)	1.07 (0.63-1.76)
Sumatriptan (50 mg) vs zolmitriptan (12.5 mg)	1	1.12 (0.87-1.45)	0.72 (0.42-1.29)
Sumatriptan (50 mg) vs frovatriptan (2.5 mg)	1	1.07 (0.56-2.04)	0.64 (0.35-1.15)
Almotriptan (2.5 mg) vs zolmitriptan (12.5 mg)	1	0.89 (0.69-1.15)	0.70 (0.41-1.19)
Zolmitriptan (12.5 mg) vs frovatriptan (2.5 mg)	1	0.73 (0.52-1.02)	0.86 (0.47-1.62)
Naratriptan (12.5 mg) vs frovatriptan (2.5 mg)	1	0.82 (0.51-1.20)	0.90 (0.49-1.79)

[a]Odds ratio estimates and 95% confidence intervals for all treatment comparisons from the direct pairwise meta-analysis of head-to-head trials and indirect comparison meta-analysis using placebo as the common comparator.

HOW CAN I APPLY THE RESULTS TO PATIENT CARE?

Were All Patient-Important Outcomes Considered?

Many NMAs report only 1 or a few outcomes of interest. For example, a recent NMA that compared the efficacy of antihypertensive treatments reported only heart failure and mortality,[40] whereas an older NMA of antihypertensive treatments also considered coronary heart disease and stroke.[41] Adverse events are infrequently assessed in meta-analysis and in NMAs, reflecting poor reporting in the *primary studies*.[42,43] Network meta-analyses conducted in the context of health technology assessment submissions and *evidence-based practice* reports are more likely to include multiple outcomes and assessments of harms than the less lengthy NMAs published in clinical medical journals.[20]

USING THE GUIDE

The authors assessed outcomes (pain-free response at 2 and 24 hours) that are important to patients. The major omission is adverse

events—if triptans differed substantially in adverse events, this would be an important consideration for patients. Fortunately, the drug that appears as or more effective than other triptans, eletriptan, also appears to be at least as well tolerated as other triptans.[44]

Were All Potential Treatment Options Considered?

Network meta-analyses may place restrictions on what treatments are examined. For example, for irritable bowel syndrome, an NMA may focus on pharmacologic agents, neglecting RCTs of diet, peppermint oil, and counseling.[45] Decisions to focus on subclasses of drugs may also be problematic. For example, in rheumatoid arthritis, biologics are used for patients in whom conventional drugs fail. Five of the 9 available biologics are anti–tumor necrosis factor (TNF) agents. One recent NMA only considered anti-TNF agents and excluded other biologics.[46] To the extent that the other biologic agents are equivalent or superior to the anti-TNF agents, their exclusion risks misleading clinicians regarding the best biologic agents.

FIGURE 24-4

Forest Plot of the Primary Multiple-Treatment Comparison Meta-analysis Results, Triptans vs Placebo

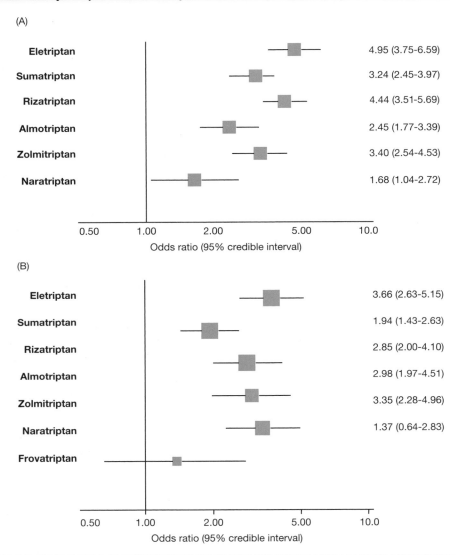

A, Pain-free response at 2 hours; B, 24 hours of sustained pain-free response.

Are Any Postulated Subgroup Effects Credible?

There are very few situations in which investigations have convincingly established important differences in the relative effect of treatment according to patient characteristics.[47] Criteria exist for determining the credibility of subgroup analyses.[47] These criteria include whether the comparisons are within-study

(subgroup A and subgroup B both participated in the same study, the stronger comparison) or between-study (one study enrolled subgroup A and another subgroup B, the weaker comparison), chance is an unlikely explanation of the differences in effect between subgroups, and the investigators made a small number of a priori subgroup hypotheses with an accurately specified direction (see Chapter 25.2, How to Use a Subgroup Analysis). Network meta-analyses allow a greater number of RCTs to be evaluated and may offer more opportunities for subgroup analysis—but with due skepticism and respect for credibility criteria.

For example, in an NMA that examined inhaled drugs for COPD, the authors examined whether severity of airflow obstruction measured by forced expiratory volume in 1 second (FEV_1) influenced patients' response.[48] If the FEV_1 was 40% or less of predicted, long-acting anticholinergics, inhaled corticosteroids, and combination treatment, including inhaled corticosteroids, reduced exacerbations significantly compared with long-acting β-agonists alone but not if the FEV_1 was greater than 40% of predicted. This difference was significant for inhaled corticosteroids ($P = .02$ for interaction) and combination treatment ($P = .01$) but not for long-acting anticholinergics ($P = .46$). The fact that these analyses were based on an a priori hypothesis, including a correctly hypothesized direction with a strong biologic rationale (greater inflammation in more severe airway disease) and a low P value for the test of interaction (ie, chance is an unlikely explanation), strengthens the credibility of the subgroup effect. It is, however, based on a between-group comparison. A reasonable judgment would be moderate to high credibility of the subgroup effect, and a clinical policy of restricting inhaled corticosteroid use to patients with more severe airflow obstruction.

CLINICAL SCENARIO RESOLUTION

You conclude that there is convincing evidence for the role of triptans in aborting migraine headaches at 2 and 24 hours. However, because triptans are a class of drugs you choose to assess whether this *class effect* is real or not (see Chapter 28.4, Understanding Class Effects). There are data available from direct and indirect comparisons that suggest that eletriptan is superior to several other triptans. You opt to discuss with the patient the benefits of starting treatment with eletriptan and will seek evidence for adverse events.

CONCLUSION

Although an NMA can provide extremely valuable information in choosing among multiple treatments offered for the same condition, it is important to determine the confidence one can place in the estimates of effect of the treatments considered and the extent to which that confidence differs across comparisons. If authors provide these confidence ratings themselves using criteria such as those suggested by *GRADE* (*Grading of Recommendations Assessment, Development and Evaluation*), the task is straightforward—simply survey the confidence ratings. Those rated as high or moderate are trustworthy and those rated low or very low much less so. If the authors do not provide these ratings themselves, you need to make your own assessments, which can be challenging.

The confidence for any comparison will be greater if individual studies are at low risk of bias and publication bias is unlikely; results are consistent in individual direct comparisons and individual comparisons with no-treatment controls and also consistent between direct and indirect comparisons; sample size is large and CIs are correspondingly narrow; and most comparisons have some direct evidence. If all of these hallmarks are present and the differences in effect sizes are large, high confidence in estimates may be warranted. However, in most cases, confidence in some key estimates is likely to warrant only moderate or low confidence. Most concerning, if authors do not provide the necessary information, it is difficult to judge which comparisons are trustworthy and which less so—and in such cases, clinicians may be best served by reviewing systematic reviews and meta-analyses of the direct comparisons and using these to guide their patient management.

References

1. Thorlund K, Mills EJ, Wu P, et al. Comparative efficacy of triptans for the abortive treatment of migraine: a multiple treatment comparison meta-analysis. *Cephalalgia*. 2014;34(4):258-267.

2. Lau J, Ioannidis JP, Schmid CH. Summing up evidence: one answer is not always enough. *Lancet*. 1998;351(9096):123-127.

3. Sacks HS, Berrier J, Reitman D, Ancona-Berk VA, Chalmers TC. Meta-analyses of randomized controlled trials. *N Engl J Med*. 1987;316(8):450-455.

4. Estellat C, Ravaud P. Lack of head-to-head trials and fair control arms: randomized controlled trials of biologic treatment for rheumatoid arthritis. *Arch Intern Med*. 2012;172(3):237-244.

5. Lathyris DN, Patsopoulos NA, Salanti G, Ioannidis JP. Industry sponsorship and selection of comparators in randomized clinical trials. *Eur J Clin Invest*. 2010;40(2):172-182.

6. Salanti G, Higgins JP, Ades AE, Ioannidis JP. Evaluation of networks of randomized trials. *Stat Methods Med Res*. 2008;17(3):279-301.

7. Lu G, Ades AE. Combination of direct and indirect evidence in mixed treatment comparisons. *Stat Med*. 2004;23(20):3105-3124.

8. Bucher HC, Guyatt GH, Griffith LE, Walter SD. The results of direct and indirect treatment comparisons in meta-analysis of randomized controlled trials. *J Clin Epidemiol*. 1997;50(6):683-691.

9. Song F, Xiong T, Parekh-Bhurke S, et al. Inconsistency between direct and indirect comparisons of competing interventions: meta-epidemiological study. *BMJ*. 2011;343:d4909.

10. Mills EJ, Bansback N, Ghement I, et al. Multiple treatment comparison meta-analyses: a step forward into complexity. *Clin Epidemiol*. 2011;3:193-202.

11. Liberati A, Altman DG, Tetzlaff J, et al. The PRISMA statement for reporting systematic reviews and meta-analyses of studies that evaluate health care interventions: explanation and elaboration. *Ann Intern Med*. 2009;151(4):W65-94.

12. Sutton A, Ades AE, Cooper N, Abrams K. Use of indirect and mixed treatment comparisons for technology assessment. *Pharmacoeconomics*. 2008;26(9):753-767.

13. Kyrgiou M, Salanti G, Pavlidis N, Paraskevaidis E, Ioannidis JP. Survival benefits with diverse chemotherapy regimens for ovarian cancer: meta-analysis of multiple treatments. *J Natl Cancer Inst*. 2006;98(22):1655-1663.

14. Mills EJ, Kanters S, Thorlund K, Chaimani A, Veroniki AA, Ioannidis JP. The effects of excluding treatments from network meta-analyses: survey. *BMJ*. 2013;347:f5195.

15. Cipriani A, Furukawa TA, Salanti G, et al. Comparative efficacy and acceptability of 12 new-generation antidepressants: a multiple-treatments meta-analysis. *Lancet*. 2009;373(9665):746-758.

16. Turner EH, Matthews AM, Linardatos E, Tell RA, Rosenthal R. Selective publication of antidepressant trials and its influence on apparent efficacy. *N Engl J Med*. 2008;358(3):252-260.

17. Ioannidis JP. Effectiveness of antidepressants: an evidence myth constructed from a thousand randomized trials? *Philos Ethics Humanit Med*. 2008;3:14.

18. Higgins JP, Whitehead A. Borrowing strength from external trials in a meta-analysis. *Stat Med*. 1996;15(24):2733-2749.

19. Ioannidis JP. Ranking antidepressants. *Lancet*. 2009;373(9677):1759-1760, author reply 1761-1762.

20. Gartlehner G, Hansen RA, Morgan LC, et al. Comparative benefits and harms of second-generation antidepressants for treating major depressive disorder: an updated meta-analysis. *Ann Intern Med*. 2011;155(11):772-785.

21. Nixon RM, Bansback N, Brennan A. Using mixed treatment comparisons and meta-regression to perform indirect comparisons to estimate the efficacy of biologic treatments in rheumatoid arthritis. *Stat Med*. 2007;26(6):1237-1254.

22. Mills EJ, Wu P, Chong G, et al. Efficacy and safety of statin treatment for cardiovascular disease: a network meta-analysis of 170,255 patients from 76 randomized trials. *QJM*. 2011;104(2):109-124.

23. Mills EJ, Wu P, Lockhart I, Thorlund K, Puhan M, Ebbert JO. Comparisons of high-dose and combination nicotine replacement therapy, varenicline, and bupropion for smoking cessation: a systematic review and multiple treatment meta-analysis. *Ann Med*. 2012;44(6):588-597.

24. Salanti G, Kavvoura FK, Ioannidis JP. Exploring the geometry of treatment networks. *Ann Intern Med*. 2008;148(7):544-553.

25. Mills EJ, Ghement I, O'Regan C, Thorlund K. Estimating the power of indirect comparisons: a simulation study. *PLoS One*. 2011;6(1):e16237.

26. Davey-Smith G, Egger MG. Going beyond the grand mean: subgroup analysis in meta-analysis of randomised trials. In: *Systematic Reviews in Health Care: Meta-analysis in context*. 2nd ed. London, England: BMJ Publishing Group; 2001:143-156.

27. Thompson SG, Higgins JP. How should meta-regression analyses be undertaken and interpreted? *Stat Med*. 2002;21(11):1559-1573.

28. Jansen J, Schmid C, Salanti G. When do indirect and mixed treatment comparisons result in invalid findings? A graphical explanation. 19th Cochrane Colloquium Madrid, Spain October 19-22, 2011. 2011:P3B379.

29. Song F, Harvey I, Lilford R. Adjusted indirect comparison may be less biased than direct comparison for evaluating new pharmaceutical interventions. *J Clin Epidemiol*. 2008;61(5):455-463.

30. Lu G, Ades A. Assessing evidence inconsistency in mixed treatment comparisons. *J Am Stat Assoc*. 2006;101(474):447-459.

31. Dias S, Welton NJ, Caldwell DM, Ades AE. Checking consistency in mixed treatment comparison meta-analysis. *Stat Med*. 2010;29(7-8):932-944.

32. Zhang WY, Li Wan Po A. Analgesic efficacy of paracetamol and its combination with codeine and caffeine in surgical pain—a meta-analysis. *J Clin Pharm Ther*. 1996;21(4):261-282.

33. Salanti G, Ades AE, Ioannidis JP. Graphical methods and numerical summaries for presenting results from multiple-treatment meta-analysis: an overview and tutorial. *J Clin Epidemiol*. 2011;64(2):163-171.

34. Golfinopoulos V, Salanti G, Pavlidis N, Ioannidis JP. Survival and disease-progression benefits with treatment regimens for advanced colorectal cancer: a meta-analysis. *Lancet Oncol*. 2007;8(10):898-911.

35. Diels J, Cure S, Gavart S. The comparative efficacy of telaprevir versus boceprevir in treatment-naive and treatment experienced patients with genotype 1 chronic hepatitis C virus infection: a mixed treatment comparison analysis. Paper presented at: 14th Annual International Society for

Pharmaceutical Outcomes Research (ISPOR) European Congress; November 5-8, 2011; Madrid, Spain.

36. Diels J, Cure S, Gavart S. The comparative efficacy of telaprevir versus boceprevir in treatment-naive and treatment-experienced patients with genotype 1 chronic hepatitis. *Value Health.* 2011;14(7):A266.

37. Higgins JP, Green S. Analysing data and undertaking meta-analyses. In: *Cochrane Handbook for Systematic Reviews of Interventions.* Oxford: Wiley & Sons; 2008.

38. Aaron SD, Fergusson D, Marks GB, et al; Canadian Thoracic Society/Canadian Respiratory Clinical Research Consortium. Counting, analysing and reporting exacerbations of COPD in randomised controlled trials. *Thorax.* 2008;63(2):122-128.

39. Mills EJ, Druyts E, Ghement I, Puhan MA. Pharmacotherapies for chronic obstructive pulmonary disease: a multiple treatment comparison meta-analysis. *Clin Epidemiol.* 2011;3: 107-129.

40. Sciarretta S, Palano F, Tocci G, Baldini R, Volpe M. Antihypertensive treatment and development of heart failure in hypertension: a Bayesian network meta-analysis of studies in patients with hypertension and high cardiovascular risk. *Arch Intern Med.* 2011;171(5):384-394.

41. Psaty BM, Lumley T, Furberg CD, et al. Health outcomes associated with various antihypertensive therapies used as first-line agents: a network meta-analysis. *JAMA.* 2003; 289(19):2534-2544.

42. Hernandez AV, Walker E, Ioannidis JP, Kattan MW. Challenges in meta-analysis of randomized clinical trials for rare harmful cardiovascular events: the case of rosiglitazone. *Am Heart J.* 2008;156(1):23-30.

43. Ioannidis JP, Evans SJ, Gøtzsche PC, et al; CONSORT Group. Better reporting of harms in randomized trials: an extension of the CONSORT statement. *Ann Intern Med.* 2004;141(10):781-788.

44. Bajwa Z, Sabahat A. Acute treatment of migraine in adults. UpToDate website. http://www.uptodate.com/contents/acute-treatment-of-migraine-in-adults. Accessed August 4, 2014.

45. Ford AC, Talley NJ, Spiegel BM, et al. Effect of fibre, antispasmodics, and peppermint oil in the treatment of irritable bowel syndrome: systematic review and meta-analysis. *BMJ.* 2008;337:a2313.

46. Schmitz S, Adams R, Walsh CD, Barry M, FitzGerald O. A mixed treatment comparison of the efficacy of anti-TNF agents in rheumatoid arthritis for methotrexate non-responders demonstrates differences between treatments: a Bayesian approach. *Ann Rheum Dis.* 2012;71(2):225-230.

47. Sun X, Briel M, Walter SD, Guyatt GH. Is a subgroup effect believable? Updating criteria to evaluate the credibility of subgroup analyses. *BMJ.* 2010;340:c117.

48. Puhan MA, Bachmann LM, Kleijnen J, Ter Riet G, Kessels AG. Inhaled drugs to reduce exacerbations in patients with chronic obstructive pulmonary disease: a network meta-analysis. *BMC Med.* 2009;7:2.

SUMMARIZING THE EVIDENCE

ADVANCED TOPICS IN SYSTEMATIC REVIEWS

Fixed-Effects and Random-Effects Models

M. Hassan Murad, Victor M. Montori, John P. A. Ioannidis,
Kameshwar Prasad, Deborah J. Cook, and Gordon Guyatt

SUMMARIZING THE EVIDENCE

IN THIS CHAPTER

MODELS FOR COMBINING DATA FOR META-ANALYSIS

In a *meta-analysis*, results from 2 or more *primary studies* are combined statistically. The meta-analyst seeking a method to combine primary study results can do so by using either a *fixed-effects model* or a *random-effects model*.[1]

We explain the differences between the 2 models based on the underlying assumptions, statistical considerations, and how the choice of model affects the results (Table 25.1-1). Note, however, that this is a controversial area within the field of meta-analysis, and expert statisticians disagree even with the characterizations in Table 25.1-1. The approach we take is, however, largely consistent with that of the Cochrane Collaboration.

A fixed-effects model considers the set of studies included in the meta-analysis and assumes that there is a single true value underlying all of the study results.[2] That is, the assumption is that if all studies that address the same question were infinitely large and completely free of *bias*, they would yield identical estimates of the effect. Thus, with the assumption that studies are free of *risk of bias*, the observed estimates of effect differ from one another only because of *random error*.[3] This assumes that any differences in the patients enrolled, the way the intervention was administered, and the way the outcome was measured have no (or minimal) impact on the magnitude of effect. The error term for a fixed-effects model comes only from within-study variation (study *variance*); the model does not consider between-study variability in results (known as *heterogeneity*) (see Chapter 23, Understanding and Applying the Results of a Systematic Review and Meta-analysis). A fixed-effects model aims to estimate this common-truth effect and the uncertainty about it.

A random-effects model assumes that the studies included are a random sample of a population of studies that address the question posed in the meta-analysis.[4] Because there are inevitably differences in the patients, interventions, and outcomes among studies that address a particular research question, each study estimates a different underlying true effect, and these effects will have a normal distribution. Thus, the *pooled estimate* in a random-effects model is not estimating a single effect of the intervention but rather the mean effect across the different populations, interventions, and methods of outcome evaluation.[3] The random-effects model takes into account both within-study variability and between-study variability.

FIXED-EFFECTS VS RANDOM-EFFECTS MODELS: AN ANALOGY

A researcher enrolls 50 teachers in a study of a new math curriculum. For each teacher, the researcher randomizes the classes so that half the classes receive the old curriculum and half receive the new curriculum. The researcher then evaluates the effectiveness of the curricula in optimizing test scores.

What is this experiment trying to answer? There is more than 1 possibility, with more than 1 underlying assumption.

1. Among these 50 teachers and no others, what is the impact of the 2 curricula on student examination scores? (Assumption: the effect of the new vs the old curriculum is the same in all teachers.)
2. Among all teachers who might ever teach this math course, of whom these 50 are a random sample, what is the impact of the 2 curricula on student examination scores? (Assumption: the effect of the new vs the old curriculum differs among teachers; ie, some teachers are better suited to the new curriculum than are others.)

The difference between these 2 scenarios:

In terms of the questions: are we interested in the effect of the curricula in these 50 teachers or the effect in all teachers?

In terms of assumptions: the relative effect of the old and new curricula is the same in each of these 50 teachers vs different across teachers.

Substitute "studies" for teachers and "therapies" for curricula and you have the questions and assumptions for fixed-effects (question 1) and random-effects (question 2) models.

TABLE 25.1-1

Comparison of Fixed-Effects and Random-Effects Models

	Fixed-Effects Models	**Random-Effects Models**
Conceptual considerations	Estimates effect in this sample of studies	Estimates effect in a population of studies from which the available studies are a random sample
	Assumes effects are the same in all studies	Assumes effects differ across studies and the pooled estimate is the mean effect
Statistical considerations	Variance is only derived from within-study variance	Variance is derived from both within-study and between-study variances
Practical considerations	Narrow CI	Wider CI
	Large studies have much more weight than small studies	Large studies have more weight than small studies, but the gradient is smaller than in fixed-effects models

Abbreviation: CI, confidence interval.

There are a variety of statistical methods used to implement fixed-effects and random-effects models. For the fixed-effects model, the "inverse variance method" means that studies are combined and weighted by the inverse of the variance. This method runs into problems when studies are small or have low event rates. Better applications of a fixed-effects model in this case are the Mantel-Haenszel method or the Peto *odds ratio*.[5] Do not worry about the details; the point here is that there are different approaches, no one knows the best approach (although some think they do), and (fortunately, rarely) choice of method can yield noticeable differences in results.

Multiple methods also exist for random-effects models that differ in how they approximate between-study variability. The most commonly used method for applying the random-effects model is the DerSimonian and Laird method,[4] although a number of alternatives exist.[6-8] Random-effects model methods also can weight studies using either the inverse variance method or the Mantel-Haenszel method.

PRACTICAL CONSIDERATIONS: DIFFERENCES IN RESULTS FROM FIXED-EFFECTS AND RANDOM-EFFECTS MODELS

Sometimes, results are similar from study to study. When it comes to statistical pooling, this will mean that the between-study variability can be fully explained by chance, and the between-study variance is estimated to be 0. This corresponds to an I^2 (which is an estimate of the variability among studies) of 0% (see Chapter 23, Understanding and Applying the Results of a Systematic Review and Meta-analysis). Under these circumstances, the fixed-effects and random-effects models will give identical results.

In approximately 40% of Cochrane meta-analyses of binary outcomes of *randomized clinical trials* (RCTs), results are sufficiently similar across trials that variability can be explained by chance and I^2 is 0.[9] This situation occurs in a smaller percentage of meta-analyses of epidemiologic studies.[10] In another 40% or so of meta-analyses of RCTs, the estimated between-study variance is not 0 but not large; thus, both fixed-effects and random-effects models provide quite similar results. In the final 20%, the between-study variability is large, and fixed-effects and random-effects models yield disparate results that may have important implications.

The Effect of Model Choice on Precision

Because the estimation of variance under the random-effects model includes between-study variability, when results vary across studies, the *confidence interval* (CI) of the combined (summary) estimate will be wider (Table 25.1-1). In this sense, the random-effects model generally produces a more conservative assessment of the precision of the summary estimate than the fixed-effects model.

FIGURE 25.1-1

Hypothetical Example of Significant Variability

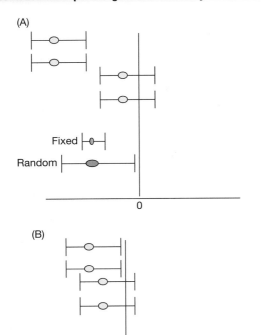

A, Random Confidence Interval (CI) Wider Than Fixed CI and
B, Hypothetical Example of Minimal Variability: Random CI Is Similar
to Fixed CI

Figure 25.1-1A shows 4 studies of equal sample size (you can tell because the width of the CI is the same in all 4 studies). There is a large amount of variability among the studies. As a result, the CI is much narrower for the fixed-effects model than for the random-effects model.

When results do not vary much among studies (ie, low heterogeneity), CIs of the 2 models become similar or the same. Figure 25.1-1B illustrates such a situation.

The Effect of Model Choice on the Point Estimate

In both models, larger studies (or studies with more events or more precise results) have larger weight. However, a random-effects model gives smaller studies proportionally greater weight in the summary estimate (Table 25.1-1). Consequently, the direction and magnitude of the summary estimate are influenced relatively more by smaller studies. Random-effects models therefore generate summary estimates closer to the *null result* (ie, no *treatment effect*) than the fixed-effects summary estimates if smaller study results are closer to the null result than those from larger studies. If the smaller studies are farther from the null result than larger studies, a random-effects model will produce larger estimates of beneficial or harmful effects than will a fixed-effects model. Therefore, the summary estimate derived from the random-effects model may be more susceptible to overestimates from small studies; this is a common phenomenon (see Chapter 23, Understanding and Applying the Results of a Systematic Review and Meta-analysis). In Figure 25.1-2, we show the effect of small studies on the summary estimate using both models.

Table 25.1-1 presents a summary of the differences between the 2 models based on conceptual, statistical, and practical considerations.

WHEN RESULTS DIFFER BETWEEN THE 2 MODELS

We all get passionate about different things, and statisticians and clinical trialists can be passionate about fixed-effects and random-effects models. Viewpoints differ, and thus the answer to which model to believe differs. Predictably, we think our approach is very sensible; be aware that others would provide different answers.

Here is a set of guidelines to follow.

1. If there is little variability among studies, fixed-effects and random-effects point estimates and CIs will vary little.

2. Intuitively, uncertainty about the accuracy and applicability of a particular point estimate

increases with increasing variability in results across studies. The random-effects model captures this uncertainty in its wider CIs and in this regard is preferable. For instance, most of us would be more comfortable with the summary estimate in Figure 25.1-1B than Figure 25.1-1A. Furthermore, the random-effects model is conceptually appealing. We are interested not just in the available studies but in applying them to a wider population. Moreover, it is likely that true effects differ across populations and thus across studies (Table 25.1-1). For these reasons, one may generally prefer the random-effects model.

3. The fixed-effects model is certainly preferable when one study is much larger and more trustworthy than one or more smaller studies that address the same question and yield quite different results.

4. The fixed-effects model also may be preferable when the number of studies included in a meta-analysis is very small (<5), leading to a concern about inaccurate estimation of between-study variance.[11]

EXAMPLES OF DIFFERENCES IN POINT ESTIMATES AND CONFIDENCE INTERVALS

Example 1

You are a surgeon evaluating a patient presenting with a localized renal tumor. You have 2 treatment options: partial or radical nephrectomy. You are interested in knowing the relative impact of each of the 2 procedures on cancer-specific mortality. A systematic review and meta-analysis[12] compared the 2 interventions (Figure 25.1-3).

The authors of the systematic review presented results using both models. Under the fixed-effects model, the results are statistically significant in favor of partial nephrectomy

FIGURE 25.1-2

Hypothetical Example of Significant Variability and Small Studies That Have Different Estimates Than Large Studies

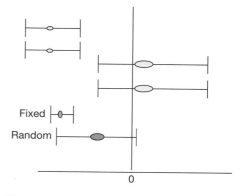

Random Confidence Interval (CI) Wider Than Fixed CI and Point Estimate of Random Closer to Small Studies

(*hazard ratio* [HR], 0.71; 95% CI, 0.59-0.85; *P* < .01). However, using the random-effects model, the results are no longer significant (HR, 0.79; 95% CI, 0.57-1.11; *P* = .17). This analysis was associated with substantial heterogeneity (I^2 = 63%; *P* for heterogeneity test <.01).

To us, the extreme differences in results (some studies appear to definitively establish benefit, and others provide a strong signal of *harm*) substantially reduce confidence in the summary estimate of effect. This reduced confidence is reflected in the wider CI of the random-effects model, which in this instance is more appropriate.

Example 2

You are evaluating a patient presenting with myocardial infarction and recall that intravenous magnesium has been used in this setting. You find a systematic review and meta-analysis[13] that evaluated the effect of magnesium on mortality for patients with myocardial infarction (Figure 25.1-4). This meta-analysis included 22 trials, and the analysis was associated with moderate heterogeneity ($I^2 = 63\%$). Most of these trials were relatively small, but 2 were not (the Medical Research Council Adjuvant Gastric Infusional Chemotherapy trial, with more than 6000 patients, and the Fourth International Study of Infarct Survival [ISIS-4] trial, with more than 50 000 patients). Many of the small trials found an apparent statistically significant reduction in mortality (eg, trials

by Gaymlani and Scechter, 1990; Shechter, 1995; and Singh, Woods, Zhu, Morton, and Raghu, 1990). The 2 largest trials, however, found no benefit. In this case, we are inclined to believe the results of the 2 large studies. The random-effects model results are therefore misleading. The figure also shows the relative weight of each trial. For example, the largest trial (ISIS-4) has a relative weight of almost 75% under the fixed-effects model but only 18% under the random-effects model.

FIGURE 25.1-3

Meta-analysis Comparing Partial and Radical Nephrectomy on Cancer-Specific Mortality[a]

Study	Hazard ratio	Lower limit	Upper limit	P value
Barbalias	1.17	0.07	19.56	.91
Becker	0.19	0.10	0.36	<.01
Bedke	0.50	0.12	2.08	.34
Breau	0.96	0.50	1.84	.90
Butler	1.37	0.50	3.75	.54
Crepel	1.96	0.72	5.34	.19
A'Armiento	1.11	0.06	20.54	.94
Hellenthal	0.39	0.26	0.58	<.01
Jeldres	2.18	0.95	5.00	.07
Kim	0.96	0.09	10.24	.97
Lau	1.33	0.30	5.90	.71
Lee	1.29	0.57	2.92	.54
Leibovich	0.63	0.19	2.07	.45
Lerner	1.31	0.80	2.15	.28
Margulis	0.41	0.15	1.12	.08
Patard	0.56	0.29	1.08	.08
Simmons	1.45	0.13	16.17	.76
Thompson	0.51	0.24	1.09	.08
Van Poppel	2.06	0.60	7.07	.25
Weight a	0.77	0.41	1.45	.42
Weight b	0.40	0.09	1.78	.23
Fixed Model	0.70	0.59	0.84	<.01
Random Model	0.79	0.57	1.11	.17

Favors partial nephrectomy — Favors radical nephrectomy

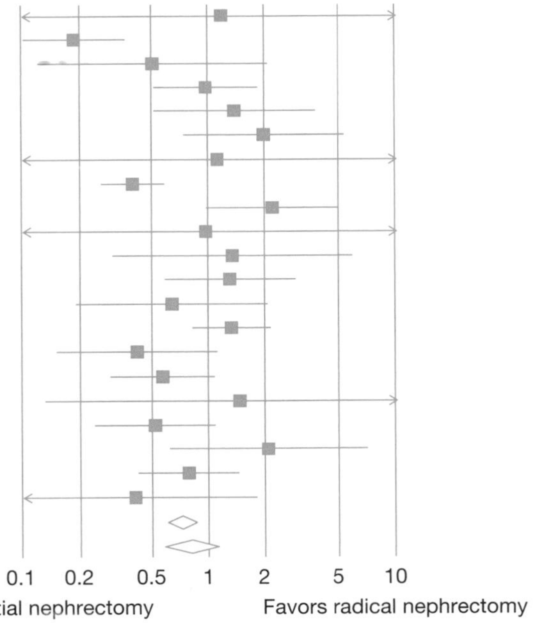

$I^2 = 63\%$

Abbreviation: CI, confidence interval.
[a]Adapted from Kim et al.[12]

FIGURE 25.1-4

Meta-analysis Comparing Magnesium to Control Therapy on Mortality in Patients With Acute Myocardial Infarction[a]

Study	Statistics for Each Study				Odds Ratio and 95% CI	Model Fixed Relative weight	Model Random Relative weight
	Odds ratio	Lower limit	Upper limit	P value			
Abraham 1987	0.96	0.06	15.77	.98		0.04	0.59
Bhargava 1995	0.95	0.18	5.00	.95		0.10	1.58
Ceremuzynzki 1989	0.28	0.03	2.88	.28		0.05	0.84
Gaymlani 2000	0.17	0.03	0.81	.03		0.12	1.75
Nakashima 2004	0.33	0.03	3.27	.35		0.06	0.88
Rasmussen 1986	0.33	0.10	1.06	.06		0.21	2.95
Santoro 2000	0.33	0.01	8.20	.50		0.03	0.45
Shechter 1990	0.10	0.01	0.82	.03		0.07	1.02
Shechter 1991	0.55	0.09	3.37	.52		0.09	1.36
Shechter 1995	0.21	0.07	0.64	.01		0.23	3.13
Singh 1990	0.51	0.18	1.45	.21		0.26	3.55
Smith 1986	0.27	0.06	1.35	.11		0.11	1.71
Thogersen 1995	0.45	0.13	1.54	.21		0.19	2.72
Urek 1996	3.00	0.12	76.58	.51		0.03	0.45
Woods 1992	0.74	0.56	0.99	.04		3.49	14.16
Wu 1992	0.31	0.11	0.92	.03		0.25	3.38
Zhu 2002	0.64	0.49	0.84	<.01		4.01	14.62
Feldstedt 1991	1.25	0.48	3.26	.65		0.31	4.08
ISIS-4 1995	1.06	1.00	1.13	.07		74.94	18.44
MAGIC 2000	1.00	0.87	1.15	.97		15.06	17.42
Morton 1984	0.44	0.04	5.02	.51		0.05	0.77
Raghu 1999	0.33	0.13	0.86	.02		0.32	4.15
Fixed Model	0.99	0.94	1.05	.80			
Random Model	0.66	0.53	0.82	<.01			

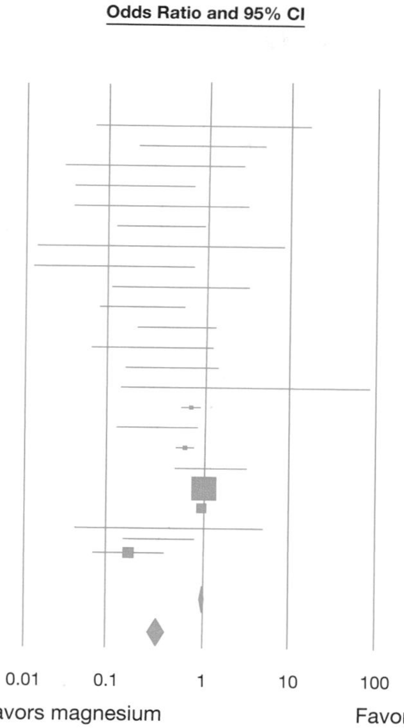

```
       0.01      0.1        1        10       100
          Favors magnesium          Favors control
```

Abbreviation: CI, confidence interval.

[a]Adapted from Li et al.[13]

CONCLUSION

There is no right answer as to which model is best, and the answer likely differs across circumstances. Table 25.1-1 presents the fundamental differences between fixed-effects and random-effects models.

Considering that table and the material in this chapter, you are now in a good position to make your own choice. Although it usually makes little difference which model data analysts choose, understanding the implications associated with the choice of the model will help clinicians make sense of situations in which large variability in study results exists.

References

1. Fleiss JL. The statistical basis of meta-analysis. *Stat Methods Med Res*. 1993;2(2):121-145.

2. Anello C, Fleiss JL. Exploratory or analytic meta-analysis: should we distinguish between them? *J Clin Epidemiol*. 1995;48(1):109-118.

3. Lau J, Ioannidis JP, Schmid CH. Summing up evidence: one answer is not always enough. *Lancet*. 1998;351(9096):123-127.

4. DerSimonian R, Laird N. Meta-analysis in clinical trials. *Control Clin Trials*. 1986;7(3):177-188.

5. Mantel N, Haenszel W. Statistical aspects of the analysis of data from retrospective studies of disease. *J Natl Cancer Inst*. 1959;22(4):719-748.

6. Smith TC, Spiegelhalter DJ, Thomas A. Bayesian approaches to random-effects meta-analysis: a comparative study. *Stat Med*. 1995;14(24):2685-2699.

7. Warn DE, Thompson SG, Spiegelhalter DJ. Bayesian random effects meta-analysis of trials with binary outcomes: methods for the absolute risk difference and relative risk scales. *Stat Med*. 2002;21(11):1601-1623.

8. Sidik K, Jonkman JN. A simple confidence interval for meta-analysis. *Stat Med*. 2002;21(21):3153-3159.

9. Higgins JP, Thompson SG, Deeks JJ, Altman DG. Measuring inconsistency in meta-analyses. *BMJ*. 2003;327(7414):557-560.

10. Ioannidis JP, Trikalinos TA, Ntzani EE, Contopoulos-Ioannidis DG. Genetic associations in large versus small studies: an empirical assessment. *Lancet*. 2003;361(9357):567-571.

11. Higgins JP, Thompson SG, Spiegelhalter DJ. A re-evaluation of random-effects meta-analysis. *J R Stat Soc Ser A Stat Soc*. 2009;172(1):137-159.

12. Kim SP, Thompson RH, Boorjian SA, et al. Comparative effectiveness for survival and renal function of partial and radical nephrectomy for localized renal tumors: a systematic review and meta-analysis. *J Urol*. 2012;188(1):51-57.

13. Li J, Zhang Q, Zhang M, Egger M. Intravenous magnesium for acute myocardial infarction. *Cochrane Database Syst Rev*. 2007;(2):CD002755.

25.2

ADVANCED TOPICS IN SYSTEMATIC REVIEWS

How to Use a Subgroup Analysis

Xin Sun, John P. A. Ioannidis, Thomas Agoritsas,
Ana C. Alba, and Gordon Guyatt

IN THIS CHAPTER

CLINICAL SCENARIO

You are a physician working at a regional trauma center. Your unit's committee, which is responsible for standardization of care, is considering using tranexamic acid to treat trauma patients who arrive 3 hours after injury. Almost all of the information on this topic is derived from a single blinded trial that randomized trauma patients to tranexamic acid or placebo.[1]

The original publication reported that 99% of the enrolled patients were followed up and there was a reduction in all-cause mortality (*relative risk* [RR], 0.91; 95% *confidence interval* [CI], 0.85-0.97) with no apparent subgroup effect.[1] A subsequent publication[2] focused on an additional analysis that addressed death from bleeding and reported a powerful subgroup effect with a large benefit for patients treated within 3 hours of injury and possible harm if treated 3 or more hours after injury. The committee's mandate is to decide whether tranexamic acid should not be given to patients 3 hours or more after injury. The *credibility* you place on the *subgroup analysis* will determine your decision.

THE CHALLENGE OF SUBGROUP ANALYSIS

Clinicians making treatment decisions use *evidence* applying most closely to the individual patient and treatment under consideration. To address this issue, clinical trialists and authors of *systematic reviews* with *meta-analyses* frequently conduct subgroup analyses to identify groups of patients (ie, sicker patients) who may respond differently to treatment than other groups (ie, less sick patients) or find more and less effective ways of administering treatment (eg, intravenous vs oral).[3,4] Although subgroup analyses may help individualize treatment, they may also mislead clinicians.

For example, the Second International Study of Infarct Survival (ISIS-2) investigators reported an apparent subgroup effect: patients presenting with myocardial infarction born under the zodiac signs of Gemini or Libra did not experience the same reduction in vascular mortality attributable to aspirin that patients with other zodiac signs had (Table 25.2-1).[5] Despite the statistical significance of the test for interaction (the probability that the difference in the effect of aspirin in Gemini and Libra patients vs those born under other zodiac signs was 3/1000), the investigators did not believe the subgroup effect, and they reported the results to indicate the dangers of subgroup analysis. Table 25.2-2 lists 19 examples in which other *randomized clinical trial* (RCT) authors have, when faced with biologically more plausible effects, claimed subgroup effects unsupported by subsequent evidence.

Clinician scientists may underestimate the extent to which chance can create imbalances (see Box 25.2-1 for another illustration). In the situations we described, the investigators were either reporting (the ISIS-2 example[5]) or being misled by (Table 25.2-2) the play of chance. When *treatment effects* are similar across patient groups or across ways of administering treatments, subgroup analyses will sometimes reveal apparently compelling but actually spurious subgroup differences.

TABLE 25.2-1

Subgroup Analysis of the Second International Study of Infarct Survival

	No. (%) of Patients		Relative Risk (95% CI)	Relative Risk Reduction or Increase, %
	Aspirin	**Placebo**		
Vascular mortality in all patients	804/8587 (9.4)	1016/8600 (11.8)	0.79 (0.73-0.87)	20.7 Reduction
Gemini or Libra	150/1357 (11.1)	147/1442 (10.2)	1.08 (0.87-1.34)	8.4 Increase
Other astrological signs	654/7228 (9.0)	868/7187 (12.1)	0.75 (0.68-0.82)	25.4 Reduction

TABLE 25.2-2

Examples of Subgroup Analyses Subsequently Found to be False[a]

Observation (Citation)	Refutation Citation
Preoperative radiotherapy improves survival in patients with Dukes' stage C rectal cancer[6,7]	8
β-Blockers are ineffective after acute myocardial infarction in elderly people and in patients with inferior myocardial infarction[9]	10
Thrombolysis is ineffective >6 hours after acute myocardial infarction[11]	12
Thrombolysis for acute myocardial infarction is ineffective or harmful in patients with a previous myocardial infarction[11]	13
Aspirin is ineffective in secondary prevention of stroke in women[14,15]	16
Antihypertensive treatment for primary prevention is ineffective in women[17,18]	19
Benefit from carotid endarterectomy for symptomatic stenosis is reduced in patients taking only low-dose aspirin because of an increased operative risk[20]	21
Angiotensin-converting enzyme inhibitors do not reduce mortality and hospital admission in patients with heart failure who are also taking aspirin[22]	23
Tamoxifen citrate is ineffective in women who have breast cancer and are younger than 50 years[24]	25
Lamifiban lowers 6-month mortality and nonfatal myocardial infarction in patients whose plasma concentrations are between 18 and 42 ng/mL but not in patients whose plasma concentrations are outside this range[26,27]	28
Mammography screening reduces mortality but not for women younger than 50 years[29]	30
Amlodipine reduces mortality in patients with chronic heart failure caused by nonischemic cardiomyopathy but not in patients with ischemic cardiomyopathy[31]	32
Ticlopidine is superior to aspirin for preventing recurrent stroke, myocardial infarction, or vascular death in blacks but not in whites[33]	34
Platelet-activating factor receptor antagonist reduces mortality in patients with gram-negative sepsis but not in other patients with sepsis[35]	36
Antihypertensive treatment is ineffective or harmful in elderly people[37]	38
Interferon reduces overall mortality in patients with idiopathic pulmonary fibrosis but only among patients with mild to moderate disease[39,40]	41
The impact of implantable cardioverter defibrillator therapy for primary prevention appears to be smaller in women[42]	43
Recombinant tissue factor pathway inhibitor does not reduce mortality in patients with severe sepsis, except in patients with community-acquired pneumonia[44,45]	46
Angiotensin receptor blockers increase mortality in patients with New York Heart Association functional class II-IV heart failure who also take both angiotensin-converting enzyme inhibitors and β-blockers but lower mortality in patients not already taking drugs in both of these classes[47]	48

[a]Examples are ordered chronologically based on the publication year of refuting citation. A number of examples originally appeared in Rothwell et al.[49]

The challenge for readers of the medical literature is to distinguish credible from less than credible reports of subgroup effects. Clinicians cannot rely on study authors to do this for them. A systematic review of 407 RCTs found 207 with subgroup analyses. Of these 207, authors claimed subgroup effects in their primary outcome in 64.[50] In most instances, the claims did not stand up to widely used guidance

---

BOX 25.2-1

The Miracle of DICE Therapy

In an imaginative investigation, Counsell et al[77] directed students in a statistics class to roll different-colored dice to simulate 44 independent clinical trials of fictitious therapies. Participants received the dice in pairs and were told that one die was an ordinary die that represented control patients, whereas the other was weighted to roll either more or fewer 6s (6 representing a patient death) than the control. Dice were colored red, white, and green, with each color representing a different treatment. The investigators simulated trials of different size (numbers of times the pair of dice were rolled), methodologic rigor (errors made in filling out the results form), and experience level of operators.

Subgroup analysis of the red dice found no statistically significantly excess mortality. When a subgroup was created by combining the white and green dice, excluding cases with errors in the forms and using data from skilled operators, there was a 39% ($P = .02$) relative risk reduction attributable to the treatments.

The participants, however, had been deliberately misled: the dice were not loaded. This study reported how a completely random phenomenon can yield statistically significant results in a subgroup analysis.

---

density lipoprotein level (40 mg/dL), and blood pressure of 130/85 mm Hg who is not receiving blood pressure treatment. Her risk of major coronary events in the next decade is 1.4%.[54] (To convert cholesterol from milligrams per deciliter to millimole per liter, multiply by 0.05259.)

Now consider a 65-year-old man, a smoker, without heart disease or diabetes, presenting with elevated total serum cholesterol level (250 mg/dL), decreased high-density lipoprotein level (30 mg/dL), and blood pressure of 165/90 mm Hg, not taking antihypertensive medication. His risk of major coronary events exceeds 38%.

These 2 individuals represent the extremes of low-risk and high-risk subgroups of candidates for lipid-lowering therapy. A systematic review and meta-analysis revealed that statin therapy reduces the RR of major coronary events by approximately 30% consistently across subgroups.[55] Thus, the 45-year-old woman could expect an absolute risk reduction of approximately 0.4% (her baseline risk of 1.4% × 30%), and the 65-year-old man could expect an absolute reduction of 10%. We would thus conclude that there is a large difference between low-risk and high-risk patients—a subgroup effect—in absolute, but not relative, terms.

In general, relative effects (eg, *risk ratio, odds ratio, hazard ratio*) have proved similar across risk groups, whereas absolute effects (eg, *absolute risk reduction, number needed to treat*) have far greater variability.[56-58] Thus, the question in subgroup analysis is not whether differences exist in absolute effects—they almost always do—but in relative effects.

The Interest Is in Subgroups Identifiable at the Start of a Study

Subgroup analysis in RCTs should focus on variables defined at the time of *randomization*. Analyses based on features that emerge during *follow-up* violate principles of randomization and are less valid.

For example, an RCT of intensive vs standard glucose management in an intensive care unit (ICU) found similar mortality in patients randomized to the intervention and the *control*

---

for the credibility of subgroup analyses.[51,52] Thus, the subgroup claims were potentially misleading.[53]

We now discuss a number of relevant general issues, followed by recommendations for how to assess subgroup analyses. Although our discussion focuses on individual RCTs and systematic reviews, the principles in this guide also apply to observational studies.

The Interest Is in Relative, Not Absolute, Subgroup Effects

Consider a 45-year-old, white, nonsmoking woman without heart disease or diabetes, elevated serum total cholesterol level (200 mg/dL), decreased high-

groups. Among patients remaining in the ICU for more than 3 days, there was an apparent reduction in death rates in the intensive glucose management group.[59] Decisions regarding length of stay may have differed between the intervention and control groups and may have been related to patients' *prognosis*. For instance, because intensive glucose management might have caused episodes of transient hypoglycemia, patients in this group might have remained longer than did similar patients in the control group. If the patients in the intervention group who stayed longer represent a group with a good prognosis, the prognostic balance that randomization initially achieved would be lost, creating a spurious treatment benefit in this subgroup.

The balance between groups achieved by randomization exists only when assessing patients in the groups to which they were initially randomized. Dividing patients into subgroups by clinical characteristics that emerge—potentially as a result of treatment—after randomization may reveal apparently statistically significant differences, but those differences arise because the patients themselves are different (ie, treatment and control patients are prognostically different), not because of a treatment effect. Subgroup claims based on characteristics arising during a study's conduct rather than on characteristics present at randomization have only low credibility.

Subgroup Claims Are Only as Credible as the Studies From Which They Arise

Consider an RCT that failed to conceal randomization, failed to undertake any *blinding*, and failed to follow up half the enrolled patients. Because of a very high *risk of bias*, clinicians would be wise to be skeptical of any subgroup claims from such a study.

Subgroup Effects Are Not All-or-Nothing Decisions

Debates about subgroup effects may be framed as absolute acceptance or rejection, yes or no with nothing in between. This approach is undesirable and destructive: it ignores the uncertainty that inevitably accompanies such judgments. It is more realistic to view the likelihood of a subgroup effect as being real on a continuum ranging from "certainly true" to "certainly false." It is better to understand where on this continuum a putative subgroup effect lies. Viewing subgroup analyses in terms of a continuum ranging from certainly true to certainly false—with the expectation that most of the time, the proper conclusion would be "probably true" or "probably false"— rather than a sharp division between true or false is the approach that we will use in this *Users' Guide*.

GUIDELINES FOR INTERPRETING SUBGROUP ANALYSES

Clinicians will encounter subgroup analyses in individual observational studies or RCTs and in systematic reviews and meta-analyses. Box 25.2-2 presents our criteria for deciding on the credibility of a subgroup analysis. Four of these criteria apply to both individual studies and systematic reviews, the fifth only to systematic reviews.

BOX 25.2-2

Credibility of Between-Study and Within-Study Comparisons

Possible explanations of difference in subgroups

Between-Study Comparisons

Hypothesized difference

Chance

Other patient differences

Different cointerventions

Different outcome measures

Different risk of bias

Within-Study Comparisons

Hypothesized difference

Chance

FIGURE 25.2-1

Inappropriate Statistical Comparison

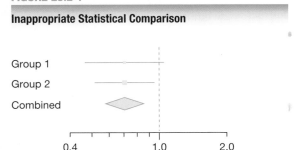

The figure presents the results of a hypothetical analysis of subgroups 1 and 2 and their pooled results. Error bars indicate 95% confidence intervals. The size of the data markers (squares) reflects the amount that each group contributes to the pooled estimates.

Can Chance Explain the Subgroup Difference?

We have emphasized the powerful and underappreciated potential for chance to mislead investigators and clinician readers. Statistical tests help determine the extent to which study results may be explained by chance alone.

Consider Figure 25.2-1, which presents the results of a hypothetical analysis of subgroups 1 and 2 and their pooled results. Assume that investigators separately test the hypothesis that chance can explain the differences between treatment and control in subgroups 1 and 2. They will conclude the answer is yes for group 1 (CIs overlap an RR of 1.0) and no for group 2 (CIs exclude an RR of 1.0). Investigators might then conclude that they have found a subgroup effect: treatment is effective in subgroup 2 but not in 1.

Such a conclusion would be misguided. Given that the *point estimates* are the same and thus the CIs completely overlap with one another, it is likely that the treatment effect is very similar in subgroups A and B. Thus, the differences in width of the CIs (overlapping no effect in 1 but not in 2) reflect differences in sample size (larger in group 2 than group 1) or number of events (more events in group 2 than in group 1). Although the example reveals exactly the same point estimates of effect for subgroups 1 and 2, the reasoning would also apply if CIs are substantially overlapping when point estimates differ considerably.

The *null hypothesis* for the appropriate statistical test is that the treatment effect is the same in the

2 subgroups. The results provide no evidence that would lead to rejecting that hypothesis. Indeed, given the identical point estimates in 1 and 2, the appropriate test, a test for interaction, would yield $P > .99$. Having conducted the appropriate test for interaction and concluded that chance explains any differences between groups, investigators should focus on the overall trial results rather than on separate subgroups 1 and 2.

Investigators made this error in logic in an RCT of angiotensin-converting enzyme (ACE) inhibitor vs diuretic-based antihypertensive therapy when they concluded that the "initiation of antihypertensive treatment involving ACE inhibitors in older subjects, particularly men, appears to lead to better outcomes than treatment with diuretic agents."[60] The investigators based their conclusion on the relative risk reductions (RRRs) of 17% (95% CI, 3%-29%) in men and 0% (95% CI, −20% to 17%) in women. The appropriate test of interaction for the subgroup effect of sex on the outcome asks the question: Can chance explain the difference between an apparent 17% RRR in men and the 0% RRR in women? The P value associated with the interaction test is 0.15. This P value tells us that if the truth were that the effect was identical in men and women, then by chance alone we would see differences between men and women as great or greater than we have observed (ie, 17% and 0%, respectively) 15% of the time. Although the difference between the ACE inhibitor and diuretic-based therapies was statistically significant in men but not women, when the 2 groups were compared directly with one another and an interaction test was performed, the data were consistent with the null hypothesis that the effect did not differ between the sexes.

Contrast this with an RCT addressing the relative effect of reamed vs unreamed nailing on subsequent operation rates in patients with tibial fractures.[61] Reamed nailing decreased subsequent operations in patients with closed fractures (RR, 0.67; 95% CI, 0.47-0.76) but increased subsequent operations in those with open fractures (RR, 1.27; 95% CI, 0.91-1.78). When investigators performed a test of interaction to address the hypothesis that reamed vs unreamed nailing had the same effect on subsequent operations in closed and open fractures, $P = .01$. Differences between groups as large or larger than observed in this study would occur by chance only 1% of the time. When chance alone is unlikely to explain subgroup differences, a subgroup effect may be present, but clinicians should also consider the other criteria that we present in this article.

A variety of statistical techniques are available to explore whether chance alone explains apparent subgroup differences.[51,62,63] When assessing the results of these tests of interaction, clinicians should note whether differences in effect are quantitative (ie, same direction but varying magnitude by treatment effects) or qualitative (ie, beneficial in one subgroup but harmful in another). Qualitative effects in subgroups are uncommon.

Clinicians should also consider that failure to find differences between subgroups does not mean that differences do not exist. An insufficient number of study participants could result in an inability to find that differences exist (ie, the test for interaction was underpowered). On other hand, if the results of an appropriate statistical test reveal that chance is an unlikely explanation for an apparent subgroup effect, it does not mean the effect is real. It means clinicians should take the possible effect seriously.

Is the Subgroup Difference Consistent Across Studies?

One may generate a hypothesis concerning differential response in a subgroup of patients by examination of data from a single study. Replication in other studies increases its credibility, and failure to replicate diminishes its credibility. Readers of trial reports should look carefully in the discussion sections for references to subgroup results in similar trials. Because investigators tend to select references related to evidence supporting their positions, statements from authors regarding a systematic search for related evidence strengthens arguments in favor of the subgroup analyses' results. Table 25.2-2 provides examples in which failure to replicate subgroup analyses undermined the subgroup claim. Subgroup claims failing replication warrant considerable skepticism.

Was the Subgroup Difference One of a Small Number of a Priori Hypotheses in Which the Direction Was Accurately Prespecified?

Embedded within any large data set are a certain number of apparent but, in fact, spurious subgroup differences. As a result, the credibility of any apparent subgroup difference that arises from post hoc rather than a priori hypotheses is questionable.

For example, in the first large trial of aspirin for patients with transient ischemic attacks, the investigators reported that aspirin had a beneficial effect in preventing stroke in men but not in women with cerebrovascular disease.[64] For many years, this led many physicians to withhold aspirin from women with cerebrovascular disease. The investigators, however, had stumbled across the finding in exploring the data rather than suspecting it beforehand. The apparent subgroup effect was subsequently found in other studies and in a meta-analysis summarizing these studies to be spurious.[65] Had clinicians been appropriately skeptical of this post hoc finding and demanded replication, they would not have missed the opportunity to prevent strokes in their female patients.

Even if investigators have prespecified their hypotheses, the strength of inference for confirmation of any hypothesis will decrease if a large number of hypotheses are tested. For example, investigators conducted an RCT of platelet-activating factor receptor antagonist in septic patients. For all 262 patients, results indicated that the small benefit for therapy failed to meet the usual threshold $P < .05$ for statistical significance. A subgroup analysis of 110 patients with gram-negative bacterial infection was found to have a large, statistically significant advantage for platelet-activating factor receptor antagonist treatment.[66]

A subsequent, larger hypothesis-testing RCT that involved 444 patients with gram-negative bacterial infection failed to replicate the apparent benefit observed in the subgroup analysis of the previous trial.[67] The disappointed investigators might have been less surprised at the result of the second trial had they fully appreciated the limitations of their first subgroup analysis: the possible differential effect of platelet-activating factor receptor antagonist in gram-negative bacterial infection was 1 of 15 subgroup hypotheses that they tested.[68]

The era of molecular medicine has increased the temptation for multiple hypothesis testing: the number of candidate subgroup analyses that can be performed for molecular analyses is enormous. Although gene-based information is often biologically fascinating, databases include information on many thousands or even millions of genetic or other molecular factors that are difficult to interpret. Testing large numbers of subgroup hypotheses will create some misleading results because of problems related to multiple comparisons.[69]

For example, although many studies have identified pharmacogenetic markers for subgroups of patients with different responses to treatment or toxicity, only a handful of these differences have proved to be true when tested in additional data sets. Given the large number of genomic and other molecular markers, statistical significance thresholds are far more stringent when testing for subgroup differences. For example, in pharmacogenomics, for which millions of gene variants are tested, researchers and readers should pay little attention to claims of important findings unless the subgroup differences (eg, between patients carrying vs those not carrying 2 copies of a putative pharmacogenetic marker) are associated with $P < 10^{-8}$.[70]

A final issue in hypothesis testing is specification of the direction of the effect. In an RCT of vasopressin vs norepinephrine in 778 patients with septic shock, the investigators specified a priori a primary subgroup analysis: reduced mortality attributable to vasopressin over norepinephrine would be greater for patients with more severe septic shock.[71] In contrast to the investigators' expectations, vasopressin appeared to benefit only patients with less severe septic shock. They reported higher 28-day mortality among the more severe cases (RR, 1.04; 95% CI, 0.83-1.3; $P = .76$) vs less severe cases (RR, 0.74; 95% CI, 0.55-1.01; $P = .05$). However, the test for the interaction between the treatment assignment and the severity-of-shock subgroup was not significant (interaction $P = .10$). The investigators' failure to correctly identify the direction of the subgroup effect appreciably weakened any inference that vasopressin was superior to norepinephrine in the less severely ill patients. Clinicians should look for explicit statements on whether subgroup hypotheses and their direction were specified a priori.

Study reports often fail to clearly identify the extent to which a hypothesis arose before, during, or after the data were collected and analyzed or the number of subgroup hypotheses tested. If the investigators withhold this information, reporting only hypotheses

that were statistically significant, the reader will be misled. When, however, the hypothesis has been clearly suggested by a different data set and investigators replicate the finding in a new RCT, clinicians can be confident regarding a priori specification.

Is There a Strong Preexisting Biologic Rationale Supporting the Apparent Subgroup Effect?

Subgroup claims are more credible if additional, external evidence (such as from laboratory studies or analogous situations in human biology) makes it plausible. Such evidence may come from 3 sources: studies of different populations (including animal studies), observations of subgroup differences for similar interventions, and results of studies of other related intermediary outcomes.

There is no shortage of biologically plausible explanations supporting almost any observation. One example of biologic evidence supporting a possible subgroup effect concerns an apparent effect described previously: a trial suggested that aspirin reduced stroke risk in men but not in women.[64] Subsequent animal research provided a biologic rationale for the observed sex differences in aspirin's effects on stroke risk.[72] However, subsequent clinical trials found that there was no sex difference in stroke response to aspirin irrespective of the biologic rationale found in laboratory animals.[73]

One of the most useful roles of biologic rationale is to raise serious questions regarding an apparent subgroup effect that is inconsistent with our current understanding of biology. The apparent interaction between birth zodiac sign and the effect of aspirin in myocardial infarction (Table 25.2-1) provides an example in which the absence of a biologic explanation seriously undermines the credibility of an apparent subgroup effect.

SUBGROUP CLAIMS IN META-ANALYSES: WITHIN- VS BETWEEN-TRIAL COMPARISONS

Up to now, this *Users' Guide* has addressed individual studies. Making inferences about subgroup effects in systematic reviews requires application of the previously discussed 4 criteria and consideration of whether the comparison among subgroups is done within or between studies. In single trials, the comparison is always within: that is, the 2 groups of patients (eg, the older and younger) or the 2 alternative ways of administering the intervention (eg, higher and lower doses) were assessed in the same RCT. Within meta-analyses, this is not necessarily the case.

Consider the controversy regarding dose effects of vitamin D on fracture reduction.[74] One meta-analysis suggesting the benefit of higher doses examined the effect of vitamin D on nonvertebral fractures and reported on results of 2 studies of lower doses (400 IU) and 5 studies of higher doses (700-800 IU).[75] The *pooled estimates* from the low-dose studies suggested no effect on fractures, whereas the higher dose studies suggest a 23% reduction in RR (Figure 25.2-2). The test for interaction, following the same principle as individual studies, addresses whether chance can explain the difference between the high-dose and low-dose studies and yielded a $P = .01$.

The inference regarding the dose effect is, however, limited because this was a between-study rather than a within-study comparison. As a result, there are a number of competing explanations for the observed differences between the high-dose and low-dose studies.

Box 25.2-2 provides the generic competing explanations present in all between-study comparisons. Aside from the hypothesized effect of vitamin D dose in the vitamin D–fracture studies, explanations for the apparent differences in study results include the following: patients in the low-dose studies were exposed to adequate sunlight (and thus did not need supplementation) whereas the high-dose study patients did not; the patients who received high dosages took calcium supplements and the patients receiving low dosages did not; the length of follow-up differed in the low-dose and high-dose studies; and the low-dose studies had a lower risk of bias than the high-dose studies.

Within-trial subgroup differences from well-designed and implemented RCTs leave only 2 likely explanations: chance and a real effect

FIGURE 25.2-2

Meta-analysis of Studies Addressing the Effect of Vitamin D on Nonvertebral Fractures

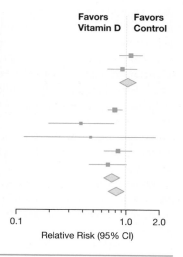

Source	No. Vitamin D	No. Control	Total Vitamin D	Total Control	Relative Risk (95% CI)
Vitamin D 400 IU/d					
Lips et al, 1996	135	122	1291	1287	1.10 (0.87-1.39)
Meyer et al, 2002	69	76	569	575	0.92 (0.68-1.24)
Pooled					1.03 (0.86-1.24)
Vitamin D 700-800 IU/d					
Chapuy et al, 1994	255	308	1176	1127	0.79 (0.69-0.92)
Dawson-Hughes et al, 1997	11	26	202	187	0.39 (0.20-0.77)
Pfeifer et al, 2000	3	6	70	67	0.48 (0.12-1.84)
Chapuy et al, 2002	97	55	393	190	0.85 (0.64-1.13)
Trivedi et al, 2003	43	62	1345	1341	0.69 (0.47-1.01)
Pooled					0.75 (0.63-0.89)
All doses					0.82 (0.69-0.98)

Abbreviation: CI, confidence interval.

The size of the data markers (squares) reflect the amount that each study contributes to the pooled estimates. This is based on Bischoff-Ferrari et al.[75]

(Box 25.2-2) Most subgroup analyses from systematic reviews are limited by between-study comparisons.[76] The exception is meta-analyses of individual patient data in which most or all studies have included patients from each relevant subgroup.

Investigators undertaking meta-analyses of individual patient data can conduct sophisticated analyses that compare the effects in subgroups within studies and then effectively pool across those studies.

CLINICAL SCENARIO RESOLUTION

Returning to our opening scenario, your committee notes that almost all of the data come from a single trial and thus reflect a within-trial comparison. The RR for death due to bleeding in patients receiving tranexamic of 1 hour or less after injury is 0.68 (95% CI, 0.57-0.82), 1 and 3 hours after injury is 0.79 (95% CI, 0.64-0.97), and more than 3 hours after injury is 1.44 (95% CI, 1.12-1.84). Chance appears a very unlikely explanation for the difference ($P < .001$). Trauma patients exhibit early fibrinolysis that could exacerbate bleeding; tranexamic acid inhibits fibrinolysis, providing a strong biologic rationale for the treatment. The fibrinolysis may be largely resolved by 3 hours, thus providing a biologic explanation for the absence of benefit after 3 hours. Prespecification is complex. The time-from-injury hypothesis was one of a small number of a priori hypotheses with a specified direction, but the analysis plan focused on all-cause mortality (in which the investigators found no subgroup effect). The analysis of cause-specific mortality represented a secondary exploration of the data. Ultimately, your committee decides that the subgroup effect, although far from completely secure, is sufficiently credible that your unit will not administer tranexamic acid to patients arriving more than 3 hours after their trauma.

CONCLUSIONS

The criteria for assessing subgroup analyses presented in this *Users' Guide* (Box 25.2-3) will help clinicians evaluating the credibility of claims of differential response to treatment in a definable subgroup of patients. These criteria are intended as core criteria that clinicians can feasibly apply when evaluating a subgroup claim. More comprehensive criteria are available for readers seeking a deeper understanding of the nuances of assessing subgroup claims.[52] Moreover, we have focused on data from randomized trials and their systematic reviews. Subgroup claims are increasingly based on observational data and these—like their estimates of effect in entire populations—warrant considerably greater skepticism.[53]

Applying these criteria, clinicians will sometimes find, at one extreme, relatively small interactions easily explained by chance and based on between-study differences generated by post hoc

BOX 25.2-3

Guidelines for Deciding Whether Apparent Differences in Subgroup Response Are Real

Issues for Individual Studies and Systematic Reviews

Can chance explain the subgroup difference?

Is the subgroup difference consistent across studies?

Was the subgroup difference one of a small number of a priori hypotheses in which the direction was accurately prespecified?

Is there a strong preexisting biologic rationale supporting the apparent subgroup effect?

An Issue for Meta-analyses Only

Is the subgroup difference suggested by comparisons within rather than between studies?

explorations. Less frequently, at the other extreme, they will find interactions with very small *P* values (for instance <.01) based on within-trial comparisons with consistent results following a limited number of subgroup hypotheses with a correctly specified direction. The former should be viewed with skepticism. The latter are more credible and can be used for clinical decision making.

Results between these extremes require consideration of a number of factors, including the risks associated with administering or avoiding treatment and patient's *values and preferences*. Judgments about the credibility of subgroup claims, based on the criteria that we have suggested, are likely to play a key part in such decisions.

References

1. Shakur H, Roberts I, Bautista R, et al; CRASH-2 trial collaborators. Effects of tranexamic acid on death, vascular occlusive events, and blood transfusion in trauma patients with significant haemorrhage (CRASH-2): a randomised, placebo-controlled trial. *Lancet*. 2010;376(9734):23-32.

2. Roberts I, Shakur H, Afolabi A, et al; CRASH-2 collaborators. The importance of early treatment with tranexamic acid in bleeding trauma patients: an exploratory analysis of the CRASH-2 randomised controlled trial. *Lancet*. 2011; 377(9771):1096-1101, e1-e2.

3. Pocock SJ, Assmann SE, Enos LE, Kasten LE. Subgroup analysis, covariate adjustment and baseline comparisons in clinical trial reporting: current practice and problems. *Stat Med*. 2002;21(19):2917-2930.

4. Sun X, Briel M, Busse JW, et al. The influence of study characteristics on reporting of subgroup analyses in randomised controlled trials: systematic review. *BMJ*. 2011;342:d1569. doi:10.1136/bmj.d1569.

5. ISIS-2 (Second International Study of Infarct Survival) Collaborative Group. Randomised trial of intravenous streptokinase, oral aspirin, both, or neither among 17,187 cases of suspected acute myocardial infarction: ISIS-2. ISIS-2 (Second International Study of Infarct Survival) Collaborative Group. *Lancet*. 1988;2(8607):349-360.

6. Roswit B, Higgins GA Jr, Keehn RJ. Preoperative irradiation for carcinoma of the rectum and rectosigmoid colon: reportof a National Veterans Administration randomized study. *Cancer*. 1975;35(6):1597-1602.

7. Rider WD, Palmer JA, Mahoney LJ, Robertson CT. Preoperative irradiation in operable cancer of the rectum: report of the Toronto trial. *Can J Surg*. 1977;20(4):335-338.

8. Duncan W, Smith AN, Freedman LS, et al. The evaluation of low dose pre-operative X-ray therapy in the management of operable rectal cancer: results of a randomly controlled trial. *Br J Surg*. 1984;71(1):21-25.

9. Andersen MP, Bechsgaard P, Frederiksen J, et al. Effect of alprenolol on mortality among patients with definite or suspected acute myocardial infarction. Preliminary results. *Lancet*. 1979;2(8148):865-868.

10. Reduction in mortality after myocardial infarction with long-term beta-adrenoceptor blockade: multicentre international study: supplementary report. *BMJ*. 1977;2(6084):419-421.

11. Yusuf S, Peto R, Lewis J, Collins R, Sleight P. β blockade during and after myocardial infarction: an overview of the randomized trials. *Prog Cardiovasc Dis*. 1985;27(5):335-371.

12. Gruppo Italiano per lo Studio della Streptochinasi nell'Infarto Miocardico (GISSI). Effectiveness of intravenous thrombolytic treatment in acute myocardial infarction. *Lancet*. 1986; 1(8478):397-402.

13. ISIS-2 Collaborative Group. Randomised trial of intravenous streptokinase, oral aspirin, both, or neither among 17,187 cases of suspected acute myocardial infarction: ISIS-2. *Lancet*. 1988;2(8607):349-360.

14. Fibrinolytic Therapy Trialists' (FTT) Collaborative Group. is Indications for fibrinolytic therapy in suspected acute myocardial infarction: collaborative overview of early mortality and major morbidity results from all randomised trials of more than 1000 patients. *Lancet*. 1994;343(8893):311-322.

15. The Canadian Cooperative Study Group. A randomized trial of aspirin and sulfinpyrazone in threatened stroke. *N Engl J Med*. 1978;299(2):53-59.

16. Fields WS, Lemak NA, Frankowski RF, Hardy RJ. Controlled trial of aspirin in cerebral ischemia. *Stroke*. 1977;8(3):301-314.

17. Antiplatelet Trialists' Collaboration. Collaborative overview of randomised trials of antiplatelet therapy, I: prevention of death, myocardial infarction, and stroke by prolonged antiplatelet therapy in various categories of patients. *BMJ*. 1994;308(6921):81-106.

18. Anastos K, Charney P, Charon RA, et al; The Women's Caucus, Working Group on Women's Health of the Society of General Internal Medicine. Hypertension in women: what is really known? *Ann Intern Med*. 1991;115(4):287-293.

19. Medical Research Council Working Party. MRC trial of treatment of mild hypertension: principal results. *Br Med J (Clin Res Ed)*. 1985;291(6488):97-104.

20. Gueyffier F, Boutitie F, Boissel JP, et al; The INDANA Investigators. Effect of antihypertensive drug treatment on cardiovascular outcomes in women and men: a meta-analysis of individual patient data from randomized, controlled trials. *Ann Intern Med*. 1997;126(10):761-767.

21. Barnett HJM, Taylor DW, Eliasziw M, et al; North American Symptomatic Carotid Endarterectomy Trial Collaborators. Benefit of carotid endarterectomy in patients with symptomatic moderate or severe stenosis. *N Engl J Med*. 1998; 339(20):1415-1425.

22. Taylor DW, Barnett HJM, Haynes RB, et al; ASA and Carotid Endarterectomy (ACE) Trial Collaborators. Low-dose and high-dose acetylsalicylic acid for patients undergoing carotid endarterectomy: a randomised controlled trial. *Lancet*. 1999;353(9171):2179-2184.

23. Cleland JGF, Bulpitt CJ, Falk RH, et al. Is aspirin safe for patients with heart failure? *Br Heart J.* 1995;74(3):215-219.

24. Flather MD, Yusuf S, Køber L, et al; ACE-Inhibitor Myocardial Infarction Collaborative Group. Long-term ACE-inhibitor therapy in patients with heart failure or left-ventricular dysfunction: a systematic overview of data from individual patients. *Lancet.* 2000;355(9215):1575-1581.

25. Early Breast Cancer Trialists' Collaborative Group. Effects of adjuvant tamoxifen and of cytotoxic therapy on mortality in early breast cancer. An overview of 61 randomized trials among 28,896 women. *N Engl J Med.* 1988;319(26):1681-1692.

26. Early Breast Cancer Trialists' Collaborative Group. Tamoxifen for early breast cancer. *Cochrane Database Syst Rev.* 2001; 1(1):CD000486.

27. Moliterno DJThe PARAGON B International Steering Committee. Patient-specific dosing of IIb/IIIa antagonists during acute coronary syndromes: rationale and design of the PARAGON B study. *Am Heart J.* 2000;139(4):563-566.

28. PARAGON Investigators. International, randomized, controlled trial of lamifiban (a platelet glycoprotein IIb/IIIa inhibitor), heparin, or both in unstable angina. *Circulation.* 1998;97(24):2386-2395.

29. Global Organization Network (PARAGON)-B Investigators. Randomized, placebo-controlled trial of titrated intravenous lamifiban for acute coronary syndromes. *Circulation.* 2002;105(3):316-321.

30. Frisell J, Lidbrink E, Hellström L, Rutqvist LE. Followup after 11 years—update of mortality results in the Stockholm mammographic screening trial. *Breast Cancer Res Treat.* 1997;45(3):263-270.

31. Nystrom L, Andersson I, Bjurstam N, Frisell J, Nordenskjold B, Rutqvist LE. Long-term effects of mammography screening: updated overview of the Swedish randomised trials. *Lancet.* 2002;359:909-919.

32. Packer M, O'Connor CM, Ghali JK, et al; Prospective Randomized Amlodipine Survival Evaluation Study Group. Effect of amlodipine on morbidity and mortality in severe chronic heart failure. *N Engl J Med.* 1996;335(15):1107-1114.

33. Wijeysundera HC, Hansen MS, Stanton E, et al; PRAISE II Investigators. Neurohormones and oxidative stress in nonischemic cardiomyopathy: relationship to survival and the effect of treatment with amlodipine. *Am Heart J.* 2003;146(2):291-297.

34. Weisberg LA. The efficacy and safety of ticlopidine and aspirin in non-whites: analysis of a patient subgroup from the Ticlopidine Aspirin Stroke Study. *Neurology.* 1993;43(1):27-31.

35. Gorelick PB, Richardson D, Kelly M, et al. Aspirin and ticlopidine for prevention of recurrent stroke in black patients: a randomized trial. *JAMA.* 2003;289:2947-2957.

36. Dhainaut JF, Tenaillon A, Le Tulzo Y, et al; BN 52021 Sepsis Study Group. Platelet-activating factor receptor antagonist BN 52021 in the treatment of severe sepsis: a randomized, double-blind, placebo-controlled, multicenter clinical trial. *Crit Care Med.* 1994;22(11):1720-1728.

37. Albrecht DM, van Ackern K, Bender HJ, et al. Efficacy and safety of the platelet-activating factor receptor antagonist BN 52021 (Ginkgolide B) in patients with severe sepsis: a randomised, double-blind, placebo-controlled, multicentre trial. *Clin Drug Investig.* 2004;24(3):137-147.

38. Amery A, Birkenhäger W, Brixko P, et al. Influence of antihypertensive drug treatment on morbidity and mortality in patients over the age of 60 years: European Working Party on High blood pressure in the Elderly (EWPHE) results: subgroup analysis on entry stratification. *J Hypertens Suppl.* 1986; 4(6):S642-S647.

39. Musini VM, Tejani AM, Bassett K, Wright JM. Pharmacotherapy for hypertension in the elderly. *Cochrane Database Syst Rev.* 2009;(4):CD000028. doi:10.1002/14651858.CD000028.pub2.

40. Raghu G, Brown KK, Bradford WZ, et al; Idiopathic Pulmonary Fibrosis Study Group. A placebo-controlled trial of interferon gamma-1b in patients with idiopathic pulmonary fibrosis. *N Engl J Med.* 2004;350(2):125-133.

41. King TE Jr, Albera C, Bradford WZ, et al; INSPIRE Study Group. Effect of interferon gamma-1b on survival in patients with idiopathic pulmonary fibrosis (INSPIRE): a multicentre, randomised, placebo-controlled trial. *Lancet.* 2009;374(9685):222-228.

42. Russo AM, Poole JE, Mark DB, et al. Primary prevention with defibrillator therapy in women: results from the Sudden Cardiac Death in Heart Failure Trial. *J Cardiovasc Electrophysiol.* 2008;19(7):720-724.

43. Santangeli P, Pelargonio G, Dello Russo A, et al. Gender differences in clinical outcome and primary prevention defibrillator benefit in patients with severe left ventricular dysfunction: a systematic review and meta-analysis. *Heart Rhythm.* 2010;7(7):876-882.

44. Abraham E, Reinhart K, Opal S, et al; OPTIMIST Trial Study Group. Efficacy and safety of tifacogin (recombinant tissue factor pathway inhibitor) in severe sepsis: a randomized controlled trial. *JAMA.* 2003;290(2):238-247.

45. Laterre PF, Opal SM, Abraham E, et al. A clinical evaluation committee assessment of recombinant human tissue factor pathway inhibitor (tifacogin) in patients with severe community-acquired pneumonia. *Crit Care.* 2009;13(2):R36.

46. Wunderink RG, Laterre PF, Francois B, et al; CAPTIVATE Trial Group. Recombinant tissue factor pathway inhibitor in severe community-acquired pneumonia: a randomized trial. *Am J Respir Crit Care Med.* 2011;183(11):1561-1568.

47. Cohn JN, Tognoni G; Valsartan Heart Failure Trial Investigators. A randomized trial of the angiotensin-receptor blocker valsartan in chronic heart failure. *N Engl J Med.* 2001;345(23):1667-1675.

48. Heran BS, Musini VM, Bassett K, Taylor RS, Wright JM. Angiotensin receptor blockers for heart failure. *Cochrane Database Syst Rev.* 2012;4:CD003040. doi:10.1002/14651858. CD003040.pub2. Review.

49. Rothwell PM. Treating individuals 2. Subgroup analysis in randomised controlled trials: importance, indications, and interpretation. *Lancet.* 2005;365(9454):176-186.

50. Sun X, Briel M, Busse JW, et al. Credibility of claims of subgroup effects in randomised controlled trials: systematic review. *BMJ.* 2012;344:e1553. doi:10.1136/bmj.e155.

51. Buyse ME. Analysis of clinical trial outcomes: some comments on subgroup analyses. *Control Clin Trials.* 1989;10(4) (suppl):187S-194S.

52. Sun X, Briel M, Walter SD, Guyatt GH. Is a subgroup effect believable? updating criteria to evaluate the credibility of subgroup analyses. *BMJ.* 2010;340:c117.

53. Wang R, Lagakos SW, Ware JH, Hunter DJ, Drazen JM. Statistics in medicine: reporting of subgroup analyses in clinical trials. *N Engl J Med.* 2007;357(21):2189-2194.

54. Goff DC Jr, Lloyd-Jones DM, Bennett G, et al. ACC/AHA Guideline on the Assessment of Cardiovascular Risk: a

report of the American College of Cardiology/American Heart Association Task Force on Practice Guidelines [published online ahead of print November 12, 2013]. *Circulation*. 2013;2013. doi:10.1016/j.jacc.2013.11.005.

55. Thavendiranathan P, Bagai A, Brookhart MA, Choudhry NK. Primary prevention of cardiovascular diseases with statin therapy: a meta-analysis of randomized controlled trials. *Arch Intern Med*. 2006;166(21):2307-2313.

56. Furukawa TA, Guyatt GH, Griffith LE. Can we individualize the 'number needed to treat'? An empirical study of summary effect measures in meta-analyses. *Int J Epidemiol*. 2002;31(1):72-76.

57. Schmid CH, Lau J, McIntosh MW, Cappelleri JC. An empirical study of the effect of the control rate as a predictor of treatment efficacy in meta-analysis of clinical trials. *Stat Med*. 1998;17(17):1923-1942.

58. Deeks JJ. Issues in the selection of a summary statistic for meta-analysis of clinical trials with binary outcomes. *Stat Med*. 2002;21(11):1575-1600.

59. Van den Berghe G, Wilmer A, Hermans G, et al. Intensive insulin therapy in the medical ICU. *N Engl J Med*. 2006;354(5):449-461.

60. Wing LM, Reid CM, Ryan P, et al; Second Australian National Blood Pressure Study Group. A comparison of outcomes with angiotensin-converting: enzyme inhibitors and diuretics for hypertension in the elderly. *N Engl J Med*. 2003;348(7):583-592.

61. Bhandari M, Guyatt G, Tornetta P III, et al; SPRINT Investigators. Study to prospectively evaluate reamed intramedually nails in patients with tibial fractures (S.P.R.I.N.T.): study rationale and design. *BMC Musculoskelet Disord*. 2008;9:91.

62. Furberg CD, Morgan TM. Lessons from overviews of cardiovascular trials. *Stat Med*. 1987;6(3):295-306.

63. Schneider B. Analysis of clinical trial outcomes: alternative approaches to subgroup analysis. *Control Clin Trials*. 1989; 10(4)(suppl):176S-186S.

64. The Canadian Cooperative Study Group. A randomized trial of aspirin and sulfinpyrazone in threatened stroke. *N Engl J Med*. 1978;299(2):53-59.

65. Antiplatelet Trialists' Collaboration. Collaborative overview of randomised trials of antiplatelet therapy, I: prevention of death, myocardial infarction, and stroke by prolonged antiplatelet therapy in various categories of patients. *BMJ*. 1994;308(6921):81-106.

66. Dhainaut JF, Tenaillon A, Le Tulzo Y, et al; BN 52021 Sepsis Study Group. Platelet-activating factor receptor antagonist BN 52021 in the treatment of severe sepsis: a randomized, double-blind, placebo-controlled, multicenter clinical trial. *Crit Care Med*. 1994;22(11):1720-1728.

67. Dhainaut JF, Tenaillon A, Hemmer M, et al; BN 52021 Sepsis Investigator Group. Confirmatory platelet-activating factor receptor antagonist trial in patients with severe gram-negative bacterial sepsis: a phase III, randomized, double-blind, placebo-controlled, multicenter trial. *Crit Care Med*. 1998;26 (12):1963-1971.

68. Natanson C, Esposito CJ, Banks SM. The sirens' songs of confirmatory sepsis trials: selection bias and sampling error. *Crit Care Med*. 1998;26(12):1927-1931.

69. Ioannidis JP. Microarrays and molecular research: noise discovery? *Lancet*. 2005;365(9458):454-455.

70. Panagiotou OA, Ioannidis JP; Genome-Wide Significance Project. What should the genome-wide significance threshold be? empirical replication of borderline genetic associations. *Int J Epidemiol*. 2012;41(1):273-286.

71. Russell JA, Walley KR, Singer J, et al; VASST Investigators. Vasopressin versus norepinephrine infusion in patients with septic shock. *N Engl J Med*. 2008;358(9):877-887.

72. Kelton JG, Hirsh J, Carter CJ, Buchanan MR. Sex differences in the antithrombotic effects of aspirin. *Blood*. 1978; 52(5):1073-1076.

73. Antiplatelet Trialists' Collaboration. Collaborative overview of randomised trials of antiplatelet therapy, III: reduction in venous thrombosis and pulmonary embolism by antiplatelet prophylaxis among surgical and medical patients. *BMJ*. 1994;308(6923):235-246.

74. *Dietary Reference Intakes for Vitamin D and Calcium*. Washington, DC: Institute of Medicine; 2011.

75. Bischoff-Ferrari HA, Willett WC, Wong JB, Giovannucci E, Dietrich T, Dawson-Hughes B. Fracture prevention with vitamin D supplementation: a meta-analysis of randomized controlled trials. *JAMA*. 2005;293(18):2257-2264.

76. Contopoulos-Ioannidis DG, Seto I, Hamm MP, et al. Empirical evaluation of age groups and age-subgroup analyses in pediatric randomized trials and pediatric meta-analyses. *Pediatrics*. 2012; 129(suppl 3):S161-S184.

77. Counsell CE, Clarke MJ, Slattery J, Sandercock PA. The miracle of DICE therapy for acute stroke: fact or fictional product of subgroup analysis? *BMJ*. 1994;309(6970):1677-1681.

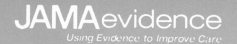

MOVING FROM EVIDENCE TO ACTION

MOVING FROM EVIDENCE TO ACTION

26

How to Use a Patient Management Recommendation: Clinical Practice Guidelines and Decision Analyses

Ignacio Neumann, Elie A. Akl, Per Olav Vandvik, Thomas Agoritsas, Pablo Alonso-Coello, David M. Rind, Nancy Santesso, Paul Elias Alexander, Reem A. Mustafa, Kameshwar Prasad, Shannon M. Bates, Holger J. Schünemann, and Gordon Guyatt

IN THIS CHAPTER

You are an obstetrician seeing a 31-year-old pregnant woman who had an unprovoked deep venous thrombosis of the leg 5 years ago that was treated with warfarin for 6 months without complication. She is no longer using antithrombotic medication and is otherwise healthy. Given a possible increased risk of thrombosis with pregnancy, you are considering discussing the possibility of low-molecular-weight heparin (LMWH) prophylaxis for the rest of the pregnancy.

To inform your discussion, you search first for an evidence-based recommendation and find the following recommendation from a practice guideline[1]: "For pregnant women at moderate to high risk of recurrent venous thromboembolism (VTE) (single unprovoked VTE, pregnancy- or estrogen-related VTE, or multiple prior unprovoked VTE not receiving long-term anticoagulation), we suggest antepartum prophylaxis with prophylactic- or intermediate-dose LMWH rather than clinical vigilance or routine care (weak recommendation, based on low confidence in effect estimates)."

The statement "weak recommendation, based on low confidence in effect estimates" leaves you uncomfortable. You decide to read further to understand the recommendation and its rationale.

DEVELOPING RECOMMENDATIONS

In general, patient management recommendations are developed in the context of *clinical practice guidelines* (see Chapter 5, Finding Current Best Evidence). However, you also may find guidance originating from a *decision analysis*. Similar criteria of credibility apply to both approaches.[2-5]

Practice Guidelines

Practice guidelines are statements that include recommendations intended to optimize patient care. They are, ideally, informed by a *systematic review* of *evidence* and an assessment of the benefits and *harms* of alternative care options.[2] To make a recommendation, guideline panelists must define clinical questions,

select the relevant *outcome variables*, retrieve and synthesize all of the relevant evidence, rate the confidence in the effect estimates, and, relying on a systematic approach but ultimately also on consensus, move from evidence to recommendations.[6] To fully inform their audience, guideline panels should provide not only their recommendations but also the key information on which their recommendations are based (see Chapter 28.1, Assessing the Strength of Recommendations: The GRADE Approach).

Decision Analysis

Decision analysis is a formal method that integrates the evidence regarding the beneficial and harmful effects of treatment options with the values or preferences associated with those effects. Clinical decision analyses are built as structured approaches (*decision trees*), and authors will usually include 1 or more diagrams showing the structure of the decision trees used for the analysis.

Figure 26-1 shows a simplified decision tree for the scenario of the pregnant woman considering thromboprophylaxis. The patient has 2 options: to use or not use prophylaxis with LMWH. The decision is represented by a square, termed "decision node." The lines that emanate from the decision node represent the clinical strategies under consideration.

Circles, called "chance nodes," symbolize the different events that can occur after each clinical strategy. Patients may or may not develop a thrombotic or bleeding event, and the decision analysis requires estimates of the probability of both events. Triangles or rectangles identify outcome states.

The decision analysis also addresses the extent to which each of the outcome events is desirable (no bleeding or thrombotic event) or undesirable (either adverse event) (in technical language, the *utility*). The combination of the probabilities and utilities allows the decision analyst to determine the relative value of each management option.

The process of decision analysis makes fully explicit all of the elements of the decision so that they are open for debate and modification.[7] When a decision analysis includes costs among the outcomes, it becomes an *economic analysis* and summarizes trade-offs between health changes and resource expenditure (see Chapter 28.2, Economic Analysis).

FIGURE 26-1

Diagram of a Simplified Decision Tree

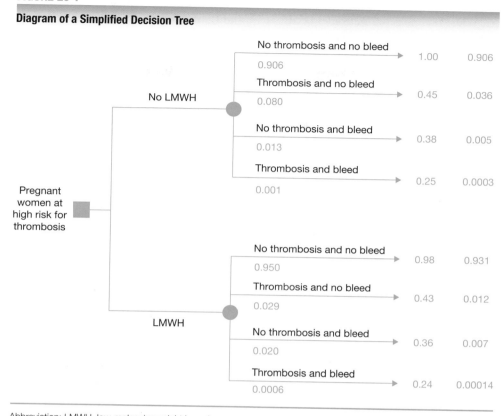

Abbreviation: LMWH, low-molecular-weight heparin.

EXAMPLE OF A DECISION TREE

Returning to Figure 26-1, each arm of the decision (no prophylaxis vs LMWH) has 1 chance node at which 4 possible outcomes could occur (the 4 possible combinations arising from bleeding or not bleeding and from having a thrombosis or not having a thrombosis). The figure depicts the probabilities associated with the decision. In the no-prophylaxis strategy, patients would have a probability of bleeding and having a thrombosis of 0.1%, a probability of bleeding and not having a thrombosis of 1.3%, a probability of not bleeding but having a thrombosis of 8%, and a probability of not bleeding and not having a thrombosis of

90.6%. With the LMWH prophylaxis strategy, the probability of bleeding and having a thrombosis is 0.06%, the probability of bleeding and not having a thrombosis is 2%, the probability of not bleeding but having a thrombosis is 2.9%, and the probability of not bleeding and not having a thrombosis is 95%.[1,8]

Figure 26-1 also presents the values associated with each health state on a scale of 0 to 1, with 1 representing the utility of full health and 0 representing the utility of death. In the no-prophylaxis strategy, the health state without any negative outcome (no thrombosis or bleeding) represents full health, a utility of 1.0. The occurrence of a thrombosis or bleeding event decreases the value of the health state to 0.45 in the case of thrombosis and to 0.38 in the case of bleeding. When both negative outcomes occur at the same time, the corresponding utility is even lower: 0.25. In the LMWH arm, the addition of the *burden of treatment* slightly decreases the utility of the 4 health states.

The final step in the decision analysis is to calculate the total expected value—the sum of the probabilities and utilities associated with each outcome—for each possible course of action. Given the particular set of probabilities and utilities we have presented, the estimated value of the no-prophylaxis branch would be $(0.906 \times 1.0) + (0.080 \times 0.45) + (0.013 \times 0.38) + (0.001 \times 0.25)$, which is 0.947. The value of the LMWH branch would be $(0.950 \times 0.98) + (0.029 \times 0.43) + (0.020 \times 0.36) + (0.0006 \times 0.24)$, which is 0.950. In this example, the prophylaxis strategy is more desirable, but the difference in the expected values between the 2 options—called "relative utility"—is relatively small.

The model presented in Figure 26-1 is over-simplified in a number of ways. For example, it does not take into account the possibility of fatal events or potential long-term morbidity (eg, after an intracranial bleeding or the development of postthrombotic syndrome). Also, it does not consider the time in the health states. For instance, having a major bleeding without any complication may appreciably reduce the utility during the episode, but almost all patients will return to a perfect health state relatively quickly. *Multistate transition models* using simulation—termed *Markov models*—permit analyses that are closer to real life. For example, an analysis using multistate transition models concluded that for patients like the one presented in the opening scenario and in the decision tree (high risk for VTE recurrence), antepartum prophylaxis with LMWH is a cost-effective use of resources.[9]

ASSESSING RECOMMENDATIONS

Box 26-1 presents our guidance for determining the extent to which a guideline or decision analysis will provide trustworthy recommendations.

Is the Clinical Question Clear and Comprehensive?

The most useful patient management recommendations from guidelines and decision analyses will use a standardized format that details precisely the recommended actions, the alternatives with which they are compared, to whom they apply, and under what circumstances.

Is the Recommended Intervention Clear and Actionable?

Recommendations are sometimes too vague to be helpful. Consider, for instance, this recommendation from a clinical practice guideline[10]: "For both outpatients and inpatients with diabetic foot infection, clinicians should attempt to provide a well-coordinated approach by those with expertise in a variety of specialties, preferably by a multidisciplinary diabetic foot care team." What remains unclear in this recommendation is the level of obligation in the "attempt," what is involved in making care "well-coordinated," and which specialties are included in the "variety."

In contrast, another guideline from the National Foundation for Health Care Excellence[11] makes clear what is being recommended: "We recommend that a multidisciplinary foot care team manage the care of patients with diabetic foot problems who require inpatient care. The multidisciplinary foot care team should include a diabetologist, a surgeon with the relevant expertise, a diabetes nurse specialist, a podiatrist and a tissue viability nurse."

Is the Alternative Clear?

When guideline panelists develop recommendations, they choose a specific course of action over others. If the alternative is not clear, the significance of the recommendation will remain obscure. For example, in the recommendation "Uterine massage is recommended for the treatment of postpartum hemorrhage,"[12] the absence of an explicit alternative may introduce challenges in the interpretation. Are the panelists suggesting performing uterine massage as a first-line treatment in preference to other therapeutic measures, or are they recommending it in addition to other concomitant measures? By comparing the recommendation with others within the guideline, it is possible to infer that panelists meant that uterine massage should be used in addition to other measures and not as a single intervention, but recommendation statements should be clear enough to be interpreted without having to read the full guideline. In contrast, the recommendation "We recommend isotonic crystalloids ... in preference to ... colloids for the initial intravenous fluid resuscitation of women with postpartum hemorrhage"[12] offers a clearer message by making the alternative explicit.

As you may have noticed, in both recommendations regarding the management of diabetic foot problems presented in the previous section, the *control group* is not clearly defined. Although the option of "no foot care team" seems to be the implicit comparator, it is not clear what this management strategy entails.

Clinicians who use a decision analysis will not face the problem of ambiguous alternatives because the options in comparison are explicit.

Were All of the Relevant Outcomes Important to Patients Explicitly Considered?

The balance between the benefits and the harms of the interventions will depend on what outcomes are considered. Clinicians should judge whether the guideline panel or the decision analysts included all *patient-important outcomes*.

For example, the eighth edition of the antithrombotic guidelines (AT8) of the American College of Chest Physicians (ACCP) recommended the use of elastic stockings for patients with stroke who have contraindications to anticoagulants.[13] The 9th edition of the antithrombotic guidelines (AT9) suggested against its use.[14] Both guideline panels considered the outcomes of mortality, pulmonary embolism, and symptomatic deep venous thrombosis, but AT9 panelists also considered that elastic stockings produce a 4-fold increase in the risk of skin complications: 39 more per 1000 patients treated for 1 month (95% *confidence interval* [CI], 17-77 more per 1000).[15] The additional consideration of skin complications is responsible for the change in recommendations.

Outcomes typically considered as patient important include mortality, morbidity (eg, major bleeding, acute exacerbation of a chronic disease, hospital admission), and patient-reported outcomes (eg, quality of life, functional status). *Surrogate outcomes* (eg, lipid levels, bone density, cognitive function tests) are variably associated with patient-important outcomes but are never important in and of themselves (see Chapter 13.4, Surrogate Outcomes).

In addition, AT8 suggested international normalized ratio (INR) monitoring at an interval of no longer than every 4 weeks in patients treated with vitamin K antagonists.[16] This recommendation was primarily based on studies that found that frequent monitoring increased the time in therapeutic INR range—a surrogate outcome. However, AT9 suggested an INR testing frequency of up to 12 weeks rather than every 4 weeks.[17] This recommendation was based on studies that found no increase in thrombotic events or major bleeding with monitoring every 12 weeks. Both recommendations were based on explicitly defined outcomes. However, the outcomes were surrogate in the first case and—more appropriately—patient important in the second.

Outcomes not plausibly influenced by the intervention are typically not relevant for decision making and therefore may not be considered. For example, mortality is a very important outcome; however, it is not relevant for the decision of whether to use intranasal antihistamines for the treatment of allergic rhinitis because the intervention does not plausibly affect the probability of dying.

Were the Recommendations Based on the Current Best Evidence?

Guideline panelists and decision analysts should base their estimates of the benefits and harms of the intervention and their evaluation of the associated confidence in effect estimates on current or updated systematic reviews, preferably those that include meta-analysis. In the absence of such meta-analytic systematic reviews, guideline panelists may conduct their own reviews or provide less systematic evidence summaries. Clinicians should look for a description of the process used to identify and summarize the relevant evidence and should judge to what extent this process is credible. Clinicians also should check the date on which the literature search was conducted (see Chapter 22, The Process of a Systematic Review and Meta-analysis).

Recommendations that do not use the best current evidence risk promoting suboptimal or even harmful care. For example, for several years guideline panels ignored a substantial body of evidence that suggested the effectiveness of prophylaxis with quinolones in patients with postchemotherapy neutropenia.[18] Only in its 2010 guidelines did the

Infectious Diseases Society of America suggest the prophylactic use of antibiotics in this population.[19] This highlights the necessity for rapid and sometimes frequent updating of guidelines in areas under active investigation (see Chapter 5, Finding Current Best Evidence).

Are Values and Preferences Appropriately Specified for Each Outcome?

Assessing treatment effects on outcomes is largely a question of measurement and a matter of science. Assigning preferences to outcomes is a matter of values. Consider, for example, the outcomes associated with routine mammographic screening in women aged 40 to 49 years: there is a very small and questionable reduction of breast cancer mortality and a relatively high probability of a false-positive result (which typically leads to unnecessary follow-up testing and sometimes to unnecessary biopsy of the breast)[20] (see Chapter 28.3, Moving From Evidence to Action: Recommendations About Screening). A guideline panel must consider the value attached to each of these 2 outcomes when trading them off to develop a recommendation. A panel that assigns a higher value to the very small reduction in cancer mortality would support the screening, whereas a panel that assigns a higher value to avoiding unnecessary procedures would not. Consequently, clinicians should look for explicit statements regarding the *values and preferences* used to inform the recommendation.

Whose values should drive recommendations? Under ideal circumstances, recommendations should be based on a systematic review of relevant studies exploring patients' values and preferences[21]; unfortunately, such evidence is still rare. In the absence of a body of empirical evidence about patients' values and preferences, guideline panels or decision analysts may fall back on the experience of clinicians who regularly engage in shared decision making. Another alternative is the involvement of representative patients and consumers in the recommendation development process.[22] However, ensuring that those involved—clinicians or patients—will be able to represent typical patients is challenging and perhaps only partly achievable.

Whatever the source of values and preferences, it is possible to make them explicit and transparent.

FIGURE 26-2

Direction and Strength of Recommendations in Different Grading Systems

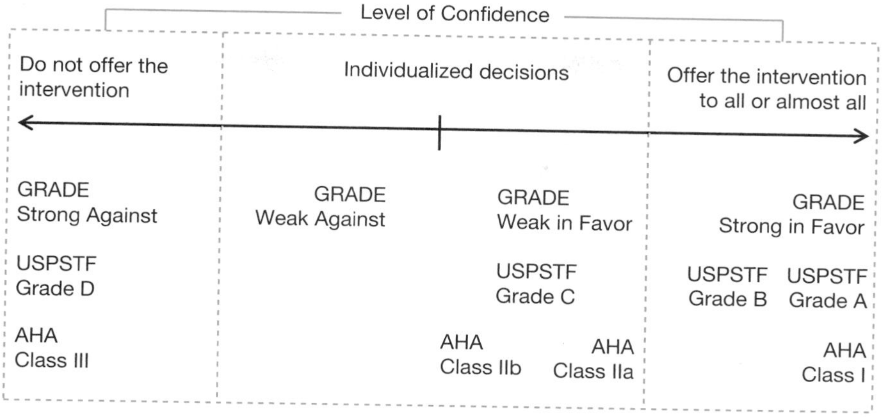

Abbreviations: AHA, American Heart Association; GRADE, Grading of Recommendations Assessment, Development and Evaluation; USPSTF, US Preventive Services Task Force.

Unfortunately, failure to do so remains the most common serious deficit in current practice guidelines. In contrast, decision analysis requires explicit and quantitative specification of values because each outcome is assigned a given health utility. However, although the values and preferences in a decision analysis may be explicit, their source may be problematic. For example, a systematic review of 54 *cost-utility analyses* (including 45 decisions analyses) in child health found that the source used for valuing health states was the authors' own judgment in 35% of the analyses, and in another 11% the source of values and preferences was not stated.[23]

Do the Authors Indicate the Strength of Their Recommendations?

Trustworthy recommendations should specify the strength of the recommendations and also a rating of the confidence in effect estimates that support the recommendations (also known as quality of evidence).[2] *Sensitivity analyses* are used to explore the strength of the conclusions that arise from a decision analysis.

Grades of Recommendation

There are dozens of grading systems for recommendations.[24] However, the 3 most commonly used approaches are *GRADE* (*Grading of Recommendations Assessment, Development and Evaluation*)[25] and those used by the American Heart Association (AHA)[26] and the US Preventive Services Task Force (USPSTF).[27] A detailed discussion of the differences among these systems is beyond the scope of this chapter; we will, however, mention 2 important similarities.

The 3 systems feature a rating for confidence in effect estimates (ie, quality of evidence). Confidence in the effect estimates represents the extent to which the estimates are sufficiently credible to support a particular recommendation (Figure 26-2). The GRADE approach specifies 4 levels of confidence: high, moderate, low, and very low (see Chapter 23, Understanding and Applying the Results of a Systematic Review and Meta-analysis). The AHA and USPSTF systems specify 3 levels of confidence: A, B, and C in the AHA approach and high, moderate, and low in the USPSTF approach.

The 3 systems share another critical feature: they differentiate between recommendations that should be applied (or avoided) in all, or almost all, patients (ie, strong recommendations) from those that require individualization to the patient's values, preferences, and circumstances (ie, weak recommendations) (Figure 26-2).

Sensitivity Analysis

Decision analysts use sensitivity analyses, the systematic exploration of the uncertainty in the data, to vary estimates for downsides, benefits, and values and to determine the impact of these varying estimates on expected outcomes. Sensitivity analysis asks the question: to what extent is the relative utility of the alternatives affected by the uncertainties in the estimates of the likelihood or value of the outcomes? To the extent that the result of the decision analysis does not change with varying probability estimates and varying values, clinicians can consider the recommendation a strong one. When the final decision shifts with different plausible values of probabilities or values, the conclusion becomes much weaker: the right choice may differ given the true probabilities, and patients' choices are likely to vary according to their preferences.

Is the Evidence Supporting the Recommendations Easily Understood?

For Strong Recommendations, Is the Strength Appropriate?

The message to the clinician from strong recommendations is "just do it." Recommendations that are inappropriately graded as strong may therefore have substantial undesirable consequences.

High confidence in the effect estimates will support a strong recommendation if the desirable consequences considerably outweigh the undesirable consequences, if there is reasonable confidence and limited variability in patients' values and preferences, and if the benefits of the proposed course of action justify its cost. When there is substantial uncertainty regarding the effects of the intervention (low confidence in the effect estimates), clinicians should generally expect weak recommendations (see Chapter 28.1, Assessing the Strength of Recommendations: The GRADE Approach).

Sometimes, guideline panels can appropriately offer strong recommendations despite low or very low confidence in effect estimates. Table 26-1 presents 5 paradigmatic situations in which this can occur. Clinicians should carefully examine a strong recommendation based on low or very low confidence. If it does not correspond to any of the situations listed in Table 26-1, it is likely that the recommendation was inappropriately graded.

For example, a systematic survey of the Endocrine Society guidelines between 2005 and 2011 found that 121 of the total of 357 recommendations identified were strong recommendations based on low or very low confidence in effect estimates. Of these 121, only 35 (29%) were consistent with one of the situations presented in Table 26-1 and thus clearly appropriate.[31] This result highlights the need for caution when facing strong recommendations based on low or very low confidence in effect estimates.

In decision analysis, the parallel to strong recommendations occurs when the relative utility of the management options changes little and the preferred alternative does not change, after varying probability estimates and varying values. Clinicians should look for a table that lists which variables were included in their sensitivity analyses, what range of values they used for each variable, and which variables, if any, altered the relative desirability of the management strategies under consideration.

Ideally, decision analysts will subject all of their probability estimates to a sensitivity analysis. The range over which they will test should depend on the source of the data. If the estimates come from large *randomized trials* with low *risk of bias* and narrow CIs, the range of estimates tested can be narrow. When risk of bias is greater or estimates of benefits and downsides less precise, sensitivity analyses testing a wide range of values become appropriate. Decision analysts also should test utility values with sensitivity analyses, with the range of values again determined by the source of the data. If large numbers of patients or knowledgeable and representative members of the general public gave similar ratings to the outcome states, investigators can use a narrow range of utility values in the sensitivity analyses. If the ratings came from a small group of raters or if the individuals provided widely varying estimates of typical utilities, then investigators should use a wider range of utility values in the sensitivity analyses.

For Weak Recommendations, Does the Information Facilitate Shared Decision Making?

Recommendations—in particular, weak recommendations—should explicitly provide the key underlying information necessary to act on the recommendation. In guidelines, this information is typically found in the remarks section, in the recommendation rationale, or in tables that accompany

TABLE 26-1

Five Paradigmatic Situations That Justify Strong Recommendations Based on Low or Very Low Confidence

Paradigmatic Situation	Confidence in Effect Estimates for Health Outcomes (Quality of Evidence)		Balance of Benefits and Harms	Values and Preferences	Resource Considerations	Recommendation	Example
	Benefits	**Harms**					
Life-threatening situation	Low or very low	Immaterial (very low to high)	Intervention may reduce mortality in a life-threatening situation; adverse events not prohibitive	A very high value is placed on an uncertain but potentially life-preserving benefit	Small incremental cost (or resource use) relative to the benefits justify the intervention	Strong recommendation in favor	Indirect evidence from seasonal influenza suggests that patients with avian influenza may benefit from the use of oseltamivir (low confidence in effect estimates). Given the high mortality of the disease and the absence of effective alternatives, the WHO made a strong recommendation in favor of the use of oseltamivir rather than no treatment in patients with avian influenza.[28]
Uncertain benefit, certain harm	Low or very low	High or moderate	Possible but uncertain benefit; substantial established harm	A much higher value is placed on the adverse events in which we are confident than in the benefit, which is uncertain	High incremental cost (or resource use) relative to the benefits may not justify the intervention	Strong recommendation against	In patients with idiopathic pulmonary fibrosis, treatment with azathioprine plus prednisone offers a possible but uncertain benefit in comparison with no treatment. The intervention, however, is associated with a substantial established harm. An international guideline made a recommendation against the combination of corticosteroids plus azathioprine in patients with idiopathic pulmonary fibrosis.[28]
Potential equivalence, one option clearly less risky or costly	Low or very low	High or moderate	Magnitude of benefit apparently similar—though uncertain—for alternatives; we are confident of less harm or cost for one of the competing alternatives	A high value is placed on the reduction in harm	High incremental cost (or resource use) relative to the benefits may not justify one of the alternatives	Strong recommendation for less harmful/less expensive	Low-quality evidence suggests that initial *Helicobacter pylori* eradication in patients with early stage extranodal marginal zone (MALT) B-cell lymphoma results in similar rates of complete response in comparison with the alternatives of radiation therapy or gastrectomy, but with high confidence of less harm, morbidity, and cost. Consequently, UpToDate made a strong recommendation in favor of *H pylori* eradication rather than radiotherapy in patients with MALT lymphoma.[29]
High confidence in similar benefits, one option potentially more risky or costly	High or moderate	Low or very low	Established that magnitude of benefit is similar for alternative management strategies; best (though uncertain)	A high value is placed on avoiding the potential increase in harm	High incremental cost (or resource use) relative to the benefits may not justify one of the alternatives	Strong recommendation against the intervention with possible greater harm	In women requiring anticoagulation and planning conception or in pregnancy, high confidence estimates suggest similar effects of different anticoagulants. However, indirect evidence (low confidence in effect estimates) suggests

MOVING FROM EVIDENCE TO ACTION

TABLE 26-1

Five Paradigmatic Situations That Justify Strong Recommendations Based on Low or Very Low Confidence *(Continued)*

Paradigmatic Situation	Confidence in Effect Estimates for Health Outcomes (Quality of Evidence)		Balance of Benefits and Harms	Values and Preferences	Resource Considerations	Recommendation	Example
	Benefits	**Harms**					
			estimate is that one alternative has appreciably greater harm				potential harm to the unborn infant with oral direct thrombin (eg, dabigatran) and factor Xa inhibitors (eg, rivaroxaban, apixaban). The AT9 guidelines recommended against the use of such anticoagulants in women planning conception or in pregnancy.[1]
Potential catastrophic harm	Immaterial (very low to high)	Low or very low	Potential important harm of the intervention, magnitude of benefit is variable	A high value is placed on avoiding potential increase in harm	High incremental cost (or resource use) relative to the benefits may not justify the intervention	Strong recommendation against the intervention	In males with androgen deficiency, testosterone supplementation likely improves quality of life. Low-confidence evidence suggests that testosterone increases cancer spread in patients with prostate cancer. The US Endocrine Society made a recommendation against testosterone supplementation in patients with prostate cancer.[30]

Abbreviations: AT9, 9th edition of the antithrombotic guidelines; MALT, mucosa-associated lymphoid tissue; WHO, World Health Organization.

the recommendation. The GRADE Working Group, in collaboration with the Cochrane Collaboration, has designed a specific table for this purpose: the *summary-of-findings table*. This table provides the confidence ratings for all important outcomes and the associated estimates of relative and absolute effects. Table 26-2 shows a summary-of-findings table relevant for the clinical scenario presented at the beginning of this chapter. As we discuss later, summary-of-findings tables can facilitate shared decision making.[33] The absolute measures of effect you will find in GRADE summary-of-findings tables are typically presented within the decisions trees in decision analyses.

Was the Influence of Conflict of Interests Minimized?

The judgments involved in the interpretation of the evidence and the decision on the final recommendation may be vulnerable to *conflicts of interest*. In medicine, guideline panelists frequently—and decision-analyst authors sometimes—report financial ties with the pharmaceutical industry.[34-36] Nonfinancial conflicts of interests are also common and may have even greater effect than financial conflicts.[37,38] These conflicts include intellectual conflicts (eg, previous publication of studies relevant to a recommendation) and professional conflicts (eg, radiologists making recommendations about breast cancer screening or urologists recommending prostate cancer screening).[39,40]

Clinicians can check the conflict of interest statements of the guideline panelists or decision analysts, usually found at the beginning or end of a publication or in a supplementary file. Just as important, clinicians should check what strategies were implemented to manage these conflicts of interest. Guidelines or decision analyses with a large representation of panelists without conflicts of interest, that have placed nonconflicted participants in positions of authority, or that have implemented rules to limit the influence of both financial and nonfinancial conflicts of

TABLE 26-2

Summary-of-Findings Table: Antepartum and Postpartum Prevention of VTE With Prophylactic Dose of Low-Molecular-Weight Heparin vs No Prophylaxis in Pregnant Women With Prior VTE[1]

Outcome	RR (95% CI)	Anticipated Absolute Effects During Pregnancy		Confidence in the Estimates of the Effect
		Risk Without Prophylaxis	Risk Difference With LMWH	
		Low Risk		
Symptomatic VTE	0.36 (0.20-0.67)	20 VTE per 1000	13 fewer VTE per 1000 (from 16 to 7 fewer)	Low due to indirectness[b] and imprecision[c]
		Intermediate and High Risk[a]		
		80 VTE per 1000	51 fewer VTE per 1000 (from 65 to 30 fewer)	
		Antepartum Period		
Major bleeding	1.57 (1.32-1.87)[d]	3 bleeds per 1000	1 more bleed per 1000 (from 1 to 3 more)[e]	Low due to indirectness[a] and imprecision[f]
		Postpartum Period		
		10 bleeds per 1000	6 more bleeds per 1000 (from 3 to 8 more)[d]	
Burden of treatment	...	No incremental burden	Daily injections	High

Abbreviations: CI, confidence interval; LMWH, low-molecular-weight heparin; RR, relative risk; VTE, venous thromboembolism.

[a]Single unprovoked VTE, pregnancy-related or estrogen-related VTE, or multiple prior unprovoked VTE not receiving long-term anticoagulation.

[b]Population is indirect (ie, did not include pregnant women).

[c]95% confidence interval includes marginal benefit.

[d]Relative effect estimate based on the systematic review by Collins et al.[32]

[e]Absolute risk estimates for major bleeding in women using LMWH based on the systematic review by Greer et al.[8]

[f]95% confidence interval includes marginal harm.

Adapted from Bates et al.[1]

interest are more credible than those that have not. Guidelines that excluded conflicted experts are likely to have limited the influence of conflicts of interest but may have compromised the credibility of the guidelines and possibly threatened their acceptability. Clinicians also can check whether recommendations were collected and managed for the whole guideline or on a recommendation-by-recommendation basis. The influence of potential conflicts of interest may be diminished with the latter approach.

The AT9 guidelines provide an example of implementation of a number of these strategies.[38] A nonconflicted methodologist was chosen as the chair of each of the 14 panels making recommendations and was primarily responsible for that chapter. The chair and 2 other members of the executive committee ultimately responsible for the whole guideline were nonconflicted methodologists. Both financial and intellectual conflicts of interest were assessed on a recommendation-by-recommendation basis. Panelists with major conflicts were in principle excluded from participation in decision making. Challenges in implementing this approach highlight the efforts required to arrive at an optimal strategy for managing conflict of interest.[41,42]

USING THE GUIDE

Is the Clinical Question Clear and Comprehensive?

The recommendation presented at the beginning of this chapter clearly specifies what is being proposed ("antepartum prophylaxis with prophylactic- or intermediate-dose LMWH") and what was the comparison ("rather than clinical vigilance or routine care").[1]

As we can see in Table 26-2, guideline panelists considered the outcomes of symptomatic thromboembolism, major bleeding, and burden of treatment—the outcomes likely important to patients.

Was the Recommendation Based on the Best Current Evidence?

In the methods section of the published AT9 guidelines, we find the following description: "To identify the relevant evidence, a team ... conducted literature searches of Medline, the Cochrane Library, and the Database of Abstracts of Reviews of Effects ... for systematic reviews and another for original studies" and "The quality of reviews was assessed ... and wherever possible, current high-quality systematic reviews were used as the source of summary estimates."[43] This strategy ensured that estimates were based on best current evidence at the time the recommendation was issued.

Are Values and Preferences Associated With Outcomes Appropriately Specified?

Guideline authors noted that a systematic review of patient preferences for antithrombotic treatment did not identify any studies of pregnant women. A rating exercise of different outcomes among experienced clinicians participating on the guideline suggested that 1 episode of VTE (deep venous thrombosis or pulmonary embolism) is more or less equivalent to 1 major extracranial bleed. Panelists' clinical experience suggested that most women, but not all, would choose long-term prophylaxis when confronted with the burden of self-injecting with LMWH for several months, suggesting a relatively high value on preventing VTE and a relatively high tolerance for self-injection. These values and preferences were used to develop the recommendation.

Do the Authors Indicate the Strength of Their Recommendations?

The recommendation was classified as "weak" using the GRADE approach.

Is the Evidence Supporting the Recommendation Easily Understood?

The recommendation was accompanied by a summary-of-findings table (Table 26-2) that provides absolute estimates for the outcomes important to patients. We discuss subsequently how this information can help with shared decision making.

Was the Influence of Conflict of Interests Minimized?

As we described earlier, the AT9 guidelines implemented a number of the strategies to diminish the influence of conflict of interest on recommendations.

HOW SHOULD YOU USE RECOMMENDATIONS?

Strong Recommendations

If the panel's assessment is astute, clinicians can apply strong recommendations to all or almost all of the patients in all or almost all circumstances without thorough—or even cursory—review of the underlying evidence and without a detailed discussion with the patient. The same is true for decision analysis when the utility of one alternative is substantially greater than the other and this relative utility is robust to sensitivity analyses. Whether discussion of the evidence with patients might sometimes still be helpful in such circumstances—for instance, whether it may increase adherence to treatment—remains uncertain.

For example, the Allergic Rhinitis and its Impact on Asthma guideline recommended intranasal glucocorticoids rather than intranasal antihistamines for treatment of allergic rhinitis in adults (strong recommendation).[44] This recommendation was based on an important reduction of *symptoms* with glucocorticoids (rhinorrhea, nasal blockage and itching) with no important adverse events. The effect estimates came from a systematic review of randomized trials with low risk of bias, consistent results across trials, precise effects (narrow CIs), and results applicable to the population. The guideline panel's inference that all, or almost all, informed patients would choose the glucocorticoids is eminently reasonable. Therefore, a detailed discussion with the patients about the benefits and potential harms of intranasal glucocorticoids over intranasal antihistamines will not be necessary.

There will always be idiosyncratic circumstances in which clinicians should not adhere to even strong recommendations. For instance, aspirin in the context of myocardial infarction warrants a strong recommendation, but it would be a mistake to administer the treatment to a patient who is allergic to aspirin. Such idiosyncratic situations are, fortunately, unusual.

Weak Recommendations

With careful consideration of the evidence, as well as of patient's values and preferences, many recommendations are weak, even in clinical fields with a large body of randomized trials and systematic reviews. For instance, two-thirds of more than 600 recommendations issued in AT9 were weak.[17]

Because weak recommendations are typically sensitive to patients' values and preferences, a shared decision-making approach that involves a discussion with the patient addressing the potential benefits and harms of the proposed course of action is the optimal way to ensure that decisions reflect both the best evidence and patients' values and preferences (see Chapter 27, Decision Making and the Patient). To use weak recommendations, clinicians need to understand the underlying evidence.

For example, the American College of Physicians suggested the use of cholinesterase inhibitors or memantine in patients with dementia (weak recommendation).[45] This recommendation is based on evidence from randomized trials warranting high confidence in a small benefit of the drugs in slowing the deterioration of cognition and global function. Guideline panelists pointed out that, if quality of life is judged as poor—in particular, with more advanced dementia—family members may not view the limited slowing of dementia progression as a desirable goal. Moreover, the magnitude of the effect is small, and there are adverse effects associated with the drugs. The panel then reasonably expected that informed patients (or their families) would make different choices.

CLINICAL SCENARIO RESOLUTION

After reviewing this guide, and specifically the information in Table 26-2, you decide that the recommendation is trustworthy and you plan to engage patients like the one presented in the opening scenario in shared decision making. When you meet with the patient, you start by discussing the benefits of LMWH during pregnancy vs no treatment (51 fewer cases of symptomatic VTE per 1000 women), followed by information about adverse effects (7 more maternal bleeds per 1000 women followed up during the pregnancy and post partum), and you mention the potential burden of treatment that daily injections for several months will represent (low confidence in effect estimates for all outcomes aside from the burden of injections). If the guideline panel is correct, most patients will place a higher value in lowering the risk of a thrombotic event and less on the uncertain small increase in the risk of bleeding and the certain burden of treatment. Such patients will choose prophylaxis. If the panel is correct, however, some patients will decline therapy.

Thus, shared decision making is required to ensure the patient understands the best evidence available and the decision is consistent with the patient's values and preference. You are not surprised when the patient chooses VTE prophylaxis.

References

1. Bates SM, Greer IA, Middeldorp S, Veenstra DL, Prabulos AM, Vandvik PO. VTE, thrombophilia, antithrombotic therapy, and pregnancy: Antithrombotic Therapy and Prevention of Thrombosis, 9th ed: American College of Chest Physicians Evidence-Based Clinical Practice Guidelines. *Chest.* 2012;141(2 suppl):e691S-736S.

2. Graham R, Mancher M, Wolman DM, Greenfield S, Steinberg E, eds. *Clinical Practice Guidelines We Can Trust.* Washington, DC: National Academies Press; 2011.

3. Laine C, Taichman DB, Mulrow C. Trustworthy clinical guidelines. *Ann Intern Med.* 2011;154(11):774-775.

4. Qaseem A, Forland F, Macbeth F, Ollenschläger G, Phillips S, van der Wees P; Board of Trustees of the Guidelines International Network. Guidelines International Network: toward international standards for clinical practice guidelines. *Ann Intern Med.* 2012;156(7):525-531.

5. Shekelle P, Woolf S, Grimshaw JM, Schünemann HJ, Eccles MP. Developing clinical practice guidelines: reviewing, reporting, and publishing guidelines; updating guidelines; and the emerging issues of enhancing guideline implementability and accounting for comorbid conditions in guideline development. *Implement Sci.* 2012;7:62.

6. Schünemann HJ, Wiercioch W, Etxeandia I, et al. Guidelines 2.0: systematic development of a comprehensive checklist for a successful guideline enterprise. *CMAJ.* 2014;186(3):E123-E142.

7. Kassirer JP, Moskowitz AJ, Lau J, Pauker SG. Decision analysis: a progress report. *Ann Intern Med.* 1987;106(2):275-291.

8. Greer IA, Nelson-Piercy C. Low-molecular-weight heparins for thromboprophylaxis and treatment of venous thromboembolism in pregnancy: a systematic review of safety and efficacy. *Blood.* 2005;106(2):401-407.

9. Johnston JA, Brill-Edwards P, Ginsberg JS, Pauker SG, Eckman MH. Cost-effectiveness of prophylactic low molecular weight heparin in pregnant women with a prior history of venous thromboembolism. *Am J Med.* 2005;118(5):503-514.

10. Lipsky BA, Berendt AR, Cornia PB, et al; Infectious Diseases Society of America. 2012 Infectious Diseases Society of America clinical practice guideline for the diagnosis and treatment of diabetic foot infections. *Clin Infect Dis.* 2012;54(12):e132-e173.

11. National Institute for Health and Care Excellence. *Diabetic foot problems: Inpatient management of diabetic foot problems (CG119).* London, England: National Institute for Health and Care Excellence; 2011.

12. World Health Organization. WHO recommendations for the prevention and treatment of postpartum haemorrhage. Geneva, Switzerland: World Health Organization; 2012.

13. Albers GW, Amarenco P, Easton J, Sacco RL, Teal P. Antithrombotic and thrombolytic therapy for ischemic stroke: American College of Chest Physicians Evidence-Based Clinical Practice Guidelines (8th Edition). *Chest.* 2008;133(6 suppl):630S-669S.

14. Lansberg MG, O'Donnell MJ, Khatri P, et al. Antithrombotic and thrombolytic therapy for ischemic stroke: antithrombotic therapy and prevention of thrombosis, 9th ed: American College of Chest Physicians Evidence-Based Clinical Practice Guidelines. *Chest.* 2012;141(2 suppl):e601S-36S.

15. Dennis M, Sandercock PA, Reid J, et al; CLOTS Trials Collaboration. Effectiveness of thigh-length graduated compression stockings to reduce the risk of deep vein thrombosis after stroke (CLOTS trial 1): a multicentre, randomised controlled trial. *Lancet.* 2009;373(9679):1958-1965.

16. Ansell J, Hirsh J, Hylek E, Jacobson A, Crowther M, Palareti G; American College of Chest Physicians. Pharmacology and management of the vitamin K antagonists: American College of Chest Physicians Evidence-Based Clinical Practice Guidelines (8th Edition). *Chest.* 2008;133(6 suppl):160S-198S.

17. Holbrook A, Schulman S, Witt DM, et al; American College of Chest Physicians. Evidence-based management of anticoagulant therapy: Antithrombotic Therapy and Prevention of Thrombosis, 9th ed: American College of Chest Physicians Evidence-Based Clinical Practice Guidelines. *Chest.* 2012;141(2 suppl):e152S-84S.

18. Hughes WT, Armstrong D, Bodey GP, et al. 2002 guidelines for the use of antimicrobial agents in neutropenic patients with cancer. *Clin Infect Dis.* 2002;34(6):730-751.

19. Freifeld AG, Bow EJ, Sepkowitz KA, et al; Infectious Diseases Society of America. Clinical practice guideline for the use of antimicrobial agents in neutropenic patients with cancer: 2010 update by the Infectious Diseases Society of America. *Clin Infect Dis.* 2011;52(4):e56-e93.

20. US Preventive Services Task Force. Screening for breast cancer: U.S. Preventive Services Task Force recommendation statement. *Ann Intern Med.* 2009;151(10):716-26, W-236.

21. MacLean S, Mulla S, Akl EA, et al; American College of Chest Physicians. Patient values and preferences in decision making for antithrombotic therapy: a systematic review: Antithrombotic Therapy and Prevention of Thrombosis, 9th ed: American College of Chest Physicians Evidence-Based Clinical Practice Guidelines. *Chest.* 2012;141(2 suppl):e1S-23S.

22. Nilsen ES, Myrhaug HT, Johansen M, Oliver S, Oxman AD. Methods of consumer involvement in developing healthcare policy and research, clinical practice guidelines and patient information material. *Cochrane Database Syst Rev.* 2006;(3):CD004563.

23. Griebsch I, Coast J, Brown J. Quality-adjusted life-years lack quality in pediatric care: a critical review of published cost-utility studies in child health. *Pediatrics.* 2005;115(5):e600-e614.

24. Atkins D, Eccles M, Flottorp S, et al; GRADE Working Group. Systems for grading the quality of evidence and the strength of recommendations I: critical appraisal of existing approaches *BMC Health Serv Res.* 2004;4(1):38.

25. Guyatt GH, Oxman AD, Schünemann HJ, Tugwell P, Knottnerus A. GRADE guidelines: a new series of articles in the Journal of Clinical Epidemiology. *J Clin Epidemiol.* 2011;64(4):380-382.

26. American College of Cardiology Foundation and American Heart Association. Methodology Manual and Policies From the ACCF/AHA Task Force on Practice Guidelines (2010). http://my.americanheart.org/professional/StatementsGuidelines/PoliciesDevelopment/Development/Methodologies-and-Policies-from-the-ACCAHA-Task-Force-on-Practice-Guidelines_UCM_320470_Article.jsp. Accessed August 4, 2014.

27. US Preventive Services Task Force. Grade definitions. http://www.uspreventiveservicestaskforce.org/uspstf/grades.htm. Accessed August 4, 2014.

28. Schünemann HJ, Hill SR, Kakad M, et al; WHO Rapid Advice Guideline Panel on Avian Influenza. WHO Rapid Advice Guidelines for pharmacological management of sporadic human infection with avian influenza A (H5N1) virus. *Lancet Infect Dis*. 2007;7(1):21-31.

29. Freedman AS, Lister A, Connor RF. Management of gastrointestinal lymphomas. UpToDate. http://www.uptodate.com. Accessed March 27, 2014.

30. Bhasin S, Cunningham GR, Hayes FJ, et al; Task Force, Endocrine Society. Testosterone therapy in men with androgen deficiency syndromes: an Endocrine Society clinical practice guideline. *J Clin Endocrinol Metab*. 2010;95(6):2536-2559.

31. Brito JP, Domecq JP, Murad MH, Guyatt GH, Montori VM. The Endocrine Society guidelines: when the confidence cart goes before the evidence horse. *J Clin Endocrinol Metab*. 2013;98(8):3246-3252.

32. Collins R, Scrimgeour A, Yusuf S, Peto R. Reduction in fatal pulmonary embolism and venous thrombosis by perioperative administration of subcutaneous heparin. Overview of results of randomized trials in general, orthopedic, and urologic surgery. *N Engl J Med*. 1988;318(18):1162-1173.

33. Treweek S, Oxman AD, Alderson P, et al; DECIDE Consortium. Developing and Evaluating Communication Strategies to Support Informed Decisions and Practice Based on Evidence (DECIDE): protocol and preliminary results. *Implement Sci*. 2013;8:6.

34. Norris SL, Holmer HK, Ogden LA, Burda BU. Conflict of interest in clinical practice guideline development: a systematic review. *PLoS One*. 2011;6(10):e25153.

35. Neuman J, Korenstein D, Ross JS, Keyhani S. Prevalence of financial conflicts of interest among panel members producing clinical practice guidelines in Canada and United States: cross sectional study. *BMJ*. 2011;343:d5621.

36. Choudhry NK, Stelfox HT, Detsky AS. Relationships between authors of clinical practice guidelines and the pharmaceutical industry. *JAMA*. 2002;287(5):612-617.

37. Ioannidis JP. Why most published research findings are false. *PLoS Med*. 2005;2(8):e124.

38. Guyatt G, Akl EA, Hirsh J, et al. The vexing problem of guidelines and conflict of interest: a potential solution. *Ann Intern Med*. 2010;152(11):738-741.

39. Norris SL, Burda BU, Holmer HK, et al. Author's specialty and conflicts of interest contribute to conflicting guidelines for screening mammography. *J Clin Epidemiol*. 2012;65(7):725-733.

40. Dahm P, Kunz R, Schünemann H. Evidence-based clinical practice guidelines for prostate cancer: the need for a unified approach. *Curr Opin Urol*. 2007;17(3):200-207.

41. Neumann I, Karl R, Rajpal A, Akl EA, Guyatt GH. Experiences with a novel policy for managing conflicts of interest of guideline developers: a descriptive qualitative study. *Chest*. 2013;144(2):398-404.

42. Neumann I, Akl EA, Valdes M, et al. Low anonymous voting compliance with the novel policy for managing conflicts of interest implemented in the 9th version of the American College of Chest Physicians antithrombotic guidelines. *Chest*. 2013;144(4):1111-1116.

43. Guyatt GH, Norris SL, Schulman S, et al. Methodology for the development of antithrombotic therapy and prevention of thrombosis guidelines: Antithrombotic Therapy and Prevention of Thrombosis, 9th ed: American College of Chest Physicians Evidence-Based Clinical Practice Guidelines. *Chest*. 2012;141(2 suppl):53S-70S.

44. Brozek JL, Bousquet J, Baena-Cagnani CE, et al; Global Allergy and Asthma European Network; Grading of Recommendations Assessment, Development and Evaluation Working Group. Allergic Rhinitis and its Impact on Asthma (ARIA) guidelines: 2010 revision. *J Allergy Clin Immunol*. 2010;126(3):466-476.

45. Qaseem A, Snow V, Cross JT Jr, et al; American College of Physicians/American Academy of Family Physicians Panel on Dementia. Current pharmacologic treatment of dementia: a clinical practice guideline from the American College of Physicians and the American Academy of Family Physicians. *Ann Intern Med*. 2008;148(5):370-378.

MOVING FROM EVIDENCE TO ACTION

27

Decision Making and the Patient

Victor M. Montori, Glyn Elwyn, PJ Devereaux, Sharon E. Straus, R. Brian Haynes, and Gordon Guyatt

IN THIS CHAPTER

MOVING FROM EVIDENCE TO ACTION

INTRODUCTION

One of the 3 key principles of *evidence-based medicine* (EBM) is that the *evidence* alone is never sufficient to make a clinical decision (see Chapter 2, What Is Evidence-Based Medicine?). Clinicians require expertise in interpreting the patient dilemma (in its clinical, social, and economic contexts) and in identifying the body of evidence that bears on optimal patient treatment. These considerations, however, are not enough. Evidence-based medicine requires that clinical decisions be consistent with the informed *values and preferences* of the patient.

We use values and preferences as an overarching term that includes patients' perspectives, priorities, beliefs, expectations, values, and goals for health and life. We also use this phrase, more precisely, to mean the processes that individuals use in considering the potential benefits, *harms*, costs, and inconveniences of the management options in relation to one another.

Consideration of patient values and preferences often enables clinicians to understand the patient who declines lifesaving treatment and the patient who seeks active treatment even when, from a clinician's perspective, the hope of any gain is lost and palliation may seem a wiser path. Differences in values and preferences also may explain policy decisions and *practice guidelines* that, despite relying on the same evidence, differ across settings and contexts. Patient values and preferences become more crucial when confidence in the estimates of a beneficial effect is low and when the balance is close between important benefits and similarly important downsides.

What Approaches to Decision Making Are Available?

Box 27-1 summarizes decision-making approaches theoretically available to the clinician and patient facing an important decision.

Paternalistic Approach

When clinicians offer patients minimal information about the options and make the decision without patient input, a style commonly referred to as a paternalistic or parental approach, they are not considering patient values and preferences. This does not mean that patients do not have an opportunity to express their wishes, but they may do so in a delayed fashion and through actions. For instance, if the treatment choice is not consistent with their values and preferences, patients may not act on the decision or may abandon the plan shortly after the visit with the clinician. Evidence-based medicine requires respecting and incorporating patient values and preferences in the process of decision. Thus, this parental approach, in its violation of patient autonomy, is inconsistent with EBM.

Clinician-as-Perfect-Agent Approach

In theory, one can ensure that decisions are consistent with patient values and preferences without actively involving the patient in the decision. To do so, clinicians must assess the patient's values and preferences and then place these in the context of the evidence about the benefits and risks of alternative courses of action.

Some experts consider this approach, sometimes called the clinician-as-perfect-agent model, impossible

---

BOX 27-1

Decision-Making Approaches

Minimal or no attempt to ensure decision consistent with patient values and preferences

> Paternalistic or parental approaches: Clinician makes minimal effort to establish patient values and preferences, makes decision on behalf of patient

Approaches that attempt to ensure decision consistent with patient values and preferences

> Clinician-as-perfect-agent approach: Clinician ascertains patient's values and preferences, makes decision on behalf of patient

> Informed decision making: Clinician provides patient with the information; patient makes the decision

> Shared decision making: Patient and clinician both bring information/evidence and values and preferences to the decision

to implement.[1] Their position is based on the absence of effective approaches that would confidently yield a deep understanding of the processes that patients use in considering the potential benefits, harms, costs, and inconveniences of the options in relation to one another.

Other experts offer tools for eliciting patient values and preferences, an approach that relies on what is called expected utility theory. Along with these tools, these experts offer models—*decision analyses*—for eliciting the numerical value (utility) that patients might put on a particular outcome and then integrating these values with a calculation of the likelihood of each important outcome for alternative management strategies (see Chapter 26, How to Use a Patient Management Recommendation: Clinical Practice Guidelines and Decision Analyses). These models are limited in that (1) psychologists have found that patients do not consistently make decisions compatible with the underlying assumptions of decision analyses,[2,3] and (2) the models are difficult to use in day-to-day practice.[4] Moreover, there is limited empirical support for the assumptions supporting these tools,[5] and decisions from these analyses may not be the ones reasonable patients would make even after understanding the issues.

Informed Decision-Making Approach

In a very different decision-making style, empowered patients may obtain all of the information pertinent to the decision, consider the options, and make a decision with minimal clinician input. This approach, often referred to as the informed decision-making style, recognizes that patients and clinicians have their own expertise. Patients are experts in their values and preferences and in their personal contexts (personal and social factors—such as working the night shift, lacking a caregiver to help with pill taking and attending laboratory testing, and undisclosed use of alternative medicine agents—that may affect their *adherence* to or tolerance of a treatment or that may affect the effectiveness of a treatment). Clinicians are experts in the technical aspects of the decision (ie, the evidence base informing the pros and cons of each of the options and the experience concerning implementation). The clinician's role with patients choosing this approach is primarily to present information with completeness and clarity.[6]

Shared Decision-Making Approach

In this approach, patients and clinicians engage in a bidirectional exchange. The clinician shares the evidence from clinical research, and the patient shares the evidence accessible in the "patient space" acquired through personal experience, social interaction, and consultation of lay sources, technical references, or the Internet. The bidirectional interaction also includes personal information (ie, sharing the basis for values and preferences). Both the patient and clinician deliberate about the options, explicitly acknowledging the values and preferences they are using, and together arrive at an agreement about the best course of action. The label offered for this model is the shared decision-making process.[6,7]

There are numerous descriptions of shared decision making.[8] One model uses the idea of clinicians having 3 types of "talk" with their patients: team talk, option talk, and decision talk.[9] Box 27-2 describes the 3 types of talk, and Figure 27-1 illustrates the suggested sequence, supporting the patients in gaining understanding about alternative courses of action and, in so doing, constructing informed preferences and, in due course, coming to good decisions.

Some clinicians might interpret shared decision making as requiring clinicians to present their own values and preferences that may then influence the decision. Evidence-based practitioners may find this undesirable for 2 reasons. The first reason is philosophical: although clinicians may experience consequences of these choices through empathy, by experiencing regret when patients experience bad outcomes, or by getting sued, it is patients who endure the treatments and bear the burdens of the outcomes of the choices made. The second reason relates to how patients and clinicians have historically related to each other. Patients may not be willing to reveal their values and preferences if they seem at odds with those the clinician reveals. This concern is made more important by evidence, particularly in preventive care decisions, that patients and clinicians sometimes have values and preferences that differ, although neither party is aware of the differences (Box 27-3).

BOX 27-2

Talk Model of Shared Decision Making

Team Talk

Team talk facilitates patients' awareness that reasonable options exist and that the clinician will help the patient understand how to consider these options in more detail. Components of team talk include:

Stepping back. Summarize and say: "Now that we have identified the problem, it's time for us as a team to think about what to do next."

Offering the choices. Be aware that patients can misconstrue the presentation of choice and think that the clinician is incompetent, uninformed, or both. Reduce this risk by saying: "There is good information about how these treatments differ that I'd like to discuss with you so that we can work together to consider them."

Justifying the choices. Emphasize the importance of respecting individual values and preferences and the role of uncertainty.

For individual values and preferences, explaining that different issues matter more to some people than to others should be easily grasped. Say: "Treatments have different consequences. Some will matter more to you than to other people."

As for uncertainty, patients are often unaware of the extent of uncertainty in medicine—that evidence may be lacking and that individual outcomes are unpredictable at the individual level. Say: "Treatments are not always effective, and the chances of experiencing adverse effects vary."

Checking the patient's reaction. The choice of options may be disconcerting, and some patients may express concern. Suggested phrases to use: "Shall we go on?" "Shall I tell you about the options?"

Postponing closure. Some patients react by asking clinicians to tell them what to do. We suggest postponing or deferring closure if this occurs, reassuring the patient that you are willing to support the process. Say: "I'm happy to share my views and help you get to a good decision. But before I do so, may I describe the options in more detail so that you understand what is at stake?"

Option Talk

Option talk is the act of being clear about reasonable treatment alternatives and helping patients compare them. Components of option talk include:

Checking the patient's knowledge. Even well-informed patients may only be partially aware of their options and the associated harms and benefits, or they be misinformed. Check by asking, "What have you heard or read about the treatment of your condition?"

Listing the options. Make a clear list of the options because it provides good structure. Jot them down and say: "Let me list the options before we get into more detail." If appropriate, include the option of watchful waiting, or use positive terms such as active surveillance.

Describing the options. Generate dialogue and explore values and preferences. Describe the options in practical terms. If there are 2 medical treatments, say: "Both options similarly involve taking medication on a regular basis." Point out when there are clear differences (surgery vs medication), where postponement is possible, and where decisions are reversible. Say: "These options will have different implications for you as compared with other people, so I want to describe...."

Explaining harms and benefits. Being clear about the pros and cons of different options is at the heart of shared decision making. Learn about effective risk communication, such as framing effects and the importance of providing risk data in absolute as well as relative terms. Try giving information in chunks and then checking to see whether the patient understands, a process known as "chunking and checking."

Providing patient decision aids. These tools make options visible and may save time. Some are sufficiently concise to use in clinical encounters. Say: "These tools have been designed to help you understand options in more detail and help us make a decision together. Let's review these together."

Summarizing the options. List the options again and assess understanding by asking for reformulations. This is called the "teach-back" method and is a good check for misconceptions.

Decision Talk

Make an effort here to ask about "what matters most" to the patients, now that they better understand how to compare the alternatives. Help them form their own views, and try to work with patients to see how best to take the next steps—to make a wise and well-considered decision. Components of decision talk include:

Focusing on values and preferences. Guide the patient to form preferences. A suggested phrase: "What, from your point of view, matters most to you?" Help patients consider which aspects of the options will lead them to choose one option over another, according to their own priorities.

Eliciting a preference. Be prepared with a backup plan by offering more time or being willing to guide patients, if they indicate that this is their wish.

Moving to a decision. Try checking for the need to either defer a decision or make a decision. Suggested phrases: "Are you ready to decide?" "Do you want more time? Do you have more questions?" "Are there more things we should discuss?"

Offering review. A good point of closure is to remind the patient, when feasible, that decisions may be reviewed.

In contrast, one might argue that all decision-making approaches incorporate clinician preferences if only to the extent that it is clinicians who decide the range of options that they are willing to offer to the patient. If one takes this position, then shared decision making has the merit of explicitly considering clinicians' values and preferences rather than doing so implicitly. Furthermore, patients appear to be interested in clinicians' preferences. Our guess is that every clinician who has tried to encourage

FIGURE 27-1

Decision-Making Approaches and Evidence-Based Medicine

Approaches	Parental	Clinician as Perfect Agent	Shared Decision Making	Informed
Direction and amount of information flow about options	Clinician ▶ Patient	Clinician ▶ Patient	Clinician ◀▶ Patient	Clinician ▶ Patient
Direction of information flow about values and preferences	Clinician ▶ Patient	Clinician ◀ Patient	Clinician ◀▶ Patient	Clinician ◀ Patient
Deliberation	Clinician	Clinician	Clinician, patient	Patient
Decider	Clinician	Clinician	Clinician, patient	Patient
Consistent with EBM principles	No, when decision is not purely technical and there are options	Yes	Yes	Yes

Abbreviation: EBM, evidence-based medicine. Modified from Charles et al.[7]

BOX 27-3

Do Patients and Their Clinicians Share Similar Values and Preferences?

Devereaux et al[10] used a technique called probability tradeoff to determine the relative strength of aversion to stroke and gastrointestinal bleeding in the context of anticoagulation to prevent stroke in 61 at-risk patients and 63 physicians who treated patients with atrial fibrillation. The figure in this box shows the maximum number of excess upper gastrointestinal tract bleeding episodes per 100 patients treated to prevent 8 additional strokes (4 major and 4 minor) that patients and physicians found acceptable. The figure shows the following: (1) there is variability in stroke aversion among patients and among physicians; (2) patients were much more stroke averse than

physicians; and (3) physicians seem more averse to adverse outcomes that they "cause" with their prescription (eg, bleeding) than to adverse outcomes that result from clinical course (eg, strokes). If one believes that patient preferences should guide treatment, these data suggest the following: if clinicians fail to incorporate patient values and preferences in the decision-making process, they will recommend against anticoagulation more often than is appropriate and, depending on which physician patients see, they will or will not get the treatment they would prefer.

Reproduced from Devereaux et al,[10] with permission from the BMJ.

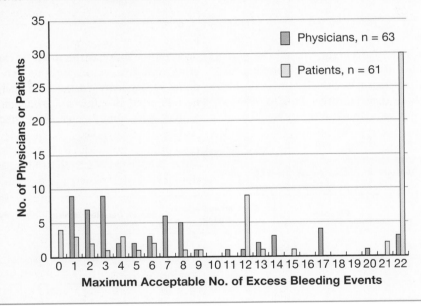

patient autonomy has faced some form of the question, "What would you do?" Finally, because shared decision making espouses the incorporation of patient values and preferences into the decision-making process, it responds to patients' desires to be cared for by their clinician.

These considerations suggest that for shared decision making to work well, the power gradient between clinicians and patients needs to decrease substantially. Only a minimal gradient will ensure

that informed patients can confidently choose an option inconsistent with the clinician's preferences; in reality, many report their clinician's opinion as the most important factor that drives their decision to undergo an invasive procedure.[11] Also, there is evidence that even well-educated patients fear conflict that may arise if they were to engage in decision making and prefer an approach distinct from one their clinicians recommend.[12] A reduced power gradient implies that clinicians will act according

FIGURE 27-2

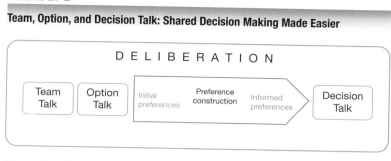

Team, Option, and Decision Talk: Shared Decision Making Made Easier

to patients' informed values and preferences even when the decisions are not those they would have made for themselves (or that will enhance their income).

Figure 27-2 describes our current understanding of decision-making approaches. According to this understanding, clinicians can be aware of clues that patients give during the encounter about their values and preferences for involvement in a decision. All forms of participatory decision making, including its extremes of patient and clinician participation, involve clinicians offering patients evidence-based information about the available options.

What Decision-Making Approach Should I Choose With This Patient?

Although surveys consistently reveal that patients are willing to receive information relevant to the decision at hand,[13] many patients prefer clinicians to take decisional responsibility.[14,15] Reasons include intense emotions surrounding the decision, lack of understanding, impaired physical or cognitive function, lack of self-confidence, and the general human tendency to prefer other people to take responsibility. More problematic reasons, however, exist: patients may not participate in decision making because clinicians do not communicate information in ways that are accessible to the patient (ie, use of technical language that requires health literacy and numeracy[16]), they have no experience or expectation of participating, or they fear disappointing or angering their clinician.

These considerations suggest that clinicians should present information about the options and then adapt to the decision approach patients prefer. Furthermore, these considerations suggest the need to exercise a high degree of empathy in determining what approach best accommodates the patient and the need to remain flexible as the patient's wishes change, which may occur even within the same visit and with each decision considered.

Given the variation in patients' values and preferences regarding the extent to which they wish to take responsibility for management decisions, an empathic, flexible approach within the range of participatory decision-making styles offers advantages. The extent to which clinicians' values and preferences enter the discussion and the extent to which the clinician or patient plays the most active role in the final decision-making process can reflect the patient's preferred decision-making approach. Many clinicians have the impression that poorer or less educated patients, particularly those in low-income countries, are less inclined to participate in decision making. This may be so. It is also possible, however, that if clinicians practice optimal information sharing, listening, and empathy, they will find such patients capable of and interested in participating in making decisions about their care.

In summary, EBM practitioners seeking to incorporate patient values and preferences into clinical decisions should be able to effectively communicate to patients the nature of each of the options, empathically identify and enable the maximum extent of participation that the informed patient wants to have in the decision-making process, and identify and explicitly acknowledge when their own values and preferences are affecting the process of arriving at a decision.

WHAT TOOLS CAN I USE IN MAKING CHALLENGING DECISIONS WITH THIS PATIENT?

Patient Decision Aids

To effectively communicate the nature of the options, researchers have devised and tested tools called patient *decision aids*. These tools are an alternative to the use of intuitive approaches of communicating concepts of risk and risk reduction that clinicians may have developed through clinical experience. Decision aids present, in a patient-friendly manner, descriptive and probabilistic information about the disease, treatment options, and potential outcomes.[17-19] A well-constructed decision aid is based on a *systematic review* of the literature and produces a rigorous summary of the outcomes and their probabilities. Clinicians who doubt that the summary of probabilities is rigorous can review the *primary studies* on which those probabilities are based and, using the principles in this book, determine their accuracy. Furthermore, a well-constructed decision aid offers a tested and effective way of communicating information to patients who may have little background in quantitative decision making. Most commonly, decision aids use visual props, such as icon arrays, to present the proportion of people who experience the outcomes of importance with and without the intervention (Figure 27-3).

What influence do decision aids have on clinical practice? A Cochrane review identified 86 *randomized trials* of decision aids that support screening and treatment decisions.[18] Compared with usual care, decision aids increased reported patient participation in decision making (*relative risk*, 1.4; 95% *confidence interval* [CI], 1.0-2.3), improved

FIGURE 27-3

Sample Decision Aid Developed to Help Patients Decide Whether to Take a Statin to Reduce Their Coronary Risk

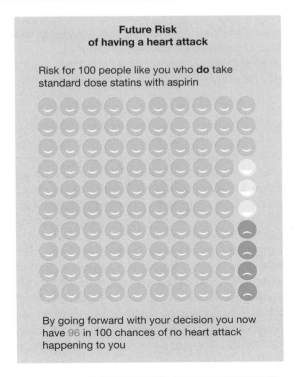

patient knowledge (19/100 points in knowledge surveys; 95% CI, 13-24), and reduced decisional conflict (−9.1/100; 95% CI, −12 to −6). The systematic reviewers concluded that decision aids did not, however, consistently improve satisfaction with the decision-making process, *health outcomes*, or adherence to treatment, or reduce health care use or costs.

Like guidelines, decision aids may be problematic when conflicted developers fail to present the evidence, options, and outcomes fairly. As in guidelines, standards are being developed to try and ensure that decision aids are safe for patient use and do not mislead patients and clinicians.[20,21]

In summary, decision aids increase patient knowledge and improve measures intended to reflect the quality of the decision-making process and its outcome. The use of decision aids in routine clinical practice remains rare, and many implementation barriers exist.[22] Simple decision aids that clinicians can integrate into regular patient care could improve adoption.[23] Randomized trials have found that simple tools for use during the clinical encounter can increase the extent of patient participation in decision making and, in turn, affect the extent to which informed patients' values determine health care decisions.[24-28] This evidence has not revealed consistent effects of using decision aids on treatment choice, adherence, clinical outcomes, or health care use or costs.

SHOULD I USE MORE TIME AND EFFORT IN DECISION MAKING WITH THIS PATIENT NOW?

Time as a Barrier

Should clinicians interested in practicing EBM and expecting to make clinical decisions that incorporate the values and preferences of the informed patient use 1 or more of the above approaches for all decisions? The ultimate constraint of clinical practice is time. Many clinicians have more to do in each encounter than they did in the past.[29-31] Attention to the patient's agenda competes with other activities that clinicians ought to do (eg, documentation, routine preventive care[32]) during visits that have not increased in duration to accommodate these

additional activities and demands. Thus, it is not surprising that clinicians frequently cite time as a key barrier to patient education about options and to enhanced patient participation in decision making.[33] Box 27-4 provides some suggestions for what to do when time is limited.

Important vs Unimportant Decisions

Many of the decisions that patients face are not crucial. Even if the patient-clinician team makes the wrong choice (ie, they do not make the choice that would result from a full discussion), the adverse consequences are minimal or at least limited. Rather than devoting time to these situations, busy clinicians may choose to focus their efforts to ensure that decisions are consistent with patients' values and preferences for choices associated with the most important consequences.

What may be unimportant for one patient, however, may be critical for another. Consider a farmer with an irritating but benign lesion on his hand and the rapidity with which the dermatologist would decide to freeze the lesion after obtaining patient consent. Now consider how the same dermatologist would consider treatment approaches for a similar skin lesion, this time in a woman working as a hand model. The dermatologist will have to engage in

> ### BOX 27-4
> ### Solutions to the Time Problem
>
> Make time for discussion of key decisions
>
> Reserve special follow-up appointments for discussion
>
> Restrict time-consuming approaches to key decisions
>
> Reserve time-consuming approaches for important problems
>
> Reserve time-consuming approaches for difficult decisions
>
> Get help
>
> If possible, refer patient to colleagues with time and expertise for decision-making discussions
>
> Use decision aids

much more than a cursory consent procedure to care for this patient, who is likely to place a much greater value on avoiding a visible scar than on avoiding costly cosmetic procedures compared with almost all other patients with the same lesion.

Straightforward vs Difficult Decisions

When the decision is straightforward (ie, there is an option that almost all informed patients would choose because it is highly effective in achieving *patient-important outcomes*, easy to administer, inexpensive, and safe), decision making can be expeditious. This is the case for aspirin use in a patient in the emergency department who has an acute coronary syndrome. Under these circumstances, a single sentence explaining the rationale and plan can suffice.

In other situations, the benefits and downsides of an intervention are more closely balanced. For instance, clinicians should have a discussion regarding use of low-dose aspirin for coronary prevention. Use of this agent is associated with bleeding, a risk that increases as the coronary risk increases. This downside must therefore be considered against the potential benefits, including the favorable effects of aspirin on coronary risk and colon cancer.[34]

These 2 situations—a clear decision that virtually all informed patients would endorse vs a close call—should correspond to strong and weak recommendations that guideline panels offer (see Chapter 26, How to Use a Patient Management Recommendation: Clinical Practice Guidelines and Decision Analyses, and Chapter 28.1, Assessing the Strength of Recommendations: The GRADE Approach). If guideline panels function appropriately, clinicians can interpret a strong recommendation as "just do it" and a weak recommendation as an invitation to engage patients in shared decision making. Sometimes, clinicians and patients need to spend more time making decisions that, when initially considered, appear straightforward. Some decisions, such as lifestyle and pharmacologic treatments for chronic conditions, require review—and reaffirmation or revision. The need for review may occur every time patients learn about or experience a potential adverse effect, renew the prescription and pay for it, or learn about an alternative solution.

Time and resources spent exploring these decisions may help patients remember why they started using these interventions in the first place and enhance their adherence to these treatments (this was the motivation behind the decision aid about statin use in patients with diabetes, described in Figure 27-3).

Misinformed Participants

Clinicians may have a distorted perception of the evidence. Distortions can be the result of misleading marketing messages that reach clinicians informally through colleagues or formally through industry-funded continuing medical education and office detailing. Misleading presentations of research findings in primary reports of research can distort clinicians' understanding of the evidence (see Chapter 13.3, Misleading Presentations of Clinical Trial Results). Panels that develop guidelines may include experts whose recommendations are influenced by their conflicts of interest. This is particularly problematic when adherence to guidelines becomes linked to monetary incentives (ie, pay-for-performance programs). Patients may perceive something amiss when clinicians make treatment recommendations that are too expensive, too invasive, or too new. Such patients, if unable to participate fully, may forgo these treatments after the visit, lose trust in the clinician, or seek attention elsewhere.

Patients also may be misinformed. Distorted evidence reaches patients through advertisements in traditional media, lay medical or health publications, social networks, and the Internet and through misinformed or conflicted clinicians. Consider the more than 75% of patients who received a coronary stent for stable angina who, after receiving this treatment, reported their belief (contradicted by evidence warranting high confidence) that this treatment will reduce their risk of myocardial infarction and death.[35] Patients convinced of what they see in print may feel empowered to request a prescription from their clinician for interventions that they do not need or would not want if they were adequately informed. Given time and skill constraints, patients who seek attention knowing what they want may leave clinician offices with their wishes satisfied, whereas clinicians are left feeling uncomfortable about the course of action chosen.[36]

Clinicians should spend more time with information sources when they suspect their own understanding is limited or inaccurate and more time with their patients when they suspect their patients have a distorted knowledge base. Strategies to calibrate the clinicians' knowledge base may include the review of the evidence that supports claims of effectiveness and strong recommendations from a variety of information sources (see Chapter 5, Finding Current Best Evidence) using the skills taught in the *Users' Guides to the Medical Literature*. Strategies to calibrate patients' knowledge are less clear but may include involving the patient in such evidence reviews. An alternative approach is, when they are available, to use evidence-based decision aids.

The Patient With Multiple Chronic Conditions

Straightforward decisions about adding a new prevention or treatment intervention can become challenging in a patient with a chronic condition who is overwhelmed by health care options. This happens most often in patients who have multiple chronic conditions, a situation that is becoming increasingly common at a younger age, particularly among the disadvantaged.[37] For these patients, each option not only involves a set of potential benefits and harms inherent to that treatment but also brings an obligatory set of treatment monitoring and administration tasks that represent an incremental *burden of treatment*. The new intervention will have to compete for patient attention, energy, and time against the patient's established treatment program. The end result of this competition may include optimal or inadequate adherence to the new treatment or discontinuation of an established therapy.

Clinicians need to assess patients' capacity to face treatment burdens. Influences on this capacity include patients' resilience, literacy, physical and mental health, financial solvency, social capital, and level of support in their environment. Clinicians must consider not only the extent to which adding a new treatment is consistent with patient values and preferences but also how feasible the resulting regimen is. Treatments may need to be prioritized, with discontinuation of low-value interventions. Such treatments impose an important burden to the patient (difficult to administer, expensive, disabling adverse effects) in exchange for limited or unclear benefits (improving a biochemical or physiologic measure without a small or uncertain impact on quality of life or *prognosis*). Prioritization of the treatment program is another opportunity for collaborative deliberation between clinician and patient. This effort, sometimes referred to as *minimally disruptive medicine*, seeks patient goals for health while imposing the smallest possible treatment burden on their lives.[38]

Other Solutions

Clinicians could consider delaying making a decision and ask that it be considered during another visit, designated for that purpose. This assumes that clinicians are permitted to allot this time in their schedule for these additional focused visits. Another option is to refer the patient to a specialist colleague with time and expertise in shared decision making. Primary care teams may designate members of the team—physicians, nurses, pharmacists, or care managers—to focus on making decisions with patients with whom the team has developed a partnership. In some centers, decision coaches (often nurses or other health care professionals) provide detailed exploration of important decisions.[39]

Use a Patient Decision Aid

Patients considering important decisions may benefit from educational material that they can take home and review with family, friends, and advisers. They then can return with questions and potentially with a final decision. There are more than 300 such patient decision aids in the Cochrane Inventory found at the Cochrane Decision Aid Registry (http://decisionaid.ohri.ca/cochinvent.php). This inventory, kept by investigators at the Ottawa Health Decision Centre, describes the decision aid and its purpose and offers contact information about each tool's developer and availability. Unfortunately, almost 80% of these tools have not been evaluated clinically.[40]

A more promising approach is to use decision aids in the clinical encounter. Such tools are optimally designed (often using user-centered approaches) for the specific context to be time sensitive and efficient. The number and nature of these tools (eg, issue cards, option grids) are now expanding as evidence accumulates of their effectiveness and feasible use in routine care.[24-28] This evidence suggests that simple tools for use during the clinical encounter add, on average, approximately 3 minutes to a primary care consultation (examples are available at http://shared decisions.mayoclinic.org and http://www.option grid.org).

CONCLUSION

Evidence-based medicine maintains that patient management decisions should reflect both the best available evidence and the patients' values and preferences (see Chapter 2, What Is Evidence-Based Medicine?). It follows that choices should be those that patients would make in collaboration with clinicians who ensure that both they and their patients are optimally informed and who respect what is most important to patients. Achieving that goal represents a major challenge and a fruitful area for clinical research. Clinicians should be aware of the different approaches to clinical decision making and the need to tailor the approach to the individual patient. They should understand how evidence and preferences fit together in the decision-making process and use the limited evidence available to find the approaches that are right for them and for their patients.

References

1. Gafni A, Charles C, Whelan T. The physician-patient encounter: the physician as a perfect agent for the patient versus the informed treatment decision-making model. *Soc Sci Med*. 1998;47(3):347-354.

2. Gafni A. When does a competent patient make an irrational choice [letter]? *N Engl J Med*. 1990;323(19):1354.

3. Kahneman D, Tversky A. Prospect theory: an analysis of decisions under risk. *Econometrica*. 1979;47(2):263-292.

4. Elwyn G, Edwards A, Eccles M, Rovner D. Decision analysis in patient care. *Lancet*. 2001;358(9281):571-574.

5. Gafni A, Birch S. Preferences for outcomes in economic evaluation: an economic approach to addressing economic problems. *Soc Sci Med*. 1995;40(6):767-776.

6. Charles C, Gafni A, Whelan T. Decision-making in the physician-patient encounter: revisiting the shared treatment decision-making model. *Soc Sci Med*. 1999;49(5):651-661.

7. Charles C, Gafni A, Whelan T. Shared decision-making in the medical encounter: what does it mean? (or it takes at least two to tango). *Soc Sci Med*. 1997;44(5):681-692.

8. Makoul G, Clayman ML. An integrative model of shared decision making in medical encounters. *Patient Educ Couns*. 2006;60(3):301-312.

9. Elwyn G, Tsulukidze M, Edwards A, Légaré F, Newcombe R. Using a 'talk' model of shared decision making to propose an observation-based measure: Observer OPTION 5 Item. *Patient Educ Couns*. 2013;93(2):265-271.

10. Devereaux PJ, Anderson DR, Gardner MJ, et al. Differences between perspectives of physicians and patients on anticoagulation in patients with atrial fibrillation: observational study. *BMJ*. 2001;323(7323):1218-1222.

11. Mazur DJ, Hickam DH, Mazur MD, Mazur MD. The role of doctor's opinion in shared decision making: what does shared decision making really mean when considering invasive medical procedures? *Health Expect*. 2005;8(2):97-102.

12. Frosch DL, May SG, Rendle KA, Tietbohl C, Elwyn G. Authoritarian physicians and patients' fear of being labeled 'difficult' among key obstacles to shared decision making. *Health Aff (Millwood)*. 2012;31(5):1030-1038.

13. Gaston CM, Mitchell G. Information giving and decision-making in patients with advanced cancer: a systematic review. *Soc Sci Med*. 2005;61(10):2252-2264.

14. Levinson W, Kao A, Kuby A, Thisted RA. Not all patients want to participate in decision making: a national study of public preferences. *J Gen Intern Med*. 2005;20(6):531-535.

15. Beaver K, Bogg J, Luker KA. Decision-making role preferences and information needs: a comparison of colorectal and breast cancer. *Health Expect*. 1999;2(4):266-276.

16. Montori VM, Rothman RL. Weakness in numbers. The challenge of numeracy in health care. *J Gen Intern Med*. 2005;20(11):1071-1072.

17. Whelan T, Gafni A, Charles C, Levine M. Lessons learned from the Decision Board: a unique and evolving decision aid. *Health Expect*. 2000;3(1):69-76.

18. Stacey D, Légaré F, Col NF, et al. Decision aids for people facing health treatment or screening decisions. *Cochrane Database of Syst Rev*. 2014;1:CD001431. doi: 10.1002/14651858. CD001431.pub4.

19. Charles C, Gafni A, Whelan T, O'Brien MA. Treatment decision aids: conceptual issues and future directions. *Health Expect*. 2005;8(2):114-125.

20. Elwyn G, O'Connor A, Stacey D, et al; International Patient Decision Aids Standards (IPDAS) Collaboration. Developing a quality criteria framework for patient decision aids: online international Delphi consensus process. *BMJ*. 2006;333(7565):417.

21. Joseph-Williams N, Newcombe R, Politi M, et al. Toward minimum standards for certifying patient decision aids: a modified delphi consensus process. *Med Dec Making*. 2013;34(6):699-710.

22. Elwyn G, Scholl I, Tietbohl C, et al. "Many miles to go ..." a systematic review of the implementation of patient decision support interventions into routine clinical practice. *BMC Med Inform Decis*. 2013;13(suppl 2):S14. doi: 10.1186/1472-6947-13-S2-S14.

23. Elwyn G, Frosch D, Volandes AE, Edwards A, Montori VM. Investing in deliberation: a definition and classification of decision support interventions for people facing difficult health decisions. *Med Decis Making*. 2010;30(6):701-711.

24. Weymiller AJ, Montori VM, Jones LA, et al. Helping patients with type 2 diabetes mellitus make treatment decisions: statin choice randomized trial. *Arch Intern Med*. 2007;167(10):1076-1082.

25. Mullan RJ, Montori VM, Shah ND, et al. The diabetes mellitus medication choice decision aid: a randomized trial. *Arch Intern Med*. 2009;169(17):1560-1568.

26. Montori VM, Shah ND, Pencille LJ, et al. Use of a decision aid to improve treatment decisions in osteoporosis: the osteoporosis choice randomized trial. *Am J Med*. 2011;124(6):549-556.

27. Hess EP, Knoedler MA, Shah ND, et al. The chest pain choice decision aid: a randomized trial. *Circ Cardiovasc Qual Outcomes*. 2012;5(3):251-259.

28. Branda ME, LeBlanc A, Shah ND, et al. Shared decision making for patients with type 2 diabetes: a randomized trial in primary care. *BMC Health Serv Res*. 2013;13:301. doi:10.1186/1472-6963-13-301.

29. Zuger A. Dissatisfaction with medical practice. *N Engl J Med*. 2004;350(1):69-75.

30. Yarnall KS, Pollak KI, Østbye T, Krause KM, Michener JL. Primary care: is there enough time for prevention? *Am J Public Health*. 2003;93(4):635-641.

31. Mechanic D, McAlpine DD, Rosenthal M. Are patients' office visits with physicians getting shorter? *N Engl J Med*. 2001;344(3):198-204.

32. Getz L, Sigurdsson JA, Hetlevik I. Is opportunistic disease prevention in the consultation ethically justifiable? *BMJ*. 2003;327(7413):498-500.

33. Légaré F, Ratté S, Gravel K, Graham ID. Barriers and facilitators to implementing shared decision-making in clinical practice: update of a systematic review of health professionals' perceptions. *Patient Educ Couns*. 2008;73(3):526-535.

34. Vandvik PO, Lincoff AM, Gore JM, et al; American College of Chest Physicians. Primary and secondary prevention of cardiovascular disease: Antithrombotic Therapy and Prevention of Thrombosis, 9th ed: American College of Chest Physicians Evidence-Based Clinical Practice Guidelines. *Chest*. 2012;141 (2 suppl):e637S-e668S.

35. Rothberg MB, Sivalingam SK, Ashraf J, et al. Patients' and cardiologists' perceptions of the benefits of percutaneous coronary intervention for stable coronary disease. *Ann Intern Med*. 2010;153(5):307-313.

36. Mintzes B, Barer ML, Kravitz RL, et al. Influence of direct to consumer pharmaceutical advertising and patients' requests on prescribing decisions: two site cross sectional survey. *BMJ*. 2002;324(7332):278-279.

37. Barnett K, Mercer SW, Norbury M, Watt G, Wyke S, Guthrie B. Epidemiology of multimorbidity and implications for health care, research, and medical education: a cross-sectional study. *Lancet*. 2012;380(9836):37-43.

38. May C, Montori VM, Mair FS. We need minimally disruptive medicine. *BMJ*. 2009;339:b2803.

39. Woolf SH, Chan EC, Harris R, et al. Promoting informed choice: transforming health care to dispense knowledge for decision making. *Ann Intern Med*. 2005;143(4):293-300.

40. Ottawa Hospital Research Institute. Decision Aid Library Inventory (DALI). Patient Decision Aids website. http://decisionaid.ohri.ca/cochinvent.php. Updated June 25, 2012. Accessed August 4, 2014.

MOVING FROM EVIDENCE TO ACTION

28.1

ADVANCED TOPICS IN MOVING FROM EVIDENCE TO ACTION

Assessing the Strength of Recommendations: The GRADE Approach

Ignacio Neumann, Elie A. Akl, Per Olav Vandvik, Pablo Alonso-Coello, Nancy Santesso, M. Hassan Murad, Frederick Spencer, Holger J. Schünemann, and Gordon Guyatt

IN THIS CHAPTER

Clinical Scenario

Direction and Strength of Recommendations

Developing GRADE Recommendations

From Evidence to Recommendations

Overall Confidence in Effect Estimates

Balance Between Benefits and Harms

Uncertainty and Variability in Patients' Values and Preferences

Resource Considerations

Clinical Scenario Resolution

You are a primary care practitioner considering the possibility of the use of aspirin for primary *prevention* of serious cardiovascular events and cancer in a 60-year-old man. He has hypertension, adequately controlled with thiazides, but he is otherwise healthy; he does not have diabetes or dyslipidemia, does not smoke, and has no family history of heart disease.

To inform your decision, you search first for an evidence-based recommendation and find the following: "In many adults, the benefits of aspirin exceed the risks (principally bleeding). For individuals 50 years or older without excess bleeding risk, we suggest low-dose daily aspirin (75-100 mg) (weak recommendation based on moderate confidence in *effect estimates*)."[1]

After reading the corresponding *Users' Guide* (see Chapter 26, How to Use a Patient Management Recommendation: Clinical Practice Guidelines and Decision Analyses), you know that weak recommendations reflect the judgment of a specific group (eg, a guideline panel) that an individualized decision is necessary. You are curious, however, about the rationale for a weak recommendation for aspirin use and decide that this is a good opportunity to understand more about the *GRADE* (*Grading of Recommendations Assessment, Development and Evaluation*) approach to move from *evidence* to recommendations.

DIRECTION AND STRENGTH OF RECOMMENDATIONS

Like recommendations based on other evidence-rating systems, recommendations developed with the GRADE approach specify the direction of the recommendation (in favor or against the intervention) and are classified as strong or weak.

Strong recommendations apply to all or almost all patients and indicate that clinicians do not (if they are ready to trust the judgment of the panel) require

thorough (or even cursory) review of the underlying evidence or a discussion of benefits and risks with the patient.

Weak recommendations, in contrast, apply to most patients but not to everyone. To effectively use weak recommendations, clinicians need to understand and consider the key factors that drive the direction and strength of the recommendation. Given that weak recommendations are usually sensitive to patients' *values and preferences*, they require that one be prepared to engage the patient in shared decision making (see Chapter 27, Decision Making and the Patient).

DEVELOPING GRADE RECOMMENDATIONS

GRADE provides a structure for assessing confidence in estimates from evidence summaries (eg, *systematic reviews* and *meta-analyses*) and, in the context of guidelines, also for moving from evidence to recommendations. Figure 28.1-1 presents the steps involved in developing a GRADE recommendation, including evidence synthesis and moving from evidence to recommendations. In the first step, guideline panelists formulate a clinical question, which involves specifying the target population, the intervention of interest, and an appropriate comparator. Conceptually, the final recommendation represents the answer to this question. Having formulated the question, guideline panelists select the relevant outcomes and rate their importance as critical, important, or not important for decision making; the panel considers the critical or important outcomes in making their recommendation. Guideline panelists then consider all of the relevant studies, using existing systematic reviews and meta-analyses or conducting their own reviews, including summaries that provide estimates of both relative and absolute effect of the intervention vs the comparator for these outcomes.

Using the evidence summaries, guideline panelists then rate the confidence in the effect estimates for each outcome as high, moderate, low, or very low

FIGURE 28.1-1

Steps Involved in Developing a GRADE Recommendation

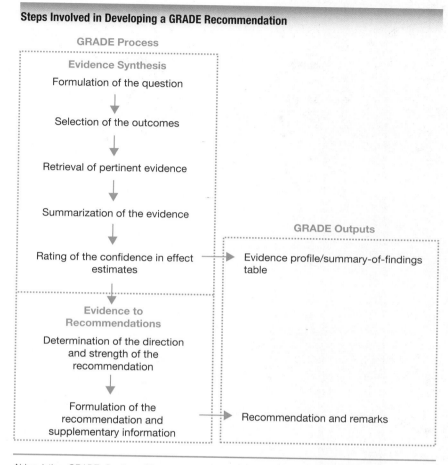

Abbreviation: GRADE, Grading of Recommendations Assessment, Development and Evaluation.

MOVING FROM EVIDENCE TO ACTION

(see Chapter 23, Understanding and Applying the Results of a Systematic Review and Meta-analysis). The GRADE Working Group has developed 2 standardized tabular formats for evidence summaries: the *evidence profile* and the *summary-of-findings table*. The evidence profile provides a detailed record of the judgments made in the evaluation of the confidence in the estimates of effect and presents both relative and absolute estimates of the effect (Table 28.1-1). The summary-of-findings table provides a more concise summary of the same information (Table 28.1-2).[2]

The next step is to move from the evidence to the recommendation. Panelists consider 4 factors as

they ponder the direction and strength of a GRADE recommendation: (1) the overall confidence in effect estimates, (2) the balance between benefits and *harms*, (3) the uncertainty and variability in patients' values and preferences, and (4) resource considerations (Table 28.1-3). The recommendation and associated remarks are the final products of the GRADE process (Figure 28.1-1). As we highlight, the process implies that although confidence in estimates of effect has an important influence on strength of recommendations, the 2 are quite separate: both high and low confidence in estimates can be associated with either strong or weak recommendations.

TABLE 28.1-1

Evidence Profile: Aspirin (75 to 100 mg) Compared With No Aspirin in the Primary Prevention of Cardiovascular Disease[a]

Quality Assessment							Effect		Confidence	Importance
No. of Studies (No. of Participants)	Study Design	Risk of Bias	Inconsistency	Indirectness	Imprecision	Other Considerations	Relative Effect (95% CI)	Absolute Risk During 10 Years		
Mortality										
9 (100076)	RCTs	Not serious	Not serious	Not serious	Serious[b]	Not serious	RR, 0.94 (0.88-1.00)	6 fewer deaths per 1000 (from 12 fewer to 0 fewer)	⊕⊕⊕◯ MODERATE	CRITICAL
Myocardial Infarction (Nonfatal Events)										
9 (100076)	RCTs	Not serious	Not serious	Not serious	Not serious	Not serious	RR 0.80 (0.67-0.96)	17 fewer MI per 1000 (from 27 fewer to 3 fewer)	⊕⊕⊕⊕ HIGH	CRITICAL
Stroke (Includes Nonfatal Ischemic and Hemorrhagic Strokes)										
9 (95000)	RCTs	Not serious	Not serious	Not serious	Serious[b]	Not serious	RR, 0.95 (0.85-1.06)	No significant difference, fewer strokes per 1000 (from 10 fewer to 4 more)	⊕⊕⊕◯ MODERATE	CRITICAL

Major Extracranial Bleeding

6 (95 000)	RCTs	Not serious	Not serious	Not serious	Not serious	RR, 1.54 (1.30-1.82)	16 more bleeds per 1000 (from 7 more to 20 more)	⊕⊕⊕⊕ HIGH	CRITICAL

Cancer Incidence

6 (35 535)	RCTs	Serious[c]	Not serious	Not serious	Serious[d]	HR, 0.88 (0.80-0.98)	6 fewer cancers per 1000 (from 10 fewer to 1 fewer)	⊕⊕○○ LOW	IMPORTANT

Abbreviations: CI, confidence interval; HR, hazard ratio; MI, myocardial infarction; RCTs, randomized clinical trials; RR, relative risk.

[a]Baseline risks included in the table are from medium-risk patients according to the Framingham Score. These risks correspond to the patient presented in the opening scenario.

[b]The 95% CI included both appreciable benefit and no benefit or harm.

[c]Two large studies were arbitrarily excluded from the original meta-analysis.

[d]The absolute estimates included a substantial benefit and a marginal effect.

Data from Vandvik PO, Lincoff AM, Gore JM, et al. Primary and Secondary Prevention of Cardiovascular Disease: Antithrombotic Therapy and Prevention of Thrombosis, 9th ed: American College of Chest Physicians Evidence-Based Clinical Practice Guidelines. *Chest* 2012; 141:e637S.

TABLE 28.1-2

Summary of Findings Table: Aspirin (75 to 100 mg) Compared With No Aspirin in the Primary Prevention of Cardiovascular Disease[a]

Outcome	No. of Patients (No. of Studies)	Relative Effect (95% CI)	Anticipated Absolute Effects During 10 Years		Confidence in Effect Estimates (GRADE)
			Without Aspirin	Risk Difference With Aspirin (95% CI)	
Mortality	100 076 (9)	RR, 0.94 (0.88-1.00)	100 deaths per 1000	6 fewer deaths per 1000 (from 12 fewer to 0 fewer)	⊕⊕⊕O MODERATE due to imprecision[b]
MI (nonfatal events)	100 076 (9)	RR 0.80 (0.67-0.96)	83 MI per 1000	17 fewer MI per 1000 (from 27 fewer to 3 fewer)	⊕⊕⊕⊕ HIGH
Stroke (nonfatal ischemic and hemorrhagic strokes)	95 000 (9)	RR, 0.95 (0.85-1.06)	65 strokes per 1000	No significant difference, 3 fewer strokes per 1000 (from 10 fewer to 4 more)	⊕⊕⊕O MODERATE due to imprecision
Major extracranial bleeding	95 000 (6)	RR, 1.54 (1.30-1.82)	24 bleeds per 1000	16 more bleeds per 1000 (from 7 more to 20 more)	⊕⊕⊕⊕ HIGH
Cancer (incidence)	35 535 (6)	HR, 0.88 (0.80-0.98)	50 cancers per 1000	6 fewer cancers per 1000 (from 10 fewer to 1 fewer)	⊕⊕OO LOW due to imprecision and risk of bias[c,d]

Abbreviations: CI, confidence interval; GRADE, Grading of Recommendations Assessment, Development and Evaluation; HR, hazard ratio; MI, myocardial infarction; RR, relative risk.

[a]Baseline risks included in the table are from medium-risk patients according to the Framingham Score. These risks correspond to the patient presented in the opening scenario.

[b]The 95% CI included both appreciable benefit and no benefit or harm.

[c]Two large studies were arbitrarily excluded from the original meta-analysis.

[d]The absolute estimates included a substantial benefit and a marginal effect.

Data from Vandvik PO, Lincoff AM, Gore JM, et al. Primary and Secondary Prevention of Cardiovascular Disease: Antithrombotic Therapy and Prevention of Thrombosis, 9th ed: American College of Chest Physicians Evidence-Based Clinical Practice Guidelines. *Chest* 2012; 141:e637S.

FROM EVIDENCE TO RECOMMENDATIONS

Overall Confidence in Effect Estimates

Confidence in estimates of effect (also known as quality of evidence) usually varies across outcomes. For instance, we are almost always more confident in estimates of the benefits of new interventions than in the frequency with which rare serious adverse effects occur. Therefore, systematic review authors and guideline panelists must present their confidence in estimates for each outcome (see Chapter 23, Understanding and Applying the Results of a Systematic Review and Meta-analysis). The GRADE guidelines also present an overall confidence in effect estimates, which represents the lowest rating among the outcomes considered critical to decision making.

High and moderate confidence in effect estimates reflects the panel's judgment that the effect

TABLE 28.1-3

Factors That Determine the Strength of the Recommendation

	A Strong Recommendation May Be Justified If	In General, We Should Expect a Weak Recommendation When
Overall confidence in effect estimates	There is high or moderate confidence in effect estimates (or in special circumstances when the confidence is low or very low)	There is low or very-low confidence in effect estimates
	AND	OR
Balance between benefits and harms	The benefits clearly outweigh the harms or vice versa	The balance between benefits and harms is close
	AND	OR
Uncertainty and variability in patients' values and preferences	All or almost all fully informed patients will make the same choice	There is variability or uncertainty in what fully informed patients may choose
	AND	OR
Resource considerations (optional)	The benefits of the intervention are clearly justified (or not) in all or almost all of the circumstances	The benefit of the intervention may not be justified in some circumstances

estimates are sufficiently credible to support a particular recommendation. High and moderate confidence will justify strong recommendations in favor of or against a particular course of action if the desirable consequences (benefits) clearly outweigh the undesirable consequences (harms, *burden*, and costs). If desirable and undesirable consequences are closely balanced, however, even high confidence in estimates will not lead to a strong recommendation (Table 28.1-3).

For example, evidence from a systematic review of *randomized trials* with low *risk of bias,* consistent results across trials, and results applicable to the population (moderate confidence due to *imprecision*) reveals that, in people with nonvalvular atrial fibrillation, the use of warfarin, as compared with aspirin, reduces the risk of stroke but increases the risk of bleeding and the *burden*

of treatment. In people at high risk of stroke (eg, congestive heart failure, hypertension, age ≥ 75 years, diabetes mellitus, prior stroke or transient ischemic attack [Cardiac failure, Hypertension, Age, Diabetes Stroke system $(CHADS_2)$] score of 3-6 points), the desirable consequences—a reduction of 40 strokes per 1000 patients treated for a year (95% *confidence interval* [CI], from 23 to 51 fewer)—clearly outweighs the undesirable consequences— an increase of 8 bleeds per 1000 patients treated for a year (95% CI, from 1 fewer to 10 more) and the need for laboratory monitoring and lifestyle changes. Consequently, a strong recommendation in favor of warfarin is appropriate.[3]

However, in persons at moderate risk of stroke (eg, $CHADS_2$ score of 1 point), the balance between desirable and undesirable consequences is closer: the use of warfarin over aspirin reduces the risk of stroke by 9 events per 1000 patients treated for a year (95% CI, from 5 to 11 fewer) and produces the same increase in bleeding and burden of treatment as in people at high risk of stroke. In this situation, despite the moderate confidence in effect estimates, a weak recommendation in favor of warfarin is more appropriate.[3]

Low and very low confidence in effect estimates reflect the guideline panel's judgment that there is considerable uncertainty regarding the outcomes associated with the alternative courses of action under consideration. In these circumstances, different attitudes toward uncertain benefits and harms are likely to lead to variability in what informed patients may choose, and guideline panels appropriately using the GRADE approach will most often issue weak recommendations.

For example, evidence from *observational studies* suggests that a diet rich in potassium might decrease cardiovascular risk. However, the confidence in effect estimates is low (coming from observational studies).[4] Although the intervention has no known adverse effects and almost no additional cost, some people are likely to judge that the uncertain benefit does not warrant the effort of changing their diet, whereas others will be prepared to do so. In this case, the uncertainty regarding the benefits of the intervention is responsible for variability in what informed patients will choose. Therefore, a weak recommendation (either for or against, depending on the panel's judgment about whether most informed individuals, in response to the evidence, would change or not change their diet) is appropriate.[4]

In general, we should expect weak recommendations when the overall confidence in effect

estimates is low or very low. Therefore, if you find a panel providing a strong recommendation on the basis of evidence warranting only low or very low confidence, you should be suspicious about that panel's judgment. Such situations warrant a careful look at why the recommendation was graded as strong.

Sometimes, however, guideline panels may appropriately offer strong recommendations despite low or very low confidence in effect estimates. Table 28.1-4 presents 5 paradigmatic situations in which strong recommendations may be warranted despite low confidence in key effect estimates.

For example, evidence warranting low confidence suggests that in males with androgen deficiency, testosterone supplementation improves well-being. However, *indirect evidence* (low confidence in effect estimates) suggests that testosterone might contribute to the spread of hormone-dependent cancers, including prostate cancer. If a guideline panel believes (as it reasonably might) that all or virtually all informed men with androgen deficiency and prostate cancer would opt not to take the risk of accelerated dissemination for the modest benefits of testosterone in well-being, a strong recommendation against testosterone will be appropriate.[5]

Balance Between Benefits and Harms

The balance between benefits and harms is a crucial determinant of both the direction and strength of a recommendation. If the net benefit (desirable vs undesirable consequences) of an intervention vs a comparator is small, guideline panels will generally issue weak recommendations (Table 28.1-3).

Two factors are involved in a panel's judgment of this balance: the magnitude of the benefits vs harms (including the burden of treatment), and the relative importance that typical patients place in the benefits and harms.

TABLE 28.1-4

Five Paradigmatic Situations That Justify Strong Recommendations Based on Low or Very-Low Confidence

Paradigmatic Situation	Confidence in Effect Estimates for Health Outcomes (Quality of Evidence)		Balance of Benefits and Harms	Values and Preferences	Resource Considerations	Recommendation	Example
	Benefits	Harms					
Life-threatening situation	Low or very low	Immaterial (very low to high)	Intervention may reduce mortality in a life-threatening situation; adverse events not prohibitive	A very high value is placed on an uncertain but potentially life-preserving benefit	Small incremental cost (or resource use) relative to the benefits justify the intervention	Strong recommendation in favor	Indirect evidence from seasonal influenza suggests that patients with avian influenza may benefit from the use of oseltamivir (low confidence in effect estimates). Given the high mortality of the disease and the absence of effective alternatives, the WHO made a strong recommendation in favor of the use of oseltamivir rather than no treatment in patients with avian influenza.[12]
Uncertain benefit, certain harm	Low or very low	High or moderate	Possible but uncertain benefit; substantial established harm	A much higher value is placed on the adverse events in which we are confident than in the benefit, which is uncertain	High incremental cost (or resource use) relative to the benefits may not justify the intervention	Strong recommendation against	In patients with idiopathic pulmonary fibrosis, treatment with azathioprine plus prednisone offers a possible but uncertain benefit in comparison with no treatment. The intervention, however, is associated with a substantial established harm. An international guideline made a recommendation against the combination of corticosteroids plus azathioprine in patients with idiopathic pulmonary fibrosis.[13]
Potential equivalence, one option clearly less risky or costly	Low or very low	High or moderate	Magnitude of benefit apparently similar—though uncertain—for alternatives; we are confident of less harm or cost for one of the competing alternatives	A high value is placed on the reduction in harm	High incremental cost (or resource use) relative to the benefits may not justify one of the alternatives	Strong recommendation for less harmful/less expensive	*Helicobacter pylori* eradication in patients with early stage extranodal MALT lymphoma who are *H pylori* positive. Low-quality evidence suggests that initial *H pylori* eradication results in similar rates of complete response in comparison to the alternatives of radiation therapy or gastrectomy but with high confidence of less harm, morbidity, and cost. Consequently, UpToDate made a strong recommendation in favor of *H pylori* eradication rather than radiotherapy in patients with MALT lymphoma.[14]
High confidence in similar benefits, one option potentially more risky or costly	High or moderate	Low or very low	Established that magnitude of benefit similar for alternative management strategies; best (though uncertain)	A high value is placed on avoiding the potential increase in harm	High incremental cost (or resource use) relative to the benefits may not justify one of the alternatives	Strong recommendation against the intervention with possible greater harm	In women requiring anticoagulation and planning conception or in pregnancy, high confidence estimates suggest similar effects of different anticoagulants. However, indirect evidence (low confidence in effect estimates) suggests

(Continued)

TABLE 28.1-4

Five Paradigmatic Situations That Justify Strong Recommendations Based on Low or Very-Low Confidence *(Continued)*

Paradigmatic Situation	Confidence in Effect Estimates for Health Outcomes (Quality of Evidence)		Balance of Benefits and Harms	Values and Preferences	Resource Considerations	Recommendation	Example
	Benefits	Harms					
			estimate is that one alternative has appreciably greater harm				potential harm to the unborn infant with oral direct thrombin (eg, dabigatran) and factor Xa inhibitors (eg, rivaroxaban, apixaban). The AT9 guidelines recommended against the use of such anticoagulants in women planning conception or in pregnancy.[7]
Potential catastrophic harm	Immaterial (very low to high)	Low or very low	Potential important harm of the intervention; magnitude of benefit is variable	A high value is placed on avoiding the potential increase in harm	High incremental cost (or resource use) relative to the benefits may not justify the intervention	Strong recommendation against the intervention	In males with androgen deficiency, testosterone supplementation likely improves quality of life. Low confidence evidence suggests that testosterone increases cancer spread in patients with prostate cancer. The Endocrine Society made a recommendation against testosterone supplementation in patients with prostate cancer.[5]

Abbreviations: AT9, antithrombotic guidelines (9th edition); MALT, mucosa-associated lymphoid tissue; WHO, World Health Organization.

For example, the use of warfarin in comparison with no therapy in people with nonvalvular atrial fibrillation and low risk of stroke (eg, CHADS$_2$ score of 0) results in a reduction of 5 strokes per 1000 patients treated for a year (95% CI, 4 fewer to 6 fewer per 1000) but in an increase of 8 major bleeds per 1000 patients treated for a year (95% CI, from 1 more to 25 more per 1000)[3] and an associated burden of treatment. The decision regarding net benefit is critically dependent on the relative value that patients place in the stroke, burden, and bleeding outcomes. Typical patients place a very high value in avoiding a stroke and its long-term consequences. The best available estimate suggests that for informed patients, avoiding a stroke is 3 times more important than avoiding a bleeding event.[6] If we take this factor into account, in patients with atrial fibrillation and low risk of stroke, the reduction of strokes is more important than the increase of bleeding:

a reduction of 5 strokes per 1000 patients (multiplied by 3) vs an increase of 8 major bleeds per 1000 patients (multiplied by 1). However, the net benefit is small and the burden of treatment substantial, particularly considering that patients with atrial fibrillation and low risk of stroke are typically young and without comorbidities. Consequently, most informed patients may choose to not use warfarin in this scenario; however, some might decide the opposite. A weak recommendation against warfarin in this circumstance is therefore appropriate.[3]

Clinicians who use GRADE to evaluate specific recommendations should expect that guideline panels will not only present the absolute effects of interventions considered when balancing the benefits and harms of the intervention but also explain the judgment of typical values and preferences they used to make the trade-off.

Uncertainty and Variability in Patients' Values and Preferences

Our discussion has emphasized the crucial role of values and preferences. If a guideline panel is very uncertain about patients' values and preferences or believes these are extremely variable, a weak recommendation is likely (Table 28.1-3).

For example, vitamin K antagonists (VKAs) have been associated with fetal wastage, bleeding in the fetus, and teratogenicity if used after 8 weeks of gestation.[7] Women using long-term VKA treatment who are attempting pregnancy face the choice of performing frequent pregnancy tests and substituting parental anticoagulants for warfarin when pregnancy is achieved or replacing VKA with parental anticoagulants before conception is attempted. Both options have limitations. Small observational studies provide low confidence estimates suggesting that VKAs are safe during the first 6 to 8 weeks of gestation.[8] This provides some, but limited, reassurance to women who, considering the burden and cost of injections, would prefer to continue using warfarin until pregnancy is achieved. What informed patients prefer in this scenario remains uncertain, but it is likely to be variable. Consequently, a weak recommendation is appropriate, and even the direction is questionable. The 9th edition of the antithrombotic guidelines issued a weak recommendation in favor of using VKA until pregnancy is achieved.[7]

Resource Considerations

The health budget—whether of a family, an organization, or a country—should be distributed fairly. Even if we focus only on interventions that lead to an important benefit on *patient-important outcomes*, depending on resource constraints, it may not be possible to offer them to all who might benefit. The existence of competing health needs and scarce resources suggests that to be optimally helpful, guideline panels may recommend against beneficial treatments when the gain is modest and the cost high.

Health *economic analysis* provides guidance for making these decisions (see Chapter 28.2, Economic Analysis). Economic analyses present the benefits and harms of the candidate interventions and their associated resource use. The analyses facilitate selection of the interventions that offer the greater benefits in relation to the amount of resources used.

Strong recommendations reflect a panel's judgment that the benefits of the recommended course of action justify its resource use in all or almost all circumstances. If there is variability in the resource use across modes of delivery (eg, well-child visits can be performed by physicians, nurses, and nurse practitioners) or variability in resource availability (eg, high-income vs low-income countries) across the settings in which the recommendation will be applied, guideline panels are likely to issue weak recommendations (Table 28.1-3).

For example, the balance between the benefits and harms of using inhaled glucocorticoids in people with stable chronic obstructive pulmonary disease (COPD) is very close: evidence from randomized trials suggests that the use of inhaled glucocorticoids may reduce symptoms and the risk of exacerbations but also may increase the risk of pneumonia.[9] This evidence has led some guideline developers to suggest the use of inhaled glucocorticoids in people with COPD, especially in those with more symptoms or with frequent exacerbations despite an optimal long-acting inhaled bronchodilator regimen.[10] However, high doses of the drug for long periods are required to achieve an appreciable effect, and the cost of the intervention is relatively high. A guideline panel from the World Health Organization considered that, for resource-limited settings, the small benefit of inhaled glucocorticoids does not justify its relative high cost in most circumstances and consequently issued a strong recommendation against the intervention.[11] If the target audiences of the guideline are in settings with different availability of resources, a weak recommendation is more appropriate, or different recommendations are needed for the different settings.

Learning how resources issues affect recommendations will help you to assess whether and how the recommendation is relevant to your setting. Resource use issues are, however, not always included in guideline panel deliberations, and some panels may legitimately choose to not consider resources to develop their recommendations.

CLINICAL SCENARIO RESOLUTION

You decide to explore the influence of the 4 factors discussed on the direction and strength of the recommendations. To do this, you look at the guideline text and Tables 28.1-1 and 28.1-2.

Overall Confidence in Effect Estimates
As the tables indicate, the guideline panelists considered 5 outcomes: mortality, myocardial infarction, stroke, major extracranial bleeding, and incidence of cancer. The first 4 were considered critical for decision making, whereas the last was considered important. The confidence in effect estimates was rated as high for myocardial infarction and major extracranial bleeding because the effect estimates came from a systematic review of randomized trials with low risk of bias, consistent results across trials, precise effects (narrow CIs), and results applicable to the population. For the outcomes of mortality and stroke, however, the 95% CIs included both appreciable benefit and no benefit or harm, and hence panelists decreased the confidence to moderate. Finally, the confidence was judged as low for the outcome of incidence of cancer because the absolute estimates included a substantial benefit and a marginal effect (imprecision), and there was concern regarding the exclusion of 2 large studies from the original meta-analysis reporting this outcome (risk of bias). Typically, the overall confidence in effect estimates is the lowest rating among the outcomes considered as critical, which in this case is moderate because the outcome of incidence of cancer (rated as low) was considered important but not critical for decision making (see Chapter 23, Understanding and Applying the Results of a Systematic Review and Meta-analysis).

Balance Between Benefits and Harms
Considering the *baseline risk* of individuals at 60 years of age and at average risk for coronary artery disease (10% to 20% during 10 years) and at average risk of malignancy (approximately 5%), the use of aspirin prevents 6 deaths per 1000 (95% CI, from 12 to 0 fewer), 19 nonfatal myocardial infarctions (95% CI, from 26 to 12 fewer), and 6 new cancers (95% CI, from 10 to 1 fewer) during a 10-year period. However, it produces 16 extracranial major bleeds (95% CI, from 7 to 20 more) during the same period (Tables 28.1-1 and 28.1-2). It is likely that most informed patients will place a higher value on avoiding mortality, vascular events, and cancer than on the possibility of bleeding, and the use of aspirin will be perceived as a net benefit by informed patients. The absolute magnitude of this benefit, however, is small because all of the events considered are infrequent in primary prevention populations.

Uncertainty and Variability in Patients' Values and Preferences
The net benefit of aspirin is very small in absolute terms. Some informed patients will be willing to tolerate the long-term medication use to gain a small reduction in the risks of death, vascular events, and cancer and will tolerate the risk of bleeding. Others, however, are likely to consider that the effect is not of sufficient magnitude to warrant the inconvenience and small risk of bleeding, and consequently, they will not be willing to use aspirin. Therefore, we can expect variability in what informed patients may choose.

Resource Considerations
Resource use was not explicitly considered in this recommendation. However, with aspirin's minimal

expense, cost issues are unlikely to play an important part in this recommendation.

Integrating the Factors

The benefits of aspirin (reduction of mortality, myocardial infarction, and incidence of cancer) outweigh the risks (increase of bleeding and burden), and hence, the guideline panel issued a recommendation in favor of aspirin.

Regarding the strength of the recommendation, the moderate overall confidence in effect estimates may have warranted a strong recommendation. However, the small magnitude of the benefit and the likely variability in patients' values and preferences appropriately led the panel to grade the recommendation as weak.

Now that you understand the panel's rationale for the recommendation, you are in a position to engage in shared decision making with the 60-year-old man considering use of aspirin for primary prevention.

References

1. Spencer FA, Guyatt GH. Aspirin in the primary prevention of cardiovascular disease and cancer. In: Basow DS, ed). *UpToDate*. Waltham, MA: UpToDate; 2013. http://www.uptodate.com/contents/aspirin-in-the-primary-prevention-of-cardiovascular-disease-and-cancer. Accessed April 10, 2014.

2. Guyatt G, Oxman AD, Akl E, et al. GRADE guidelines, 1: introduction-GRADE evidence profiles and summary of findings tables. *J Clin Epidemiol*. 2011;64(4):383-394.

3. You JJ, Singer DE, Howard PA, et al; American College of Chest Physicians. Antithrombotic therapy for atrial fibrillation: Antithrombotic Therapy and Prevention of Thrombosis, 9th ed: American College of Chest Physicians Evidence-Based Clinical Practice Guidelines. *Chest*. 2012;141(2)(suppl):e531S-e575S.

4. World Health Organization. *Potassium intake for adults and children*. Geneva, Switzerland: World Health Organization (WHO); 2012. http://www.who.int/nutrition/publications/guidelines/potassium_intake_printversion.pdf. Accessed April 10, 2014.

5. Bhasin S, Cunningham GR, Hayes FJ, et al; Task Force, Endocrine Society. Testosterone therapy in men with androgen deficiency syndromes: an Endocrine Society clinical practice guideline. *J Clin Endocrinol Metab*. 2010;95(6):2536-2559.

6. Devereaux PJ, Anderson DR, Gardner MJ, et al. Differences between perspectives of physicians and patients on anticoagulation in patients with atrial fibrillation: observational study. *BMJ*. 2001;323(7323):1218-1222.

7. Bates SM, Greer IA, Middeldorp S, Veenstra DL, Prabulos AM, Vandvik PO; American College of Chest Physicians. VTE, thrombophilia, antithrombotic therapy, and pregnancy: Antithrombotic Therapy and Prevention of Thrombosis, 9th ed: American College of Chest Physicians Evidence-Based Clinical Practice Guidelines. *Chest*. 2012;141(2)(suppl):e691S-e736S.

8. Schaefer C, Hannemann D, Meister R, et al. Vitamin K antagonists and pregnancy outcome: a multi-centre prospective study. *Thromb Haemost*. 2006;95(6):949-957.

9. Yang IA, Clarke MS, Sim EH, Fong KM. Inhaled corticosteroids for stable chronic obstructive pulmonary disease. *Cochrane Database Syst Rev*. 2012;7:CD002991. doi: 10.1002/14651858.CD002991.pub3.

10. Erbland ML. Role of inhaled glucocorticoid therapy in stable COPD. In: Basow DS, ed. *UpToDate*. Waltham, MA: UpToDate; 2013. http://www.uptodate.com/contents/role-of-inhaled-glucocorticoid-therapy-in-stable-copd#H14. Accessed April 10, 2014.

11. World Health Organization. *Prevention and control of NCDs: Guidelines for primary health care in low-resource settings*. Geneva, Switzerland: World Health Organization; 2012. http://apps.who.int/iris/bitstream/10665/76173/1/9789241548397_eng.pdf. Accessed April 10, 2014.

12. Schünemann HJ, Hill SR, Kakad M, et al; WHO Rapid Advice Guideline Panel on Avian Influenza. WHO Rapid Advice Guidelines for pharmacological management of sporadic human infection with avian influenza A (H5N1) virus. *Lancet Infect Dis*. 2007;7(1):21-31.

13. Raghu G, Collard HR, Egan JJ, et al; ATS/ERS/JRS/ALAT Committee on Idiopathic Pulmonary Fibrosis. An official ATS/ERS/JRS/ALAT statement: idiopathic pulmonary fibrosis: evidence-based guidelines for diagnosis and management. *Am J Respir Crit Care Med*. 2011;183(6):788-824.

14. Freedman AS, Lister A, Connor RF. Management of gastrointestinal lymphomas. In: Basow DS, ed. *UpToDate*. Waltham, MA: UpToDate; 2013. http://www.uptodate.com/contents/management-of-gastrointestinal-lymphomas. Accessed April 10, 2014.

MOVING FROM EVIDENCE TO ACTION

28.2

ADVANCED TOPICS IN MOVING FROM EVIDENCE TO ACTION

Economic Analysis

Ron Goeree, Michael F. Drummond, Paul Moayyedi, and Mitchell Levine

IN THIS CHAPTER

You are a gastroenterologist on the staff of a large community hospital in which there is considerable pressure on the endoscopy service to provide more colonoscopy *screening* to reduce colorectal cancer mortality, but no funds are available to increase endoscopy facilities. Approximately 50% of the workload is devoted to upper gastrointestinal tract endoscopy for patients with dyspepsia. One possibility is to reduce upper gastrointestinal tract endoscopy demand by providing a *Helicobacter pylori* test-and-treat service as the preferential management strategy for patients younger than 55 years with dyspepsia without alarm symptoms. This strategy involves giving patients a noninvasive test for *H pylori* (eg, a serologic test or urea breath test), treating patients with positive results with antibiotic therapy, and reassuring patients with negative results that they are unlikely to have peptic ulcer disease.

You are hesitant to recommend the new approach. Some physicians believe that prompt endoscopy for all helps select the most effective treatment. Moreover, the *H pylori* test-and-treat strategy will save no resources if patients all undergo endoscopy anyway. Before providing your advice, you decide to seek a formal *economic analysis* of the *H pylori* test-and-treat approach compared with prompt endoscopy.

FINDING THE EVIDENCE

Having recently attended a short workshop on *economic evaluation*, you are aware that a good source of information is the UK National Health Service Economic Evaluation Database (NHS EED). This database contains *structured abstracts* of full economic evaluations, plus references to methodology articles and cost studies, and is available through the advanced search Cochrane Library by selecting "Economic Evaluations" as a search limit (http://onlinelibrary.wiley.com/cochranelibrary/search). Your hospital does not subscribe to the database, but you have free access through the website of the Centre for Reviews and Dissemination of the University of York (http://www.crd.york.ac.uk/crdweb).

You first select the box next to "NHS EED," then select the drop-down option "Any field" and enter the following 3 search terms: "dyspepsia AND endoscopy AND helicobacter." Note that the interface allows you to enter each term separately and link them with different operators, such as "AND," "OR," or "NOT," to form more complex searches (see Chapter 5, Finding Current Best Evidence). This search generates 56 results in the NHS EED database. You scan the results and find that the structured abstract of the 16th citation on the list is an article by Ford et al,[1] which reports that the economic analysis is based on a *meta-analysis* of 5 *randomized clinical trials* (RCTs), including 1924 patients, comparing the test-and-treat approach with prompt endoscopy. This strikes you as the highest quality *evidence* you are likely to find, and you retrieve the article.

WHY ECONOMIC ANALYSIS?

Clinicians not only make decisions about the care of individual patients but also help establish clinical policy. Some clinicians also help to set health policy at a broader level (addressing questions such as whether more resources should be made available for the treatment of peptic ulcer disease).

When making decisions for patient groups, clinicians need to not only weigh the benefits and *risks* but also consider whether these benefits will be worth the health care costs. Increasingly, clinicians must persuade colleagues and health policymakers that the benefits of their interventions justify the resources consumed.

In general, economic analysis can help justify allocation of scarce resources by providing a set of formal, quantitative methods to compare 2 or more treatments, programs, or strategies with respect to their resource use and their expected outcomes.[2-4] A comparison of 2 treatments or strategies that considers only costs informs only the resource-use half of the decision and is termed a *cost analysis*. Comparing only the consequences of 2 or more strategies (such as in an RCT of treatment efficacy) informs only the health benefit portion of the decision. A full economic comparison addresses both the costs and consequences of the strategies being compared.

Economic evaluations seek to inform resource allocation decisions rather than to make them. Economic analyses, widely applied in the health care field, have informed decisions at different levels of the health care system, including managing major institutions such as hospitals and determining regional or national policy.[4]

COST: JUST ANOTHER OUTCOME?

In one sense, cost is like physiologic function, *quality of life*, morbid events (eg, stroke and myocardial infarction), and death—simply another *outcome variable* for clinicians to consider when assessing the effects of therapy. Although there are fundamental similarities between cost and other outcomes, there are also important differences that we will now describe.

The Role of Costs in Clinical Decision Making Remains Controversial

Although few would deny the importance of cost considerations in setting health care policy, the relevance of costs in individual patient decision making remains controversial. Some would argue—taking an extreme of what can be called a *deontologic* approach to distributive justice—that clinicians' only responsibilities are to best meet the needs of the individuals under their care. An alternate view—philosophically *consequentialist* or *utilitarian*—would contend that even in individual decision making, clinicians should take a broader social view. In this broader view, the effect on others of allocating resources to a particular patient's care should bear on the decision.

As health care technologies proliferate, their potential benefits and their costs increase, but their marginal benefits over less resource-intensive approaches are often small. In such a world, the arguments for bedside rationing become more compelling.[5] Our own belief is that although individual clinicians should attend primarily to the needs of the patients under their care, they should not neglect the resource implications of the advice they offer their patients. Neglect of resource issues in one patient may, after all, affect resource availability for other patients under their care. That is, there is always an *opportunity cost* in making any resource allocation decision. For those who disagree, this section remains relevant for consideration of health policy decisions.

Costs Are More Variable Than Other Outcomes

Whether clinicians administer the *H pylori* test-and-treat approach to a patient with dyspepsia in Toronto or Singapore, the relative effect on dyspepsia is likely to be similar. Indeed, *treatment effects* of drug therapy on conventional outcomes of quality of life, morbidity, and mortality have proved on most occasions to be similar across geographic locations and also across patient groups and ways of administering the intervention (see Chapter 25.2, How to Use a Subgroup Analysis).

In contrast to clinical *end points*, costs vary hugely across jurisdictions, both in absolute terms and in the relative costs of different components of care, including physicians, other clinicians and health care workers, hospitalizations, drugs, services, and medical devices.

For example, outpatient treatment of deep venous thrombosis (DVT) with low-molecular-weight heparin (LMWH) compared with inpatient treatment with unfractionated heparin was found to be more cost-effective in the United States than in Canada, despite the fact that LMWH was more than double the price in the United States at that time.[6] This was because the price of reduced hospital days relative to the price of LMWH was much greater in the United States than in Canada.

One need not move across international—or even national, regional, or state—boundaries to see large cost differences. Adjacent hospitals may have different success in negotiating a contract with a drug company to purchase a large volume of a drug at a lower price. Drug prices in adjacent hospitals may therefore vary by a factor of 2 or more, and the resource implications for use of alternative agents may therefore differ substantially in the 2 institutions.

Costs also depend on how care is organized, and organization of care varies widely across jurisdictions. The same service may be delivered by a physician or a nurse practitioner, in the outpatient setting or in the hospital, and with or without administrative costs related to adjudication of patient eligibility to receive the service. If it is delivered by a physician, in the hospital, with maximal administrative costs, as our example of inpatient DVT treatment in the United States suggested, the expense will be greater than if the service is delivered on an outpatient basis or in an institution with lower administrative costs.

The substantial dependence of resource consumption on local costs and local organization of health care provision means that most cost data are specific to a particular jurisdiction and have limited transferability. An additional problem with RCTs is that their conduct may alter practice patterns in ways that further limit *generalizability* to other settings, or even to their own setting, outside the RCT context. For example, in an economic evaluation of misoprostol, a drug for prophylaxis against gastric ulcer in patients receiving high doses of nonsteroidal anti-inflammatory drugs, Hillman and Bloom[7] used data from an RCT undertaken by Graham et al.[8] This *blinded* RCT of 3 months' duration compared misoprostol (400 and 800 mg daily) with placebo. An important issue for economic analysis was that prevention of ulcers by misoprostol may generate savings in health care expenditure, savings that could balance the cost of adding the drug. In this study, however, endoscopy was performed monthly. In regular clinical practice, endoscopy would be undertaken in response to symptoms. An analysis of the results from this trial would have told clinicians of the cost implications of misoprostol administration when patients undergo routine monthly endoscopy, information that would be useless, given how different such circumstances are from regular clinical practice.

Using Cost Information Raises Questions of Distributive Justice

In health care policy decisions, we must use cost information to allocate scarce resources efficiently. Let us assume that 2 treatments both cost, in comparison to conventional treatment and after consideration of all their consequences, $1 million for each of the 1000 patients treated for 1 year. For treatment A, the benefits achieved by this expenditure are the prevention of 200 patients from having symptoms of dyspepsia. For treatment B, the benefit is avoiding a single case of gastric cancer. If, in a resource-constrained environment, one had to choose between A and B, what would be the better choice?

If the choice makes you feel uncomfortable, you are in good company. Choosing between competing beneficial treatments presents daunting logistic, ethical, and political challenges. The example indicates how, when using economic analysis, we must trade off costs against benefits and how we must deal with very different outcomes that accrue to very different people—in this case, the prevention of dyspepsia in one patient group and prevention of a case of gastric cancer in another—in deciding on allocation of resources.

ECONOMIC ANALYSIS OFFERS SOLUTIONS TO ITS SPECIAL CHALLENGES

Problems of Cost Variability

As for other outcomes, there are 2 fundamental strategies for discovering the effect of alternative management strategies on resource consumption. One is to conduct a single study, ideally an RCT, comparing 2 or more interventions. Such an approach asks what happens (on average and limited by the precision of the estimate) when clinicians choose management strategy A vs strategy B.

The second approach is to construct a decision analytic model of events that flow from a clinical decision, using all of the available evidence to estimate the probabilities of all possible outcomes, including the costs generated. This second approach asks what might happen if clinicians choose management strategy A vs strategy B. The what-might-happen modeling approach of *decision analysis* allows investigators to deal with problems such as the idiosyncrasies of care provided in the RCT context and the variability in costs across jurisdictions.

Refer to the example of the unnecessary endoscopies conducted in the RCT performed by Graham et al[8] of misoprostol for prevention of gastric ulcers in patients taking high doses of nonsteroidal anti-inflammatory drugs. In the subsequent analysis, Hillman and Bloom[7] adjusted observed ulcer rates to reflect the fact that 40% of endoscopically determined lesions did not produce any symptoms. Observing that *adherence* of patients in the trial was greater than one might expect in clinical practice, they also adjusted for lower adherence by using the ulcer rates in the evaluable cohort and assuming that only 60% of this efficacy would be achieved in practice.

Modeling through decision analysis allows investigators to deal with other problems such as inadequate length of *follow-up* by using available data to estimate what will happen in the long term. Decision analysts also can examine a variety of cost assumptions and ways of organizing care and calculate the sensitivity of their results to these alternate assumptions (see Chapter 26, How to Use a Patient Management Recommendation: Clinical Practice Guidelines and Decision Analyses).

The key limitation of the decision analytic approach is that if its assumptions are flawed, it will not give us an accurate picture. For example, in a review of 326 pharmacoeconomic analyses submitted to the Australian Department of Health by the pharmaceutical industry, 218 (67%) included significant problems, many of which required a detailed review to detect.[9]

Even rigorous economic analyses without *conflict of interest* will yield misleading results if the underlying assumptions are inaccurate. A *cost-effectiveness analysis* using pristine decision-analysis methods concluded that trying to achieve rhythm control in older patients with atrial fibrillation was more cost-effective than a strategy based on controlling only the heart rate.[10] Unfortunately, subsequent RCTs found that the assumptions the authors made about the benefits of rhythm control were inaccurate.[11] A subsequent economic analysis based on more valid assumptions revealed the unequivocal superiority of the rate-control approach.[12]

The ideal way forward may be a melding of the 2 approaches, in which the analysis rests on data from RCTs, with adjunctive analytic decision–based modeling to adapt the results to the actual situations in which they will be applied.[13] Even the melding approach, however, must use average patient values. These averages may be different from the *values and preferences* of the individual patient, and different values may lead to different decisions (see Chapter 27, Decision Making and the Patient). Looking at the underlying assumptions of an economic analysis may provide clinicians with insight into application of results to their patients. Thus, the extent to which the authors make their assumptions transparent will add to the *credibility* of any economic analysis.

There is another aspect to solving a component of the cost-variability problem. If authors present resources used by the alternative management strategies, users of the research can consider how much those resources would cost in their own setting. Indeed, cost is really shorthand for resource consumption, a point that clinicians can usefully bear in mind when considering economic issues.

Trading Off Benefits, Risks, and Costs

As we have mentioned, economic analysis must deal with the problem of the relative value of different outcomes and the tradeoff of dollar values against health. Typically, health economists use 3 strategies. One is to report *patient-important outcomes* in physical or natural units, such as life-years gained, patients symptom-free, or gastric cancers prevented (*cost-effectiveness analysis*).

In another approach, health economists weigh different types of outcomes to produce a composite index of outcome, such as the *quality-adjusted life-year* (QALY) (we call this *cost-utility analysis*, sometimes classified as a subcategory of cost-effectiveness analysis). Quality adjustment involves placing a lower value on time spent with impaired physical and emotional function than time spent in full health. On a scale in which 0 represents death and 1.0 represents full health, the greater the impairment, the lower the utility value of a particular *health state*.

Finally, investigators may put a dollar value on additional life gained, cases of dyspepsia prevented, or gastric cancers prevented. In these *cost-benefit analyses*, health care consumers consider what they would be willing to pay for programs or products that achieve particular outcomes, such as prolonging life or preventing adverse events.

USING THE GUIDE

In the study from our scenario, Ford et al[1] chose cost-effectiveness as their primary analysis, using the outcome "patients symptom-free of dyspepsia." The strength of this approach is that the outcome data are generated directly from the individual patient data meta-analysis that they conducted. The main disadvantage is that the outcome measure relates to dyspepsia only. Therefore, it is difficult to make any comparisons of cost-effectiveness, or value for money, with other interventions in gastroenterology or health care more generally.

A more generic outcome measure, such as QALYs gained, would have facilitated these comparisons. Small changes in dyspepsia symptoms may, however, not even register on a metric such as a QALY. Therefore, it may not be a good approach for detecting small differences in benefits between 2 treatment strategies for dyspepsia. It also may fail to represent adequately large differences in benefits that are limited to a brief period, such as the value of a local anesthetic when having root canal dental treatment. However, when it comes to the broader aspects of resource allocation in health care, we need a measure such as the QALY to compare the benefits of improvements in dyspepsia symptoms with outcomes in other fields of health care.

BOX 28.2-1

Users' Guides for an Article About Economic Analyses

Are the results valid?

Did the recommendations consider all relevant patient groups, management options, and possible outcomes?

- Did investigators adopt a sufficiently broad viewpoint?
- Are results reported separately for relevant patient subgroups?

Is there a systematic review and summary of evidence linking options to outcomes for each relevant question?

- Were costs measured accurately?
- Did investigators consider the timing of costs and consequences?

What are the results?

- What were the incremental costs and effects of each strategy?
- Do incremental costs and effects differ between subgroups?
- How much does allowance for uncertainty change the results?

How can I apply the results to patient care?

- Are the treatment benefits worth the risks and costs?
- Can I expect similar costs in my setting?

Using an Economic Analysis

Having outlined some of the challenges of economic analysis, we offer our traditional structure for guides to the medical literature: Are the results valid (which includes *risk of bias*)? What are the results? How can I apply the results to patient care? Our key criteria from Chapter 26, How to Use a Patient Management Recommendation: Clinical Practice Guidelines and Decision Analyses, also apply to economic analyses: Do the recommendations consider all relevant patient groups, management options, and possible outcomes? Is there a *systematic review* of evidence linking options to each relevant outcome? Is there an appropriate specification of values and preferences associated with outcomes? The issues we present in Box 28.2-1 are those specific to economic analysis.

ARE THE RESULTS VALID?

Limitations in design of economic analyses include issues beyond risk. Therefore, in this chapter, we continue to use the term *validity* to address risk of bias and these other issues.

Did Investigators Adopt a Sufficiently Broad Viewpoint?

Investigators can evaluate costs and consequences from a number of viewpoints: the patient, a health care institution such as a hospital, the third-party payer (insurer, drug benefit program, or national or local government in some countries), or society at large. Each viewpoint may be relevant, depending on the question being asked, but broader viewpoints are most relevant to those allocating health care resources. For example, an evaluation adopting the viewpoint of the hospital will be useful in estimating the budgetary effect of alternative therapies for that institution. However, economic evaluation is usually directed at informing policy from a broader perspective. For example, in an evaluation of an early-discharge program, reporting only hospital costs is insufficient because patients discharged early may consume substantial community resources.

One of the main reasons for considering narrower viewpoints in conducting an economic analysis is to assess the influence of change on the main budget holders because budgets may need to be adjusted before a new therapy can be adopted, often termed the *silo effect*. For instance, Feldman et al[14] reported that donepezil therapy in moderate to severe Alzheimer disease was worthwhile from the perspective of society as a whole because of the reduced demands on caregivers. Nevertheless, it would be more costly to the organization responsible for paying for the medication. Even within the same institution, narrow budgetary viewpoints can prevail. In an economic analysis comparing 2 drug regimens, it would be wrong to focus exclusively on the relative costs of the drugs, which are included in the pharmacy budget, if there are also effects on other hospital resource use. In the DVT example we used earlier, use of outpatient LMWH will decrease hospital cost, but whoever pays the drug budget will find their costs increasing. The patient's perspective also may merit specific consideration if costs (eg, travel-related costs or time off work) reduce access to care. Also, some patients may not be able to participate in community care programs if these impose major costs in terms of informal nursing support in the home. In general, however, economic analyses integrate the patient's perspective by measuring the consequences of therapy, such as income losses or the effect on quality of life.

From a societal viewpoint, determination of costs should include the therapy's effect on the patients' ability to work and hence their contribution to the nation's productivity. The issue of inclusion or exclusion of productivity changes (sometimes known as *indirect costs and benefits*) remains a frequent topic of debate. On one hand, productivity changes represent resource-use changes, such as those occurring in the health care system. On the other hand, production may not actually be lost if a worker is absent for a short period. Also, for longer periods of absence, employers may hire a previously unemployed worker. Furthermore, inclusion of productivity changes biases evaluations in favor of programs for individuals who are in full-time employment. Therefore, clinicians should be skeptical about any economic analysis that includes productivity changes without clearly presenting the implications.

USING THE GUIDE

Table 28.2-1, which outlines the costs used by Ford et al[1] in calculating the total cost per patient for the 2 alternative treatment strategies, reveals that the costs span both primary and secondary care. If you work in health care, depending on your setting, some of the costs might strike you as unrealistic. This emphasizes the important issue of the lack of portability of unit costs across jurisdictions. Table 28.2-1 reflects the authors' decision to adopt the perspective of someone making decisions for the whole health care system. In publicly funded systems, this would be the government or national health insurance agency. In privately funded systems, the relevant perspective would be that of an insurer providing coverage for health care costs.

Are Results Reported Separately for Relevant Patient Subgroups?

Costs and consequences may differ among patients of different age, sex, or illness severity. The most likely

MOVING FROM EVIDENCE TO ACTION

TABLE 28.2-1

Costs Used in Obtaining a Total Cost per Patient for *Helicobacter pylori* Test-and-Treat vs Endoscopy

Variable	Cost, $ (2003)
General practitioner visit	170
Outpatient visit	232
Inpatient day	550
PPI (1-mo single dose)	99.99
H₂RA (1 mo)	112.29
Prokinetic (1 mo)	70
Antacid (1 mo)	8.49
Eradication therapy	152
Urea breath test	80
Endoscopy	450
Barium meal	99.69
Abdominal ultrasonographic scan	118

Abbreviations: H₂RA, histamine₂-receptor antagonist; PPI, proton-pump inhibitors.

This article was published in *Gastroenterology*, Vol. 128, Ford AC et al. *Helicobacter pylori* "test and treat" or endoscopy for managing dyspepsia: an individual patient data meta-analysis. pp 1838-1844.[1] Copyright Elsevier 2005.

differences are those related to the *baseline risk* of the adverse outcome that the treatment is designed to *prevent*. For example, the cost-effectiveness of drug therapy for elevated cholesterol level will improve compared with no drug intervention as patient risk increases. Cost-effectiveness will be superior in men vs women; older vs younger patients; and those with higher cholesterol level, hypertension, diabetes, and family history of heart disease vs those without these risk factors.[15]

A study that compared drug-eluting stents to bare metal stents for treatment of coronary artery disease reports that differences across patient groups can be substantial. The authors found that the cost-utility of drug-eluting stents varied substantially from CAD$420 000 per QALY to more than CAD$9 million per QALY, depending on patient baseline risk factors.[16]

The impact of baseline risk factors on cost-effectiveness findings is apparent when comparing primary vs secondary prevention. For instance, in a study of the cost-effectiveness of screening

for proteinuria to slow the progression of chronic renal disease, Boulware et al[17] found that the cost per QALY gained was $283 000 for all individuals older than 50 years but was only $19 000 for those individuals older than 50 years with hypertension. The differences in the cost-effectiveness ratios were driven primarily by the patient's risk of developing chronic renal disease (ie, if you are unlikely to develop chronic renal disease, you have a limited capacity to benefit).

Were Costs Measured Accurately?

Although the viewpoint determines the relevant range of costs and consequences in an economic evaluation, there are many issues relating to their measurement and evaluation. First, clinicians should look for the physical quantities of resources consumed or released by the treatments separately from their prices or unit costs. Not only does this allow them to scrutinize the method of assigning monetary values to resources, it also helps to extrapolate the results of a study from one setting to another because prices vary by location.

Second, there are different approaches to valuing costs or cost savings. One approach is to use published charges. Charges, however, may differ from true opportunity costs, depending on the sophistication of accounting systems and the relative bargaining power of health care institutions and third-party payers.[18] Where there is a systematic deviation between costs and charges, the analyst may adjust the latter by a *cost-to-charge ratio*. The association between charges and costs may, however, vary markedly by institution, so simple adjustments may not suffice. From the third-party payer's perspective, charges will bear some relation to the amounts actually paid, although in some settings payments vary by payer. From a societal perspective, we would like the true opportunity costs because these reflect what society is forgoing in benefits elsewhere to provide a given treatment.

For example, Taira et al[19] compared the costs and charges for 2 methods of percutaneous coronary revascularization. When hospital charges were used, the difference in the mean cost between the 2 methods was $21 311. When itemized procedure costs and departmental cost-to-charge ratios were used, however, the difference was only $5454. Thus, clinicians may have been dissuaded from using one of the therapies because of the high "cost," when the apparent cost difference may have been an artifact of hospital accounting systems or bargaining power, rather than a reflection of the real value to society of the resources consumed by those procedures.

USING THE GUIDE

Ford et al[1] presented costs for the US setting for each of the 2 treatment strategies. Drug costs were obtained from the average retail prices for pharmaceuticals. Physician costs, including procedures, were obtained from the American Medical Association procedural code book and the 2003 Medicare fee schedule. The quantities of resources used (eg, number of outpatient visits, number of barium meals) were obtained from 1771 of 1924 patients enrolled in the 5 RCTs that were included in the individual patient data meta-analysis. Therefore, the accuracy of the cost estimates is likely to be more dependent on the accuracy of the unit costs than the resource-use data.

There are a number of reasons why published prices or costs that are readily available may differ from those actually incurred. One can resolve this issue only through considering the relevance of study results to a particular setting, an issue to which we shall return.

Did Investigators Consider the Timing of Costs and Consequences?

A final issue in the measurement and valuation of costs and consequences relates to the adjustment for differences in their timing. Generally, people prefer benefits sooner and prefer to postpone costs because of uncertainty about the future and because resources, if invested, usually yield a positive return.

The accepted way of allowing for this in economic evaluations is to discount costs and consequences that occur in the future to present values by assigning a lower weight to future costs and benefits. The US Panel on Cost-Effectiveness in Health and Medicine[17] proposed a 3% annual discount rate based on the inflation-adjusted rate of return on US government bonds, and this rate is the one most often used in studies undertaken in North America. There remain debates about whether health outcomes should be discounted at the same rate as costs.[20-23]

USING THE GUIDE

Ford et al[1] did not discount because the period of the analysis was only 12 months, and making adjustments for differential timing of costs and benefits within this period would have minimally affected the results. The authors point out that there are few data on the effects of the 2 strategies on the long-term history of dyspepsia, although one study with a 6-year follow-up found that the difference in resource use at 12 months appears to continue thereafter, with no difference in the symptom status. The other longer-term issue is whether the choice of strategy has any effect on the costs of, or the rate of, survival from gastric carcinoma. In the absence of long-term clinical trials, the rates of gastric cancer would have to be estimated by the use of models. If there were such an influence, the costs and effects would need to be considered formally and, being mainly in the future, they would be discounted.

WHAT ARE THE RESULTS?

What Were the Incremental Costs and Effects of Each Strategy?

Consider the costs for each treatment option, remembering that costs are the product of the quantity of a resource used and its unit cost or price. These costs should include those incurred to "produce" the treatment, such as the physician's time, nurses' time, diagnostic tests, drugs, and so forth, which we might term the up-front costs, as well as the downstream costs because of resources consumed in the future and associated with clinical events that are attributable to the therapy.

USING THE GUIDE

Ford et al[1] state that they considered both primary and secondary care costs (including primary care and outpatient consultations with dyspepsia and inpatient admissions as a consequence of dyspepsia), costs of prescribed drugs for dyspepsia (using total defined doses of acid-suppression drugs and number of courses of eradication therapy), and investigation rates (number of barium meals, upper gastrointestinal tract endoscopies, abdominal ultrasonographic scans, and breath tests). Resource use was tracked during a 1-year period, which was the follow-up time for the clinical trials included in the analysis.

The authors presented results as weighted mean difference, with a 95% *confidence interval* (CI). Endoscopy was more expensive than the test-and-treat approach by $389 (95% CI, $276-$502). The authors observed that most of this increased burden resulted from the cost of investigations in the prompt endoscopy group (weighted mean difference, $318; 95% CI, $285-$350).

The difference in the effectiveness of the 2 strategies was measured in 2 ways: total dyspepsia symptoms score and absence of dyspepsia at 12 months (expressed as a *relative risk*). Overall, 82% of the endoscopy group still had dyspepsia at 12 months compared with 86% of the test-and-treat group, corresponding to a relative risk of 0.95 (95% CI, 0.92-0.99).

A visual representation of the association between costs and effects, the cost-effectiveness plane, can highlight implications of the results (Figure 28.2-1). The horizontal axis in the plane represents the difference in effect between the experimental intervention (ie, endoscopy) and the control management strategy (ie, test and treat), and this points to the right of control, indicating superior effectiveness of the intervention. The vertical axis,

showing the difference in costs, points above control and indicates that the intervention is more costly than control. We can designate the *point estimate* of the effect and cost of our intervention as point A on the cost-effectiveness plane.

If point A is in quadrant 2, the intervention of interest is both more effective and less costly than the control strategy and therefore is *dominant* over the alternative. In quadrant 4, the opposite is true; the control is both more effective and less costly and dominates the experimental intervention. In quadrant 1, the choice depends on the maximum incremental costs (per unit of effect) one is willing to pay. In quadrant 3, the choice depends on the decrease in effectiveness one is willing to accept, given less resource consumption with the experimental intervention.

When (as is the case with endoscopy vs test and treat) the experimental intervention is both more effective and more costly (ie, in quadrant 1), one can calculate the *incremental cost-effectiveness ratio* (ICER; ie, the cost per unit benefit gained with the experimental intervention; in this case, the incremental cost per additional patient symptom-free at 12 months). In Figure 28.2-1, the slope of the line from the origin to point A represents the ICER. Choice of a threshold (the maximum one is willing to pay to gain a single unit of benefit; in this case, how much one would be willing to pay to have a single patient symptom-free at 12 months) allows one to designate the experimental intervention as cost-effective (costs do not cross the threshold) or not cost-effective (costs are greater than the threshold). In this case, the authors point out that even if one were willing to pay $1000 per patient symptom-free (which the authors consider quite a high threshold), endoscopy would still not be the preferred strategy.

FIGURE 28.2-1

The Cost-effectiveness Plane

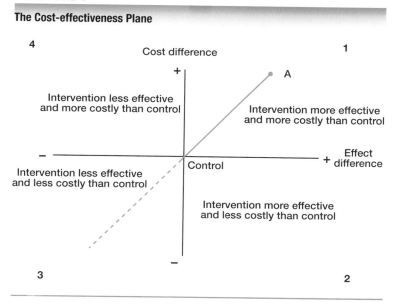

Do Incremental Costs and Effects Differ Between Subgroups?

One of our validity criteria for an economic analysis is to consider the possibility that cost-effectiveness differs across subgroups of patients. As we have observed, of particular relevance are patient groups that vary, to a large degree, in their risk of the adverse outcome that the experimental intervention is designed to prevent.

USING THE GUIDE

Ford et al[1] conducted prespecified *subgroup analyses*, examining symptom status at 12 months for patients according to sex, age (younger than 50 years or 50 years and older), predominant symptom at trial entry (epigastric pain or heartburn), and initial *H pylori* status. The analyses revealed that there was a small but *statistically significant* effect on symptoms in favor of prompt endoscopy in patients 50 years and older compared with no difference in effect in those younger than 50 years. There appeared to be no overall difference in effect between the 2 strategies for patients with predominant epigastric pain,

predominant heartburn, or initial *H pylori* status. The investigators failed to report differences in cost or cost-effectiveness by subgroup, so we do not know, for example, whether the higher effectiveness of the prompt endoscopy strategy in patients older than 50 years would make this strategy cost-effective. In the other subgroups, it is unlikely that there would be differences in cost-effectiveness, given the similarities in effectiveness.

In a climate of fiscal constraints and with many treatments providing only marginal health improvements at often substantially higher costs, it is increasingly common for researchers to conduct (and reimbursement agencies to request) subgroup analyses of the cost-effectiveness results. Such analyses can inform funding decisions overall and whether specific conditions or restrictions should be imposed.[16]

How Much Does Allowing for Uncertainty Change the Results?

The primary output of an economic analysis uses the investigators' best estimates of each of the key variables that bear on the costs and effects of the alternative management strategies (often referred to as the *base case*). Inevitably, however, there is uncertainty that arises from choices concerning the data used in the analysis, the main methodologic assumptions used in the analysis, and the desire to generalize the results to other settings. Exploring the effect of these sources of uncertainty complements consideration of possible heterogeneity of cost-effectiveness across patient subgroups that we dealt with in the previous section.

The conventional approach for handling uncertainty in economic analyses is to undertake *sensitivity analyses* in which investigators vary estimates of key variables one at a time (1-way sensitivity analysis) or together (multiway sensitivity analysis) to assess the effect on study results. However, during the last decade, there has been increasing attention devoted to identifying and analyzing different types of uncertainty (eg, methodologic, structural, parameter).[24] Investigators continue to use conventional sensitivity analysis (often called deterministic sensitivity analysis), in which variables are altered one at a time or in combination with other variables, to explore uncertainty related to methodologic assumptions (eg, discount rates or the way of estimating the cost of a test or procedure), to issues of applicability (eg, applying results to another geographic location with different practice patterns or unit costs), and for structural assumptions in a decision analytic model (eg, the number of treatment comparators or the number of dyspeptic episodes permitted per year in a model).

To illustrate how investigators address parameter uncertainty (ie, uncertainty around variables in an economic model), we draw on another economic evaluation of alternative approaches for treating patients with gastroesophageal reflux disease (GERD).[25] Gastroesophageal reflux disease is a chronic relapsing-remitting-type disease and thus has both initial treatment and secondary prevention (ie, maintenance) components. There are different drugs (eg, histamine$_2$-receptor antagonists [H$_2$RAs], proton-pump inhibitors [PPIs]), doses of drugs, and combinations of drugs that a clinician can use for long-term patient treatment. For example, although PPIs are more effective in relieving symptoms and preventing recurrence, they are considerably more expensive than H$_2$RAs. As a result, experts often advocate strategies such as step-up therapy for relapses and step-down therapy for maintenance treatment.

In this study, the authors estimated the costs and effects of 6 alternative management strategies.[25] The primary measure of effectiveness in this study was the number of weeks free of GERD symptoms during the year. An advantage of this type of outcome measure for chronic relapsing-remitting-type diseases is that it combines the probability of treatment success, the speed of treatment success, and the probability of recurrence of GERD in a single measure. Table 28.2-2 presents a summary of the cost, effects, and cost-effectiveness from this analysis.

When comparing multiple alternatives in economic evaluations, investigators begin by making their base case estimates of the costs and effects for each alternative and determining whether any of the alternatives are dominated by another or if any combination of alternatives dominates another. As indicated in Table 28.2-2, in this example, one alternative (D) was dominated by C, A, and E, and another (F) was dominated by a combination of E and B. The next step is to rank-order the nondominated strategies according to effectiveness and then calculate the ICERs of moving from one strategy to the next (see the last column of Table 28.2-2). Authors can display these cost and effectiveness results graphically on the cost-effectiveness plane (Figure 28.2-2) and also display the ICERs (shown as the sloped line segments joining strategies C, A, E, and B). Taken together, the line segments in Figure 28.2-2 are referred to as the *efficiency frontier* for treating patients with GERD. Any treatment or strategy that has a base case cost-effectiveness that is above the efficiency frontier would be considered dominated.

To explore uncertainty related to methodologic assumptions or for structural assumptions in a decision analytic model, analysts use conventional deterministic sensitivity analyses and compare the results from these analyses with the base case results (ie, Table 28.2-2 and Figure 28.2-2) to observe how sensitive the results are to changes in these model input assumptions. For parameter uncertainty, analysis of uncertainty involves generating a distribution of the possible underlying true values associated with each key variable. The investigators then allow all of these variables to vary simultaneously in the analysis. Computerized random generators repeatedly draw a random point from each distribution and for each draw generate a single cost-and-effect pair for each treatment alternative. Repeated simulations (Monte Carlo simulations) generate a large number of cost-and-effect pairs that provide estimates of the underlying uncertainty.[26] The term applied to this approach is probabilistic analysis of uncertainty or *probabilistic sensitivity analysis* (PSA). Patient-level trial data from RCTs usually provide the source for the distributions defined in a PSA model, although investigators can also use registries, administrative databases, surveys, and even expert opinion. However, the risk of bias associated with these data sources increases

TABLE 28.2-2

Base Case Cost, Effectiveness, and Cost-effectiveness Results for Alternative Strategies for Treating Patients With GERD

Strategy	Expected 1-Year Cost per Patient	Expected Weeks With (Without) GERD per Patient in 1 Year	Incremental Cost, $ (ΔC)	Incremental Effects (ΔE, No. of Weeks GERD Averted)	ΔC/ΔE
C, Maintenance H₂RA	657	10.41 (41.59)	—[a]	—[a]	—[a]
A, Intermittent PPI	678	7.778 (44.22)	21	2.63	
E, Step-down maintenance H₂RA	748	6.17 (45.83)	70[b]	1.61[b]	44[b]
B, Maintenance PPI	1093	4.82 (47.18)	345[c]	1.35[c]	256[c]
D, Step-down maintenance PA	805	12.60 (39.40)	NA[d]	NA[d]	Dominated
F, Step-down maintenance PPI	955	5.54 (46.46)	NA[d]	NA[d]	Dominated

Abbreviations: GERD, gastroesophageal reflux disease; H₂RA, histamine₂-receptor antagonist; PA, prokinetic agent; PPI, proton-pump inhibitor; NA, not available.
[a]Reference indicates the reference strategy and incremental costs, incremental effects, and cost-effectiveness are not relevant.
[b]Relative to strategy A.
[c]Relative to strategy E.
[d]Incremental costs and incremental effects are not calculated for these strategies due to dominance.

FIGURE 28.2-2

Cost-effectiveness Plane and Sensitivity Analysis on Price of H₂RAs

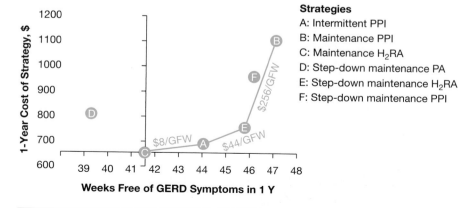

Strategies
A: Intermittent PPI
B: Maintenance PPI
C: Maintenance H₂RA
D: Step-down maintenance PA
E: Step-down maintenance H₂RA
F: Step-down maintenance PPI

Abbreviations: GERD, gastroesophageal reflux disease; GFW, GERD-free week; H₂RA, histamine₂-receptor agonist; PA, prokinetic agent; PPI, proton-pump inhibitor. Dollar amounts are Canadian dollars.

FIGURE 28.2-3

Probabilistic Sensitivity Analysis and Cost-effectiveness Acceptability Curves for GERD Management

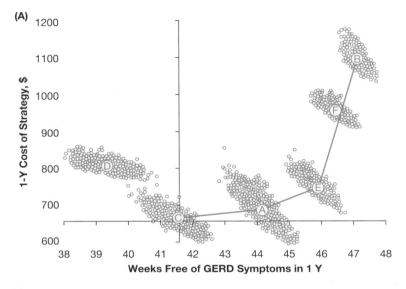

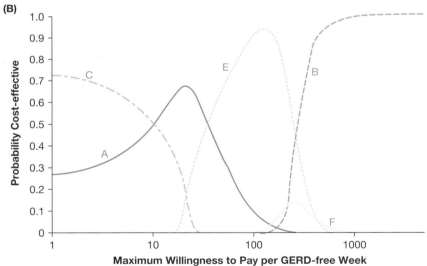

A, Probabilistic sensitivity analysis for GERD management. B, Cost-effectiveness acceptability curves for GERD management. The line segments in A represent the base case cost-effectiveness of alternative ways of treating patients with heartburn using best estimates of treatment success rates, event rates, and costs. The dots represent possible underlying true values of cost-effectiveness when fully accounting for uncertainty in these costs and outcomes. Dollar amounts are Canadian dollars. In both A and B, inset graph labels A through F represent the following test groups: A, Intermittent PPI; B, Maintenance PPI; C, Maintenance H_2RA; D, Step-down maintenance PA; E, Step-down maintenance H_2RA; F, Step-down maintenance PPI.

Abbreviations: GERD, gastroesophageal reflux disease; H_2RA, histamine$_2$-receptor agonist; PA, prokinetic agent; PPI, proton-pump inhibitor.

progressively as investigators move away from RCTs to lower-quality sources of evidence.

The results of the PSA for the GERD example by Goeree et al[25] are shown in Figure 28.2-3A. Although the representation of uncertainty in Figure 28.2-3A provides a visual image of the sampling variation in a trial-based analysis or the parameter uncertainty in a decision analytic model, this method of display is difficult to interpret for public-policy decision making. To overcome the problem for summarizing all uncertainty on a single cost-effectiveness plane, the effect of sampling variation (trials) or parameter uncertainty (models) can be expressed using *cost-effectiveness acceptability curves* (CEACs). The formula for the ICER can be rearranged into incremental net benefits (INBs) (INB = $\lambda \Delta E - \Delta C$), where λ (ceiling ratio) is the maximum amount a third-party payer or patient would be willing to pay per GERD week averted. Incremental net benefits can be applied to the sampling variation in trials or simulation results in models to estimate the probability a treatment or strategy is cost-effective for any given ceiling ratio (λ).

Figure 28.2-3B shows the CEACs for the GERD example. The CEACs are useful because all of the sampling variation or parameter uncertainty is simultaneously expressed in a single diagram, and decision makers can use their own criteria for how much they would be willing to pay to avoid a week of GERD symptoms. For example, in Figure 28.2-3B, if decision makers were willing to pay only up to $10 per GERD-free week, the preferred option would be strategy C. Between $10 and $80, the preferred option would be strategy A; between $80 and $250, strategy E; and above $250, strategy B.

HOW CAN I APPLY THE RESULTS TO PATIENT CARE?

Having established the results of the economic study and the precision of the estimates, we now turn to 2 important issues of interpretation. The first is how clinicians can interpret ICERs to help in decision making; the second is the extent to which they can apply the cost or effects from the study in their practice settings.

Are the Treatment Benefits Worth the Risks and Costs?

Having estimated the incremental effectiveness of the endoscopy strategy (in terms of dyspepsia status at 1 year) and the incremental costs and assuming for the moment that these data apply to your practice setting, how do you decide whether the extra benefits are worth the extra costs? One approach would be to compare the ICER for endoscopy vs the test-and-treat approach to other funded health care interventions. However, the specificity of the outcome—proportion of patients free of dyspeptic symptoms at 12 months—precludes such a comparison.

Another approach would be to explore what level of *willingness to pay*, per patient symptom-free of dyspepsia, would make the endoscopy strategy potentially cost-effective. The authors conduct this analysis and find the required willingness to pay to be approximately $180 000. They argue that this is not a reasonable amount and so conclude that the extra costs of the endoscopy strategy are not worth the small additional effect.

When results are not available in units that can be applied across different diseases and conditions (such as QALYs) and investigators fall back on willingness-to-pay approaches and choose a willingness-to-pay threshold (such as the amount one is willing to pay for a single patient to be symptom-free), one may disagree with the authors' threshold. In such instances, plotting of the CEAC allows one to apply one's own threshold value for willingness to pay. The decision maker can see immediately the probability that a given treatment strategy is cost-effective for different values of the willingness-to-pay threshold, as shown in Figure 28.2-3B.

Investigators have debated the validity of such interpretive strategies for ICERs and CEACs at both theoretical[27,28] and practical levels.[29] Although some health economists[27] maintain that prioritizing resource allocations based on rank-orderings of interventions by incremental cost-effectiveness leads to an efficient allocation of resources, many—citing practical problems that include different methods, data, and underlying assumptions—disagree.

Clinicians should therefore exercise caution when drawing conclusions from ICERs. The ultimate criterion is one of local opportunity cost: If the money for a new program will result in decreased ability to provide other health care interventions, what other services will be compromised and what are the consequences? For instance, what other programs' quality (such as screening colonoscopy) will decrease to use the prompt endoscopy strategy for all? One practical difficulty in choosing between alternative local programs is that many existing programs or services may not have been evaluated; therefore, the opportunity cost of reducing or removing them is unknown or speculative.

Can I Expect Similar Costs in My Setting?

If costs or consequences differ in your setting, the cost-effectiveness, utility, and benefit ratios from the study will not apply. We deal with issues of whether you can anticipate the same consequences of treatment in detail in Chapter 13.1, Applying Results to Individual Patients, and we focus here on costs.

USING THE GUIDE

In the endoscopy study by Ford et al,[1] the investigators used data from 5 pragmatic clinical trials in which the inclusion and exclusion criteria were sufficiently broad that patients likely reflect the mix of those with dyspepsia in many clinical settings. Further, given that the unit costs are presented, you should be able to judge their applicability to your own setting. Relevant prices that may vary from place to place include drugs and endoscopy (prices for which will be higher in the United States than in other jurisdictions). The authors recognized this and undertook a sensitivity analysis in which the unit cost of endoscopy is reduced from $450 to $80, a price more typical of European countries. They found that even in this situation, prompt endoscopy became cost-effective only when the willingness to pay per patient symptom-free of dyspepsia at 12 months reached $40 000. An assessment of whether the resource

use in this study applies in your own setting is more difficult. The 5 trials were conducted in England, Scotland, Wales, Denmark, and the Netherlands. Patterns of resource use might vary from country to country because of various clinical practice patterns, the availability of resources, the financial incentives faced by health care professionals and institutions, and the relative prices of resources (if one item is particularly inexpensive in a given country, it might more often be used). Ford et al[1] recognized the potential for such cross-country differences, but they argue that it is unlikely to be substantial. Reporting similar resource use across the 5 country settings would have bolstered this argument, although this would still leave doubts about applicability to the United States. At the same time, if clinicians were to follow the same management protocols tested in the trials, the result is likely to be similar resource use.

CLINICAL SCENARIO RESOLUTION

The economic analysis based on the meta-analysis suggests upper gastrointestinal tract endoscopy is more effective than the *H pylori* test-and-treat approach in curing dyspepsia symptoms at 1 year, but it is also more expensive. You decide that the costs and effects found in this article are likely to be applicable to your institution. All committee members agree that $180 000 per patient free of symptoms at 1 year is too expensive for the local hospital to fund (in fact, likely for anybody). This committee finds the practical choice they confront

even more compelling: adopting the test-and-treat approach will permit more screening colonoscopies, which studies suggest will provide greater health benefits and superior cost-effectiveness to screening endoscopy.[30] The committee decides to endorse the *H pylori* test-and-treat service for patients younger than 55 years with dyspepsia in the absence of alarm symptoms. The local hospital agrees to provide funds for 13C-urea breath-test kits and analysis so that *H pylori* can be diagnosed noninvasively.

References

1. Ford AC, Qume M, Moayyedi P, et al. *Helicobacter pylori* "test and treat" or endoscopy for managing dyspepsia: an individual patient data meta-analysis. *Gastroenterology*. 2005;128(7):1838-1844.

2. Eisenberg JM. Clinical economics. A guide to the economic analysis of clinical practices. *JAMA*. 1989;262(20):2879-2886.

3. Detsky AS, Naglie IG. A clinician's guide to cost-effectiveness analysis. *Ann Intern Med*. 1990;113(2):147-154.

4. Elixhauser A, Luce BR, Taylor WR, Reblando J. Health care CBA/CEA: an update on the growth and composition of the literature. *Med Care*. 1993;31(7 Suppl):JS1-JS11, JS18-JS149.

5. Ubel P. *Pricing Life: Why It's Time for Health Care Rationing*. Cambridge, MA: MIT Press; 2000.

6. O'Brien B, Levine M, Willan A, et al. Economic evaluation of outpatient treatment with low-molecular-weight heparin for proximal vein thrombosis. *Arch Intern Med*. 1999;159(19):2298-2304.

7. Hillman AL, Bloom BS. Economic effects of prophylactic use of misoprostol to prevent gastric ulcer in patients taking nonsteroidal anti-inflammatory drugs. *Arch Intern Med*. 1989;149(9):2061-2065.

8. Graham DY, Agrawal NM, Roth SH. Prevention of NSAID-induced gastric ulcer with misoprostol: multicentre, double-blind, placebo-controlled trial. *Lancet*. 1988;2(8623):1277-1280.

9. Hill SR, Mitchell AS, Henry DA. Problems with the interpretation of pharmacoeconomic analyses: a review of submissions to the Australian Pharmaceutical Benefits Scheme. *JAMA*. 2000;283(16):2116-2121.

10. Catherwood E, Fitzpatrick WD, Greenberg ML, et al. Cost-effectiveness of cardioversion and antiarrhythmic therapy in nonvalvular atrial fibrillation. *Ann Intern Med*. 1999;130(8):625-636.

11. de Denus S, Sanoski CA, Carlsson J, Opolski G, Spinler SA. Rate vs rhythm control in patients with atrial fibrillation: a meta-analysis. *Arch Intern Med*. 2005;165(3):258-262.

12. Marshall DA, Levy AR, Vidaillet H, et al; AFFIRM and CORE Investigators. Cost-effectiveness of rhythm versus rate control in atrial fibrillation. *Ann Intern Med*. 2004;141(9):653-661.

13. O'Brien B. Economic evaluation of pharmaceuticals. Frankenstein's monster or vampire of trials? *Med Care*. 1996;34(12)(suppl):DS99-DS108.

14. Feldman H, Gauthier S, Hecker J, et al; Donepezil MSAD Study Investigators Group. Economic evaluation of donepezil in moderate to severe Alzheimer disease. *Neurology*. 2004;63(4):644-650.

15. Mihaylova B, Briggs A, Armitage J, Parish S, Gray A, Collins R; Heart Protection Study Collaborative Group. Cost-effectiveness of simvastatin in people at different levels of vascular disease risk: economic analysis of a randomised trial in 20,536 individuals. *Lancet*. 2005;365(9473):1779-1785.

16. Goeree R, Bowen JM, Blackhouse G, et al. Economic evaluation of drug-eluting stents compared to bare metal stents using a large prospective study in Ontario. *Int J Technol Assess Health Care*. 2009;25(2):196-207.

17. Boulware LE, Jaar BG, Tarver-Carr ME, Brancati FL, Powe NR. Screening for proteinuria in US adults: a cost-effectiveness analysis. *JAMA*. 2003;290(23):3101-3114.

18. Finkler SA. The distinction between cost and charges. *Ann Intern Med*. 1982;96(1):102-109.

19. Taira DA, Seto TB, Siegrist R, Cosgrove R, Berezin R, Cohen DJ. Comparison of analytic approaches for the economic evaluation of new technologies alongside multicenter clinical trials. *Am Heart J*. 2003;145(3):452-458.

20. Parsonage M, Neuburger H. Discounting and health benefits. *Health Econ*. 1992;1(1):71-76.

21. Cairns J. Discounting and health benefits: another perspective. *Health Econ*. 1992;1(1):76-79.

22. van Hout BA. Discounting costs and effects: a reconsideration. *Health Econ*. 1998;7(7):581-594.

23. Smith DH, Gravelle H. The practice of discounting in economic evaluations of healthcare interventions. *Int J Technol Assess Health Care*. 2001;17(2):236-243.

24. Bilcke J, Beutels P, Brisson M, Jit M. Accounting for methodological, structural, and parameter uncertainty in decision-analytic models: a practical guide. *Med Decis Making*. 2011;31(4):675-692.

25. Goeree R, O'Brien BJ, Blackhouse G, Marshall J, Briggs A, Lad R. Cost-effectiveness and cost-utility of long-term management strategies for heartburn. *Value Health*. 2002;5(4):312-328.

26. Briggs A. Handling uncertainty in economic evaluation. In: Drummond M, McGuire A, eds. *Economic Evaluation in Healthcare: Merging Theory With Practice*. Oxford, England: Oxford University Press; 2001:172-214.

27. Johannesson M, Weinstein MC. On the decision rules of cost-effectiveness analysis. *J Health Econ*. 1993;12(4):459-467.

28. Birch S, Gafni A. Changing the problem to fit the solution: Johannesson and Weinstein's (mis) application of economics to real world problems. *J Health Econ*. 1993;12(4):469-476.

29. Drummond M, Torrance G, Mason J. Cost-effectiveness league tables: more harm than good? *Soc Sci Med*. 1993;37(1):33-40.

30. Sonnenberg A, Delcò F, Inadomi JM. Cost-effectiveness of colonoscopy in screening for colorectal cancer. *Ann Intern Med*. 2000;133(8):573-584.

28.3

ADVANCED TOPICS IN MOVING FROM EVIDENCE TO ACTION

Recommendations About Screening

Kirsten Jo McCaffery, Gemma Louise Jacklyn, Alexandra Barratt, John Brodersen, Paul Glasziou, Stacy M. Carter, Nicholas R. Hicks, Kirsten Howard, and Les Irwig

IN THIS CHAPTER

MOVING FROM EVIDENCE TO ACTION

You are a primary care physician advising a 50-year-old woman who is concerned because a friend of hers was recently diagnosed as having breast cancer and has urged her to undergo mammography *screening* because "it's better to be safe than sorry."

The woman does not have a family history of breast or ovarian cancer or a breast lump. She asks whether you agree that she should undergo screening. You know that trials of mammography screening support both a mortality reduction from breast cancer and the existence of *overdetection* and *false-positive* results, which may result in unnecessary investigations and overtreatment. You are unsure of the magnitude of these effects, which you know are crucial in helping your patient to make her decision. To help, you need to know how screening can be evaluated, how screening test results should be interpreted, and whether there are any valid, relevant, and up-to-date *clinical practice guidelines* or recommendations about screening for breast cancer.

In this chapter, we probe specific issues introduced in Chapter 26, How to Use a Patient Management Recommendation: Clinical Practice Guidelines and Decision Analyses, focusing on those that are specific to screening (Box 28.3-1).

BOX 28.3-1

Issues for Consideration

How serious is the risk of bias?

Is there randomized trial evidence that the intervention benefits people with asymptomatic disease?

What are the recommendations, and will they help you in caring for patients?

Were the data identified, selected, and combined in an unbiased fashion?

What are the benefits?

What are the harms?

How do benefits and harms compare in different people and with different screening strategies?

What is the effect of individuals' values and preferences?

What is the effect of uncertainty associated with the evidence?

What is the cost-effectiveness?

FINDING THE EVIDENCE

Clinical practice guidelines by the US Preventive Services Taskforce (USPSTF)[1,2] are available online. You obtain the full version of the 2002 USPSTF guidelines, including the *systematic review* on which the recommendations are based, from their website, as well the 2009 update.

SCREENING TEST RESULTS AND THEIR ASSOCIATION WITH UNDERLYING DISEASE

Table 28.3-1 presents the association between screening test results and the underlying disease or *risk* state. In group A are the people who receive *true-positive* results and have a patient-important disease. Some of this group will benefit from screening: those who receive effective treatment. For instance, children found on screening to have phenylketonuria will experience large, long-lasting benefits because treating asymptomatic disease is more effective than treating the disease once *symptoms* develop. Other people in group A will not benefit, despite having a true-positive result: this occurs when finding and treating the disease early do not provide benefit

TABLE 28.3-1

Summary of the Relation of Screening Test Results to Underlying Disease State

Screening Test Result	Reference Standard Results		
	Disease or Risk Factor Present		Disease or Risk Factor Absent
Positive	A: True positive: disease or risk factor that will cause symptoms in the future	B: True positive (inconsequential disease): disease or risk factor asymptomatic until death from another cause	C: False positive
Negative	D: False negative: missed disease that will be symptomatic in the future	E: False negative (inconsequential disease): missed disease that will be inconsequential in the future	F: True negative

Sensitivity = A + B / A + B + D + E. Specificity = F / C + F.

compared with finding and treating it later. In such cases, screening has been described as extending "disease time" rather than extending life-time.

In group B are people who have true-positive results but for a disease that will not influence their future health. These people meet current pathologic criteria for the disease, but their disease is destined not to become clinically manifest within their lifetime; in other words, they have experienced overdetection (sometimes referred to as overdiagnosis). Had they not been screened, these individuals would never have experienced symptoms, would have died of causes unrelated to the condition for which they were screened, and would never have known that they had the *target disease.*

Consider, for instance, a man in his 50s in whom screening reveals low-grade prostate cancer. He is treated for prostate cancer, develops urinary incontinence and impotence as adverse effects of treatment, and then dies in his early 80s from coronary artery disease. Unbeknown to him, he was not destined to have symptoms or die of prostate cancer. The cancer would never have been found if not for screening, and his lifespan would have been the same regardless of whether he had the screening test. Because of screening, this man had to cope with a prostate cancer diagnosis and the adverse effects of the treatment for 30 years. This is an example of overdetection with overtreatment. Such an outcome is neither hypothetical nor rare; approximately 50% of the prostate cancers found by screening in men aged 50 to 70 years would have remained clinically silent in the men's lifetimes had they not been detected by screening.[3]

In breast cancer screening, detection of some, perhaps even most, ductal carcinoma in situ (DCIS) may represent overdetection.[4] Estimates of the extent of overdetection of invasive breast cancer range from 1.7% to 54%.[5] Overdetection is especially important in breast and prostate cancer screening because the harms are immediate, whereas there is a long gap between detection and possible mortality benefits (7 to 10 years).

Screening for *risk factors* (such as high blood pressure or elevated cholesterol level) increases the likelihood of overdetection compared with screening for diseases (such as heart disease, cerebrovascular disease, and kidney disease). When screening is for risk factors, large numbers of people must be screened and treated for many years to *prevent* 1 patient-important adverse event years later.[6]

In group C are people with false-positive results (ie, a positive test result but no underlying disease, pathologic findings, or risk factors). These people may be adversely affected by the *harm* associated with investigation of the screen-detected abnormality, such as the anxiety and complications of biopsy after an abnormal mammogram result.

In group D are people with *false-negative* results of patient-important disease: these people have a negative test result despite having a disease that will later manifest itself in symptoms and possibly in reduced lifespan. They may experience harm if false reassurance results in delayed presentation or investigation of symptoms. They may feel emotional distress and anger if they discover they have a disease despite having negative screening test results, and their experience has the potential to undermine their trust in health care.

The people in group E may be considered to have a false-negative test result, but in practice they are not harmed by the incorrect result because the disease that was missed was destined to never become clinically manifest. From empirical data collected in *randomized clinical trials* (RCTs) and *cohort studies*, it is possible to get values of groups A + B, C, D, and F. However, we cannot currently say with precision what the values of groups A, B, or E are in most screening programs because of our very limited ability, at present, to distinguish inconsequential (nonprogressive) disease from biologically important disease.

Finally, in group F, people with true-negative results may experience benefit associated with an accurate reassurance of being disease free, although they may also experience inconvenience and anxiety and incur personal costs to achieve this accurate result.

HOW SERIOUS IS THE RISK OF BIAS?

To evaluate the USPSTF guidelines and update, you need to know the extent of *risk of bias*. The best way to think about screening is as a therapeutic intervention. Doing so immediately clarifies the *evidence* required to support a policy of screening: RCTs examining the effect of screening vs no screening on *patient-important outcomes*.[5,7]

Is There Randomized Trial Evidence That the Intervention Benefits People With Asymptomatic Disease?

A serious problem to consider is the possibility of bias in the evidence that screening is beneficial. One can be much more confident in guidelines recommending screening if they are based on RCTs in which screening is compared with conventional care. This is because RCTs are less likely to be biased than *observational studies* (see Chapter 6, Why Study Results Mislead: Bias and Random Error).

In the past, some screening programs have been appropriately introduced (eg, screening for phenylketonuria) on the basis of observational data because their very large *effect sizes* warranted high confidence in their impact on patient-important outcomes (see Chapter 23, Understanding and Applying the Results of a Systematic Review and Meta-analysis). However, mistakes have been made in other screening programs where the effect size was smaller than the biases introduced by observational methods. For example, neuroblastoma screening was implemented in some jurisdictions based on evidence from observational studies but was subsequently withdrawn because, in practice, harms of false-positive results and overdiagnosis far outweighed the benefits that had been overestimated in the observational studies.[8]

There are several reasons observational studies may be misleading. As noted above, survival, as measured from the time of diagnosis, may be increased not because patients live longer but because screening lengthens the time that they know they have disease (*lead-time bias*). Furthermore, people whose disease is discovered by screening may appear to do better or live longer than patients whose disease presents clinically with symptoms because screening tends to detect disease that is destined to progress slowly and that therefore has a good *prognosis* (*length-time bias*).[9]

We argue that today no screening program should be implemented without providing comprehensive evidence from RCTs about the intended benefits and the unintended harms so that an assessment of benefit vs harm can be made.

Study Designs for Randomized Trials of Screening

Investigators may choose 1 of 2 study designs to test the effect of screening. One design addresses the entire screening process (early detection and early intervention; see Figure 28.3-1) by *randomization* of people invited to screening and subsequently treated if an abnormality is detected or not screened and therefore treated only if symptomatic disease occurs. Trials of cancer screening (eg, screening for breast, colorectal, prostate, lung, and ovarian cancer) use this design.[10-14]

FIGURE 28.3-1

Designs for Randomized Clinical Trials of Screening

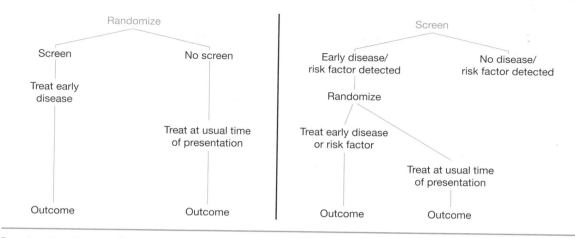

Reproduced from Barratt et al[6] with permission from *JAMA*.

Alternatively, all participants may undergo screening, and investigators randomize those with positive results to be treated or not treated (Figure 28.3-1). If those who receive treatment do better, then one can conclude that early treatment has provided benefit. Investigators usually use this study design when screening detects not the disease itself but factors that increase the risk of disease. Tests of screening programs for hypertension and high cholesterol level have used this design.[15] The principles outlined in this chapter apply to both of the study designs used in addressing screening issues (Figure 28.3-1).

Regardless of which design investigators use, RCTs of screening are always testing the combined effect of early detection plus early treatment. For a fair comparison, it is important that the follow-up diagnostic tests applied to people who screen positive and the treatment they undergo if the screening results are true positive are of the same standard and quality as the diagnostic tests and treatments available to people in the *control group*, just given earlier because of early detection. If they are better (eg, more sensitive diagnostic tests are used) then outcomes will be biased in favor of screening.

In practice, this issue has been encountered in cancer screening trials.[16]

Guidelines, to be credible, must appropriately collect, critically appraise, and analyze the evidence (or use someone else's rigorous process) (see Chapter 22, The Process of a Systematic Review and Meta-analysis). After reviewing the evidence, guideline developers should provide a summary of the evidence about benefits and harms; for example, in a balance sheet.[17] Ideally, they should also provide information about how these benefits and harms can vary in subgroups of the population and under different screening strategies. Furthermore, they should provide their judgment of the confidence in estimates of effect, which may vary from high to very low. These may differ across outcomes, and the authors should therefore provide their confidence in estimates for each outcome (see Chapter 23, Understanding and Applying the Results of a Systematic Review and Meta-analysis).

Were the Data Identified, Selected, and Combined in an Unbiased Fashion?

As is true for all guidelines, developers must specify the *inclusion criteria* and *exclusion criteria* for the

MOVING FROM EVIDENCE TO ACTION

studies they choose to consider, conduct a comprehensive search, and assess the risk of bias in the studies they include.

USING THE GUIDE

The USPSTF recommendation[1,2] is based on an assessment of the benefit of mammography screening from a systematic review of RCTs and information on the harms of screening obtained from multiple sources, including systematic reviews, *meta-analyses*, and recently published literature. Data from the Breast Cancer Surveillance Consortium from 2000 to 2005 were also used for mammography outcomes and follow-up testing. In addition, the USPSTF requested a report from the Cancer Intervention and Surveillance Modeling Network Breast Cancer Modeling Group on optimal starting and stopping ages for breast screening.

The USPSTF uses a standardized and comprehensive approach to rate evidence about screening based on its quality and the size of any net benefit. Ratings range from A (high certainty that net benefit is substantial) to B (high certainty that the net benefit is moderate or moderate certainty that the net benefit is moderate to substantial) to C (moderate certainty that the net benefit is small) to D (moderate or high certainty that harms outweigh benefit). A rating of I indicates that the current evidence is insufficient to assess the balance of benefits and harms of the service because the evidence is lacking, of poor quality, or conflicting.

The USPSTF assigned a B rating to evidence about breast cancer screening for women aged 50 to 74 years, indicating moderate certainty that the net benefit is moderate. A similar rating is obtained using *GRADE* (*Grading of Recommendations Assessment, Development and Evaluation*): There are RCTs with minimal risk of bias showing benefit, but this could be downgraded to moderate quality because of variability in risk of bias among trials, some *inconsistency* of results, *imprecision* in estimates, and incomplete assessment of harms.

WHAT ARE THE RECOMMENDATIONS, AND WILL THEY HELP IN CARING FOR PATIENTS?

USING THE GUIDE

The next step in advising the woman is to consider the balance of benefits and harms that she may experience if she proceeds with mammographic screening.

What Are the Benefits?

What outcomes must investigators measure to estimate the benefits of a screening program? If treatment is effective, some of those who test positive will experience a reduction in mortality or an increase in quality of life. One can estimate the benefit as an *absolute risk reduction* or a *relative risk reduction* (RRR) in adverse outcomes. The *number of people needed to invite to screening* (NNI) to prevent an adverse outcome provides another way of presenting benefit (see Chapter 9, Does Treatment Lower Risk? Understanding the Results).

When the benefit is a reduction in mortality, it is better if decisions are based on an understanding of reduction in both disease-specific and total mortality (ie, mortality from any and all possible causes). Because the target condition is typically only one of many causes of death, and particularly when the treatment of the screen-detected disease can have life-threatening complications (eg, aortic aneurysm repair), very large studies may be required to reveal reductions in all-cause and disease-specific mortality. So for the most part, policymakers have had to be satisfied with demonstrated reductions in disease-specific mortality only. At a minimum, investigators should collect data on all deaths in screening trials so that any increase in deaths in the screened group can be detected and explored.

In addition to *prevention* of adverse outcomes, people may also regard knowledge of the presence of an abnormality as a benefit, as in antenatal screening for Down syndrome.

Another potential benefit of screening is the reassurance afforded by a negative test result if a person is experiencing anxiety because a family member or friend has developed the target condition. However, if the screening program itself has generated the anxiety—for instance, through extensive publicity—then claiming reduction in that anxiety as a benefit of screening is very questionable.[18,19]

USING THE GUIDE

The 2002 USPSTF systematic review includes a meta-analysis of 7 mammography (plain radiographs) trials among women aged 39 to 75 years.[1] The authors report an RRR of 16% (95% CI, 9%-23%) after a mean of 14 years of *follow-up*. This is equivalent to an NNI of 1224 to prevent 1 death due to breast cancer.

There is always uncertainty about the benefits of screening. Evaluation of screening generally requires very large-scale trials to reveal a *statistically significant* effect because we are dealing with asymptomatic individuals who are at low risk of developing a relatively rare disease.

As noted earlier, most of the screening trials use disease-specific mortality as their primary outcome, so we are often left with uncertainty about the impact on all-cause mortality.[20]

USING THE GUIDE

There is also uncertainty about the *generalizability* of this evidence base to the clinical scenario in this chapter. Most of the mammography trials were conducted in the 1960s to 1980s. Since then, mammography techniques have improved,[21] and the treatments for clinically detected and screen-detected breast cancer have become much more effective, which may reduce the benefit of screening.[22] The *incidence* of DCIS has increased because of screening,[23] and the overall mortality rate from breast cancer has decreased.[1,2,24] There are also differences between the trials and international screening programs with respect to target age, screening intervals, mammography views, and follow-up time.

In general, the benefits of screening are not fixed in time and decrease as the effectiveness, safety, and availability of treatment for more advanced disease increases. If there is a safe, effective, affordable treatment for advanced disease that is readily available with few adverse effects, then the mortality benefits of screening reduce to near zero. This occurred in the case of testicular cancer, with few countries now continuing to screen. Benefits of screening also decrease as *prevalence* of the risk factor or disease decreases. In several cases, screening was originally useful but is no longer worthwhile because of reduced underlying prevalence, such as with tuberculosis screening because of the reduction in tuberculosis infections and in abdominal aortic aneurism screening when smoking rates have been substantially reduced.

What Are the Harms?

False-positive results: The USPSTF *review*[1,2] observed that test accuracy data are conventionally reported for a test at a single point, whereas for a screening program, cumulative test-positive data over time are more relevant. The cumulative risk of a false-positive result after 10 mammography examinations was reported to range from 21% to 49%. More recently, a study using Breast Cancer Surveillance Consortium data from the United States found that for women who begin screening at 40 years of age, the cumulative probability of receiving at least 1 false-positive recall after 10 years was 61.3% with annual screening compared with 41.6% with biennial screening.[25] The cumulative risk of a false-positive biopsy recommendation was 7.0% with annual screening and 4.8% with biennial screening.

Results are similar in women who begin screening at 50 years of age. The US study[25] cited above also estimated a false-positive rate of 16.3% in the initial screening round and 9.6% in subsequent rounds. This compares to the lower estimated cumulative risk of false-positive screening results in European women aged 50 to 69 years undergoing 10 biennial screening tests of 19.7%.[26]

The adverse effects associated with false-positive results are one of the main risks of mammography screening. For example, in a *qualitative study* of women with false-positive results, participants reported negative psychosocial consequences (eg, anxiety, negative effect on sleep and behavior) in the period after their abnormal screening result until they were declared free of cancer suspicion.[27] Negative effects persisted into the longer term.[26] In a quantitative *longitudinal study*, 1, 6, 18, and 36 months after their screening, women who had false-positive screening results had significantly ($P < .01$) higher (worse) mean scores than women who had not screened positive on, respectively, 12, 6, 9, and 4 of 12 dimensions of a validated questionnaire specific to psychological consequences of breast cancer screening.[28,29] There are also physical harms associated with a biopsy for a benign breast lump, including pain and scarring.[30,31]

Overdetection and overtreatment: A major harm associated with mammography screening is overdetection and the resulting overtreatment of disease that is destined to never manifest clinically. For example, a recent meta-analysis of 3 RCTs of mammography screening found that for women invited to screening, there is a 19% probability that a cancer diagnosed during the screening period is overdetected.[32] An observational study based on 30 years of US data reported a 100% increase in early-stage breast cancer, with only a very small (8%) reduction in advanced cancer, strongly suggesting that overdetection is a major consequence of mammography screening (Figure 28.3-2).[33] The removal and treatment of breast cancers that were destined to never cause symptoms or death lead to unnecessary surgery, radiotherapy, adjuvant hormone therapy, and chemotherapy, all of which carry important adverse consequences.

Harms of overdetection also include negative psychological consequences, such as increased anxiety, heightened sense of cancer risk, and negative effect on sleep behavior and sexuality. There are also adverse effects of being labeled as a cancer patient, including feelings of stigma, shame, and guilt, and wider ramifications, such as effects on relationships, family members, and insurance status.

False-negative results (missed cancers): As noted previously, among those who test negative, adverse consequences may include false reassurance and delayed presentation of later symptomatic disease. Mammography screening will detect between 61% and 89% of the cancers that occur in a population of regularly screened women.[1,2] Thus, the interval cancer rate (which includes both missed cancers

and cancers that develop de novo in the screening interval) is 11% to 39%.

Other harms: The USPSTF review[2] reports data from a systematic review of radiation-induced breast cancer. In low-dose radiation *exposure,* risk was inconsistent, whereas high-dose exposure was associated with increased risk of breast cancer.[34] A Canadian analysis found that for every 100 000 women screened annually from ages 40 to 55 years, then biennially to age 74 years, radiation exposure due to mammography would cause 86 breast cancers and 11 breast cancer deaths.[35] The introduction of digital mammography (which uses a lower radiation dose and is currently the main form of screening in the United States) should reduce the risk.[25]

People found by screening to have clinically important disease may experience a benefit from early detection and treatment, but they can also experience earlier physical and psychosocial adverse effects of treatment. Health economists have found that we often consider present benefits, harms, and costs to be more important than those that will occur in the future. That is, we discount future outcomes and costs.[36] The preference for the present over the future is more pronounced as people age.[37] There is also the societal harm of the *opportunity costs* of screening if the money could be more cost-effectively spent elsewhere in health. We address cost-effectiveness considerations later in this discussion.

Balancing Benefits and Harms

Now that you are aware of the possible benefits and harms, if the woman proceeds with screening mammography, how can these benefits and harms be balanced against one another, and how can they be evaluated for her particular situation?

Unfortunately, the USPSTF guideline[1,2] does not include information about breast cancer screening in a user-friendly format, such as a balance sheet of benefits and harms for people aged 40, 50, and 60 years who are regularly screened or not.[38] Such data[38] can be obtained by applying the rates of benefits and harms reported in RCTs to local populations and then used to develop *decision aids* for women considering screening mammography.[39,40] We have recently updated earlier estimates[38] using this approach for Australian women, and a

FIGURE 28.3-2

Effect of 3 Decades of Screening Mammography on Breast Cancer Incidence

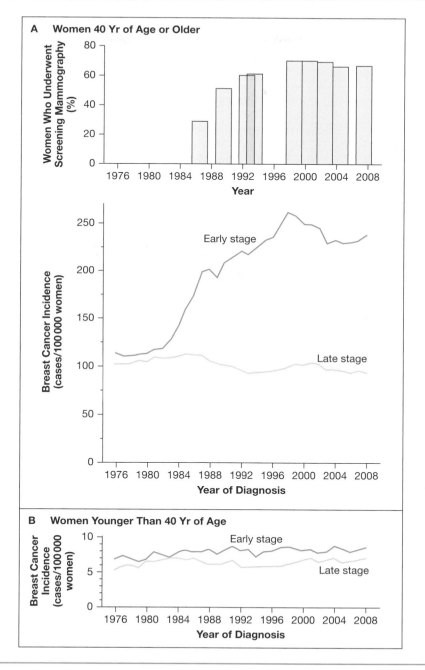

A, Self-reported use of screening mammography and the incidence of stage-specific breast cancer among women 40 years or older. B, Incidence of stage-specific breast cancer among women who generally did not have exposure to screening mammography: those younger than 40 years.

MOVING FROM EVIDENCE TO ACTION

TABLE 28.3-2

Estimates of Number of Women Among 1000 Screened Every 2 Years Who Will be Recalled, Number Diagnosed With Breast Cancer, and Number of Deaths and Confidence in Estimates

Event During 20 Years	No. of Events Among 1000 50-Year-Old Women Screened Every 2 Years for 20 Years	No. of Events Among 1000 50-Year-Old Women Who Do Not Receive Screening	Confidence in Estimates
Recalled	467		High
False-positive results	412		High
Have a biopsy	122		High
All breast cancers	73	44	High
Cancers found by screening	55		High
Invasive cancers	62	43	High
DCIS	11	1	High
Interval cancers	18		High
Overdetected cancers	19		Moderate
Total deaths	86	89	Moderate
Breast cancer deaths	8	12	Moderate

Abbreviation: DCIS, ductal carcinoma in situ.

balance sheet of outcomes for 20 years is given in Table 28.3-2 for women who begin biennial screening at 50 years of age. For example, of 1000 50-year-old women screened every 2 years for 20 years, 467 will be recalled at least once, and of those, 412 will have a false-positive and 122 will have a biopsy. Of the screened women, 73 will have a diagnosis of breast cancer as will 44 who are not screened. In the screened women, of the 73 with diagnosed breast cancer, 55 will have their cancer found by screening. Guideline committees could commission balance sheets like this when making local recommendations about screening to help in discussions with patients about screening.

The balance sheet provides perspective on the benefits and harms of breast cancer screening. It shows that screening 1000 women biennially with mammography from 50 years of age will prevent approximately 4 deaths from breast cancer during 20 years but will lead to about 412 women experiencing a false-positive result and 19 women having an overdetected cancer during the same period. We can have high confidence in most of the estimates in the table because they are obtained directly from recent screening program statistics from records of

hundreds of thousands of women. However, the estimates of the number of overdetected cancers and the estimates of the number of deaths among screened women are based on RCTs of mammography screening. Although these were reasonably good trials, they were conducted 20 to 50 years ago, and their applicability to current screening practice is uncertain.

When interpreting such balance sheets you need to consider that, unlike the presentation above, they often do not include all relevant benefits and harms that might be important to the patient. For instance, in a recent review, the most important harms of screening—overdetection and false-positive findings—were reported in only 7% and 4% of 57 cancer screening trials, respectively.[41]

We have already considered the advantage of RCT data: a reduced likelihood of bias. However, there is also a difficulty in applying trial data to real-world settings. Randomized trials often provide a better-quality screening program and subsequent intervention than are available in practice. If screening and interventions in the real world are not of the same quality as those in the trials, the benefits will be smaller and the harms will be greater than the ones calculated from trial data.

How Do Benefits and Harms Compare in Different People and With Different Screening Strategies?

The USPSTF update[2] recommends screening for women aged 50 to 74 years but does not assign any rating (strong to weak) to that recommendation. Using the GRADE approach, one would lean toward a weak recommendation because of variability in trial quality and results, uncertainty about the balance of benefit to harm, and variability in women's *values and preferences* in relation to the benefit and harms of screening. This suggests that informed, individual decision making could be appropriate.

Because breast cancer incidence and mortality increase substantially with age, the magnitude of benefits and harms will vary for women according to their age. Indeed, the USPSTF[2] recommends that the decision to start before the age of 50 years should be an individual one and take the woman's context into account, including the woman's values regarding specific benefits and harms. The balance of benefit to harm also depends on other factors, such as screening interval, screening test, and strategy, as the following discussion reveals.

It is important to keep in mind that the benefits of screening are experienced at some point in the future, whereas harms may be experienced at any time, including immediately after the first screening.

Risk of Disease

The probability that the woman will benefit from screening depends on her underlying risk of disease. Assuming that the RRR is constant over a broad range of risk of disease, benefits will be greater for people at higher risk of disease. For example, mortality from breast cancer increases with age, and the mortality benefit achieved by screening increases accordingly.[2] However, the life-years lost to breast cancer are related both to the age at which mortality is highest and the length of life still available.

Factors such as a family history may increase risk of disease and therefore increase the benefits from screening. The USPSTF[1,2] focuses only on average-risk people without an identified BRCA1 or BRCA2 mutation. Assessment of the benefits vs harms of screening in women from families at very high risk because of known mutations is very different. Such

women, who may have a lifetime risk of breast cancer of 26% to 84%,[42] may be referred to genetic counseling clinics or a clinical geneticist for testing and advice on prophylactic options, such as prophylactic mastectomy and oophorectomy. However, BRCA1 and BRCA2 mutations are very rare in the population (identified in less than 1% of the population overall and approximately 5% of women diagnosed as having breast cancer). Guidance on assessment of risk is available for women in this category. See, for example, the US National Cancer Institute's Breast Cancer Risk Assessment Tool.[43] This is not relevant to the woman who has asked your advice because she has no family history of breast or ovarian cancer.

Screening Interval

The probability that this woman will obtain a net benefit from screening depends on when she begins screening and how often she is screened (the screening interval). As the screening interval gets shorter, the detection rate (*sensitivity*) of a screening program and hence its potential effectiveness at cancer detection will improve.

Benefits, however, rarely increase in direct inverse proportion to reductions in screening interval. For example, one might expect screening twice as often to potentially double the relative mortality reduction obtainable by screening. In practice, however, the effect is usually much less. Cervical cancer screening, for instance, may reduce the incidence of invasive cervical cancer among women aged 55 to 69 years by 83%, 87%, and 87% if screening is conducted at 5-year, 3-year, and 2-year intervals, respectively.[44]

In contrast, the frequency of harms tends to increase in direct proportion to the number of screening tests a person receives. The consequence is that the marginal return (if any) of increasing screening intervals decreases as the screening interval is shortened. Ultimately, the marginal harms will outweigh the marginal benefit of further reductions in the screening interval. For example, modeling performed for the USPSTF assessment of the benefits and harms of mammography screening revealed that biennial screening maintained most (80%) of the mortality benefits of annual screening, but with fewer false-positive results and less overdetection.[45]

Extending the screening interval and/or changing the starting age of screening have been used in some screening programs to reduce the potential harms of screening, including overdetection and overtreatment. For example, the UK National Screening Committee increased the starting age for cervical screening to 25 years to reduce the overdetection of high-grade lesions in young women that would otherwise spontaneously regress. A large, population-based study in the United Kingdom found that screening women aged 20 to 24 years made virtually no difference in cancer rates among women up to aged 30 years when comparing women who were screened with those who were not.[46] However, there is evidence of long-term psychosocial harm (eg, worry, anxiety, guilt, and concerns about infertility and relationships), economic costs (eg, treatment and sick leave), and potential physical harm with the treatment of the cervix linked to perinatal mortality and adverse pregnancy outcomes.[47-50]

Test Characteristics

Even with the same underlying risk, starting age, and screening interval, the woman seeking your advice will obtain a different net benefit, depending on the sensitivity and *specificity* of the test used to screen her for breast cancer. This is a particular issue as new tests are released and marketed for screening purposes. If the apparent sensitivity of a new test is greater than that of the test used in existing trials and if it is detecting significant disease earlier, the benefit of screening will increase (see Chapter 18, Diagnostic Tests). It may be, however, that the new, more sensitive test is detecting more cases of clinically irrelevant disease—for example, by detecting more low-grade prostate cancers or more low-grade cervical epithelial abnormalities[51]—which will increase the potential for harm.[51] This increased sensitivity will be misleading if it does not increase the sensitivity to disease that is destined to become clinically manifest. If specificity is improved and testing produces fewer false-positive results, the net benefit will increase and the test may now be useful in groups in which the old test was not as useful.[52]

A relatively new technology that may improve breast cancer detection (by improving both sensitivity and specificity compared with mammography) is digital breast tomosynthesis or 3-dimensional mammography.[53] As yet, however, we do not know how much the increase in sensitivity is related to cancers that will never become clinically manifest (overdetection) vs those that will.[53,54] In screening for breast cancer in selected high-risk women, magnetic resonance imaging (MRI) has been found to have increased sensitivity (but lower specificity) compared with mammography. However, there is also emerging evidence that MRI may contribute to overdetection and may not improve patient outcomes.[55-57]

USING THE GUIDE

For an average-risk woman like the woman who has sought your advice, you would likely not recommend other screening modalities at this time.[55,56]

The benefits and harms of screening may also change if the threshold used to identify an abnormal result is increased or reduced. For example, in abdominal aortic aneurysm (AAA) screening, authorities have proposed lowering the threshold from 30 to 25 mm in the screening program.[58] However, only 15% of the men initially identified as having an aortic diameter of 25 to 29 mm develop an aortic diameter sufficient to require surgery (>54 mm) in 10 years.[59] This indicates that lowering the threshold will lead to a substantial increase of overdetection of harmless AAAs, resulting in more than a doubling of the incidence of AAA. This changes the number of individuals identified in groups A through E (Table 28.3-1) and the net balance of benefits and harms.

What Is the Effect of Values and Preferences?

Different people hold different values and preferences (see Chapter 27, Decision Making and the Patient). For example, couples considering fetal screening for Down syndrome may make different choices, depending on the value they place on knowing if their child will have Down syndrome vs the risk of iatrogenic abortion from amniocentesis.[60]

The woman's values about the range of potential breast screening benefits and harms will inform her own assessment of the best decision. She will also have a preference for the method of decision making and may want to analyze information and choose for herself. She may find decision making challenging and prefer to trust a physician to advise her on what to do, or she may want to engage in shared decision making with support from her physician.[61]

If she wants to understand the probabilities of harm or benefit in detail and make an independent or shared decision, a high-quality decision aid can provide balanced information about difficult decisions in a format that is easy for her to understand.[61] Decision aids have already been widely evaluated for treatment decisions and have been found to increase knowledge and reduce decisional conflict without increasing anxiety (see Chapter 27, Decision Making and the Patient). Increasingly, investigators are developing patient decision aids for screening decisions.[39,40,62]

What if the woman prefers to be helped by a trusted person to consider an offer of screening? Entwistle and colleagues,[63] who developed the Consider an Offer approach, suggest that such a conversation might include the following:

- Who made the recommendation or offer?
- What is the basis of the recommendation, and what are the main benefits and harms of screening?
- Are there any factors that make the screening test more appropriate for some people than others?
- Who might gain from screening and how are people protected?
- Does this person need more information?

This conversation would provide less detailed epidemiologic information than a decision aid. However, it would help patients guard against screening offers that may not be in their best interests by, for example, contrasting offers made by unscrupulous commercial providers with those made by reputable professional providers or by determining whether the patient is in an age group for which the test is not recommended. The Consider an Offer approach has recently influenced population screening programs in the United Kingdom.[64] Consider an Offer invitations for screening do not encourage screening or simply offer information about benefits and harms. Rather, as shown in the list above, the information provided acknowledges other drivers of decision making and recognizes that not accepting the offer of screening can be a reasonable choice.

What Is the Cost-Effectiveness?

Although clinicians will be most interested in the balance of benefits and harms for the individual screening participant, policymakers must consider issues of cost-effectiveness and local resources in their decisions (see Chapter 28.2, Economic Analysis).

Early cost-effectiveness estimates for mammography screening were very favorable—the UK Forrest Report (1987) estimated that screening would cost £3309 per *quality-adjusted life-year* (QALY) gained (approximately equivalent to £8094 today).[65] US cost-effectiveness estimates were $15 000 to $20 000 per life-year saved (LYS) for annual screening for women aged 50 to 69 years in the 1990s.[66,67]

Incremental cost-effectiveness ratios were higher (ie, less cost-effective) for screening younger women (because of lower incidence and lower effectiveness) and older women (because of competing mortality). These estimates compared favorably with cost-effectiveness estimates for other preventive and therapeutic interventions at the time (eg, the cost-effectiveness estimate for antihypertension medication was $15 000 per LYS[67,68]; for coronary artery bypass surgery, $28 000 per LYS; and for car seat belts and airbags, $32 000 per LYS).

These early estimates did not, however, include costs of overdetection and overtreatment plus the potential cost from negative psychosocial consequences of false-positive results. They were based on screening delivering large mortality benefits, whereas more recent estimates[1,2] have been much more modest. A recent study, including overdetection and overtreatment and a current estimate of mortality reduction, reported a cost-effectiveness ratio for triennial screening (compared with no screening) at £20 800 per QALY gained,[65] still a generally acceptable cost-effectiveness ratio (see Chapter 28.2, Economic Analysis).[65]

CLINICAL SCENARIO RESOLUTION

Returning to our opening clinical scenario, you inform the woman that the USPSTF guidelines recommend biennial screening mammography for women aged 50 to 74 years but that it would be very reasonable to either follow the guidelines and choose to be screened or make an informed decision considering the benefit and harms herself.

The task facing you and her in shared decision making—should she decide to take the second option—is to weigh the benefit of reduced risk of death from breast cancer against the risks of potentially adverse consequences. These adverse consequences include the high probability of a false-positive result arising from the screening, the risk of an overdetected breast cancer and the adverse effects of treatment for the cancer, as well

as the cost and anxiety generated by the investigations and treatment.

You could consider helping her clarify her values about the possible outcomes. For example, if the patient is not bothered by the prospect of regular mammograms and is happy to be screened knowing that if an abnormality is detected there is a risk that it could be overdetected and overtreated, she would probably choose to be screened. However, if she places a high value on avoiding unnecessary investigations and treatment, she may prefer to reconsider screening in a few years' time when the benefits will be greater or decrease altogether. Guiding her to online resources to support informed decision making about breast cancer screening is also an option.[69,70]

References

1. Humphrey LL, Helfand M, Chan BK, Woolf SH. Breast cancer screening: a summary of the evidence for the U.S. Preventive Services Task Force. *Ann Intern Med*. 2002;137(5, pt 1):347-360.

2. Nelson HD, Tyne K, Naik A, et al. Screening for breast cancer: an update for the U.S. Preventive Services Task Force. *Ann Intern Med*. 2009;151(10):727-737.

3. Barry MJ, Mulley AJ Jr. Why are a high overdiagnosis probability and a long lead time for prostate cancer screening so important? *J Natl Cancer Inst*. 2009;101(6):362-363.

4. Ernster VL, Ballard-Barbash R, Barlow WE, et al. Detection of ductal carcinoma in situ in women undergoing screening mammography. *J Natl Cancer Inst*. 2002;94(20):1546-1554.

5. Biesheuvel C, Barratt A, Howard K, Houssami N, Irwig L. Effects of study methods and biases on estimates of invasive breast cancer overdetection with mammography screening: a systematic review. *Lancet Oncol*. 2007;8(12):1129-1138.

6. Khaw KT, Rose G. Cholesterol screening programmes: how much potential benefit? *BMJ*. 1989;299(6699):606-607.

7. Sackett DL, Haynes RB, Tugwell P. *Clinical Epidemiology: A Basic Science for Clinical Medicine*. 2nd ed. Boston, MA: Little, Brown & Co; 1991.

8. Evans I, Thornton H, Chalmers I, Glasziou P. *Testing Treatments: Better Research for Better Healthcare*. 2nd ed. London, England: Pinter & Martin; 2011.

9. American College of Physicians. Finding and redefining disease. *Effective Clinical Practice*. March/April 1999. http://www.acponline.org/clinical_information/journals_publications/ecp/marapr99/primer.htm. Accessed March 31, 2014.

10. Anttila A, Koskela J, Hakama M. Programme sensitivity and effectiveness of mammography service screening in Helsinki, Finland. *J Med Screen*. 2002;9(4):153-158.

11. Zahl PH, Strand BH, Maehlen J. Incidence of breast cancer in Norway and Sweden during introduction of nationwide screening: prospective cohort study. *BMJ*. 2004;328(7445):921-924.

12. Hewitson P, Glasziou P, Watson E, Towler B, Irwig L. Cochrane systematic review of colorectal cancer screening using the fecal occult blood test (hemoccult): an update. *Am J Gastroenterol*. 2008;103(6):1541-1549.

13. Prorok PC, Andriole GL, Bresalier RS, et al; Prostate, Lung, Colorectal and Ovarian Cancer Screening Trial Project Team. Design of the Prostate, Lung, Colorectal and Ovarian (PLCO) Cancer Screening Trial. *Control Clin Trials*. 2000;21(6)(suppl):273S-309S.

14. Schröder FH, Hugosson J, Roobol MJ, et al; ERSPC Investigators. Screening and prostate-cancer mortality in a randomized European study. *N Engl J Med*. 2009;360(13):1320-1328.

15. Frick MH, Elo O, Haapa K, et al. Helsinki Heart Study: primary-prevention trial with gemfibrozil in middle-aged men with dyslipidemia: safety of treatment, changes in risk factors, and incidence of coronary heart disease. *N Engl J Med*. 1987;317(20):1237-1245.

16. Riboe DG, Dogan TS, Brodersen J. Potential biases in colorectal cancer screening using faecal occult blood test. *J Eval Clin Pract*. 2013;19(2):311-316.

17. Eddy DM. Comparing benefits and harms: the balance sheet. *JAMA*. 1990;263(18):2493-2505, 2498, 2501 passim.

18. Brodersen J, Siersma V, Ryle M. Breast cancer screening: "reassuring" the worried well? *Scand J Public Health*. 2011;39(3):326-332.

19. Ostero J, Siersma V, Brodersen J. Breast cancer screening implementation and reassurance. *Eur J Public Health*. 2014;24(2):258-263.

20. Sigurdsson JA, Getz L, Sjönell G, Vainiomäki P, Brodersen J. Marginal public health gain of screening for colorectal cancer: modelling study, based on WHO and national databases in the Nordic countries. *J Eval Clin Pract*. 2013;19(2):400-407.

21. Pisano ED, Gatsonis C, Hendrick E, et al; Digital Mammographic Imaging Screening Trial (DMIST) Investigators Group. Diagnostic performance of digital versus film mammography for breast-cancer screening. *N Engl J Med*. 2005;353(17):1773-1783.

22. Peto R, Davies C, Godwin J, et al; Early Breast Cancer Trialists' Collaborative Group (EBCTCG). Comparisons between different polychemotherapy regimens for early breast cancer: meta-analyses of long-term outcome among 100,000 women in 123 randomised trials. *Lancet*. 2012;379(9814):432-444.

23. Kerlikowske K. Epidemiology of ductal carcinoma in situ. *J Natl Cancer Inst Monogr*. 2010;2010(41):139-141.

24. Siegel R, Naishadham D, Jemal A. Cancer statistics, 2012. *CA Cancer J Clin*. 2012;62(1):10-29.

25. Hubbard RA, Kerlikowske K, Flowers CI, Yankaskas BC, Zhu W, Miglioretti DL. Cumulative probability of false-positive recall or biopsy recommendation after 10 years of screening mammography: a cohort study. *Ann Intern Med*. 2011;155(8):481-492.

26. Hofvind S, Ponti A, Patnick J, et al; EUNICE Project and Euroscreen Working Groups. False-positive results in mammographic screening for breast cancer in Europe: a literature review and survey of service screening programmes. *J Med Screen*. 2012;19(suppl 1):57-66.

27. Brodersen J, Thorsen H. Consequences of Screening in Breast Cancer (COS-BC): development of a questionnaire. *Scand J Prim Health Care*. 2008;26(4):251-256.

28. Brodersen J, Thorsen H, Kreiner S. Validation of a condition-specific measure for women having an abnormal screening mammography. *Value Health*. 2007;10(4):294-304.

29. Brodersen J, Siersma VD. Long-term psychosocial consequences of false-positive screening mammography. *Ann Fam Med*. 2013;11(2):106-115.

30. Yazici B, Sever AR, Mills P, Fish D, Jones SE, Jones PA. Scar formation after stereotactic vacuum-assisted core biopsy of benign breast lesions. *Clin Radiol*. 2006;61(7):619-624.

31. Zagouri F, Sergentanis TN, Gounaris A, et al. Pain in different methods of breast biopsy: emphasis on vacuum-assisted breast biopsy. *Breast*. 2008;17(1):71-75.

32. Independent UK Panel on Breast Cancer Screening. The benefits and harms of breast cancer screening: an independent review. *Lancet*. 2012;380(9855):1778-1786.

33. Bleyer A, Welch HG. Effect of three decades of screening mammography on breast-cancer incidence. *N Engl J Med*. 2012;367(21):1998-2005.

34. Armstrong K, Moye E, Williams S, Berlin JA, Reynolds EE. Screening mammography in women 40 to 49 years of age: a systematic review for the American College of Physicians. *Ann Intern Med*. 2007;146(7):516-526.

35. Yaffe MJ, Mainprize JG. Risk of radiation-induced breast cancer from mammographic screening. *Radiology*. 2011;258(1):98-105.

36. Shiell A, Donaldson C, Mitton C, Currie G. Health economic evaluation. *J Epidemiol Community Health*. 2002;56(2):85-88.

37. Peters E, Diefenbach MA, Hess TM, Västfjäll D. Age differences in dual information-processing modes: implications for cancer decision making. *Cancer*. 2008;113(12)(suppl):3556-3567.

38. Barratt A, Howard K, Irwig L, Salkeld G, Houssami N. Model of outcomes of screening mammography: information to support informed choices. *BMJ*. 2005;330(7497):936-940.

39. Mathieu E, Barratt A, Davey HM, McGeechan K, Howard K, Houssami N. Informed choice in mammography screening: a randomized trial of a decision aid for 70-year-old women. *Arch Intern Med*. 2007;167(19):2039-2046.

40. Mathieu E, Barratt AL, McGeechan K, Davey HM, Howard K, Houssami N. Helping women make choices about mammography screening: an online randomized trial of a decision aid for 40-year-old women. *Patient Educ Couns*. 2010;81(1):63-72.

41. Heleno B, Thomsen MF, Rodrigues DS, Jørgensen KJ, Brodersen J. Quantification of harms in cancer screening trials: literature review. *BMJ*. 2013;347:f5334.

42. Malone KE, Daling JR, Doody DR, et al. Prevalence and predictors of BRCA1 and BRCA2 mutations in a population-based study of breast cancer in white and black American women ages 35 to 64 years. *Cancer Res*. 2006;66(16):8297-8308.

43. US National Cancer Institute. Breast cancer risk assessment tool. http://www.cancer.gov/bcrisktool. Updated March 16, 2011. Accessed March 31, 2014.

44. Sasieni P, Adams J, Cuzick J. Benefit of cervical screening at different ages: evidence from the UK audit of screening histories. *Br J Cancer*. 2003;89(1):88-93.

45. Mandelblatt JS, Cronin KA, Bailey S, et al; Breast Cancer Working Group of the Cancer Intervention and Surveillance Modeling Network. Effects of mammography screening under different screening schedules: model estimates of potential benefits and harms. *Ann Intern Med*. 2009;151(10):738-747.

46. Sasieni P, Castanon A, Cuzick J. Effectiveness of cervical screening with age: population based case-control study of prospectively recorded data. *BMJ*. 2009;339:b2968.

47. Arbyn M, Kyrgiou M, Simoens C, et al. Perinatal mortality and other severe adverse pregnancy outcomes associated with treatment of cervical intraepithelial neoplasia: meta-analysis. *BMJ*. 2008;337:a1284.

48. Ferenczy A, Choukroun D, Arseneau J. Loop electrosurgical excision procedure for squamous intraepithelial lesions of the cervix: advantages and potential pitfalls. *Obstet Gynecol*. 1996;87(3):332-337.

49. Kyrgiou M, Koliopoulos G, Martin-Hirsch P, Arbyn M, Prendiville W, Paraskevaidis E. Obstetric outcomes after conservative treatment for intraepithelial or early invasive cervical lesions: systematic review and meta-analysis. *Lancet*. 2006;367(9509):489-498.

50. International Agency for Research on Cancer. Cervix cancer screening. In: *Handbooks of Cancer Prevention*. Lyon, France: International Agency for Research on Cancer; 2005.

51. Raffle AE. New tests in cervical screening. *Lancet*. 1998;351(9098):297.

52. Irwig L, Houssami N, Armstrong B, Glasziou P. Evaluating new screening tests for breast cancer. *BMJ*. 2006;332(7543):678-679.

MOVING FROM EVIDENCE TO ACTION

53. Ciatto S, Houssami N, Bernardi D, et al. Integration of 3D digital mammography with tomosynthesis for population breast-cancer screening (STORM): a prospective comparison study. *Lancet Oncol*. 2013;14(7):583-589.

54. Houssami N, Skaane P. Overview of the evidence on digital breast tomosynthesis in breast cancer detection. *Breast*. 2013;22(2):101-108.

55. Irwig L, Houssami N, van Vliet C. New technologies in screening for breast cancer: a systematic review of their accuracy. *Br J Cancer*. 2004;90(11):2118-2122.

56. Morrow M, Waters J, Morris E. MRI for breast cancer screening, diagnosis, and treatment. *Lancet*. 2011;378(9805):1804-1811.

57. Brennan ME, Houssami N, Lord S, et al. Magnetic resonance imaging screening of the contralateral breast in women with newly diagnosed breast cancer: systematic review and meta-analysis of incremental cancer detection and impact on surgical management. *J Clin Oncol*. 2009;27(33):5640-5649.

58. Thompson SG, Ashton HA, Gao L, Buxton MJ, Scott RA; Multicentre Aneurysm Screening Study (MASS) Group. Final follow-up of the Multicentre Aneurysm Screening Study (MASS) randomized trial of abdominal aortic aneurysm screening. *Br J Surg*. 2012;99(12):1649-1656.

59. Darwood R, Earnshaw JJ, Turton G, et al. Twenty-year review of abdominal aortic aneurysm screening in men in the county of Gloucestershire, United Kingdom. *J Vasc Surg*. 2012;56(1):8-13.

60. Fletcher J, Hicks NR, Kay JD, Boyd PA. Using decision analysis to compare policies for antenatal screening for Down's syndrome. *BMJ*. 1995;311(7001):351-356.

61. O'Connor AM, Rostom A, Fiset V, et al. Decision aids for patients facing health treatment or screening decisions: systematic review. *BMJ*. 1999;319(7212):731-734.

62. Smith SK, Trevena L, Simpson JM, Barratt A, Nutbeam D, McCaffery KJ. A decision aid to support informed choices about bowel cancer screening among adults with low education: randomised controlled trial. *BMJ*. 2010;341:c5370.

63. Entwistle VA, Carter SM, Trevena L, Flitcroft K, Irwig L, McCaffery K, et al. Communicating about screening. *BMJ*. 2008;337:a1591.

64. National Health Service. *Approach to developing information about NHS Cancer Screening Programmes UK*. London, England: National Health Service; 2012.

65. Pharoah PD, Sewell B, Fitzsimmons D, Bennett HS, Pashayan N. Cost effectiveness of the NHS breast screening programme: life table model. *BMJ*. 2013;346:f2618.

66. Rosenquist CJ, Lindfors KK. Screening mammography in women aged 40-49 years: analysis of cost-effectiveness. *Radiology*. 1994;191(3):647-650.

67. Feig S. Cost-effectiveness of mammography, MRI, and ultrasonography for breast cancer screening. *Radiol Clin North Am*. 2010;48(5):879-891.

68. Tengs TO, Adams ME, Pliskin JS, et al. Five-hundred life-saving interventions and their cost-effectiveness. *Risk Anal*. 1995;15(3):369-390.

69. Gøtzsche PC, Hartling OJ, Neilsen M, Brodersen J. *Screening for Breast Cancer with Mammography*. 2nd ed. København, Denmark: The Nordic Cochrane Centre; 2012.

70. National Health Service. Informed choice about cancer screening. In: *NHS breast screening: helping you decide*. London, England: National Health Services; 2013.

28.4

ADVANCED TOPICS IN MOVING FROM EVIDENCE TO ACTION

Understanding Class Effects

Edward J. Mills, David Gardner, Kristian Thorlund, Matthias Briel, Heiner C. Bucher, Stirling Bryan, Brian Hutton, and Gordon Guyatt

IN THIS CHAPTER

CLINICAL SCENARIO

As a cost-cutting strategy, your hospital's Pharmacy and Therapeutics Committee is recommending a strategy wherein drugs within the same class can be substituted at the level of the pharmacy for the generic or least costly within-class option. As a physician dealing predominantly with cardiovascular prevention, this would have important implications on your practice. Your clinical team questions the new policy, and several members argue that assuming that drugs with a similar chemical structure exert similar effect on *patient-important outcomes* without direct *evidence* is misguided. Statins are the most widely prescribed drug within your practice, and you wonder whether there is a therapeutic *class effect* for statins.

LOOKING FOR EVIDENCE OF A CLASS EFFECT

Determining whether drugs within a class exhibit similar or different therapeutic profiles can be challenging. Typically, a decision on whether a drug acts similarly to other agents with a similar biological makeup is based on an evaluation of the empirical data and pharmacopathophysiologic reasoning. Because of the inadequacies of the former and the subjective nature of the latter, a rigorous and reproducible process is required to support the establishment of whether biologically similar drugs exert a class effect.

An underlying assumption when examining class effects—an assumption that may or may not be accurate—is that each drug offers similar therapeutic efficacy and safety. However, the methods for determining this are not well established.[1] Determining whether a drug is sufficiently similar to another drug should be based on its evidence profile rather than on its name or biological mechanism of action alone.

Using a series of methodologic questions, we review the clinical example of 3-hydroxy-methyl-3-methylglutaryl coenzyme A reductase

inhibitors (statins) to determine whether therapeutic substitution offers patients a sufficiently similar efficacy-safety profile to justify interchangeable use of different statins. We chose statins as the example because they have been well evaluated in more than 80 *randomized clinical trials* (RCTs) addressing patient-important outcomes,[2] they are one of the most widely prescribed drugs in the history of modern medicine, and they are used for both primary and secondary cardiovascular disease (CVD) *prevention*.[3,4]

ARE THE AGENTS BIOLOGICALLY SIMILAR?

There is no uniformly accepted definition of a class effect.[1] Although the exact mechanism of action of drugs is rarely known, the biological target of a drug may be well established. For example, although all pharmacologic antihypertensives reduce blood pressure, there are several unrelated putative mechanisms involved (such as natriuresis with diuretics, inhibition of vascular cellular calcium influx with calcium channel blockers, and impaired synthesis of the vasoconstrictor angiotensin II with angiotensin-converting enzyme inhibitors). Although these different mechanisms may result in similar changes in blood pressure, their ultimate effect on cardiovascular morbidity and mortality may—and, in this case, do—differ.[5,6] Clinical effects may differ even when 2 medications share the same primary pharmacologic action. For example, different β-blockers may not be equivalent in their ability to limit cardiovascular event risk despite their shared mechanism of action.[7]

THE BIOLOGICAL AGENT

Previously, statins were understood to derive their beneficial effects from their ability to lower low-density lipoprotein (LDL) levels—the greater the LDL reduction, the greater the clinical benefit in terms of risk reduction for CVD events.[8,9] Subsequently, other actions have been associated with statin benefits, including reduced vascular inflammation, improved endothelial function, and decreased thrombus formation.[10-12] How different statins compare regarding these effects is less well established, raising uncertainties about a class effect and clinical interchangeability.

Differences in drug interactions, via cytochrome P450 (CYP) metabolism, have been well established and may result in differing effects on patient-important outcomes.[13] Cytochrome P3A4 is predominantly responsible for metabolism of lovastatin, simvastatin, atorvastatin, and cerivastatin, whereas CYP2C9 predominantly metabolizes fluvastatin (as do CYP3A4 and CYP2C8).[14] Rosuvastatin uses mostly CYP2C9, and pravastatin is not predominantly metabolized by any CYP isoenzymes.[14] An automatic therapeutic substitution for the statin with the lowest drug interaction risk would be desirable to avoid the dose-related adverse effects of the statin when combined with, for example, selected protease inhibitors, which are potent CYP3A4 metabolic pathway inhibitors, in patients with human immunodeficiency virus (HIV) and AIDS.[15]

If one statin automatically replaces another when an individual is hospitalized, for example, determining the equivalent dose is often a challenge. The approved dosing ranges across statins may not offer equal efficacy, tolerability, or safety moving from the lowest to the highest approved (or clinically used) doses.[16] For example, although the Pravastatin or Atorvastatin Evaluation and Infection Therapy (PROVE-IT) trial[17] found better outcomes with atorvastatin at 80 mg/d (its maximum recommended dose), compared with pravastatin at 40 mg/d (its usual but not maximum dose), it is not known how these 2 statins compare at their respective maximum doses of 80 mg/d.

IS THERE POTENTIALLY COMPELLING EVIDENCE FOR A CLASS EFFECT?

What Is the Geometry of Evidence for Your Evaluation?

Determining whether a drug exerts a therapeutic or harmful effect compared with no treatment or another treatment is often complex (see Chapter 28.3, Recommendations About Screening).[2] Multiple sources inform our decision making, and one or even a few RCTs are often insufficient to provide irrefutable evidence of a drug's comparative safety or effectiveness.[18] The amount of information available for the different potential interventions will vary, and *indirect evidence* from RCTs may provide the best evidence for some comparisons (see Chapter 24, Network Meta-analysis). For instance, one way of showing that a drug is superior to another is to conduct a head-to-head comparison (direct comparison) choosing an optimal dose of the favored drug and a suboptimal dose of the less favored drug.[19,20] Under such circumstances, an indirect comparison of optimal doses of both drugs in comparison with a *placebo* may provide a more accurate picture of their relative effect.[19] Figure 28.4-1 displays an example geometric distribution of the available randomized trials of therapies used for chronic obstructive pulmonary disease.[21] The figure displays the complexity of the network and also illustrates where connections within a network may be weak, moderate, or strong.

Are There Head-To-Head (Direct) Comparisons Warranting High Confidence?

Evidence of the therapeutic similarity of drugs rarely comes from a single trial.[22] Rather, a large body of evidence, including multiple RCTs with placebo and active comparators, needs to be considered.[23] The best evidence comes from head-to-head (direct) evidence from large RCTs evaluating the agents at their usual doses. However, when considering multiple alternative agents for a target condition, the availability of this type of information is the exception rather than the rule. Available data generally involve comparisons with placebo, in fixed-dose and flexible-dose trials, in which demonstrating *statistical significance*

FIGURE 28.4-1

Complex Network of Trials Evaluating COPD Medications

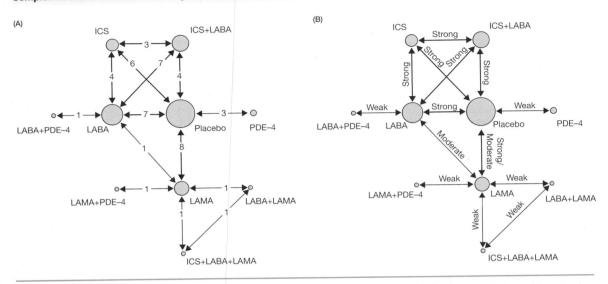

A, Example of a complex network for the evaluation of COPD medications. B, The same network displaying the connectedness of the network. In this figure, the lines represent where there is direct evidence from head-to-head comparisons in randomized clinical trials. The size of each node represents the relative number of patients per node. The number of trials, the connectedness of the network, and the number of patients in each comparison will determine whether the comparisons will provide strong, moderate, or weak inferences.

Abbreviations: COPD, chronic obstructive pulmonary disease; ICS, inhaled corticosteroids; LABA, long-acting β-agonists; LAMA, long-acting muscarinic agents; PDE-4, phosphodiesterase type 4 inhibitor.

is easier (ie, less costly and less risky) than establishing *noninferiority, equivalency,* or *superiority* to the standard medical management strategy.[24]

Findings of nonsignificance between agents in a head-to-head trial need to be interpreted with caution. Often, a nonsignificant finding results from a study's lack of *power.* Nonsignificance is not the same as equivalence, which typically requires much higher statistical precision (see Chapter 10, Confidence Intervals: Was the Single Study or Meta-analysis Large Enough?).[24]

How Can We Use Indirect Evidence?

In the past, indirect comparisons across medications were performed by simply comparing individual arms between different trials as if they were from a single trial.[25] This naive approach ignores differences in prognostic factors (eg, illness severity) at baseline.[25] A method called the *adjusted indirect comparison*

provides a formal test for differences among pooled indirect estimates.[26] The adjusted indirect comparison requires that 2 medications use a similar control (eg, medication A vs placebo and medication B vs placebo). A limitation of this method is that it evaluates only 2 interventions at a time and uses only indirect evidence.

A more recently developed method called *network meta-analysis* (also called multiple treatment comparison meta-analysis) allows the comparison of multiple interventions, including head-to-head evaluations at the same time as indirect comparisons, in a connected network of comparisons (see Figure 28.4-1 and Chapter 24, Network Meta-analysis). This is particularly relevant as fields of medicine that are rapidly evaluating new interventions may avoid head-to-head trials and newer agents may all have a similar comparator.[27] Determining the *credibility* of a network meta-analysis may itself be a challenge (see Chapter 24, Network Meta-analysis).[28]

Are the End Points in Randomized Clinical Trials Important to Patients?

End points used in RCTs range from measures of clear importance to the patient to measures of questionable importance. *Binary outcomes* (yes/no outcomes) may be extremely important (eg, all-cause or disease-specific mortality) or only moderately important (eg, visits to the emergency department or hospitalization) to patients. *Patient-reported outcomes,* such as *health-related quality of life,* may be of primary importance. *Surrogate outcomes* chosen because of a belief that modifying the surrogate will predict effects on patient-important outcomes are not necessarily important themselves (see Chapter 13.4, Surrogate Outcomes).

Pharmacy and therapeutics committees can accept differing levels of evidence for outcomes, depending on the severity of the disease and the strength of evidence that a surrogate marker will translate to a clinical event. Surrogate measures range in value from strong (eg, viral load in HIV infection or adherence to antipsychotics in schizophrenia) to weak (eg, high-density lipoprotein and triglycerides in cardiovascular disease prediction) to negligible (eg, prostate-specific antigen as a predictor of prostate cancer outcomes) (see Chapter 13.4, Surrogate Outcomes). Initial RCTs often address surrogates and are followed by large RCTs evaluating major patient-important end points, and these large RCTs are then followed by trials used to determine the applicability of a medication within specific populations.[29] The first large trials addressing patient-important outcomes establish effectiveness in an area that does not have a well-established and effective standard of care. Once standard of care is established, newer interventions may need to be evaluated in the presence of the standard of care (eg, a medication plus standard of

care vs placebo plus standard of care).[30] During the process of establishing standard of care, the mechanism of action of a medication may become better understood and a surrogate marker of disease progression may become accepted.[31-34]

For example, early RCTs evaluating the effectiveness of antiretroviral treatments for HIV/AIDS originally used progression to AIDS or death as the primary end point.[35] Subsequent trials have used the surrogate end point of suppression of the HIV RNA viral load as the end point because a large number of RCTs addressing different medications have found a reduction in viral load paralleled both delay in progression to AIDS and mortality.

FIGURE 28.4-2

Studies Identified Using Different Statins for the Prevention of CVD Events[2]

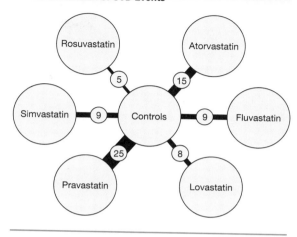

Geometric distribution of included randomized clinical trials in mixed-treatment analysis. Each node in the network represents a drug treatment, and each arm is weighted by the number of trials of that intervention vs the common control comparator. CVD indicates cardiovascular disease.

MOVING FROM EVIDENCE TO ACTION

USING THE GUIDE

In a network meta-analysis, 76 RCTs evaluating statins for both primary and secondary prevention of CVD events were analyzed[2]; the trials ranged from small investigations that involved as few as 38 participants to large studies that involved as many as 20 536 participants.[2,16,36] Twenty-five percent of patients in these trials were women. Six individual statins were included, with the number of RCTs for each comparison agent ranging from 5 for rosuvastatin vs control (n = 30 245) to 25 for pravastatin vs control/placebo (n = 51 011). Figure 28.4-2 displays the network.[2]

The doses used in the trials ranged from lower doses to higher doses of each statin. In a network meta-analysis, investigators examined whether doses changed the results using a meta-regression technique and found borderline significance (*odds ratio*, 1.42; 95% *confidence interval* [CI], 0.99-1.95) that higher doses were associated with increased treatment effects on CVD death. There was no useful head-to-head comparison evidence identified because no large equivalent-dose, head-to-head comparison trials have been conducted for statins.[16] Therefore, the best available evidence comes from indirect comparisons using placebo or no treatment as the comparator.

The end points used across clinical trials varied. However, most clinical trials provided information on CVD death. Because additional evidence would narrow the CIs in any analysis, the addition of new RCTs as listed in Table 28.4-1 could change our interpretation of the existing evidence.

TABLE 28.4-1

Pairwise Meta-analysis Results for Statin vs Control Comparison

Comparison	OR (95% CI)		
	Original Network Meta-analysis	**Trials With 5000 Patient Arms**	**Trials With 10000 Patient Arms**
Pravastatin vs control	**0.78 (0.65-0.93)**	**0.78 (0.68-0.89)**	**0.78 (0.70-0.87)**
Atorvastatin vs control	**0.80 (0.65-0.96)**	**0.80 (0.70-0.92)**	**0.80 (0.72-0.89)**
Fluvastatin vs control	**0.61 (0.41-0.88)**	**0.61 (0.51-0.73)**	**0.61 (0.53-0.70)**
Simvastatin vs control	**0.74 (0.56-0.98)**	**0.74 (0.63-0.87)**	**0.74 (0.65-0.84)**
Lovastatin vs control	0.73 (0.43-1.22)	**0.73 (0.61-0.88)**	**0.73 (0.64-0.83)**
Rosuvastatin vs control	0.88 (0.73-1.06)	0.88 (0.77-1.00)	**0.88 (0.79-0.98)**
Atorvastatin vs pravastatin	1.03 (0.79-1.33)	1.03 (0.85-1.24)	1.03 (0.88-1.20)
Fluvastatin vs pravastatin	0.79 (0.51-1.19)	**0.79 (0.63-0.98)**	**0.79 (0.66-0.93)**
Simvastatin vs pravastatin	0.95 (0.68-1.33)	0.95 (0.77-1.17)	0.95 (0.81-1.12)
Lovastatin vs pravastatin	0.94 (0.55-1.60)	0.94 (0.75-1.17)	0.94 (0.79-1.11)
Rosuvastatin vs pravastatin	1.13 (0.87-1.46)	1.13 (0.94-1.36)	1.13 (0.97-1.31)
Fluvastatin vs atorvastatin	0.76 (0.50-1.18)	**0.76 (0.61-0.96)**	**0.76 (0.64-0.91)**
Simvastatin vs atorvastatin	0.93 (0.66-1.31)	0.93 (0.75-1.14)	0.93 (0.78-1.12)
Lovastatin vs atorvastatin	0.91 (0.53-1.58)	0.91 (0.73-1.15)	0.91 (0.77-1.11)
Rosuvastatin vs atorvastatin	1.10 (0.84-1.44)	1.10 (0.91-1.33)	1.10 (0.94-1.28)
Simvastatin vs fluvastatin	1.21 (0.76-1.97)	1.21 (0.95-1.54)	**1.21 (1.01-1.46)**
Lovastatin vs fluvastatin	1.20 (0.63-2.27)	1.20 (0.93-1.55)	1.20 (0.99-1.45)
Rosuvastatin vs fluvastatin	1.44 (0.94-2.20)	**1.44 (1.15-1.80)**	**1.44 (1.21-1.72)**
Lovastatin vs simvastatin	0.99 (0.55-1.76)	0.99 (0.77-1.26)	0.99 (0.82-1.18)
Rosuvastatin vs simvastatin	1.19 (0.85-1.66)	1.19 (0.97-1.46)	**1.19 (1.01-1.40)**
Rosuvastatin vs lovastatin	1.21 (0.69-2.09)	1.21 (0.96-1.51)	**1.21 (1.02-1.43)**

A 5% control risk is assumed for the placebo arm in each hypothetical trial. Bolded results indicate statistical significance. Data derived from the original network meta-analysis estimate and the original estimate plus 1 large placebo-controlled trial where the effect is held constant added for each statin. Patients per arm in each added (hypothetical) trial are presented in the column titles.

Abbreviations: CI, confidence interval; OR, odds ratio.

WHAT ARE THE RESULTS?

Do the Number of Trials Testing Each Agent Differ?

There are usually large differences in the number of RCTs available for agents in a putative drug class. Interventions that have been evaluated in a large number of patients enrolled in multiple RCTs will provide stronger inferences than less studied interventions.[37] As we pool results across trials, we hope that trials with a high *risk of bias* will have much less influence on the pooled result than will multiple RCTs at low risk of bias.[19,38] Putting aside risk of bias, the *pooled estimate*, including large amounts of data, should provide a more precise estimate of effect.

When, however, evidence for a medication comes only from a small number of RCTs of limited sample size, small trials at high risk of bias may have an unfortunately large influence on the pooled estimate.[37] When there are many more RCTs that address one drug and few that address an alternative in the same class, the comparison of medications may therefore spuriously indicate superiority of a newer medication with a limited amount of information compared with an older and more thoroughly evaluated medication. This is of particular concern when there is selective publication of the limited number of trials (see Chapter 22, The Process of a Systematic Review and Meta-analysis).

Are Treatment Effects Similar Across Agents?

Even among RCTs of the same medication with the same control among similar populations, we would expect *heterogeneity* of *point estimates* and CIs simply due to chance. In pairwise meta-analysis, I^2 is the most commonly used statistic to evaluate whether RCTs appear to exhibit treatment effects that differ beyond the play of chance (see Chapter 23, Understanding and Applying the Results of a Systematic Review and Meta-analysis).[39] The I^2 statistic provides an estimate of heterogeneity on a scale of 0% to 100%, with lower estimates suggesting less

heterogeneity. No such measure exists with indirect comparisons or network meta-analyses.

In determining whether different medications within a class display similar effects, clinicians may examine whether CIs overlap or whether hypothesis tests are significant. It is possible for a medication within a class to display a treatment effect that is convincing (eg, simvastatin for prevention of CVD death; *relative risk* [RR], 0.74; 95% CI, 0.56-0.98). Lovastatin, within the same class, exhibits a nonsignificant treatment effect that is very similar in magnitude of effect but less precise (eg, RR, 0.73; 95% CI, 0.43-1.22).

In such a situation, a clinician who does not believe the class effect may recommend the use of simvastatin but not recommend the use of lovastatin. A clinician who accepts the class effect may be convinced of the effect of simvastatin and be willing to accept that lovastatin is likely similar (ie, with more participants, the CI for lovastatin would narrow to the point of looking similar to simvastatin). However, this inference may weaken if another statin, say cerivastatin (now withdrawn from the market), exhibited no treatment effects (eg, RR, 1.00; 95% CI, 0.90-1.20).

In the example in the preceding paragraphs, the CIs overlap among all 3 statins and would be consistent with no difference among the 3 treatments. The evidence does not, however, exclude an underlying true difference. This example reveals that confidence in a class effect diminishes if new evidence is inconsistent with prior evidence of treatment efficacy. This example includes statistically significant and nonsignificant findings; the same issues will apply when findings are statistically significant across all medications but one appears to offer a much larger treatment effect than the rest.

Would the Addition of Sufficiently Powered Evidence Change the Results of Direct or Indirect Evidence?

It is unlikely that evidence from head-to-head comparison trials will be solely responsible for informing decisions regarding class effects. Indirect evidence is very likely to be necessary for fully informed inferences.[40]

As indicated in Table 28.4-1, in the absence of heterogeneity of the new trials, the point estimates remain stable but the CIs narrow. In the original, RCT-driven meta-analysis, the differences among medications were nonsignificant. When an additional 5000 patients are added to each comparison (with the same event rates), significant differences are found among fluvastatin, pravastatin, atorvastatin, and rosuvastatin. When an additional 10 000 patients are added, the differences are significant between fluvastatin and pravastatin, atorvastatin, simvastatin, and rosuvastatin and also between rosuvastatin vs simvastatin and lovastatin. The message is that even in a very large database of RCTs that fail to show differences among drugs in a class, true differences may still exist and remain undetected because investigators have enrolled an insufficient number of patients.

Are Adverse Events Similar Across Agents?

Interpretation of class effects needs to give as much consideration to the tolerability and safety of the replacement medication as it does to its comparative effectiveness. Tolerability can be crudely assessed by comparing rates of adverse events and medication use discontinuation reported in clinical trials. However, safety, especially for uncommon and serious adverse effects, usually requires consideration of other forms of research with inherently higher risks of bias,

including *observational studies* (eg, *case-control* and *cohort* studies) and pharmacovigilance surveillance systems based on spontaneous reporting of adverse events. Although much of the profile of adverse effects may be similar among medications of the same chemical and pharmacologic class, serious idiosyncratic adverse effects may be considerably more frequent with one agent in a class (eg, liver failure with troglitazone vs pioglitazone).[42]

Safety profiles are generally better characterized for older vs newer medications, which supports therapeutic substitutions of older medications. If the older medication has convincingly fewer adverse effects, the decision is easy. The substitution decision becomes more complicated when the 2 medications appear similarly tolerable and the potential substitute medication, usually the older medication, has been well characterized with very low rates of serious adverse effects, whereas the link between the newer agent and its putative idiosyncratic serious adverse effects remains tenuous.

Another challenge occurs when both agents have known but quite different adverse effect profiles. For example, nevirapine, a nonnucleoside reverse transcriptase inhibitor (NNRTI) medication used as a component of HIV therapy, is associated with chronic toxicity, resulting in hepatopathy, severe rash, and fatigue.[43] Efavirenz, an alternative NNRTI, is typically much better tolerated but is associated more commonly with psychiatric symptoms that are not seen with nevirapine.[43] Nevirapine offers a substitute for efavirenz for people with an active mental illness, but this preference may not apply to all patients affected by such a therapeutic substitution policy because different patients may vary in their susceptibility to particular adverse events.

What Are the Overall Quality and Limitations of the Evidence?

The following aspects are hallmarks of high-quality evidence for class effects: individual studies are at low risk of bias and *publication bias* is unlikely; studies are well powered and sample sizes are large, with CIs that are correspondingly narrow; the findings have been replicated in a number of similarly well-designed RCTs; and the biology of the candidate drugs is very similar. In most cases of putative class effects, the evidence meets some, but not all, of these criteria.

USING THE GUIDE

Returning to our opening scenario, there is imbalance in the number of RCTs included in the network meta-analysis of statins, with as few as 5 RCTs for rosuvastatin and 25 for pravastatin. Therefore, we should suspect a possible bias against the more studied drugs. Treatments revealed variability in the magnitude of their effect (see column 1 in Table 28.4-1). Rosuvastatin had nonsignificant treatment effects for reducing CVD deaths. Given our understanding of different statins, we wonder whether this is a true null effect or an artifact of the predominantly primary prevention trials involved with the use of rosuvastatin (thus with lower power due to the reduced number of events).[44]

Certain statins exhibit different adverse events than others. For example, an older statin, cerivastatin, was withdrawn from the market because of serious rhabdomyolysis.[45] For currently available statins, indirect comparisons suggest that specific statins have slightly different safety profiles.[36] Atorvastatin significantly elevated aspartate aminotransferase levels compared with pravastatin (OR, 2.21; 95% CI, 1.13-4.29), and simvastatin significantly increased creatine kinase levels when compared with rosuvastatin (OR, 4.39; 95% CI, 1.01-19.07).

CLINICAL SCENARIO RESOLUTION

In resolving our scenario, we are left with weak inferences that statins exhibit a constant class effect. We know that there are different biological mechanisms of how the medications are metabolized. Evidence comes in part from indirect comparisons of medications that are imbalanced in the number of patients and RCTs involved. Finally, the medications appear to exhibit different treatment effects that are not entirely explained by their differing patient populations. This leaves us with uncertainty that all statins are the same and can be used interchangeably. We provide these results to the formulary committee and state that we cannot blindly implement the new policy of drug substitution when class effects are uncertain.

CONCLUSION

In this chapter, we address several questions necessary for evaluating whether different medications are exhibiting a class effect. Evidence will seldom securely support an inference of a class effect (ie, any differences in both benefits and adverse effects are too small to be important). Therefore, clinicians should apply caution before concluding broad class effects and assuming therapeutic and adverse effect equivalence.

MOVING FROM EVIDENCE TO ACTION

References

1. Furberg CD, Psaty BM. Should evidence-based proof of drug efficacy be extrapolated to a "class of agents"? *Circulation.* 2003;108(21):2608-2610.

2. Mills EJ, Wu P, Chong G, et al. Efficacy and safety of statin treatment for cardiovascular disease: a network meta-analysis of 170,255 patients from 76 randomized trials. *QJM.* 2011;104(2):109-124.

3. Mills EJ, Rachlis B, Wu P, Devereaux PJ, Arora P, Perri D. Primary prevention of cardiovascular mortality and events with statin treatments: a network meta-analysis involving more than 65,000 patients. *J Am Coll Cardiol.* 2008;52(22):1769-1781.

4. Briel M, Nordmann AJ, Bucher HC. Statin therapy for prevention and treatment of acute and chronic cardiovascular disease: update on recent trials and metaanalyses. *Curr Opin Lipidol.* 2005;16(6):601-605.

5. ALLHAT Officers and Coordinators for the ALLHAT Collaborative Research Group. The Antihypertensive and Lipid-Lowering Treatment to Prevent Heart Attack Trial. Major outcomes in

high-risk hypertensive patients randomized to angiotensin-converting enzyme inhibitor or calcium channel blocker vs diuretic: The Antihypertensive and Lipid-Lowering Treatment to Prevent Heart Attack Trial (ALLHAT). *JAMA*. 2002;288(23):2981-2997.

6. Dahlöf B, Sever PS, Poulter NR, et al; ASCOT Investigators. Prevention of cardiovascular events with an antihypertensive regimen of amlodipine adding perindopril as required versus atenolol adding bendroflumethiazide as required, in the Anglo-Scandinavian Cardiac Outcomes Trial-Blood Pressure Lowering Arm (ASCOT-BPLA): a multicentre randomised controlled trial. *Lancet*. 2005;366(9489):895-906.

7. Lindholm LH, Carlberg B, Samuelsson O. Should beta blockers remain first choice in the treatment of primary hypertension? A meta-analysis. *Lancet*. 2005;366(9496):1545-1553.

8. Baigent C, Keech A, Kearney PM, et al; Cholesterol Treatment Trialists' (CTT) Collaborators. Efficacy and safety of cholesterol-lowering treatment: prospective meta-analysis of data from 90,056 participants in 14 randomised trials of statins. *Lancet*. 2005;366(9493):1267-1278.

9. Bucher HC, Griffith LE, Guyatt GH. Systematic review on the risk and benefit of different cholesterol-lowering interventions. *Arterioscler Thromb Vasc Biol*. 1999;19(2):187-195.

10. Colivicchi F, Tubaro M, Mocini D, et al. Full-dose atorvastatin versus conventional medical therapy after non-ST-elevation acute myocardial infarction in patients with advanced non-revascularisable coronary artery disease. *Curr Med Res Opin*. 2010;26(6):1277-1284.

11. Rajpathak SN, Kumbhani DJ, Crandall J, Barzilai N, Alderman M, Ridker PM. Statin therapy and risk of developing type 2 diabetes: a meta-analysis. *Diabetes Care*. 2009;32(10):1924-1929.

12. Colivicchi F, Guido V, Tubaro M, et al. Effects of atorvastatin 80 mg daily early after onset of unstable angina pectoris or non-Q-wave myocardial infarction. *Am J Cardiol*. 2002;90(8):872-874.

13. Zhong HA, Mashinson V, Woolman TA, Zha M. Understanding the molecular properties and metabolism of top prescribed drugs. *Curr Top Med Chem*. 2013;13(11):1290-1307.

14. Willrich MA, Hirata MH, Hirata RD. Statin regulation of CYP3A4 and CYP3A5 expression. *Pharmacogenomics*. 2009;10(6):1017-1024.

15. Ray GM. Antiretroviral and statin drug-drug interactions. *Cardiol Rev*. 2009;17(1):44-47.

16. Mills EJ, O'Regan C, Eyawo O, et al. Intensive statin therapy compared with moderate dosing for prevention of cardiovascular events: a meta-analysis of >40 000 patients. *Eur Heart J*. 2011;32(11):1409-1415.

17. Cannon CP, Braunwald E, McCabe CH, et al; Pravastatin or Atorvastatin Evaluation and Infection Therapy-Thrombolysis in Myocardial Infarction 22 Investigators. Intensive versus moderate lipid lowering with statins after acute coronary syndromes. *N Engl J Med*. 2004;350(15):1495-1504.

18. Atkins D, Best D, Briss PA, et al; GRADE Working Group. Grading quality of evidence and strength of recommendations. *BMJ*. 2004;328(7454):1490.

19. Song F, Harvey I, Lilford R. Adjusted indirect comparison may be less biased than direct comparison for evaluating new pharmaceutical interventions. *J Clin Epidemiol*. 2008;61(5):455-463.

20. Gardner DM, Baldessarini RJ, Waraich P. Modern antipsychotic drugs: a critical overview. *CMAJ*. 2005;172(13):1703-1711.

21. Mills EJ, Druyts E, Ghement I, Puhan MA. Pharmacotherapies for chronic obstructive pulmonary disease: a multiple treatment comparison meta-analysis. *Clin Epidemiol*. 2011;3:107-129.

22. Guyatt GH, Mills EJ, Elbourne D. In the era of systematic reviews, does the size of an individual trial still matter. *PLoS Med*. 2008;5(1):e4.

23. Song F, Altman DG, Glenny AM, Deeks JJ. Validity of indirect comparison for estimating efficacy of competing interventions: empirical evidence from published meta-analyses. *BMJ*. 2003;326(7387):472.

24. Piaggio G, Elbourne DR, Altman DG, Pocock SJ, Evans SJ; CONSORT Group. Reporting of noninferiority and equivalence randomized trials: an extension of the CONSORT statement. *JAMA*. 2006;295(10):1152-1160.

25. Glenny AM, Altman DG, Song F, et al; International Stroke Trial Collaborative Group. Indirect comparisons of competing interventions. *Health Technol Assess*. 2005;9(26):1-134, iii-iv.

26. Bucher HC, Guyatt GH, Griffith LE, Walter SD. The results of direct and indirect treatment comparisons in meta-analysis of randomized controlled trials. *J Clin Epidemiol*. 1997;50(6):683-691.

27. Ioannidis JP. Perfect study, poor evidence: interpretation of biases preceding study design. *Semin Hematol*. 2008;45(3):160-166.

28. Mills EJ, Thorlund K, Ioannidis JP. Demystifying trial networks and network meta-analysis. *BMJ*. 2013;346:f2914.

29. Food and Drug Administration. Dose-Response Information to Support Drug Registration. ICH-E4. http://www.fda.gov/downloads/Drugs/GuidanceComplianceRegulatoryInformation/Guidances/ucm073115.pdf. Accessed August 4, 2014.

30. Prasad V, Cifu A, Ioannidis JP. Reversals of established medical practices: evidence to abandon ship. *JAMA*. 2012;307(1):37-38.

31. Buyse M, Molenberghs G. Criteria for the validation of surrogate endpoints in randomized experiments. *Biometrics*. 1998;54(3):1014-1029.

32. Buyse M, Molenberghs G, Burzykowski T, Renard D, Geys H. The validation of surrogate endpoints in meta-analyses of randomized experiments. *Biostatistics*. 2000;1(1):49-67.

33. Buyse M, Piedbois P. On the relationship between response to treatment and survival time. *Stat Med*. 1996;15(24):2797-2812.

34. Buyse M, Sargent DJ, Grothey A, Matheson A, de Gramont A. Biomarkers and surrogate end points—the challenge of statistical validation. *Nat Rev Clin Oncol*. 2010;7(6):309-317.

35. Kent DM, Mwamburi DM, Bennish ML, Kupelnick B, Ioannidis JP. Clinical trials in sub-Saharan Africa and established standards of care: a systematic review of HIV, tuberculosis, and malaria trials. *JAMA*. 2004;292(2):237-242.

36. Alberton M, Wu P, Druyts E, Briel M, Mills EJ. Adverse events associated with individual statin treatments for cardiovascular disease: an indirect comparison meta-analysis. *QJM*. 2012;105(2):145-157.

37. Pereira TV, Horwitz RI, Ioannidis JP. Empirical evaluation of very large treatment effects of medical interventions. *JAMA*. 2012;308(16):1676-1684.

38. Mills EJ, Thorlund K, Ioannidis JP. Calculating additive treatment effects from multiple randomized trials provides useful estimates of combination therapies. *J Clin Epidemiol*. 2012;65(12):1282-1288.

39. Higgins JP, Thompson SG, Deeks JJ, Altman DG. Measuring inconsistency in meta-analyses. *BMJ*. 2003;327(7414):557-560.

40. Madan J, Stevenson MD, Cooper KL, Ades AE, Whyte S, Akehurst R. Consistency between direct and indirect trial evidence: is direct evidence always more reliable? *Value Health*. 2011;14(6):953-960.

41. Yusuf S, Collins R, Peto R. Why do we need some large, simple randomized trials? *Stat Med*. 1984;3(4):409-422.

42. Rajagopalan R, Iyer S, Perez A. Comparison of pioglitazone with other antidiabetic drugs for associated incidence of liver failure: no evidence of increased risk of liver failure with pioglitazone. *Diabetes Obes Metab*. 2005;7(2):161-169.

43. Drake SM. NNRTIs-a new class of drugs for HIV. *J Antimicrob Chemother*. 2000;45(4):417-420.

44. Ridker PM, Danielson E, Fonseca FA, et al; JUPITER Study Group. Rosuvastatin to prevent vascular events in men and women with elevated C-reactive protein. *N Engl J Med*. 2008;359(21):2195-2207.

45. Staffa JA, Chang J, Green L. Cerivastatin and reports of fatal rhabdomyolysis. *N Engl J Med*. 2002;346(7):539-540.

MOVING FROM EVIDENCE TO ACTION

28.5

ADVANCED TOPICS IN MOVING FROM EVIDENCE TO ACTION

Evidence-Based Practitioners and Evidence-Based Care

Gordon Guyatt, Maureen O. Meade, Jeremy Grimshaw, R. Brian Haynes, Roman Jaeschke, Deborah J. Cook, Mark C. Wilson, and W. Scott Richardson

IN THIS CHAPTER

Top-quality health care implies the practice of medicine that is consistent with the best evidence (*evidence-based health care*). An intuitively appealing way to achieve *evidence-based practice* is to train clinicians who can independently find, appraise, and judiciously apply the best *evidence* (*evidence-based experts*). Indeed, our fondest hope for this book is that it will help you become an evidence-based expert. The following discussion, however, illustrates that training evidence-based experts is not, by itself, an optimal strategy for ensuring patients receive evidence-based care.[1]

In this chapter, we acknowledge the challenges in developing expertise in *evidence-based medicine* (EBM). Next, we highlight an alternative approach to providing evidence-based care, which is training clinicians who can use evidence-based summaries and recommendations; we call such clinicians *evidence-based practitioners*. We then acknowledge the limitations of this strategy and suggest a solution. Finally, we present some of the reasons you might wish to pursue development of more advanced EBM skills, although these skills are not prerequisites for practicing EBM.

BECOMING AN EVIDENCE-BASED MEDICINE EXPERT TAKES TIME AND EFFORT

The skills needed to provide an evidence-based solution to a clinical dilemma include precisely defining the problem, conducting an efficient search to locate the best evidence, critically appraising the evidence, and considering that evidence—and its implications—in the context of patients' circumstances and values. Although attaining these skills at a basic level is relatively easy, developing the expertise to allow efficient and sophisticated critical appraisal and application to the individual patient requires (as with developing expertise in any area) time, effort, and deliberate practice.

The advanced topics chapters of this book highlight the challenges of becoming an EBM expert. You must have a deep understanding of

and be alert to violations of the principles of valid scientific inquiry (issues such as *stopped early trials*, analyzing according to the *intention-to-treat principle*, and selective reporting of *outcome variables*). In addition, you must be aware of how even studies at low *risk of bias* may mislead (note the strategies to avoid being misled in Chapter 13.3, Misleading Presentations of Clinical Trial Results, and additional issues, such as the use of *surrogate end points* and *composite end points*). In short, you must be motivated to continue learning about new developments in clinical research methods and to explore their effect on clinical decision making. Becoming an EBM expert is gratifying, but it is not for everyone.

ALL CLINICIANS CAN BECOME EVIDENCE-BASED PRACTITIONERS

Considering the challenges of becoming an EBM expert, it comes as no surprise that most internal medicine residents at McMaster University, even in a program explicitly committed to systematic training in EBM,[2] are not interested in attaining an advanced level of EBM skills. Our trainees' responses mirror those of general practitioners in the United Kingdom, who often use evidence-based summaries generated by others (72%) and evidence-based practice guidelines or protocols (84%) but who overwhelmingly (95%) believe that "learning the skills of EBM" is not the most appropriate method for "moving … to EBM."[3]

At McMaster and in other residency programs,[4] we have observed that even the trainees who are less interested in critically appraising evidence develop an appreciation for and an ability to track down, recognize, and use secondary sources of preappraised evidence (evidence-based resources) to solve their patient management problems. Having mastered this more restricted set of EBM skills, these trainees can become highly competent and regularly updated practitioners who provide evidence-based care—evidence-based practitioners.

A WORLD OF EVIDENCE-BASED PRACTITIONERS DOES NOT GUARANTEE EVIDENCE-BASED CARE

Unfortunately, even the availability of evidence-based resources and recommendations and practitioners trained to use them will be insufficient to produce consistent evidence-based care because of barriers working at different levels of health care systems, many of which operate at levels beyond the control of an individual practitioner. These barriers include structural barriers (eg, financial disincentives), organizational barriers (eg, inappropriate skill mix, lack of facilities or equipment), peer group barriers (eg, local standards of care not in line with desired practice), professional barriers (eg, knowledge, attitudes, skills), and cognitive barriers (most clinical practice is based on habitual behaviors and heuristics with information overload in busy settings, leading to acts of omission).[5] Furthermore, evidence-based practitioners are subject to external product marketing (in particular, pharmaceutical industry marketing). These barriers are often stronger determinants of practice than current best evidence. Traditional continuing education activities are insufficient to optimize evidence-based care.

BEHAVIOR CHANGE STRATEGIES CAN HELP TO ACHIEVE EVIDENCE-BASED CARE

Achieving evidence-based care often requires active strategies (beyond training in EBM) to promote practitioner behavior change. There are a wide range of possible strategies, including continuing education meetings[6]; one-to-one conversations with an expert (*academic detailing*)[7]; *computer decision support systems*, including alerting systems and reminders[8,9]; preceptorships; advice from *opinion leaders*[10]; and targeted *audit and feedback*.[11] Administrative strategies that can potentially help to achieve evidence-based care include the availability of restricted drug formularies and the application of financial incentives[12] (eg, pay for performance) and institutional *clinical practice guidelines*.[13]

All of these strategies are effective under some circumstances (although the improvements in behavior are modest), but none are effective under all circumstances.[14] This has led to the recognition of the need to design and tailor behavior change strategies to address local barriers and facilitators. For example, academic detailing may be useful if the key barriers involve practitioners' knowledge and attitudes relating to simple behaviors in the individual physician's control (eg, choice of drugs to prescribe). Audit and feedback will be useful if the key barrier relates to practitioners' awareness of their performance. Thus, achieving evidence-based care requires a variety of strategies that focus on behavior change. Currently, the evidence about different knowledge translation and implementation strategies is incomplete, and we encourage evidence-based practitioners to participate in knowledge translation and implementation research projects.

ADVANTAGES OF EVIDENCE-BASED MEDICINE EXPERTISE

We hope that the previous discussion has not dissuaded you from continuing to read and study the *Users' Guides to the Medical Literature*. Powerful reasons remain for achieving the highest possible skill level in evidence-based practice.

First, attempts to change physician practice will sometimes be directed to objectives, such as increasing specific drug use or reducing health care costs, which have little to do with evidence-based care. Only those with advanced skills in interpreting the medical literature will be able to determine the extent to which studies of pharmaceutical interventions, or restricted drug formularies, are consistent with the best evidence. Second, a high level of EBM skills will allow you to use the original literature effectively, regardless of whether preappraised *synopses* and evidence-based recommendations are available. Third, sophisticated EBM skills facilitate taking an effective leadership role in the medical community. In particular, evidence-based experts will have the key skills to help develop clinical policies and pathways in their health care setting and to be useful members of clinical practice guideline committees.

References

1. Guyatt G, Meade M, Jaeschke R, Cook D, Haynes R. Practitioners of evidence-based care: not all clinicians need to appraise evidence from scratch but all clinicians need some EBM skills [editorial]. *BMJ.* 2000;320(7240):954-955.

2. Evidence-Based Medicine Working Group. Evidence-based medicine: a new approach to teaching the practice of medicine. *JAMA.* 1992;268(17):2420-2425.

3. McColl A, Smith H, White P, Field J. General practitioner's perceptions of the route to evidence based medicine: a questionnaire survey. *BMJ.* 1998;316(7128):361-365.

4. Akl EA, Izuchukwu IS, El-Dika S, Fritsche L, Kunz R, Schünemann HJ. Integrating an evidence-based medicine rotation into an internal medicine residency program. *Acad Med.* 2004;79(9):897-904.

5. Grimshaw JM, Eccles MP, Walker AE, Thomas RE. Changing physicians' behaviour: what works and thoughts on getting more things to work. *J Contin Educ Health Prof.* 2002;22(4):237-243.

6. Forsetlund L, Bjørndal A, Rashidian A, et al. Continuing education meetings and workshops: effects on professional practice and health care outcomes. *Cochrane Database Syst Rev.* 2009;(2):CD003030.

7. O'Brien MA, Rogers S, Jamtvedt G, et al. Educational outreach visits: effects on professional practice and health care outcomes. *Cochrane Database Syst Rev.* 2007;(4):CD000409.

8. Garg AX, Adhikari NK, McDonald H, et al. Effects of computerized clinical decision support systems on practitioner performance and patient outcomes: a systematic review. *JAMA.* 2005;293(10):1223-1238.

9. Shojania KG, Jennings A, Mayhew A, Ramsay CR, Eccles MP, Grimshaw J. The effects of on-screen, point of care computer reminders on processes and outcomes of care. *Cochrane Database Syst Rev.* 2009;(3):CD001096.

10. Flodgren G, Parmelli E, Doumit G, et al. Local opinion leaders: effects on professional practice and health care outcomes. *Cochrane Database Syst Rev.* 2011;(8):CD000125.

11. Ivers N, Jamtvedt G, Flottorp S, et al. Audit and feedback: effects on professional practice and healthcare outcomes. *Cochrane Database Syst Rev.* 2012;6:CD000259.

12. Flodgren G, Eccles MP, Shepperd S, Scott A, Parmelli E, Beyer FR. An overview of reviews evaluating the effectiveness of financial incentives in changing healthcare professional behaviours and patient outcomes. *Cochrane Database Syst Rev.* 2011;(7):CD009255.

13. Grimshaw J, Eccles M, Tetroe J. Implementing clinical guidelines: current evidence and future implications. *J Contin Educ Health Prof.* 2004;24(Suppl 1):S31-S37.

14. Grimshaw JM, Eccles MP, Lavis JN, Hill SJ, Squires JE. Knowledge translation of research findings. *Implement Sci.* 2012;7(1):50.

29

Teachers' Guides to the Users' Guides

Peter Wyer, Deborah J. Cook, Per Olav Vandvik, W. Scott Richardson, Mahmoud Elbarbary, Regina Kunz, and Mark C. Wilson

IN THIS CHAPTER

CLINICAL SCENARIOS

Scenario 1

You are an attending physician in your hospital's intensive care unit (ICU) doing morning rounds on a patient with septic shock. The resident notes that the patient is still hypotensive after receiving 5 L of intravenous Ringer's lactate solution and asks if starch solution should be administered.

Scenario 2

You are awaiting the noon conference in the ICU where a patient admitted that week will be discussed in detail with 2 attending physicians, a fellow, 2 senior residents, and 2 junior residents. The fellow is now addressing preventive interventions as part of admission orders, noting that this patient did not receive heparin thromboprophylaxis when first admitted because his admitting diagnosis was ruptured abdominal aortic aneurysm. Now, 2 days after the patient's surgery, the fellow is wondering which type of heparin to prescribe.

Scenario 3

You are the faculty adviser for journal club in your surgical residency program. The resident assigned to lead this month's session attended the patient admitted from the emergency department with ruptured aortic aneurysm from scenario 2. She proposes to review the literature on the choice of low-molecular-weight heparin vs other prophylactic alternatives for postoperative patients.

These 3 scenarios raise issues related to teaching *evidence-based clinical practice* (EBCP) to practicing clinicians and clinicians in training. Readers of the *Users' Guides to the Medical Literature* (*Users' Guides*) who are clinical educators have doubtless already begun to ponder how to incorporate its concepts into their teaching. In this chapter, we provide

some suggestions. A theme that will pervade this discussion is our increasing emphasis on *systematic reviews* and practice guidelines as bread-and-butter content for EBCP teaching on all levels. The scope of EBCP is rapidly evolving, and the settings for EBCP teaching are broadening. In this chapter, we identify some related challenges to educators and provide examples of innovative responses. We then return to the opening scenarios and to some additional examples.

TEACHING EBCP IN AN EXPANDING UNIVERSE OF EVIDENCE AND EDUCATION

During the more than 2 decades since it was introduced as an educational intervention at the residency and house officer level, EBCP has been widely accepted as an important component of medical education. Evidence-based clinical practice skills are included in competency-based frameworks for graduate medical education, including the Outcome Project of the US Accreditation Council for Graduate Medical Education (ACGME)[1] and the Canadian Royal College of Physicians' CanMEDS program.[2,3] These frameworks, in turn, have been widely adopted as guides for clinical education at other levels, including undergraduate education. In some cases, they have undergone further transformation.[4]

The competency-based frameworks have served to reinforce a practice-based orientation, further shifting emphasis away from the predominant emphasis on critical appraisal and toward what have been termed "initiation skills" (ie, skills required to initiate exploration of research literature in response to actual clinical encounters).[5,6] Published approaches to teaching EBCP have been criticized for inadequate attention to the cognitive processes and relational skills that generate recognition of information needs.[7,8] A recent systematic review of reports of teaching EBCP to undergraduates included learner identification of information needs as a required skill category and found that it was considered in only a small number of such reports.[9] An emerging literature addresses the need to wed EBCP with both narrative and relational skills.[10-12]

Despite widening acceptance and increasing clinical relevance, routine incorporation of EBCP into clinical training faces resource challenges. It places a demand not only on faculty development but also on curricular time, when calls are being voiced to make medical education shorter and more efficient.[13] Shorter resident work hours are compounding this problem. Finally, relevant curricular efforts may be variable in content duration and quality. Under such circumstances, Web-based distance learning approaches have increasing appeal. Results of a *randomized trial* suggested that computer-based EBCP courses may be equally effective as lecture frameworks in increasing relevant knowledge and attitudes.[14]

A particularly impressive example of a computer-based EBCP program was initially sponsored by the European Union (EU) as the EU-EBM (Evidence-Based Medicine) Unity Project[15,16] and was subsequently expanded to encompass trials in 7 Central and South American, African, and Asian countries.[17] The program combines e-learning and on-site facilitation and involves a set of teaching and learning modules covering a broad range of EBCP skills. On-site facilitation helps to integrate the learning activities with practitioners' own daily tasks and roles. This e-learning is Internet based[15] and may be accessed on the Monash University website (http://ebm-unity.med.monash.edu). Studies performed in Europe[16,18] and developing nations[17] have uniformly observed gains in EBCP knowledge and related attitudes with application of the EU-EBM Unity Project program.

Emphasis on incorporation of *clinical practice guidelines* into standard teaching of EBCP is relatively recent and has gained momentum with the advent of the *GRADE* (*Grading of Recommendations Assessment, Development and Evaluation*) system[19] and other systems used to rate the quality of *evidence* and with a recent report on standards for trustworthy practice guidelines from the US Institute of Medicine[20] and the Guidelines International Network.[21] In 2005, David Eddy warned of the pitfalls of fragmentation between the teaching of "evidence-based medicine," largely restricted to applications to care of individual patients, and of "evidence-based guidelines," concerned with health care recommendations for populations.[22] Eddy

referred to these 2 dimensions of *evidence-based health care* as evidence-based guidelines and evidence-based individual decision making.[22] Teaching evidence-based guidelines requires educators to emphasize guidelines as integrated sources of evidence and to teach the skills that allow differentiation of trustworthy from untrustworthy guidelines (see Chapter 26, How to Use a Patient Management Recommendation: Clinical Practice Guidelines and Decision Analyses).[20]

The GRADE system provides a structure for teaching critical appraisal of the best available body of evidence, whether it be from a systematic review or a report of a single study (see Chapter 23, Understanding and Applying the Results of a Systematic Review and Meta-analysis). The structure of GRADE provides a closely related, attractive alternative to the regular *Users' Guide* structure of assessment of *risk of bias*, results, and applicability. The GRADE approach focuses on quality of evidence, defined as confidence in the estimates of effect for purposes of decision making.[23] Assessing quality of evidence involves considering the fundamental study design (eg, randomized trials or *observational studies*) and a number of factors that may undermine confidence: risk of bias, *inconsistency, indirectness, imprecision,* and *publication bias*.[24] For example, when faced with a *forest plot* reporting a *meta-analysis*, educators might ask: What is the best estimate of the effect of the intervention and what factors might result in reduced confidence in the estimate of effect? Our experience is that even beginners, with a little bit of coaching, can generate the 5 categories of factors that reduce confidence.

Clinical learners undergoing structured experiences related to EBCP deserve exposure to evolving standards for development of health care recommendations and the challenges of reconciling such recommendations with the needs of individual patients.[25] For example, when faced with a recommendation developed with the GRADE system, educators can probe understanding of weak and strong recommendations and factors that the guideline panel should consider and make explicit when moving from evidence to recommendations (see Chapter 28.1, Assessing the Strength of Recommendations: The GRADE Approach). A conceptual understanding of strong and weak recommendations is necessary to apply guidelines in practice.

A third dimension of EBCP, supplementing guidelines and individual decision making, that has emerged in recent years is the challenge of adapting and implementing externally developed guidelines, as well as homegrown clinical policies, in specific health care systems and settings.[26] From an educational perspective, this poses new challenges. For example, the Carnegie Foundation report[13] identified lack of emphasis on systems-level care, *quality improvement*, and team-based care as major deficiencies within current medical education. Some international EBCP teaching efforts are beginning to integrate principles of knowledge translation[26] and implementation science into their curricular approaches.[27,28] The curricular design developed by the European and international e-learning initiative previously cited includes an implementation module.[15,17] E-learning frameworks may well emerge as flagship solutions to yet another important demand on today's overburdened medical education agenda.

EVIDENCE-BASED CLINICAL PRACTICE AND CLINICAL TEACHING: MORE THAN JUST JOURNAL CLUB

Returning now to the challenges of teaching EBCP in clinical settings, how might learning and teaching EBCP differ from learning and teaching any other complex set of skills? For instance, although EBCP is becoming incorporated into undergraduate medical curricula in the United States, priorities and interpretations of EBCP-related skill sets may be highly variable across different programs.[9] Practitioners not familiar with EBCP may continue to perceive demands on them to learn new approaches as unwanted intrusions. As a result, teachers may face considerable challenges in effectively communicating the practical relevance of EBCP to their learners.

Our 3 scenarios illustrate different aspects of these challenges. In the first scenario, time pressure on rounds may result in a cursory and nontransparent response on the part of the physician, such as "The evidence favors crystalloids over starch for septic shock, so we use crystalloids." Similarly, in the slightly less time-pressed context of the second scenario, the resident, left to her own devices and lacking appropriate mentorship, may be tempted to limit the presentation to pronouncements from sources such as standard textbooks and *narrative reviews*. The third scenario presents a setting in which some elaboration of EBCP concepts is likely to be perceived as pertinent. In all cases, the challenge is to persuasively link awareness of research evidence to the process of making clinical decisions. In the following section, we offer suggestions for effectively incorporating EBCP teaching into these and other settings.

Interactive teaching approaches, generally more effective than conventional didactic approaches to teaching and updating clinical skills,[29-31] are particularly well suited to teaching EBCP.[31] Table 29-1 summarizes interactive techniques not unique to EBCP but highly relevant to its teaching.[34]

Modes of Teaching

Straus et al[34] and Richardson[35] describe 3 modes of teaching EBCP that may help incorporate EBCP into routine clinical teaching (Table 29-2). They are largely distinguished by the degree of emphasis on communicating and discussing the knowledge basis for decision making, including knowledge of research evidence.

The opening 3 scenarios correspond to the above 3 modes. When role modeling, the teacher demonstrates the use of clinical practice guidelines and summarized clinical evidence as a routine aspect of communicating clinical practice and decision making. During integrated teaching of EBCP, the teacher adds summarized clinical evidence to the mixture of knowledge taught about a clinical topic, weaving it in where it fits naturally. In cases where clinical practice guidelines exist, the teacher can raise issues regarding their trustworthiness[20] and applicability to the local context (see Chapter 26, How to Use a Patient Management Recommendation: Clinical Practice Guidelines and Decision Analyses).

Direct teaching of specific EBCP skills involves communicating about specific ways to seek, appraise, or use evidence in clinical decision making. We will refer to these modes throughout the rest of this chapter.

TABLE 29-1

Interactive Approaches to Teaching Evidence-Based Clinical Practice (EBCP)

Interactive and Self-Learning Techniques for Teaching EBCP	
Individual	Educational prescription[a]
	Identify patient-important problems calling for EBCP skills
Smaller group presentations	Role playing
	Team learning interludes[b]
	Establish roles and guidelines as appropriate
	—Timekeeper
	—Chalkboard scribe
	—Discourage distracting conversations
	—Use timeouts to discuss process and refocus discussion
	Interjected teaching tips
	Poll group members on key questions and practice decisions prior to giving suggested answers
	Avoid answering questions before involving group
Larger group presentations	Team learning interludes[b]
	Buzz group interludes[c]
	Poll audience on key questions and practice decisions before giving suggested answers
	Avoid answering questions before involving group

[a]Encourage the learner to take on an assignment that requires use of EBCP skills to complete.

[b]Team learning involves breaking a larger group into a set of smaller groups and assigning them 1 or more identical or related tasks, followed by sharing of solutions between the groups.[32,33]

[c]Buzz groups may be seen as a variant of the team learning technique in which the smaller groups consist of only 2 or 3 individuals.

MATCHING CONTENT AND CONTEXT: EVIDENCE-BASED TEACHING SCRIPTS

Learning is more effective and more likely to lead to change in behavior when it takes place in the context in which it will be applied.[36,37] It is particularly important to center as much of the teaching of EBCP in clinical teaching settings as possible.[29,35] This requires the teacher to be skilled in each of the 3 teaching modes.

The clinical teacher will find it advantageous to present the content of the *Users' Guides* in small, discrete segments woven into discussions of clinical problems. These constitute a type of teaching script that Irby,[38] Schmidt et al,[39] and Wyer et al[40] have described: well-prepared, structured, interactive presentations of key concepts. Schmidt et al[39] identified "illness scripts" as bundled constructs, specific to particular

clinical presentations, that embodied practitioner theoretical and practical knowledge of medical conditions embedded in the memory in a form that could be brought into the conscious mind in response to clinical triggers. Irby[38] found that educators identified as outstanding by clinical learners quite consciously accessed preexisting "teaching scripts" in response to scenarios simultaneously involving both patient care and skill development within clinical learners. In many cases, the teachers in question had written down prepared teaching scripts and could describe the process through which they were modified and adapted to the needs of specific patients and learners.[38]

Later in this chapter, we provide examples of short instructional segments that may be incorporated into such scripts. We encourage clinical teachers, as they read through this book, to ponder the development of their own scripts incorporating

TABLE 29-2

Modes of Teaching

Mode	Description	Goal	Example Venues	Example Content
Role modeling	Demonstrating the incorporation of evidence into patient care decisions	Communicating clinical decisions and recommendations to health care team members and/or patients	Abbreviated work rounds Sign-out rounds Clinical supervision and bedside teaching	Summary of a guideline, systematic review, or meta-analysis relevant to the care of an active patient or results of a related quick literature search during a work rounds sign out
Integrated teaching	Combining consideration of relevant clinical evidence with clinical teaching	Teaching clinical skills, principles of assessment, and disease-oriented management	Morning report or full work rounds Clinical topic sessions Morbidity and mortality case reviews Quality improvement meetings	Interactive discussion of relevant study or synopsis during extended case discussion
Direct skills teaching	Teaching in which EBCP skills constitute the direct subject	Enhancing learners' independent capacity to bring EBCP skills to bear on their decisions	Journal club EBCP "carve outs"[a] within integrated teaching sessions	Systematic examination of process of solving a problem using EBCP skills

Abbreviation: EBCP, evidence-based clinical practice.

[a]Pertinent guidelines or evidence summaries may be used as a stimulus for relevant explanatory digressions. For example, reference to the performance of a diagnostic test, as demonstrated in a cited study, may be supplemented by a quick explanation of the interpretation of likelihood ratios.

EBCP skills and concepts and to consider where they might apply these scripts. This book includes the material for several hundred EBCP teaching scripts of varying duration and complexity.

Learner Needs and Interests

An effective teaching script encompasses content adapted to the teaching venue, period, and competing demands, as well as the learners' previous knowledge, readiness, and inclination to absorb new content. Irby[41] posited that the ability to modify and adapt a teaching script to learner needs and knowledge level while being attentive to the needs posed by the patient problem at hand is the hallmark of a master clinical teacher.

Learner level and the degree of incorporation of EBCP within a teaching program or practice environment may shape learner priorities. A medical student

is likely to be preoccupied with connecting her developing knowledge of disease to patient evaluation and management. A senior resident doing a rotation in her specialty will be ready to contemplate specific diagnostic and therapeutic choices and the guidelines or body of evidence available to inform those choices. When EBCP is not routinely modeled and is quite new to the learner, the most fruitful initial focus may be asking questions and choosing appropriate online resources to answer them (see Chapter 4, What Is the Question? and Chapter 5, Finding Current Best Evidence). On the other hand, in a graduate medical education environment in which EBCP has matured and is commonly modeled by the clinical faculty, entry-level residents might be primarily interested in the process of routine incorporation of clinical evidence into decision making. The teaching focus in this context would be how to interpret and apply to clinical practice the recommendations within clinical practice guidelines and the results of systematic reviews and relevant *primary studies.*[42]

The effective clinical teacher will ensure that all learners achieve skills adequate to routinely access and consider relevant preappraised resources for decision making. At the same time, they will identify a smaller number of learners who are motivated to deepen their appraisal skills and inspire them to gain a much greater level of expertise. Such individuals may ultimately build the expertise to develop and implement evidence-based clinical policies in their health care settings[26,43] and contribute to the development of EBCP resources and clinical practice guidelines in their specialties (see Chapter 28.5, Evidence-Based Practitioners and Evidence-Based Care).[44]

Verbal Synopses

Verbal synopses of critically appraised articles can facilitate incorporation of key evidence into practice.

For example, several days after a critical appraisal session, participants may experience difficulty recapturing the essential information from articles addressing clinical issues. Practicing short structured oral summaries immediately after the completion of the exercise may serve to sharpen perception of the take-home messages and facilitate point-of-care recall. We believe that both students and teachers will benefit from practicing this skill.

Figure 29-1 summarizes 3 key components of a verbal study synopsis: context, content, and comments. Teachers can emphasize specific context points or content issues, such as the magnitude of effect on the *patient-important outcomes* about which the patient was most concerned. They can also engage learners by highlighting the landmark nature of the article or its potential to change practice. Final comments at the end can underscore key features of the article, such as a recent, classic, or controversial contribution, its exceptional quality, or its relevance given the burden of illness it addresses.

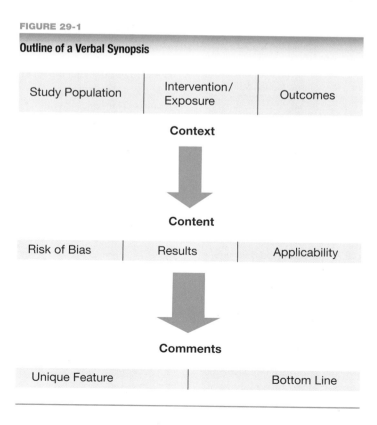

FIGURE 29-1

Outline of a Verbal Synopsis

| Study Population | Intervention/ Exposure | Outcomes |

Context

Content

| Risk of Bias | Results | Applicability |

Comments

| Unique Feature | Bottom Line |

MOVING FROM EVIDENCE TO ACTION

The following examples illustrate the use of synopses in practice. The first 2 correspond to scenarios provided at the outset of this chapter. The third is drawn from the clinical example used to frame the chapter on therapy in this book (see Chapter 7, Therapy [Randomized Trials]). The scripts provided here are simulated excerpts of communications between practitioners and staff in the course of bedside care. They neither represent the entirety of such transactions nor capture the narrative dimensions of clinical care, such as the patient's experience of illness and the relational process that ultimately determines all health care decisions.[45]

Verbal synopses constitute one format that teachers and learners may use to summarize their own evidence appraisals. Synopses can also be useful as a written exercise for learners. Early in the development of EBCP, as an educational initiative, written

---

USING THE GUIDE

Example 1

Context

ICU resident: "Mrs Richardson is in septic shock from her community-acquired pneumonia and is still hypotensive after receiving 5 L of Ringer's lactate. Should starch be administered now?" The underlying question is, "In critically ill patients with septic shock, what is the effect of starch for volume resuscitation vs crystalloid?"

Content

ICU attending physician: "Several randomized clinical trials, summarized in a recent well-conducted meta-analysis, tested starches for volume resuscitation and provide high-quality evidence that starch resuscitation is associated with increased risk of death in severe sepsis.[46] The results of this meta-analysis apply to Mrs Richards, and I suggest we avoid starches for her."

Example 2

Context

ICU resident: "Mr Jones is 2 days postoperation for ruptured abdominal aortic aneurysm. His risk of bleeding has decreased, but his risk of venous thromboembolism is on my mind because 5 years ago, after hip surgery, he developed a pulmonary embolism. I think it is safe to start heparin thromboprophylaxis today. Which type of heparin should we use?"

Underlying question: "In critically ill patients, what is the effect of low-molecular-weight heparin vs unfractionated heparin on the risk of venous thromboembolism and major bleeds?"

Content and Comments

ICU attending physician: "It has been unclear whether low-molecular-weight heparin is any better than unfractionated heparin for preventing venous thromboembolism. A recent meta-analysis of randomized trials in medical/surgical critically ill patients revealed that the risk of deep vein thrombosis is not significantly different between these 2 drugs, but the risk of symptomatic pulmonary embolism is significantly lower with low-molecular-weight heparin. There is no increased risk of major bleeding and a trend toward a lower risk of heparin-induced thrombocytopenia with low-molecular-weight heparin.[47] Only 2 trials with low risk of bias contributed to this comparison, resulting in low confidence in the effect estimates due to imprecision—a small number of participants and events—and heterogeneity. The drug costs are currently similar, and the choice of low-molecular-weight heparin for thromboprophlyaxis is reasonable."

Example 3

Context

Mr Smith has previously diagnosed peripheral vascular disease, controlled hypertension, hyperlipidemia, and no history of coronary artery disease. He has presented to you, his primary care physician, with intermittent claudication that limits his physical function and quality of life. He is already being treated with an antiplatelet agent, pentoxifylline, a statin, and 2 antihypertensive agents. He has previously undergone a physical therapy program but still finds he cannot walk far enough to complete his activities of daily living without pain or assistance. You would like to help improve his ability to walk and his quality of life. You have been in touch with his vascular specialist, who is a member of your group, and she has recommended a switch of his medicine from pentoxifylline to aspirin according to a recent trustworthy guideline providing a strong recommendation for antiplatelet therapy in patients with symptomatic peripheral vascular disease. She also suggests he should use ramipril.

Underlying question: "In patients with hypertension and intermittent claudication, does treatment with ramipril result in superior exercise tolerance and quality of life?"

Content and Comments

Primary care physician: "A recently published trial constitutes the best evidence available on this question. It included more than 200 patients with stable claudication and no history of vascular surgery or treatment with ACE [angiotensin-converting enzyme] inhibitors and suggests that ramipril increased pain-free walking distance by treadmill test as well as patient-perceived walking tolerance and quality of life by previously existing instruments.[48] The trial was randomized, *concealed*, and well *blinded*, with a 94% 6-month *follow-up* and with analysis adhering to the *intention-to-treat* principle—thus, low risk of bias. Patients receiving ramipril experienced, on average, 1 to 2 minutes increased pain-free and total walking time and reported improvements of 13 to 25 on a scale of 100 in the disease-specific, patient-reported functional status scale and of 5 on a scale of 100 in the physical components of the SF-36 quality-of-life scale. Changes of 5 or more on the latter scale are considerate 'moderate' in magnitude. Fewer than 10% of patient receiving ramipril had mild dizziness and cough. There were no other adverse outcomes reported in the active treatment group.

"Evidence from this single trial suggests that ramipril may be worth trying for Mr Smith, and we should discuss it with him. Because of concerns of the small total number of patients and risk of publication bias, we would classify this as low-quality to moderate-quality evidence, and additional trials will be needed before we can strongly recommend ramipril to such patients."

summaries of educational prescriptions[34] were introduced in the form of critically appraised topics (CATS).[49] These can provide a vehicle for independent literature searches and appraisals by learners to be reviewed by experienced faculty. Written summaries of learner-initiated exercises, including those related to EBCP, have become a key part of the evaluation and assessment tools of accredited medical education programs in the United States and elsewhere.

The Outcomes Project of the US ACGME strongly advocates the use of learner portfolios as vehicles for evaluation, assessment, and documentation.[50-52] A novel use of learner-driven written summaries has been reported from Norway.[53] "Work files" are used as a vehicle for exercise of skills and learner evaluation in a distance learning framework.

The framework has been evaluated in the context of undergraduate medical education but could also be used as part of residency training or in continuing medical education.[53]

Review of portfolio entries may, in turn, present the teacher with useful opportunities for direct EBCP skills teaching. Here, the teacher gains a direct glimpse of a resident-learner's ability to apply EBCP principles to the care of actual patients. The components of a resident portfolio entry might include a summary of the patient presentation, documentation of a search, an evidence summary, and a plan for self-improvement that addresses not only the patient in question but also similar future patients. Both resident learner and faculty preceptor may make use of relevant chapters of the *Users' Guides* for the purpose of preparing and reviewing portfolio entries.

Portfolio entries hold the potential for valuable opportunities for direct EBM skills teaching and integrated teaching of EBM and general clinical practice. A potential danger of such summaries (the equivalent of CATS), which on occasion have been freely posted online, is that they may be misconstrued as reflecting rigorous and trustworthy syntheses.[54,55] We therefore urge that they be understood strictly as tools of education and assessment and not disseminated further.

CLINICAL SCENARIO RESOLUTIONS

We have seen how synopses of relevant bodies of evidence constitute an effective vehicle for role modeling evidence-based clinical practice. Let us briefly examine how our 3 scenarios lend themselves to the 3 teaching modes we identified earlier in this chapter.

Scenario 1

Scenario 1 illustrated how the evidence bearing on the choice of starch vs crystalloid fluid resuscitation of patients with severe sepsis can be summarized to communicate the essential features of cases under active management and the decisions yet to be made. On occasion, such abbreviated summaries can spawn more extended discussions in the context of integrated teaching or in settings such as journal clubs, where direct EBCP skill acquisition may constitute the learning focus. Clinical teachers can set these applications in motion via educational prescriptions given to learners during bedside rounds.

Scenario 2

As we have pointed out, scenario 2, a discussion of thromboprophylaxis in the ICU while waiting for a noon conference to start, provides an opportunity for role modeling. In a setting such as full work rounds or a case review conference, the discussion of the relevant evidence may be extended. In such contexts, the discussion could consider aspects of the body of evidence reflected in the relevant systematic review[47] in more depth, perhaps referencing the GRADE criteria of risk of bias, precision, consistency of results across studies, and, particularly, the directness of the evidence relative to the context at hand.

In addition to the particular patient, the clinical question pertains to thromboprophylaxis for a population of postoperative patients. Hence, the choice between low-molecular-weight heparin vs unfractionated heparin may emerge from the discussion as an issue for which a clinical policy is called for on your service or throughout your institution and lead to engagement of the quality review committee. Clinical learners could fruitfully be assigned to follow this process, thereby participating in a dimension of systems-based care that constitutes an important deficit in today's medical education.[13]

Scenario 3

As a mentor for journal club, teachers can steer learners to draw on experience or issues that arise from their clinical care. The resident's proposal to use journal club to review evidence regarding surgical thromboprophylaxis provides the opportunity to close the gap between journal club and issues of clinical care. As already noted, the clinical question suggests an issue of clinical policy for which a clinical guideline would be an appropriate source of both evidence and recommendations. Journal clubs or other venues for direct teaching and acquisition of EBCP skills are well advised to seek opportunities to introduce learners to the different aspects of guideline development, adaptation, and implementation. In this case, a guideline relevant to the question at hand is available[56] and conveniently uses the GRADE framework[23] for summarizing and evaluating evidence and moving from evidence to recommendations. The guideline includes a methods section, and although it does not include primary evidence tables, it offers citations of included studies and, separately, a summary of the reasons for the evidence ratings assigned to specific comparisons and outcomes. Hence, this guideline could be used as a problem-based vehicle for learner engagement with the GRADE system and other important aspects of the guideline development and reporting process.

TEACHING CONTENT FROM THE USERS' GUIDES

The *Users' Guides* is replete with demonstrations and illustrations suitable for incorporation into teaching scripts or worksheets and other adjuncts to teaching. Indeed, in many cases, the text reflects approaches that were originally developed as interactive teaching scripts. A series of EBCP teaching tips have been published in *CMAJ*[57-62] and the *Journal of General Internal Medicine*.[63-67] A summary of these tips by topic is available in Table 29-6.[40]

The articles in the *CMAJ* and the *Journal of General Internal Medicine* present teaching approaches to commonly encountered issues in interpreting and using the medical literature to solve patient problems. They vary by level of EBCP expertise and by the time required for their use. Abbreviated approaches are most suitable when one is teaching in the role-modeling or integrated mode. More extended and detailed demonstrations, involving some simple calculations, are appropriate when more time is available and direct skills teaching is feasible. Clinically oriented learners appreciate bite-sized aliquots of EBCP skills teaching selected as directly relevant to clinical problems at hand. Some will be inclined to seek knowledge beyond that required by the immediate circumstance, and seasoned teachers are prepared with extended scripts that meet such needs.

Teaching Materials From the Users' Guides

For purposes of direct teaching of EBCP skills, you will find many examples in the *Users' Guides*. For example, as an adjunct to skills teaching regarding asking answerable questions, the teacher might convert the framework illustrated in Box 4-1 (see Chapter 4, What Is the Question?) into a worksheet, such as that provided in Table 29-3. Many variations on this table are possible to accommodate the needs and goals of different situations. For example, depending on the context, intended uses, and learning goals, one might add rows conforming to the designation of the clinical question type and the preferred study design. In a setting in which these domains are pertinent, the teacher might augment this even further by asking the learners to specify their preferred choice of online resource for doing a search for articles, syntheses, or synopses meeting these specifications (see Chapter 5, Finding Current Best Evidence).

Similarly, creating worksheets for individual study and skills-based seminars from the *Users' Guides* chapters that address questions of therapy, harm, diagnosis, prognosis, and others is straightforward. As an example, one can convert Box 22-1 (see Chapter 22, The Process of a Systematic Review and Meta-analysis) into the worksheet provided in Table 29-4.

TABLE 29-3

Worksheet for Formulating a Clinical Question

Context	Comments and Clinical Questions
Patients	
Intervention or exposure and comparator	
Outcomes	
Clinical question type[a]	
Relevant study designs[a]	

[a]Optional.

TABLE 29-4

Worksheet for Assessment of Credibility of the Process of a Systematic Review

Guide	Comments
Was the process credible? How serious was the risk of bias?	
Did the review explicitly address a sensible clinical question?	
Was the search for relevant studies detailed and exhaustive?	
Was the risk of bias of the primary studies assessed?	
Did the review address possible explanations of between-study differences in results?	
Did the review present results that are ready for clinical application?	
Were selection and assessments of studies reproducible?	
Did the review address confidence in effect estimates?	

MOVING FROM EVIDENCE TO ACTION

The worksheets provided in Tables 29-3 and 29-4 might be appropriate for use in an extended direct skills teaching session that involves an adaptation of a team-learning interactive exercise with learner subgroups working on similar designated tasks.[32,33]

A Directory of Teaching Tips From the Users' Guides

Table 29-5 provides a roadmap of selected content segments across the *Users' Guides*, many of which are included in the aforementioned articles.[40,69] Table 29-6

TABLE 29-5

Teachers' Roadmap of Potential Teaching Tips in the *Users' Guides to the Medical Literature*[a]

Content Issue	*Users' Guides* Chapter	Figure/Table	Learner Stumbling Block
Sources of bias and ways of reducing bias in studies addressing questions of therapy and harm	Chapter 6, Why Study Results Mislead: Bias and Random Error	Table 6-1	Understanding categories of bias and bias reduction strategies in randomized trials and observational studies
When does loss to follow-up seriously threaten validity?	Chapter 7, Therapy (Randomized Trials)	Table 7-1	Provides criteria for assessing importance of loss to follow-up
Relative vs absolute risk[b]	Chapter 9, Does Treatment Lower Risk? Understanding the Results	Figure 9-1	Understanding effect of baseline risk on absolute risk reduction
Confidence intervals and study size[b]	Chapter 10, Confidence Intervals: Was the Single Study or Meta-analysis Large Enough?	Table 10-1	Understanding how confidence intervals vary with study size
Clinical interpretation of confidence intervals[b]	Chapter 10, Confidence Intervals: Was the Single Study or Meta-analysis Large Enough?	Figure 10-1	Understanding how treatment thresholds determine whether a result is definitive
Bias and random error	Chapter 11.1, An Illustration of Bias and Random Error	Figure 11.1-1	Understanding bias as systematic error, independent of study size
Why early stopping for benefit is a problem	Chapter 11.3, Randomized Trials Stopped Early for Benefit	Figure 11.3-1	Apparent credibility of point estimates and confidence intervals from trials stopped early for benefit
Intention to treat	Chapter 11.4 (and Montori and Guyatt[68]), The Principle of Intention to Treat and Ambiguous Dropouts	Figure 11.4-1	Understanding how postrandomization exclusions may undermine randomization
P values and hypothesis testing[b]	Chapter 12.1, Hypothesis Testing	Figure 12.1-1	Understanding the limitations of *P* values as yes/no answers to effectiveness
Odds	Chapter 12.2, Understanding the Results: More About Odds Ratios	Table 12.2-3	Understanding odds and when odds are close to risk
Regression	Chapter 15.1, Correlation and Regression	Figures 15.1-2, 15.1-4, and 15.1-5	Regression analysis intimidating to most clinicians

(Continued)

TABLE 29-5

Teachers' Roadmap of Potential Teaching Tips in the *Users' Guides to the Medical Literature*[a] (Continued)

Content Issue	*Users' Guides* Chapter	Figure/Table	Learner Stumbling Block
Thresholds in diagnostic decision making	Chapter 16, The Process of Diagnosis	Figure 16.2	Determinants of diagnostic and therapeutic thresholds
Spectrum and bias in studies of diagnostic tests[b]	Chapter 19.1, Spectrum Bias	Figures 19.1-1 to 19.1-3	Understanding why lack of clinical uncertainty in a study population introduces systematic error in performance estimates of diagnostic tests
Measuring agreement[b]	Chapter 19.3, Measuring Agreement Beyond Chance	Figure 19.3-1	Understanding how chance contributes to measured agreement
Calculating κ value[b]	Chapter 19.3, Measuring Agreement Beyond Chance	Figures 19.3-2 to 19.3-4	Understanding how chance agreement is influenced by prevalence
Appraising prediction rules	Chapter 19.4, Clinical Prediction Rules	Figure 19.4-2	Understanding the difference among derivation, clinical validation, and impact analysis

[a]In each case, the cited figures and immediately associated text may be adapted into an interactive teaching tip.
[b]Topics have been dealt with in the EBCP Teaching Tips series (Table 29-6).

provides references to these open access publications. In addition to these materials, many useful teaching materials and tools are available on the JAMAevidence website (http://www.jamaevidence.com). These include online versions for worksheets such as the one provided in Table 29-4.

EVALUATING TEACHING AND ASSESSING LEARNER SKILLS

The development of tools for skill assessment and evaluation of EBCP teaching efforts remains a frontier area in the development of EBCP.[70-72] Reviews of studies that evaluated the teaching of EBCP and critical appraisal report heavy reliance on self-assessment and other unvalidated measures,[73,74] with only a few undergoing credible psychometric evaluation.[75-77] Multiple systematic reviews and meta-analyses have attested to a lack of rigorously developed and validated assessment tools for EBCP[9,78,79] or for the related practice-based competency.[80] Furthermore, among the very few psychometrically sound instruments in the literature, only an even smaller number have

attempted to cover the full range of EBCP knowledge and skills.[6,9] One recent report describes the validation of a tool derived from a rigorous approach to defining the EBCP domain from the perspective of practice-based learning and improvement.[81] Large-scale validation studies would be required for this or other such instruments to fully mature.

FURTHER READING

We have provided examples that illustrate how concepts and derived materials drawn from the *Users' Guides* may bear on a variety of settings and contexts for the purpose of stimulating the learning of EBCP skills. Much literature is directly and indirectly relevant to our offering. We mention a few that have caught our attention.

The concept of the 3 modes of teaching EBCP was introduced and articulated in a chapter in another EBCP text.[3] Approaches to teaching EBCP have been heavily influenced by problem-based learning and by related concepts pertaining to small-group learning settings. The ABC of Learning and

TABLE 29-6

Links to Evidence-Based Clinical Practice Teaching Tips Installments by Topic

Topic	Description	Reference
Relative and absolute risk, NNT	Understanding the relationship between measures of association	Barratt A, Wyer PC, Hatala R, et al. Tips for teachers of evidence-based medicine, 1: relative risk reduction, absolute risk reduction and number needed to treat. *CMAJ.* 2004;171(4):1-8.
NNT for studies with long-term follow-up	Interpreting hazard ratios for decision making	Barratt A, Wyer PC, Guyatt G, Simpson JM. NNT for studies with long-term follow-up. *CMAJ.* 2005;172(5):613.
Confidence intervals and *P* values	Clinical interpretation of confidence intervals and the limitations of *P* values	Montori VM, Kleinbart J, Newman TB, et al. Tips for teachers of evidence-based medicine, 2: confidence intervals and *p* values. *CMAJ.* 2004;171(6):1-12.
κ value	Understanding and calculating agreement above chance	McGinn T, Wyer PC, Newman TB, et al. Tips for teachers of evidence-based medicine, 3: understanding and calculating kappa. *CMAJ.* 2004;171(11):1-9.
Heterogeneity	Assessment of variation in trial results and when it is acceptable to pool results	Hatala R, Keitz S, Wyer PC, Guyatt G. Tips for teachers of evidence-based medicine, 4: assessing heterogeneity of primary studies in systematic reviews and whether to combine their results. *CMAJ.* 2005:172(5):1-8.
Spectrum bias	Lack of diagnostic uncertainty as source of systematic error in estimates of test performance	Montori VM, Wyer P, Newman TB, Keitz S, Guyatt G. Tips for teachers of evidence-based medicine, 5: the effect of spectrum of disease on the performance of diagnostic tests. *CMAJ.* 2005:173(4):1-7.
Decision analysis	Using decision analysis and trees to teach clinical reasoning	Lee A, Joynt GM, Ho AMH, et al. Tips for teachers of evidence-based medicine: making sense of decision analysis using a decision tree. *J Gen Intern Med.* 2009;24(5):642-648.
Likelihood ratios	Deriving and using likelihood ratios for decision making	Richardson WS, Wilson, MC, Keitz SA, Wyer PC. Tips for teachers of evidence-based medicine: making sense of diagnostic test results using likelihood ratios. *J Gen Intern Med.* 2008;23(1):87-92.
Adjusting for prognostic imbalance	Understanding confounding and adjustment	Kennedy CC, Jaeschke R, Keitz S. Tips for teachers of evidence-based medicine: adjusting for prognostic imbalances (confounding variables) in studies on therapy or harm. *J Gen Intern Med.* 2008;23(3): 337-343.
Odds ratios	Understanding relationships between odds and risk	Prasad K, Jaeschke R, Wyer P, Keitz S. Tips for teachers of evidence-based medicine: understanding odds ratios and their relationship to risk ratios. *J Gen Intern Med.* 2008;23(5):635-640.
Clinical prediction rules	Understanding pretest probabilities and the role of prediction rules	McGinn T, Ramiro J, Wisnivesky J, Keitz S, Wyer PC. Tips for teachers of evidence-based medicine: clinical prediction rules (CPRs) and estimating pretest probability. *J Gen Intern Med.* 2008;23(8):1261-1268.

Abbreviation: NNT, number needed to treat.

Teaching Medicine series published in *BMJ* offers a convenient set of articles on these and related topics and is available via open access at http://annietv600.wordpress.com/2006/05/13/the-abc-of-learning-and-teaching-in-medicine-bmj-series-2003.[82] Likewise, adult learning theory and related concepts have potential bearing on the concepts we have elaborated here,[83] as do classic articles on the development of expertise.[84-86] A useful series on "microteaching" (teaching on the run) is available from the *Medical Journal of Australia*.[87]

In this chapter, we largely addressed undergraduate and graduate medical training settings. Direct teaching of EBCP skills to practitioners who have finished formal clinical training poses its own challenges and frequently requires an even more explicit negotiation of learning and teaching goals. Evidence-based clinical practice workshops, continuing medical education programs, and the integration of article reviews as items in division meetings can be useful in this regard but are beyond the scope of our discussion.[88,89]

References

1. Batalden P, Leach D, Swing S, Dreyfus H, Dreyfus S. General competencies and accreditation in graduate medical education. *Health Aff (Millwood)*. 2002;21(5):103-111.

2. Royal College of Physicians and Surgeons of Canada. CanMEDS 2005 Framework. http://www.royalcollege.ca/portal/page/portal/rc/canmeds/framework. Accessed August 12, 2013.

3. Frank JR, Jabbour M, Tugwell P, et al. Skills for the new millennium: report of the Societal Needs Working Group, CanMEDS 2000 Project. *Ann R Coll Physicians Surg Can*. 1996;29(4):206-216.

4. Nasca TJ, Philibert I, Brigham T, Flynn TC. The next GME accreditation system: rationale and benefits. *N Engl J Med*. 2012;366(11):1051-1056.

5. Chatterji M, Graham MJ, Wyer PC. Mapping cognitive overlaps between practice-based learning and improvement and evidence-based medicine: an operational definition for assessing resident physician competence. *J Grad Med Educ*. 2009;1(2):287-298.

6. Wyer PC, Naqvi Z, Dayan PS, Celentano JJ, Eskin B, Graham MJ. Do workshops in evidence-based practice equip participants to identify and answer questions requiring consideration of clinical research? a diagnostic skill assessment. *Adv Health Sci Educ Theory Pract*. 2009;14(4):515-533.

7. Epstein RM. Mindful practice in action (I): technical competence, evidence-based medicine, and relationship-centered care. *Fam Syst Health*. 2003;21(1):1-9.

8. Sestini P. Epistemology and ethics of evidence-based medicine: putting goal-setting in the right place. *J Eval Clin Pract*. 2010;16(2):301-305.

9. Maggio LA, Tannery NH, Chen HC, ten Cate O, O'Brien B. Evidence-based medicine training in undergraduate medical education: a review and critique of the literature published 2006-2011. *Acad Med*. 2013;88(7):1022-1028.

10. Greenhalgh T. Narrative based medicine: narrative based medicine in an evidence based world. *BMJ*. 1999;318(7179):323-325.

11. Silva SA, Charon R, Wyer PC. The marriage of evidence and narrative: scientific nurturance within clinical practice. *J Eval Clin Pract*. 2011;17(4):585-593.

12. Silva SA, Wyer PC. The Roadmap: a blueprint for evidence literacy within a Scientifically Informed Medical Practice and Learning model. *Eur J Person Centered Healthcare*. 2013;1(1):53-68.

13. Cooke M, Irby DM, O'Brien BC. *Educating Physicians: A Call for Reform of Medical School and Residency*. San Francisco, CA: Jossey-Bass; 2010.

14. Davis J, Chryssafidou E, Zamora J, Davies D, Khan K, Coomarasamy A. Computer-based teaching is as good as face to face lecture-based teaching of evidence based medicine: a randomised controlled trial. *BMC Med Educ*. 2007;7:23.

15. Coppus SFPJ, Emparanza JI, Hadley J, et al. A clinically integrated curriculum in evidence-based medicine for just-in-time learning through on-the-job training: the EU-EBM project. *BMC Med Educ*. 2007;7:46.

16. Kulier R, Hadley J, Weinbrenner S, et al. Harmonising evidence-based medicine teaching: a study of the outcomes of e-learning in five European countries. *BMC Med Educ*. 2008;8:27.

17. Kulier R, Gülmezoglu AM, Zamora J, et al. Effectiveness of a clinically integrated e-learning course in evidence-based medicine for reproductive health training: a randomized trial. *JAMA*. 2012;308(21):2218-2225.

18. Kulier R, Coppus SF, Zamora J, et al. The effectiveness of a clinically integrated e-learning course in evidence-based medicine: a cluster randomised controlled trial. *BMC Med Educ*. 2009;9:21.

19. Atkins D, Best D, Briss PA, et al; GRADE Working Group. Grading quality of evidence and strength of recommendations. *BMJ*. 2004;328(7454):1490-1494.

20. Committee on Standards for Developing Trustworthy Clinical Practice Guidelines. *Clinical Practice Guidelines We Can Trust*. Washington, DC: Institute of Medicine; 2011.

21. Qaseem A, Forland F, Macbeth F, Ollenschläger G, Phillips S, van der Wees P; Board of Trustees of the Guidelines International Network. Guidelines International Network: toward international standards for clinical practice guidelines. *Ann Intern Med*. 2012;156(7):525-531.

22. Eddy DM. Evidence-based medicine: a unified approach. *Health Aff (Millwood)*. 2005;24(1):9-17.

23. Guyatt G, Oxman AD, Akl EA, et al. GRADE guidelines, 1: introduction-GRADE evidence profiles and summary of findings tables. *J Clin Epidemiol*. 2011;64(4):383-394.

24. Guyatt GH, Oxman AD, Kunz R, Vist GE, Falck-Ytter Y, Schünemann HJ; GRADE Working Group. What is "quality of evidence" and why is it important to clinicians? *BMJ*. 2008;336(7651):995-998.

25. Eddy DM, Adler J, Patterson B, Lucas D, Smith KA, Morris M. Individualized guidelines: the potential for increasing quality and reducing costs. *Ann Intern Med*. 2011;154(9):627-634.

26. Straus SE, Tetroe JM, Graham ID. Knowledge translation is the use of knowledge in health care decision making. *J Clin Epidemiol*. 2011;64(1):6-10.

27. Lang ES, Wyer P, Tabas JA, Krishnan JA. Educational and research advances stemming from the Academic Emergency Medicine consensus conference in knowledge translation. *Acad Emerg Med*. 2010;17(8):865-869.

28. Wahabi HA, Al-Ansary LA. Innovative teaching methods for capacity building in knowledge translation. *BMC Med Educ*. 2011;11:85.

29. Coomarasamy A, Khan KS. What is the evidence that postgraduate teaching in evidence based medicine changes anything? a systematic review. *BMJ*. 2004;329(7473):1017-1021.

30. Davis D, O'Brien MA, Freemantle N, Wolf FM, Mazmanian P, Taylor-Vaisey A. Impact of formal continuing medical education: do conferences, workshops, rounds, and other traditional continuing education activities change physician behavior or health care outcomes? *JAMA*. 1999;282(9):867-874.

31. Ghali WA, Saitz R, Eskew AH, Gupta M, Quan H, Hershman WY. Successful teaching in evidence-based medicine. *Med Educ*. 2000;34(1):18-22.

32. Haidet P, O'Malley KJ, Richards B. An initial experience with "team learning" in medical education. *Acad Med*. 2002; 77(1):40-44.

33. Hunt DP, Haidet P, Coverdale JH, Richards B. The effect of using team learning in an evidence-based medicine course for medical students. *Teach Learn Med*. 2003;15(2):131-139.

34. Straus SE, Richardson WS, Glasziou P, Haynes RB. *Evidence-Based Medicine: How to Practice and Teach EBM*. 4th ed. Edinburgh, Scotland: Elsevier Churchill Livingstone; 2011.

35. Richardson WS. Teaching evidence-based practice on foot. *ACP J Club*. 2005;143(2):A10-A12.

36. Norman GR, Eva KW, Schmidt HG. Implications of psychology-type theories for full curriculum interventions. *Med Educ*. 2005;39(3):247-249.

37. Norman GR, Schmidt HG. Effectiveness of problem-based learning curricula: theory, practice and paper darts. *Med Educ*. 2000;34(9):721-728.

38. Irby DM. How attending physicians make instructional decisions when conducting teaching rounds. *Acad Med*. 1992; 67(10):630-638.

39. Schmidt HG, Norman GR, Boshuizen HP. A cognitive perspective on medical expertise: theory and implication. *Acad Med*. 1990;65(10):611-621.

40. Wyer PC, Keitz S, Hatala R, et al. Tips for learning and teaching evidence-based medicine: introduction to the series. *CMAJ*. 2004;171(4):347-348.

41. Irby DM. What clinical teachers in medicine need to know. *Acad Med*. 1994;69(5):333-342.

42. Weingart S, Wyer P. *Emergency Medicine Decision Making: Critical Choices in Chaotic Environments*. New York, NY: McGraw-Hill Companies; 2006.

43. Straus SE, Tetroe JM, Graham ID. *Knowledge Translation in Health Care: Moving from Evidence to Practice*. 2nd ed. Oxford, UK: Wiley Blackwell; 2013.

44. Guyatt GH, Meade MO, Jaeschke RZ, Cook DJ, Haynes RB. Practitioners of evidence based care: not all clinicians need to appraise evidence from scratch but all need some skills. *BMJ*. 2000;320(7240):954-955.

45. Charon R, Wyer P; NEBM Working Group. Narrative evidence based medicine. *Lancet*. 2008;371(9609):296-297.

46. Zarychanski R, Abou-Setta AM, Turgeon AF, et al. Association of hydroxyethyl starch administration with mortality and acute kidney injury in critically ill patients requiring volume resuscitation: a systematic review and meta-analysis. *JAMA*. 2013;309(7):678-688.

47. Alhazzani W, Lim W, Jaeschke RZ, Murad MH, Cade J, Cook DJ. Heparin thromboprophylaxis in medical-surgical critically ill patients: a systematic review and meta-analysis of randomized trials. *Crit Care Med*. 2013;41(9):2088-2098.

48. Ahimastos AA, Walker PJ, Askew C, et al. Effect of ramipril on walking times and quality of life among patients with peripheral artery disease and intermittent claudication: a randomized controlled trial. *JAMA*. 2013;309(5):453-460.

49. Sauve S, Lee HN, Meade MO, et al. The critically appraised topic: a practical approach to learning critical appraisal. *Ann R Coll Physicians Surg Can*. 1995;28(7):396-398.

50. Carraccio C, Englander R. Evaluating competence using a portfolio: a literature review and web-based application to the ACGME competencies. *Teach Learn Med*. 2004;16(4):381-387.

51. Lynch DC, Swing SR, Horowitz SD, Holt K, Messer JV. Assessing practice-based learning and improvement. *Teach Learn Med*. 2004;16(1):85-92.

52. Mathers NJ, Challis MC, Howe AC, Field NJ. Portfolios in continuing medical education: effective and efficient? *Med Educ*. 1999;33(7):521-530.

53. Kongerud IC, Vandvik PO. Work files as learning tools in knowledge management. *Tidsskr Nor Laegeforen*. 2013;133(15):1587-1590.

54. Wyer PC. The critically appraised topic: closing the evidence-transfer gap. *Ann Emerg Med*. 1997;30(5):639-640.

55. Wyer PC, Rowe BH, Guyatt GH, Cordell WH. Evidence-based emergency medicine: the clinician and the medical literature: when can we take a shortcut? *Ann Emerg Med*. 2000;36(2):149-155.

56. Gould MK, Garcia DA, Wren SM, et al. Prevention of VTE in nonorthopedic surgical patients antithrombotic therapy and prevention of thrombosis, 9th ed: American College of Chest Physicians Evidence-Based Clinical Practice Guidelines. *Chest*. 2012;141(2 Suppl):e227S–e277S.

57. Barratt A, Wyer PC, Hatala R, et al; Evidence-Based Medicine Teaching Tips Working Group. Tips for learners of evidence-based medicine, 1: relative risk reduction, absolute risk reduction and number needed to treat. *CMAJ*. 2004;171(4):353-358.

58. de Lemos ML, Wyer PC, Guyatt G, Simpson JM. NNT for studies with long-term follow-up. *CMAJ*. 2005;172(5): 613-615.

59. Montori VM, Kleinbart J, Newman TB, et al. Tips for teachers of evidence-based medicine, 2: confidence intervals and *p* values. *CMAJ*. 2004;171(6):1-12.

60. McGinn T, Wyer PC, Newman TB, et al. Tips for teachers of evidence-based medicine, 3: understanding and calculating kappa. *CMAJ*. 2004;171(11):1-9.

61. Hatala R, Keitz S, Wyer P, Guyatt G; Evidence-Based Medicine Teaching Tips Working Group. Tips for learners of evidence-based medicine, 4: assessing heterogeneity of primary studies in systematic reviews and whether to combine their results. *CMAJ.* 2005;172(5):661-665.

62. Montori VM, Wyer P, Newman TB, Keitz S, Guyatt G; Evidence-Based Medicine Teaching Tips Working Group. Tips for learners of evidence-based medicine, 5: the effect of spectrum of disease on the performance of diagnostic tests. *CMAJ.* 2005;173(4):385-390.

63. Lee A, Joynt GM, Ho AMH, Keitz S, McGinn T, Wyer PC; EBM Teaching Scripts Working Group. Tips for teachers of evidence-based medicine: making sense of decision analysis using a decision tree. *J Gen Intern Med.* 2009;24(5):642-648.

64. Richardson WS, Wilson MC, Keitz SA, Wyer PC; EBM Teaching Scripts Working Group. Tips for teachers of evidence-based medicine: making sense of diagnostic test results using likelihood ratios. *J Gen Intern Med.* 2008;23(1):87-92.

65. Kennedy CC, Jaeschke R, Keitz S, et al; Evidence-Based Medicine Teaching Tips Working Group. Tips for teachers of evidence-based medicine: adjusting for prognostic imbalances (confounding variables) in studies on therapy or harm. *J Gen Intern Med.* 2008;23(3):337-343.

66. Prasad K, Jaeschke R, Wyer P, Keitz S, Guyatt G; Evidence-Based Medicine Teaching Tips Working Group. Tips for teachers of evidence-based medicine: understanding odds ratios and their relationship to risk ratios. *J Gen Intern Med.* 2008;23(5):635-640.

67. McGinn T, Jervis R, Wisnivesky J, Keitz S, Wyer PC; Evidence-based Medicine Teaching Tips Working Group. Tips for teachers of evidence-based medicine: clinical prediction rules (CPRs) and estimating pretest probability. *J Gen Intern Med.* 2008;23(8):1261-1268.

68. Montori VM, Guyatt GH. Intention-to-treat principle. *CMAJ.* 2001;165(10):1339-1341.

69. Williams BC, Hoffman RM. Teaching Tips: a new series in JGIM. *J Gen Intern Med.* 2008;23(1):112-113.

70. Dobbie AE, Schneider FD, Anderson AD, Littlefield J. What evidence supports teaching evidence-based medicine? *Acad Med.* 2000;75(12):1184-1185.

71. Hatala R, Guyatt G. Evaluating the teaching of evidence-based medicine. *JAMA.* 2002;288(9):1110-1112.

72. Straus SE, Green ML, Bell DS, et al; Society of General Internal Medicine Evidence-Based Medicine Task Force. Evaluating the teaching of evidence based medicine: conceptual framework. *BMJ.* 2004;329(7473):1029-1032.

73. Green ML. Graduate medical education training in clinical epidemiology, critical appraisal, and evidence-based medicine: a critical review of curricula. *Acad Med.* 1999;74(6):686-694.

74. Shaneyfelt TM, Baum K, Bell DS, et al. Evaluating evidence-based medicine competence: a systematic review of instruments [Abstract]. *J Gen Intern Med.* 2005;20(S1):155.

75. Fritsche L, Greenhalgh T, Falck-Ytter Y, Neumayer HH, Kunz R. Do short courses in evidence based medicine improve knowledge and skills? Validation of Berlin questionnaire and before and after study of courses in evidence based medicine. *BMJ.* 2002;325(7376):1338-1341.

76. Ramos KD, Schafer S, Tracz SM. Validation of the Fresno test of competence in evidence based medicine. *BMJ.* 2003;326(7384):319-321.

77. Taylor R, Reeves B, Mears R, et al. Development and validation of a questionnaire to evaluate the effectiveness of evidence-based practice teaching. *Med Educ.* 2001;35(6):544-547.

78. Oude Rengerink K, Zwolsman SE, Ubbink DT, Mol BWJ, van Dijk N, Vermeulen H. Tools to assess evidence-based practice behaviour among healthcare professionals. *Evid Based Med.* 2013;18(4):129-138.

79. Shaneyfelt T, Baum KD, Bell D, et al. Instruments for evaluating education in evidence-based practice: a systematic review. *JAMA.* 2006;296(9):1116-1127.

80. Lurie SJ, Mooney CJ, Lyness JM. Measurement of the general competencies of the accreditation council for graduate medical education: a systematic review. *Acad Med.* 2009;84(3):301-309.

81. Wyer P, Chatterji M. Designing outcome measures for the accreditation of medical education programs as an iterative process combining classical test theory and Rasch measurement. *Int J Educ Psychol Assess.* 2013;13(2):35-61.

82. Prideaux D. ABC of learning and teaching in medicine: curriculum design. *BMJ.* 2003;326(7383):268-270.

83. Bransford JD, Brown AL, Cocking RR. *How People Learn: Brain, Mind, Experience and School.* Washington, DC: National Academy Press; 2000.

84. Ananthakrishnan N. Microteaching as a vehicle of teacher training: its advantages and disadvantages. *J Postgrad Med.* 1993;39(3):142-143.

85. Ericsson KA. *The Road to Excellence: The Acquisition of Expert Performance in the Arts and Sciences, Sports and Games.* Mahwah, NJ: Lawrence Erlbaum Associates; 1996.

86. Ericsson KA. Deliberate practice and the acquisition and maintenance of expert performance in medicine and related domains. *Acad Med.* 2004;79(10)(suppl):S70-S81.

87. University of Western Australia Faculty of Medicine. Dentistry and Health Sciences. Tip series. University of Western Australia website. http://www.meddent.uwa.edu.au/teaching/on-the-run/tips. Updated September 16, 2009. Accessed April 4, 2014.

88. Leipzig RM, Wallace EZ, Smith LG, Sullivant J, Dunn K, McGinn T. Teaching evidence-based medicine: a regional dissemination model. *Teach Learn Med.* 2003;15(3):204-209.

89. Murad MH, Montori VM, Kunz R, et al. How to teach evidence-based medicine to teachers: reflections from a workshop experience. *J Eval Clin Pract.* 2009;15(6):1205-1207.

MOVING FROM EVIDENCE TO ACTION

GLOSSARY

Term	Definition
Absolute Difference	The absolute difference in rates of good or harmful outcomes between experimental groups (experimental group risk [EGR]) and control groups (control group risk [CGR]), calculated as the risk in the control group minus the risk in the experimental group (CGR − EGR). For instance, if the rate of adverse events is 20% in the control group and 10% in the treatment group, the absolute difference is 20% − 10% = 10%.
Absolute Risk (or Baseline Risk or Control Event Rate [CER])	The risk of an event (eg, if 10 of 100 patients have an event, the absolute risk is 10% expressed as a percentage and 0.10 expressed as a proportion).
Absolute Risk Increase (ARI)	The absolute difference in the risk of harmful outcomes between experimental groups (experimental group risk [EGR]) and control groups (control group risk [CGR]), calculated as the risk of harmful outcomes in the experimental group minus the rate of harmful outcomes in the control group (EGR − CGR). Typically used to describe a harmful exposure or intervention (eg, if the rate of adverse outcomes is 20% in the treatment group and 10% in the control group, the absolute risk increase would be 10% expressed as a percentage and 0.10 expressed as a proportion). See also Absolute Risk Reduction; Number Needed to Harm.
Absolute Risk Reduction (ARR) (or Risk Difference [RD])	The absolute difference (risk difference) in risks of harmful outcomes between experimental groups (experimental group risk [EGR]) and control groups (control group risk [CGR]), calculated as the risk of harmful outcome in the control group minus the risk of harmful outcome in the experimental group (CGR − EGR). Typically used to describe a beneficial exposure or intervention (eg, if 20% of patients in the control group have an adverse event, as do 10% among treated patients, the ARR or risk difference would be 10% expressed as a percentage and 0.10 expressed as a proportion).
Academic Detailing (or Educational Outreach Visits)	A strategy for changing clinician behavior. Use of a trained person who meets with health care professionals in their practice settings to provide information with the intent of changing their practice. The pharmaceutical industry frequently uses this strategy, to which the term "detailing" is applied. Academic detailing is such an interaction initiated by an academic group or institution rather than the pharmaceutical industry.
Additive	In genetic association studies, this describes any trait that increases proportionately in expression when comparing those with no copy, 1 copy, or 2 copies of that allele (ie, those with 1 copy of the allele show more of the trait than those without and, in turn, those with 2 copies show more of the trait than those with 1 copy).
Adherence (or Compliance)	The extent to which patients follow health care recommendations or the extent to which clinicians follow recommendations for use of diagnostic tests, monitoring equipment, interventional requirements, and other technical specifications that define optimal patient management.
Adjusted Analysis	An adjusted analysis takes into account differences in prognostic factors (or baseline characteristics) between groups that may influence the outcome. For instance, when comparing an experimental and control intervention, if the experimental group is on average older, and thus at higher risk of an adverse outcome than the control group, the analysis adjusted for age will have a larger treatment effect than the unadjusted analysis.
Adjusted Indirect Comparison	A statistical technique that permits comparison between 2 interventions that have not been compared directly (head-to-head) but have both been compared to the same third comparator. This method preserves the principle of randomization.

Term	Definition
Alerting (or Alerting Systems)	A strategy for changing clinician behavior. A type of computer decision support system that alerts the clinician to a circumstance that might require clinical action (eg, a system that highlights out-of-range laboratory values).
Algorithm	An explicit description of an ordered sequence of steps with branching logic that can be applied under specific clinical circumstances. The logic of an algorithm is if *a*, then do *x*; if *b*, then do *y*; etc.
Allele	In genetic association studies, this is one of several variants of a gene, usually referring to a specific site within the gene
Allocation Concealment (or Concealment)	Randomization is concealed if the person who is making the decision about enrolling a patient is unaware of whether the next patient enrolled will be entered in the intervention or control group (using techniques such as central randomization or sequentially numbered opaque sealed envelopes). If randomization is not concealed, patients with differing prognoses may be differentially recruited to treatment or control groups. Of particular concern, patients with better prognoses may tend to be preferentially enrolled in the active treatment arm, resulting in exaggeration of the apparent benefit of the intervention (or even the false conclusion that the intervention is efficacious).
α Level (or type I error)	The probability of erroneously concluding that there is a difference between comparison groups when there is in fact no difference (also called a type I error). Typically, investigators decide on the chance of a false-positive result they are willing to accept when they plan the sample size for a study (eg, investigators often set α level at .05).
Anchor Based	One way to establish the interpretability of measures of patient-reported outcomes is anchor based (the other is distribution based). Anchor-based methods require an independent standard, or anchor, that is itself interpretable and at least moderately correlated with the instrument being assessed. This anchor typically helps establish a minimum important difference of instruments that measure patient-reported outcomes.
Applicability	See Generalizability.
As-Treated Analysis	Includes patients according to the intervention they received rather than the intervention to which they were randomized. Thus, intervention group patients who received the control are counted in the control group, and control group patients who received the intervention are counted in the treatment group. This analysis is very likely to destroy the prognostic balance randomization achieved and provide misleading results.
Audit and Feedback	A strategy for changing clinician behavior. Any written or verbal summary of clinician performance (eg, based on medical record review or observation of clinical practice) during a specified period. The summary may also include recommendations to improve practice.
Background Questions	These clinical questions are about physiology, pathology, epidemiology, and general management and are often asked by clinicians in training. The answers to background questions are often best found in textbooks or narrative review articles.
Base Case	In an economic evaluation, the base case is the best estimates of each of the key variables that bear on the costs and effects of the alternative management strategies.
Baseline Characteristics	Factors that describe study participants at the beginning of the study (eg, age, sex, disease severity). In comparison studies, it is important that these characteristics be initially similar between groups; if not balanced or if the imbalance is not statistically adjusted, these characteristics can cause confounding and can bias study results.

Term	Definition
Baseline Risk (or Baseline Event Rate or Control Event Rate [CER])	The proportion or percentage of study participants in the control group in whom an adverse outcome is observed.
Bayesian Analysis	A statistical method that uses prior knowledge combined with data. See also Bayesian Diagnostic Reasoning.
Bayesian Diagnostic Reasoning	The essence of Bayesian reasoning is that one starts with a prior probability or probability distribution and incorporates new information to arrive at a posterior probability or probability distribution. The approach to diagnosis presented in the *Users' Guides to the Medical Literature* assumes that diagnosticians are intuitive Bayesian thinkers and move from pretest to posttest probabilities as information accumulates.
Before-After Design (or One-Group Pretest-Posttest Design)	A study in which the investigators compare the status of a group of study participants before and after the implementation of an intervention. In a controlled before-after study, investigators identify a control population with characteristics and performance similar to those of the study population. Data are collected and outcomes measured in both the study and control populations before and after the introduction of an intervention to the study population. Observed differences between groups in the postintervention period or in change scores (from baseline in each group) are assumed attributed to the intervention. In an uncontrolled before-after study, outcomes are measured before and after the introduction of an intervention in the same study setting. Observed differences in the outcomes are assumed to be attributable to the intervention.
β Error (or Type II Error)	Otherwise known as type II error, β error is the probability that a study will fail to rule out a null hypothesis when in fact that null hypothesis (typically that the treatment effect is 0; for instance, the relative risk is 1.0) is true. In other words, it is the probability of missing a true treatment effect. In sample-size calculations, β is typically set at .2 or .1.
Bias (or Systematic Error)	Systematic deviation from the underlying truth because of a feature of the design or conduct of a research study (eg, overestimation of a treatment effect because of failure to randomize). Sometimes, authors label specific types of bias in a variety of contexts. 1. Channeling Effect or Channeling Bias: Tendency of clinicians to prescribe treatment according to a patient's prognosis. As a result of this behavior in observational studies, treated patients are more or less likely to be high-risk patients than untreated patients, leading to a biased estimate of treatment effect. 2. Data Completeness Bias: Using a computer decision support system (CDSS) to log episodes in the intervention group and using a manual system in the non-CDSS control group can create variation in the completeness of data. 3. Detection Bias (or Surveillance Bias): Tendency to look more carefully for an outcome in one of the comparison groups. 4. Differential Verification Bias: When test results influence the choice of the reference standard (eg, test-positive patients undergo an invasive test to establish the diagnosis, whereas test-negative patients undergo long-term follow-up without application of the invasive test), the assessment of test properties may be biased. 5. Expectation Bias: In data collection, an interviewer has information that influences his or her expectation of finding the exposure or outcome. In clinical practice, a clinician's assessment may be influenced by previous knowledge of the presence or absence of a disorder.

(Continued)

Term	Definition
Bias (or Systematic Error) (*Continued*)	6. Incorporation Bias: Occurs when investigators use a reference standard that incorporates a diagnostic test that is the subject of investigation. The result is a bias toward making the test appear more powerful in differentiating target-positive from target-negative patients than it actually is.
	7. Interviewer Bias: Greater probing by an interviewer of some participants than others, contingent on particular features of the participants.
	8. Lead-Time Bias: Occurs when outcomes such as survival, as measured from the time of diagnosis, may be increased not because patients live longer, but because screening lengthens the time that they know they have disease.
	9. Length-Time Bias: Occurs when patients whose disease is discovered by screening may also appear to do better or live longer than people whose disease presents clinically with symptoms because screening tends to detect disease that is destined to progress slowly and that therefore has a good prognosis.
	10. Observer Bias: Occurs when an observer's observations differ systematically according to participant characteristics (eg, making systematically different observations in treatment and control groups).
	11. Partial Verification Bias: Occurs when only a selected sample of patients who underwent the index test is verified by the reference standard, and that sample is dependent on the results of the test. For example, patients with suspected coronary artery disease whose exercise test results are positive may be more likely to undergo coronary angiography (the reference standard) than those whose exercise test results are negative.
	12. Publication Bias: Occurs when the publication of research depends on the direction of the study results and whether they are statistically significant.
	13. Recall Bias: Occurs when patients who experience an adverse outcome have a different likelihood of recalling an exposure than patients who do not experience the adverse outcome, independent of the true extent of exposure.
	14. Referral Bias: Occurs when characteristics of patients differ between one setting (such as primary care) and another setting that includes only referred patients (such as secondary or tertiary care).
	15. Reporting Bias (or Selective Outcome Reporting Bias): The inclination of authors to differentially report research results according to the magnitude, direction, or statistical significance of the results.
	16. Social Desirability Bias: Occurs when participants answer according to social norms or socially desirable behavior rather than what is actually the case (for instance, underreporting alcohol consumption).
	17. Spectrum Bias: Ideally, diagnostic test properties will be assessed in a population in which the spectrum of disease in the target-positive patients includes all those in whom clinicians might be uncertain about the diagnosis, and the target-negative patients include all those with conditions easily confused with the target condition. Spectrum bias may occur when the accuracy of a diagnostic test is assessed in a population that differs from this ideal. Examples of spectrum bias would include a situation in which a substantial proportion of the target-positive population has advanced disease and target-negative participants are healthy or asymptomatic. Such situations typically occur in diagnostic case-control studies (eg, comparing those with advanced disease with healthy individuals). Such studies are liable to yield an overly sanguine estimate of the usefulness of the test.

(Continued)

Term	Definition
Bias (or Systematic Error) (*Continued*)	18. Surveillance Bias. See Detection Bias.
	19. Verification Bias. See Differential Verification Bias.
	20. Workup Bias. See Differential Verification Bias.
Binary Outcome (or Dichotomous Outcome)	A categorical variable that can take 1 of 2 discrete values rather than an incremental value on a continuum (eg, pregnant or not pregnant, dead or alive).
Bivariable Regression Analysis	Regression when there is only 1 independent variable under evaluation with respect to a dependent variable. See also Multivariate Regression Analysis (or Multivariable Regression Analysis).
Blind (or Blinded or Masked)	Patients, clinicians, data collectors, outcome adjudicators, or data analysts unaware of which patients have been assigned to the experimental or control group. In the case of diagnostic tests, those interpreting the test results are unaware of the result of the reference standard or vice versa.
Bonferroni correction	A statistical adjustment to the threshold P value to adjust for multiple comparisons. The usual threshold for statistical significance (α) is 0.05. To perform a Bonferroni correction, one divides the critical P value by the number of comparisons being made. For example, if 10 hypotheses are being tested, the new critical P value would be $\alpha/10$, usually 0.05/10 or 0.005. The Bonferroni correction represents a simple adjustment but is very conservative (ie, less likely than other methods to give a significant result).
Boolean Operators (or Logical Operators)	Words used when searching electronic databases. These operators are AND, OR, and NOT and are used to combine terms (AND/OR) or exclude terms (NOT) from the search strategy.
Bootstrap Technique	A statistical technique for estimating parameters, such as standard errors and confidence intervals, based on resampling from an observed data set with replacement from the original sample.
Burden	The term "burden" is used in 2 ways in the *Users' Guides to the Medical Literature*. One is burden of illness, which refers to the frequency of an illness in a population and its associated effect on quality of life, morbidity, mortality, and health care costs. Another is burden of treatment, which refers to the inconvenience of attending to the treatment's optimal use, of its monitoring, the limitations in lifestyle that it entails, and the possibility of interactions with other treatments.
Burden of Illness	See Burden.
Burden of Treatment	See Burden.
Candidate Gene Study	A study that evaluates the association of specific genetic variants with outcomes or traits of interest, selecting the variants to be tested according to explicit considerations (known or postulated biology or function, previous studies, etc).
Case-Control Study	A study designed to determine the association between an exposure and outcome in which patients are sampled by outcome. Those with the outcome (cases) are compared with those without the outcome (controls) with respect to exposure to the suspected harmful agent.
Case Series	A report of a study of a collection of patients treated in a similar manner, without a control group. For example, a clinician might describe the characteristics of an outcome for 25 consecutive patients with diabetes who received education for prevention of foot ulcers.
Case Study	In qualitative research, an exploration of a case defined by some boundaries or contemporary phenomena, usually within a real-life context.

Term	Definition
Categorical Variable	A categorical variable may be nominal or ordinal. Categorical variables can be defined according to attributes without any associated order (eg, medical admission, elective surgery, or emergency surgery); these are called nominal variables. A categorical variable can also be defined according to attributes that are ordered (eg, height, such as high, medium, or low); these are called ordinal variables.
Censoring	Censoring occurs when the value of a measurement or observation is only partially known. The problem of censored data, in which the observed value of some variables is partially known, is related to the problem of missing data. Many statistical methods can be used to estimate, impute, or otherwise model censored data.
Chance-Corrected Agreement	The proportion of possible agreement achieved beyond that which one would expect by chance alone, often measured by the κ statistic.
Chance-Independent Agreement	The proportion of possible agreement achieved that is independent of chance and unaffected by the distribution of ratings, as measured by the φ statistic.
Channeling Effect or Channeling Bias	The tendency of clinicians to prescribe treatment according to a patient's prognosis. As a result of this behavior in observational studies, treated patients are more or less likely to be high-risk patients than untreated patients, leading to a biased estimate of treatment effect. See also Bias.
Checklist Effect	The improvement seen in medical decision making because of more complete and structured data collection (eg, clinicians fill out a detailed form, so their decisions improve).
χ^2 Test	A nonparametric test of statistical significance used to compare the distribution of categorical outcomes in 2 or more groups, the null hypothesis of which is that the underlying distributions are identical.
Chromosome	Self-replicating structures in the nucleus of a cell that carry genetic information.
Class Effect (or Drug Class Effect)	When similar effects are produced by most or all members of a class of drugs (eg, β-blockers or calcium antagonists).
Clinical Decision Rules (or Decision Rules, Clinical Prediction Rules, or Prediction Rules)	A guide for practice that is generated by initially examining, and ultimately combining, a number of variables to predict the likelihood of a current diagnosis or a future event. Sometimes, if the likelihood is sufficiently high or low, the rule generates a suggested course of action.
Clinical Decision Support System	A strategy for changing clinician behavior. An information system used to integrate clinical and patient information and provide support for decision making in patient care. See also Computer Decision Support System.
Clinical Practice Guidelines (or Guidelines or Practice Guidelines)	A strategy for changing clinician behavior. Systematically developed statements or recommendations to assist clinician and patient decisions about appropriate health care for specific clinical circumstances.
Cluster Analysis	A statistical procedure in which the unit of analysis matches the unit of randomization, which is something other than the patient or participant (eg, school, clinic). See also Cluster Assignment (or Cluster Randomization).
Cluster Assignment (or Cluster Randomization)	The assignment of groups (eg, schools, clinics) rather than individuals to intervention and control groups. This approach is often used when assignment by individuals is likely to result in contamination (eg, if adolescents within a school are assigned to receive or not receive a new sex education program, it is likely that they will share the information they learn with one another; instead, if the unit of assignment is schools, entire schools are assigned to receive or not receive the new sex education program). Cluster assignment is typically randomized, but it is possible (though not advisable) to assign clusters to treatment or control by other methods.

Term	Definition
Cochrane Collaboration	An international network working to help health care practitioners, policymakers, patients, patient advocates, and caregivers make well-informed decisions about health care, by preparing, updating, and promoting the accessibility of more than 5000 Cochrane Reviews, published online in the *Cochrane Database of Systematic Reviews*, as part of *The Cochrane Library*. The Cochrane Collaboration also prepares records of randomized clinical trials, in a database called CENTRAL, as part of *The Cochrane Library*.
Cochrane Q	A test for heterogeneity that assumes the null hypothesis that all of the apparent variability among individual study results is due to chance. Cochrane Q generates a probability, presented as a P value, based on a χ^2 distribution, that between-study differences in results equal to or greater than those observed are likely to occur simply by chance. See also I^2 Statistic.
Coefficient	See Correlation Coefficient.
Coherence	The agreement in treatment effect estimates between direct and indirect evidence, as in network meta-analyses.
Cohort	A group of persons with a common characteristic or set of characteristics. Typically, the group is followed for a specified period to determine the incidence of a disorder or complications of an established disorder (prognosis).
Cohort Study (or Longitudinal Study or Prospective Study)	This is an investigation in which a cohort of individuals who do not have evidence of an outcome of interest but who are exposed to the putative cause is compared with a concurrent cohort of individuals who are also free of the outcome but not exposed to the putative cause. Both cohorts are then followed forward in time to compare the incidence of the outcome of interest. When used to study the effectiveness of an intervention, it is an investigation in which a cohort of individuals who receive the intervention is compared with a concurrent cohort who does not receive the intervention, wherein both cohorts are followed forward to compare the incidence of the outcome of interest. Cohort studies can be conducted retrospectively in the sense that someone other than the investigator has followed patients, and the investigator obtains the database and then examines the association between exposure and outcome.
Cointerventions	Interventions other than the intervention under study that affect the outcome of interest and that may be differentially applied to intervention and control groups and thus potentially bias the result of a study.
Comorbidity	Diseases or conditions that coexist in study participants in addition to the index condition that is the subject of the study.
Compliance (or Adherence)	See Adherence.
Composite End Point (or Composite Outcome)	When investigators measure the effect of treatment on an aggregate of end points of various levels of importance, this is a composite endpoint. Inferences from composite end points are strongest in the rare situations in which (1) the component end points are of similar patient importance, (2) the end points that are more important occur with at least similar frequency to those that are less important, and (3) strong biologic rationale supports results that, across component end points, reveal similar relative risks with sufficiently narrow confidence intervals.
Computer Decision Support System (CDSS)	A strategy for changing clinician behavior. Computer-based information systems are used to integrate clinical and patient information and provide support for decision making in patient care. In clinical decision support systems that are computer based, detailed individual patient data are entered into a computer program and are sorted and matched to programs or algorithms in a computerized database,

(Continued)

Term	Definition
Computer Decision Support System (CDSS) (*Continued*)	resulting in the generation of patient-specific assessments or recommendations. Computer decision support systems can have the following purposes: alerting, reminding, critiquing, interpreting, predicting, diagnosing, and suggesting. See also Clinical Decision Support System.
Concealment (or Allocation Concealment)	See Allocation Concealment.
Concepts	The basic building blocks of theory.
Conceptual Framework	An organization of interrelated ideas or concepts that provides a system of relationships between those ideas or concepts.
Conditional Probabilities	The probability of a particular state, given another state (ie, the probability of A, given B).
Confidence Interval (CI)	The range of values within which it is probable that the true value of a parameter (eg, a mean, a relative risk) lies.
Conflict of Interest	A conflict of interest exists when investigators, authors, institutions, reviewers, or editors have financial or nonfinancial relationships with other persons or organizations (such as study sponsors), or personal investments in research projects or the outcomes of projects that may inappropriately influence their interpretation or actions. Conflicts of interest can lead to biased design, conduct, analysis, and interpretation of study results as well as bias in review articles and opinion-based articles.
Confounder (or Confounding Variable or Confounding)	A factor that is associated with the outcome of interest and is differentially distributed in patients exposed and unexposed to the outcome of interest.
Consecutive Sample (or Sequential Sample)	A sample in which all potentially eligible patients treated throughout a period are enrolled.
Consequentialist (or Utilitarian)	A consequentialist or utilitarian view of distributive justice contends that, even in individual decision making, the clinician should take a broad social view, favoring actions that provide the greatest good to the greatest number. In this broader view, the effect on others of allocating resources to a particular patient's care would bear on the decision. This is an alternative to the deontologic view.
Construct Validity	In measurement theory, a construct is a theoretically derived notion of the domain(s) we wish to measure. An understanding of the construct will lead to expectations about how an instrument should behave if it is valid. Construct validity therefore involves comparisons between the instrument being evaluated and other measures (eg, characteristics of patients or other scores) and the logical relationships that should exist between them.
Contamination	Occurs when participants in either the experimental or control group receive the intervention intended for the other arm of the study.
Content Validity	The extent to which a measurement instrument represents all facets of a given social construct.
Continuous Variable (or Interval Data)	A variable that can theoretically take any value and in practice can take a large number of values with small differences between them (eg, height). Continuous variables are also sometimes called interval data.
Control Event Rate (CER) (or Baseline Risk or Baseline Event Rate)	See Baseline Risk.
Control Group	A group that does not receive the experimental intervention. In many studies, the control group receives either usual care or a placebo.

Term	Definition
Control Group Risk (CGR)	The risk of an event occurring in the control group of a study.
Controlled Time Series Design (or Controlled Interrupted Time Series)	Data are collected at several times both before and after the intervention in the intervention group and at the same times in a control group. Data collected before the intervention allow the underlying trend and cyclical (seasonal) effects to be estimated. Data collected after the intervention allow the intervention effect to be estimated while accounting for underlying secular trends. Use of a control group addresses the greatest threat to the validity of a time series design, which is the occurrence of another event at the same time as the intervention, both of which may be associated with the outcome.
Convenience Sample	A sample of participants chosen primarily for their convenience to the researcher rather than for their salience to the research questions or the analysis. This is generally considered a scientifically inferior sampling approach to probability sampling in quantitative research or purposive sampling in qualitative research.
Correlation	The magnitude of the association between 2 variables. The strength of the association is described by the correlation coefficient. See also Correlation Coefficient.
Correlation Coefficient	A numeric expression (eg, r^2 or R^2) of the magnitude and direction of the association between 2 variables, which can take values from -1.0 (perfect negative relationship) to 0 (no relationship) to 1.0 (perfect positive relationship). If the analysis is bivariable, the correlation coefficient may be indicated as r and the coefficient of determination is r^2, and if the correlation coefficient is derived from multivariable (or multivariate) analysis, the correlation coefficient may be indicated as R and the coefficient of determination is R^2.
Cost Analysis	An economic analysis in which only costs of various alternatives are compared. This comparison informs only the resource-use half of the decision (the other half being the expected outcomes).
Cost-Benefit Analysis	An economic analysis in which both the costs and the consequences (including increases in the length and quality of life) are expressed in monetary terms.
Cost-Effectiveness Acceptability Curve	The cost-effectiveness acceptability is plotted on a graph that relates the maximum amount one is willing to pay for a particular treatment alternative (eg, how many dollars one is willing to pay to gain 1 life-year) on the horizontal axis to the probability that a treatment alternative is cost-effective compared with all other treatment alternatives on the vertical axis. The curves are generated from uncertainty around the point estimates of costs and effects in trial-based economic evaluations or uncertainty around values for variables used in decision analytic models. As one is willing to pay more for health outcomes, treatment alternatives that initially might be considered unattractive (eg, a high cost per life-year saved) will have a higher probability of becoming more cost-effective. Cost-effectiveness acceptability curves are a convenient method of presenting the effect of uncertainty on economic evaluation results on a single figure instead of through the use of numerous tables and figures of sensitivity analyses.
Cost-Effectiveness Analysis	An economic analysis in which the consequences are expressed in natural units (eg, cost per life saved or cost per bleeding event averted). Sometimes, cost-utility analysis is classified as a subcategory of cost-effectiveness analysis.
Cost-Effectiveness Efficiency Frontier	The cost and effectiveness results of each treatment alternative from an economic evaluation can be graphed on a figure known as the cost-effectiveness plane. The cost-effectiveness plane plots cost on the vertical axis (ie, positive infinity at the top and negative infinity at the bottom) and effects such as life-years on the horizontal axis (ie, negative infinity at the far left and positive infinity at the far right). One treatment alternative, such as usual care, is plotted at the origin (ie, 0, 0), and all other treatment alternatives are plotted relative to the treatment at the origin.

(Continued)

Term	Definition
Cost-Effectiveness Efficiency Frontier (*Continued*)	Treatment alternatives are considered dominated if they have both higher costs and lower effectiveness relative to any other. Line segments can be drawn connecting the nondominated treatment alternatives, and the combination of line segments that join these nondominated treatment alternatives is referred to as the cost-effectiveness efficiency frontier. Constructed in this way, any treatment alternative that lies above the cost-effectiveness efficiency frontier is considered to be inefficient (dominated) by a treatment alternative or combination of alternatives on the efficiency frontier.
Cost-Minimization Analysis	An economic analysis conducted in situations in which the consequences of the alternatives are identical and the only issue is their relative costs.
Cost-to-Charge Ratio	Where there is a systematic deviation between costs and charges, an economic analysis may adjust charges using a cost-to-charge ratio to approximate real costs.
Cost-Utility Analysis	A type of economic analysis in which the consequences are expressed in terms of life-years adjusted by peoples' preferences. Typically, one considers the incremental cost per incremental gain in quality-adjusted life-years (QALYs).
Cox Regression Model	A regression technique that allows adjustment for known differences in baseline characteristics or time-dependent characteristics between 2 groups applied to survival data.
Credibility (or Trustworthiness)	In qualitative research, a term used (in preference to quantitative terms such as "validity") to reflect the extent to which readers can trust researchers' empirical interpretations or descriptions as sound and insightful. Signs of credibility can be found not only in the procedural descriptions of methods but also through an assessment of the coherence and depth of the findings reported.
Credible Intervals	The Bayesian analogy to confidence intervals.
Criterion Standard (or Gold Standard or Reference Standard)	A method having established or widely accepted accuracy for determining a diagnosis that provides a standard to which a new screening or diagnostic test can be compared. The method need not be a single or simple procedure but could include patient follow-up to observe the evolution of a condition or the consensus of an adjudication committee about the patient's outcome.
Critical Theory	A qualitative research tradition focused on understanding the nature of power relationships and related constructs, often with the intention of helping to remedy systemic injustices in society.
Critiquing (or Critiquing System)	A strategy for changing clinician behavior. A decision support approach in which the computer evaluates a clinician's decision and generates an appropriateness rating or an alternative suggestion.
Cronbach α Coefficient	Cronbach α is an index of reliability, homogeneity, or internal consistency of items on a measurement instrument. The Cronbach α increases with the magnitude of the interitem correlation and with the number of items.
Cross-Sectional Study	The observation of a defined population at a single point in time or during a specific interval. Exposure and outcome are determined simultaneously.
Data Completeness Bias	Using a computer decision support system (CDSS) to log episodes in the intervention group and using a manual system in the non-CDSS control group can create variation in the completeness of data. See also Bias.
Data Dredging	Searching a data set for differences among groups on particular outcomes, or in subgroups of patients, without explicit a priori hypotheses.
Decision Aid	A tool that presents patients with the benefits and harms of alternative courses of action in a manner that is quantitative, comprehensive, and understandable.

Term	Definition
Decision Analysis	A systematic approach to decision making under conditions of uncertainty. It involves identifying all available alternatives and estimating the probabilities of potential outcomes associated with each alternative, valuing each outcome, and, on the basis of the probabilities and values, arriving at a quantitative estimate of the relative merit of each alternative.
Decision Rules (or Clinical Decision Rules)	See Clinical Decision Rules.
Decision Tree	Most clinical decision analyses are built as decision trees; articles usually will include 1 or more diagrams showing the structure of the decision tree used for the analysis.
Degrees of Freedom	A technical term in a statistical analysis that has to do with the power of the analysis. The more degrees of freedom, the more powerful the analysis. The degrees of freedom typically refer to the number of observations in a sample minus the number of unknown parameters estimated for the model. It reflects a sort of adjusted sample size, with the adjustment based on the number of unknowns that need to be estimated in a model. For example, in a 2-sample t test, the degrees of freedom is n1 + n2 − 1 − 1 because there are n1 + n2 subjects altogether and 1 mean estimated in one group and 1 mean in another, giving n1 + n2 − 2.
Deontologic	A deontologic approach to distributive justice holds that the clinician's only responsibility should be to best meet the needs of the individual under his or her care. This is an alternative to the consequentialist or utilitarian view.
Dependent Variable (or Outcome Variable or Target Variable)	The target variable of interest. The variable that is hypothesized to depend on or be caused by another variable, the independent variable.
Detection Bias (or Surveillance Bias)	The tendency to look more carefully for an outcome in one of the comparison groups. See also Bias.
Determinants of Outcome	The factors most strongly determining whether a target event will occur.
Dichotomous Outcome (or Binary Outcome)	A categorical variable that can take 1 of 2 discrete values rather than an incremental value on a continuum (eg, pregnant or not pregnant, dead or alive).
Differential Diagnosis (or Active Alternatives)	The set of diagnoses that can plausibly explain a patient's presentation.
Differential Verification Bias (or Verification Bias or Workup Bias)	When test results influence the choice of the reference standard (eg, test-positive patients undergo an invasive test to establish the diagnosis, whereas test-negative patients undergo long-term follow-up without application of the invasive test), the assessment of test properties may be biased. See also Bias.
Dimensional Analysis	One of several possible approaches to analysis in grounded theory research, in which complex phenomena are characterized in terms of component parts (attributes, context, conditions, processes or actions, meanings).
Directness	A key element to consider when grading the quality of evidence for a health care recommendation. Evidence is direct to the extent that study participants, interventions, and outcome measures are similar to those of interest.
Direct Observation	See Field Observation.
Discriminant Analysis	A statistical technique similar to logistic regression analysis that identifies variables that are associated with the presence or absence of a particular categorical (nominal) outcome.
Disease-Specific Health-Related Quality of Life	See Health-Related Quality of Life.

Term	Definition
Distribution Based	One way to establish the interpretability of measures of patient-reported outcomes is distribution based (the other is anchor based). Distribution-based methods interpret results in terms of the relation between the magnitude of observed effect and some measure of variability in instrument scores. The magnitude of effect may be the difference in patients' scores before and after treatment or the difference in end point scores. As a measure of variability, investigators may choose between-patient variability (eg, the SD of scores measured in patients at baseline) or within-patient variability (eg, the SD of change in scores that patients experienced during a study).
Document Analysis	In qualitative research, this is 1 of 3 basic data collection methods. It involves the interpretive review of written material.
Dominant	In genetic association studies, this describes any trait that is expressed in a heterozygote (ie, one copy of that allele is sufficient to manifest its effect).
Dominate	In economic evaluation, if the intervention of interest is both more effective and less costly than the control strategy, it is said to dominate the alternative.
Dose-Response Gradient (or Dose Dependence)	Exists when the risk of an outcome changes in the anticipated direction as the quantity or the duration of exposure to the putative harmful or beneficial agent increases.
Downstream Costs	Costs of resources consumed in the future and associated with clinical events in the future that are attributable to the intervention.
Drug Class Effects (or Class Effects)	See Class Effects.
Ecologic Study	Ecologic studies examine relationships between groups of individuals with exposure to a putative risk factor and an outcome. Exposures are measured at the population, community, or group level rather than at the individual level. Ecologic studies can provide information about an association; however, they are prone to bias: the ecologic fallacy. The ecologic fallacy holds that relationships observed for groups necessarily hold for individuals (eg, if countries with more dietary fat have higher rates of breast cancer, then women who eat fatty foods must be more likely to get breast cancer). These inferences may be correct but are only weakly supported by the aggregate data.
Economic Analysis (or Economic Evaluation)	A set of formal, quantitative methods used to compare 2 or more treatments, programs, or strategies with respect to their resource use and their expected outcomes.
Educational Meetings (or Interactive Workshops)	A strategy for changing clinician behavior. Participation of professionals in workshops that include interaction and discussion.
Educational Outreach Visits (or Academic Detailing)	See Academic Detailing.
Effect Size	The difference in outcomes between the intervention and control groups divided by some measure of variability, typically the standard deviation.
Efficacy Analysis (Effectiveness Analysis)	This analysis includes the subset of patients in the trial who received the intervention of interest, regardless of initial randomization, and who do not have missing data for any reason. This approach is ill-named in that it does not tell one about either efficacy or effectiveness because it compromises the prognostic balance that randomization achieves and is therefore likely to provide a biased estimate of treatment effect.
Efficiency	Technical efficiency is the relationship between inputs (costs) and outputs (in health, quality-adjusted life-years [QALYs]). Interventions that provide more QALYs for the same or fewer resources are more efficient. Technical efficiency is assessed using cost minimization, cost-effectiveness, and cost-utility analysis. Allocative efficiency recognizes that health is not the only goal that society wishes to pursue, so competing goals must be weighted and then related to costs. This is typically done through cost-benefit analysis.

Term	Definition
Efficiency Frontier	When the cost and effectiveness results of an economic evaluation are graphed on a cost-effectiveness plane along with incremental cost-effectiveness ratios, the resultant line segments are referred to as the efficiency frontier. Any strategy that has a base-case cost-effectiveness that is above the efficiency frontier would be considered dominated.
End Point	An event or outcome that leads to completion or termination of follow-up of an individual in a study (eg, death or major morbidity).
Equivalence Study (or Equivalence Trial)	Trials that estimate treatment effects that exclude any patient-important superiority of interventions under evaluation are equivalence trials. Equivalence trials require a priori definition of the smallest difference in outcomes between these interventions that patients would consider large enough to justify a preference for the superior. The confidence interval for the estimated treatment effect at the end of the trial should exclude that difference for the authors to claim equivalence. Equivalence trials are helpful when investigators want to see whether a cheaper, safer, or simpler (or, increasingly often, better method to generate income for the sponsor) intervention is neither better nor worse (in terms of efficacy) than a current intervention.
Ethnography (or Ethnographic Study)	In qualitative research, an approach to inquiry that focuses on the culture or subculture of a group of people to try to understand the world view of those under study.
Evidence	A broad definition of evidence is any empirical observation, whether systematically collected or not. The unsystematic observations of the individual clinician constitute one source of evidence. Physiologic experiments constitute another source. Clinical research evidence refers to systematic observation of clinical events and is the focus of the *Users' Guides to the Medical Literature*.
Evidence-Based Experts	Clinicians, who can, in a sophisticated manner, independently find, appraise, and judiciously apply the best evidence to patient care.
Evidence-Based Health Care (EBHC)	The conscientious, explicit, and judicious use of current best evidence in making decisions about the care of individual patients. Evidence-based clinical practice requires integration of individual clinical expertise and patient preferences with the best available external clinical evidence from systematic research and consideration of available resources.
Evidence-Based Medicine (EBM)	Evidence-based medicine can be considered a subcategory of evidence-based health care, which also includes other branches of health care practice, such as evidence-based nursing or evidence-based physiotherapy. Subcategories of EBM include evidence-based surgery and evidence-based cardiology. See also Evidence-Based Health Care.
Evidence-Based Policy Making	Policy making is evidence based when practice policies (eg, use of resources by clinicians), service policies (eg, resource allocation, pattern of services), and governance policies (eg, organizational and financial structures) are based on research evidence of benefit or cost benefit.
Evidence-Based Practice (EBP)	Evidence-based practice is clinical practice in which patient management decisions are consistent with the principles of evidence-based health care. This means that decisions will be, first of all, consistent with the best evidence about the benefits and downsides of the alternative management strategies. Second, decisions will be consistent with the values and preferences of the individual patient.
Evidence-Based Practitioners	Clinicians who can differentiate evidence-based summaries and recommendations from those that are not evidence-based and understand results sufficiently well to apply them judiciously in clinical care, ensuring decisions are consistent with patients' values and preferences.

Term	Definition
Evidence Profile	An evidence profile is a tabular or list summary of a body of evidence addressing a structured clinical question of alternative management strategies. It includes, at minimum, the number of studies and patients, the study design(s), the reasons for increasing or decreasing confidence ratings in estimates, and measures of relative and absolute effect. The evidence profile is an expanded version of the summary-of-findings table.
Evidentialism	A theory of knowledge that holds that the justification or reason of a belief is determined by the quality of the believer's evidence for the belief.
Exclusion Criteria	The characteristics that render potential participants ineligible to participate in a study or that render studies ineligible for inclusion in a systematic review.
Expectation Bias	In data collection, an interviewer has information that influences his or her expectation of finding the exposure or outcome. In clinical practice, a clinician's assessment may be influenced by previous knowledge of the presence or absence of a disorder. See also Bias.
Experimental Therapy (or Experimental Treatment or Experimental Intervention)	A therapeutic alternative to standard or control therapy, which is often a new intervention or different dose of a standard drug.
Exposure	A condition to which patients are exposed (either a potentially harmful intervention or a potentially beneficial one) that may affect their health.
Face Validity	The extent to which a measurement instrument appears to measure what it is intended to measure.
Fail-Safe N	The minimum number of undetected studies with negative results that would be needed to change the conclusions of a meta-analysis. A small fail-safe N suggests that the conclusion of the meta-analysis may be susceptible to publication bias.
False Negative	Those who have the target disorder, but the test incorrectly identifies them as not having it.
False Positive	Those who do not have the target disorder, but the test incorrectly identifies them as having it.
Federated Search Engine	A federated search engine searches several online information sources simultaneously and is especially useful when there is no single comprehensive, current, rigorous resource, as is currently the case for evidence-based health care. Examples of evidence-based federated search engines include ACCESSSS (http://plus.mcmaster.ca/accessss) and Trip (http://www.tripdatabase.com).
Feedback Effect	The improvement seen in medical decision making because of performance evaluation and feedback.
Feeling Thermometer	A feeling thermometer is a visual analog scale presented as a thermometer, typically with markings from 0 to 100, with 0 representing death and 100 full health. Respondents use the thermometer to indicate their utility rating of their health state or of a hypothetical health state.
Field Observation	In qualitative research, this is 1 of 3 basic data collection methods. It involves investigators witnessing and recording events as they occur. There are 3 approaches to field observation. With direct observation, investigators record detailed field notes from the milieu they are studying. In nonparticipant observation, the researcher participates relatively little in the interactions he or she is studying. In participant observation, the researcher assumes a role in the social setting beyond that of a researcher (eg, clinician, committee member).

Term	Definition
Fixed-Effects Model	A model to generate a summary estimate of the magnitude of effect in a meta-analysis that restricts inferences to the set of studies included in the meta-analysis and assumes that a single true value underlies all of the primary study results. The assumption is that if all studies were infinitely large, they would yield identical estimates of effect; thus, observed estimates of effect differ from one another only because of random error. This model takes only within-study variation into account and not between-study variation.
Focus Group	See Interview.
Follow-up (or Complete Follow-up)	The extent to which investigators are aware of the outcome in every patient who participated in a study. If follow-up is complete, the outcome is known for all study participants.
Foreground Questions	These clinical questions are more commonly asked by seasoned clinicians. They are questions asked when browsing the literature (eg, what important new information should I know to optimally treat my patients?) or when problem solving (eg, defining specific questions raised in caring for patients and then consulting the literature to resolve these problems).
Forest Plot	A forest plot is a graphic display that illustrates the magnitude of effect of an intervention vs a control in several studies. It provides a visual representation of the best estimate of effect and the range of plausible truth (confidence interval) for each study and for the pooled estimate combining all studies. A vertical line represents no effect. The area of each square or dot (typically representing individual studies) or diamond (typically representing the pooled estimates) is sometimes proportional to the study's weight in the meta-analysis.
Frequentist Analysis	A statistical approach that places the emphasis on available data (conventional approach to statistical analysis, contrast with Bayesian).
Funnel Plot	A graphic technique for assessing the possibility of publication bias in a systematic review. The effect measure is typically plotted on the horizontal axis and a measure of the random error associated with each study on the vertical axis. In the absence of publication bias, because of sampling variability, the graph should have the shape of a funnel. If there is bias against the publication of null results or results revealing an adverse effect of the intervention, one quadrant of the funnel plot will be partially or completely missing.
Generalizability (or Applicability)	The degree to which the results of a study can be generalized to settings or samples other than the ones studied.
Generic Health-Related Quality of Life	See Health-Related Quality of Life.
Genetic Association Study	A study that attempts to identify and characterize genomic variants underlying the susceptibility to multifactorial disease.
Genome	The entire collection of genetic information (or genes) that an organism possesses.
Genome-wide Association Study (GWAS)	A study that evaluates the association of genetic variation with outcomes or traits of interest by using 100 000 to 1 000 000 or more markers across the genome.
Genotype	The genetic constitution of an individual, either overall or at a specific gene.
Geometry of a Network	A graphic representation of the distribution of treatments and their comparisons across a network.
Gold Standard (or Reference Standard or Criterion Standard)	See Criterion Standard.

Term	Definition
GRADE (Grading of Recommendations Assessment, Development and Evaluation)	The Grading of Recommendations Assessment, Development and Evaluation (GRADE) approach is a system for rating the quality of evidence and strength of recommendations that is explicit, comprehensive, and increasingly adopted by guideline organizations. The system classifies the confidence in estimates of effect into 1 of 4 levels (high, moderate, low, or very low). Recommendations are graded as strong or weak.
Grounded Theory	In qualitative research, an approach to collecting and analyzing data with the aim of developing a theory grounded in real-world observations.
Haplotype	Alleles that tend to occur together on the same chromosome because of single-nucleotide polymorphisms being in proximity and therefore inherited together.
Harm	Adverse consequences of exposure to an intervention.
Hawthorne Effect	The tendency for human performance to improve when participants are aware that their behavior is being observed.
Hazard Ratio (HR)	The weighted relative risk of an outcome (eg, death) during the entire study period; often reported in the context of survival analysis.
Health Costs (or Health Care Costs)	Health care resources that are consumed. These reflect the inability to use the same resources for other worthwhile purposes (opportunity costs).
Health Outcomes	All possible changes in health status that may occur for a defined population or that may be associated with exposure to an intervention. These include changes in the length and quality of life, major morbid events, and mortality.
Health Profile	A type of data collection tool, intended for use in the entire population (including the healthy, the very sick, and patients with any sort of health problem), that attempts to measure all important aspects of health-related quality of life (HRQL).
Health-Related Quality of Life (HRQL)	1. Health-Related Quality of Life (HRQL): Measurements of how people are feeling or the value they place on their health state. Such measurements can be disease specific or generic. 2. Disease-Specific Health-Related Quality of Life: Disease-specific HRQL measures evaluate the full range of patients' problems and experiences relevant to a specific condition or disease. 3. Generic Health-Related Quality of Life: Generic HRQL measures contain items that cover all relevant areas of HRQL. They are designed for administration to people with any kind of underlying health problem (or no problem at all). Generic HRQL measures allow comparisons across diseases or conditions.
Health State	The health condition of an individual or group during a specified interval (commonly assessed at a particular point).
Heterogeneity	Differences among individual studies included in a systematic review, typically referring to study results; the term can also be applied to other study characteristics.
Heterozygous	An individual is heterozygous at a gene location if he or she has 2 different alleles (one on the maternal chromosome and one on the paternal) at that location.
Hierarchic Regression	Hierarchic regression examines the relation between independent variables or predictor variables (eg, age, sex, disease severity) and a dependent variable (or outcome variable) (eg, death, exercise capacity). Hierarchic regression differs from standard regression in that one predictor is a subcategory of another predictor. The lower-level predictor is nested within the higher-level predictor. For instance, in a regression predicting likelihood of withdrawal of life support in intensive care units (ICUs) participating in an international study, city is nested within country and ICU is nested within city.
Hierarchy of Evidence	A system of classifying and organizing types of evidence, typically for questions of treatment and prevention. Clinicians should look for the evidence from the highest position in the hierarchy.

Term	Definition
Historiography	A qualitative research method concerned with understanding both historical events and approaches to the writing of historical narratives.
Homogeneity	The inverse of heterogeneity.
Homozygous	An individual is homozygous at a gene location if he or she has 2 identical alleles at that location.
I^2 Statistic	The I^2 statistic is a test of heterogeneity. I^2 can be calculated from Cochrane Q according to the formula: $I^2 = 100\% \times$ (Cochrane Q − degrees of freedom). Any negative values of I^2 are considered equal to 0, so that the range of I^2 values is 0% to 100%, indicating no heterogeneity to high heterogeneity, respectively.
Imprecision	In rating the quality of evidence, GRADE (Grading of Recommendations Assessment, Development and Evaluation) suggests that examination of 95% confidence intervals (CIs) provides the optimal primary approach to decisions regarding imprecision. Decreasing the rating in the quality of evidence (ie, confidence in estimates of effect) is required if clinical action would differ if the upper vs the lower boundary of the CI represented the truth. An exception to this rule occurs when an effect is large, and consideration of CIs alone suggests a robust effect, but the total sample size is not large and the number of events is small. Under these circumstances, one should consider rating the quality of evidence down for imprecision.
Incidence	The number of new cases of disease that occur during a specified period, expressed as a proportion of the number of people at risk during that time.
Inclusion Criteria	The characteristics that define the population eligible for a study or that define the studies that will be eligible for inclusion in a systematic review.
Incoherence	The disagreement in treatment effect estimates between direct and indirect evidence, as in network meta-analyses.
Inconsistency	In the GRADE (Grading of Recommendations Assessment, Development and Evaluation) system of recommendations, a body of evidence is not rated up in quality for consistency but may be rated down in quality if inconsistent. Criteria for evaluating consistency include similarity of point estimates, extent of overlap of confidence intervals, and statistical criteria, including tests of heterogeneity and I^2. To explore heterogeneity, a small number of a priori subgroups may be examined related to the population, intervention, outcomes, and risk of bias.
Incorporation Bias	Occurs when investigators use a reference standard that incorporates a diagnostic test that is the subject of investigation. The result is a bias toward making the test appear more powerful in differentiating target-positive from target-negative patients than it actually is. See also Bias.
Incremental Cost-Effectiveness Ratio	The price at which additional units of benefit can be obtained.
Independent Association	When a variable is associated with an outcome after adjusting for multiple other potential prognostic factors (often after regression analysis), the association is an independent association.
Independent Variable	The variable that is believed to cause, influence, or at least be associated with the dependent variable.
Indicator Condition	A clinical situation (eg, disease, symptom, injury, or health state) that occurs reasonably frequently and for which there is sound evidence that high-quality care is beneficial. Indicator conditions can be used to evaluate quality of care by comparing the care provided (as assessed through medical record review or observation) to that which is recommended.

Term	Definition
Indirect Costs and Benefits	The effect of alternative patient management strategies on the productivity of the patient and others involved in the patient's care.
Indirect Evidence	Evidence bearing on the relative effect of treatments that that have not been compared directly against each other but have a common comparator. Indirect evidence may be evaluated using accepted statistical approaches, including adjusted indirect comparisons and network meta-analyses.
Indirectness	In rating confidence in estimates of effect (quality of evidence), the GRADE (Grading of Recommendations Assessment, Development and Evaluation) approach suggests examining directness. Directness in GRADE has 2 elements. The first is the extent to which the research evidence is about the patients and interventions of interest and measuring outcomes important to patients. Rating down the confidence in estimates is required if evidence is sufficiently indirect, which occurs in 4 ways: (1) if patients differ from those of interest, (2) if interventions differ from those of interest, (3) if outcomes differ from those of interest to patients (eg, surrogate outcomes), and (4) if interventions have not been tested in head-to-head comparisons and, as a result, indirect comparisons are required.
Individual Patient Data Meta-analysis	A meta-analysis in which individual patient data from each primary study are used to create pooled estimates. Such an approach can facilitate more accurate intention-to-treat analyses and informed subgroup analyses.
Informational Redundancy	In qualitative research, the point in the analysis at which new data fail to generate new themes and new information becomes redundant. This is considered an appropriate stopping point for data collection in most methods and an appropriate stopping point for analysis in some methods.
Informed Consent	A participant's expression (verbal or written) of willingness, after full disclosure of the risks, benefits, and other implications, to participate in a study.
Intention-to-Treat Analysis, Intention-to-Treat Principle	Authorities differ on the definition of an intention-to-treat analysis. All agree that it means that patients for whom data are available are analyzed in the groups to which they are randomized irrespective of what treatment they received. How one handles those patients for whom data are not available (loss to follow-up) in an intention-to-treat analysis is controversial. The authors of the *Users' Guides to the Medical Literature* believe that the term "intention-to-treat" should be restricted to patients with follow-up data. Thus, how one handles those patients lost to follow-up should be an issue separate from intention-to-treat.
Internal Validity	Whether a study provides valid results depends on whether it was designed and conducted well enough that the study findings accurately represent the direction and magnitude of the underlying true effect (ie, studies that have higher internal validity have a lower likelihood of bias/systematic error).
Interrater Reliability	The extent to which 2 or more raters are able to consistently differentiate subjects with higher and lower values on an underlying trait (typically measured with an intraclass correlation).
Interrupted Time Series Design (or Time Series Design)	See Time Series Design.
Interval Data (or Continuous Variable)	See Continuous Variable.
Intervention Effect (or Treatment Effect)	See Treatment Effect.
Interview	In qualitative research, this is 1 of 3 basic data collection methods. It involves an interviewer asking questions to engage participants in dialogue to allow interpretation of experiences and events in the participants' own terms. The 2 most common

(Continued)

Term	Definition
Interview (*Continued*)	interviews are interviews of individuals or focus groups, which are group interviews in which a researcher facilitates discussion among multiple participants. Statements and interactions are then used as data. In quantitative research, an interview is a method of collecting data in which an interviewer obtains information from a participant through conversation.
Interviewer Bias	Greater probing by an interviewer of some participants than others, contingent on particular features of the participants. See also Bias.
Intraclass Correlation Coefficient	This is a measure of reproducibility that compares variance between patients to the total variance, including both between-patient and within-patient variance.
Intrarater Reliability	The extent to which a rater is able to consistently differentiate participants with higher and lower values of an underlying trait on repeated ratings over time (typically measured with an intraclass correlation).
Inverse Rule of 3s	A rough rule of thumb that tells us the following: If an event occurs, on average, once every x days, we need to observe 3x days to be 95% confident of observing at least 1 event.
Investigator Triangulation	See Triangulation.
Isoform	Variant in the amino acid sequence of a protein.
Jackknife Technique (or Jackknife Dispersion Test)	A statistical technique for estimating the variance and bias of an estimator. It is applied to a predictive model that is derived from a study sample to determine whether the model fits different subsamples from the model equally well.
Judgmental Sampling (or Purposive Sampling or Purposeful Sampling)	See Purposive Sampling.
Kaplan-Meier Curve (or Survival Curve)	A graphical plot of the Kaplan-Meier statistical estimate of survival in a survival analysis. See also Survival Curve and Survival Analysis.
κ Statistic (or Weighted κ or κ Value)	A measure of the extent to which observers achieve agreement beyond the level expected to occur by chance alone. The value ranges from 0 to 100, with 0 indicating no agreement and typically values greater than 75 indicating excellent agreement.
Law of Multiplicative Probabilities	The law of multiplicative probabilities for independent events (where one event in no way influences the other) tells us that the probability of 10 consecutive heads in 10 coin flips can be found by multiplying the probability of a single head (1/2) 10 times over; that is, 1/2, 1/2, 1/2, and so on.
Leading Hypothesis (or Working Diagnosis)	See Working Diagnosis.
Lead Time Bias	Occurs when outcomes such as survival, as measured from the time of diagnosis, may be increased not because patients live longer but because screening lengthens the time that they know they have disease. See also Bias.
Length Time Bias	Occurs when patients whose disease is discovered by screening also may appear to do better or live longer than people whose disease presents clinically with symptoms because screening tends to detect disease that is destined to progress slowly and that therefore has a good prognosis. See also Bias.
Levels of Evidence	A hierarchy of research evidence to inform practice, usually ranging from strongest to weakest.
Likelihood Ratio (LR)	For a screening or diagnostic test (including clinical signs or symptoms), the likelihood ratio (LR) expresses the relative likelihood that a given test would be expected in a patient with, as opposed to one without, a disorder of interest. An LR of 1 means that the posttest probability is identical to the pretest probability. As LRs

(Continued)

Term	Definition
Likelihood Ratio (LR) (*Continued*)	increase above 1, the posttest probability progressively increases in relation to the pretest probability. As LRs decrease below 1, the posttest probability progressively decreases in relation to the pretest probability. An LR is calculated as the proportion of target positive with a particular test result (which, with a single cut point, would be either a positive or negative result) divided by the proportion of target negative with the same test result.
Likert Scales	Scales, typically with 3 to 9 possible values, that include extremes of attitudes or feelings (such as from totally disagree to totally agree) that respondents mark to indicate their rating.
Linear Regression	The term used for a regression analysis when the dependent variable or target variable is a continuous variable and the relationship between the dependent variable and independent variable is thought to be linear.
Linkage	The tendency of genes or other DNA sequences at specific loci to be inherited together as a consequence of their physical proximity on a single chromosome.
Linkage Disequilibrium	A measure of association between alleles at different loci.
Local Consensus Process	A strategy for changing clinician behavior. Inclusion of participating clinicians in discussions to create agreement with a suggested approach to change clinician practice.
Local Opinion Leaders (or Opinion Leaders)	A strategy for changing clinician behavior. These persons are clinician peers who are recognized by their colleagues as model caregivers or who are viewed as having particular content expertise.
Locus	The site(s) on a chromosome at which the gene for a particular trait is located or on a gene at which a particular single-nucleotide polymorphism is located.
Logical Operators (or Boolean Operators)	See Boolean Operators.
Logistic Regression	A regression analysis in which the dependent variable is binary.
Longitudinal Study (or Cohort Study or Prospective Study)	See Cohort Study.
Lost to Follow-up	Patients whose status on the outcome or end point of interest is unknown.
Markov Model (or Multistate Transition Model)	Markov models are tools used in decision analyses. Named after a 19th-century Russian mathematician, Markov models are the basis of software programs that model what might happen to a cohort of patients during a series of cycles (eg, periods of 1 year). The model allows for the possibility that patients might move from one health state to another. For instance, one patient may have a mild stroke in one 3-month cycle, continue with minimal functional limitation for a number of cycles, have a gastrointestinal bleeding episode in a subsequent cycle, and finally experience a major stroke. Ideally, data from randomized trials will determine the probability of moving from one state to another during any cycle under competing management options.
Masked (or Blind or Blinded)	See Blind.
Matching	A deliberate process to make the intervention group and comparison group comparable with respect to factors (or confounders) that are extraneous to the purpose of the investigation but that might interfere with the interpretation of the study's findings. For example, in case-control studies, individual cases may be matched with controls on the basis of comparable age, sex, or other clinical features.
Median Survival	The length of time that half the study population survives.

Term	Definition
Medical Subject Headings (MeSH)	The National Library of Medicine's controlled vocabulary used for indexing articles for MEDLINE/PubMed. Medical Subject Headings (MeSH) terms provide a consistent way to retrieve information that may use different terms for the same concepts.
Member Checking	In qualitative research, this involves sharing draft findings with the participants to get feedback on whether the findings make sense to them, whether researchers interpreted their viewpoints faithfully, or whether they perceive errors of fact. Note that any discrepancies would not necessarily indicate that the research is biased or in error but rather that the next stage of empirical analysis should interpret and account for the discrepancies.
Messenger RNA	An RNA-containing single-strand copy of a gene that migrates out of the cell nucleus to the ribosome, where it is translated into a protein.
Meta-analysis	A statistical technique for quantitatively combining the results of multiple studies that measure the same outcome into a single pooled or summary estimate.
Meta-regression Analysis	A regression in which the dependent variable is the magnitude of treatment effect in individual studies and the independent variable is study characteristics. Meta-regression is used to determine whether study characteristics can explain differences in magnitude of treatment effect across studies. Meta-regression techniques can be used to explore whether patient characteristics (eg, younger or older patients) or design characteristics (eg, studies of low or high quality) are related to the size of the treatment effect.
Meta-synthesis	A procedure for combining qualitative research on a specific topic in which researchers compare and analyze the texts of individual studies and develop new interpretations.
Minimal Important Difference	The smallest difference in a patient-important outcome that patients perceive as beneficial and that would mandate, in the absence of troublesome adverse effects and excessive cost, a change in the patient's health care management.
Minimally Disruptive Medicine	Medicine practiced to minimize the burden of treatment or intervention on the patient's life.
Mixed-Methods Study	A study that combines data collection approaches, sometimes both qualitative and quantitative, into the study methods and is commonly used in the study of service delivery and organization. Some mixed-methods studies combine study designs (eg, investigators may embed qualitative or quantitative process evaluations alongside quantitative evaluative designs to increase understanding of factors that influence a phenomenon). Some mixed-methods studies include a single overarching research design but use mixed-methods for data collection (eg, surveys, interviews, observation, and analysis of documentary material).
Model	The term "model" is often used to describe statistical regression analyses that involve more than 1 independent variable and 1 dependent variable. This is a multivariable or multiple regression (or multivariate) analysis.
Multifaceted Interventions	The use of multiple strategies to change clinician behavior. Multiple strategies may include a combination that includes 2 or more of the following: audit and feedback, reminders, local consensus processes, patient-mediated interventions, or computer decision support systems.
Multistate Transition Model	See Markov Model.
Multivariate Regression Analysis (or Multivariable Regression Analysis)	A type of regression that provides a mathematical model that attempts to explain or predict the dependent variable (or outcome variable or target variable) by simultaneously considering 2 or more independent variables (or predictor variables). Multivariable refers to multiple predictors (independent variables) for a single outcome (dependent variable). Multivariate refers to 1 or more independent variables for multiple outcomes. See also Bivariable Regression.

Term	Definition
Mutation	A rare variant in a gene, occurring in less than 1% of a population. See Polymorphism.
Narrative Review	A review article (such as a typical book chapter) that is not conducted using methods to minimize bias (in contrast to a systematic review).
Natural History	As distinct from prognosis, natural history refers to the possible consequences and outcomes of a disease or condition and the frequency with which they can be expected to occur when the disease condition is untreated.
Negative Predictive Value (NPV)	See Predictive Value.
Negative Study (or Negative Trial)	Studies in which the authors have concluded that the comparison groups do not differ statistically in the variables of interest. The research results fail to support the researchers' hypotheses.
Network Meta-analysis (or Multiple Treatment Comparison Meta-analysis)	This systematic review allows the comparison of multiple interventions, including head-to-head evaluations at the same time as indirect comparisons, in a connected network of comparisons.
Neural Network	The application of nonlinear statistics to pattern-recognition problems. Neural networks can be used to develop clinical prediction rules. The technique identifies those predictors most strongly associated with the outcome of interest that belong in a clinical prediction rule and those that can be omitted from the rule without loss of predictive power.
N-of-1 Randomized Clinical Trial (or N-of-1 RCT)	An experiment designed to determine the effect of an intervention or exposure on a single study participant. In one n-of-1 design, the patient undergoes pairs of treatment periods organized so that 1 period involves the use of the experimental treatment and 1 period involves the use of an alternate treatment or placebo. The patient and clinician are blinded if possible, and outcomes are monitored. Treatment periods are replicated until the clinician and patient are convinced that the treatments are definitely different or definitely not different.
Nomogram	A graphic scale facilitating calculation of a probability. The most used nomogram in evidence-based medicine is one developed by Fagan to move from a pretest probability, through a likelihood ratio, to a posttest probability.
Nonadherent	Patients are nonadherent if they are not exposed to the full course of a study intervention (eg, most commonly, they do not take the prescribed dose or duration of a drug or they do not participate fully in the study program).
Noninferiority Trial	Noninferiority trials address whether the effect of an experimental intervention is not worse than a standard intervention by more than a specified margin. This contrasts with equivalence trials, which aim to determine whether an intervention is similar to another intervention. Noninferiority of the experimental intervention with respect to the standard treatment may be of interest if the new intervention has some other advantage, such as greater availability, reduced cost, less invasiveness, fewer harms, or decreased burden—or a potential for increased income for the sponsor.
Nonparticipant Observation	See Field Observation.
Null Hypothesis	In the hypothesis-testing framework, this is the starting hypothesis that the statistical test is designed to consider and possibly reject, which contends that there is no association among the variables under study.
Null Result	A nonsignificant result; no statistically significant difference between groups.

Term	Definition
Number Needed to Harm (NNH)	The number of patients who, if they received the experimental intervention, would lead to 1 additional patient being harmed during a specific period. It is the inverse of the absolute risk increase (ARI), expressed as a percentage (100/ARI).
Number Needed to Screen (NNS)	The number of patients who would need to be screened to prevent 1 adverse event.
Number Needed to Treat (NNT)	The number of patients who need to be treated during a specific period to achieve 1 additional good outcome. When NNT is discussed, it is important to specify the intervention, its duration, and the desirable outcome. If an NNT calculation results in a decimal, round up as per Cochrane guidance (http://www.cochrane-net.org/openlearning/html/mod11-6.htm). It is the inverse of the absolute risk reduction (ARR), expressed as a percentage (100/ARR).
Number of People Needed to Invite to Screening (NNI)	The number of people who need to be invited to screen to prevent 1 adverse event (calculated from the absolute risk difference in intention-to-treat analyses of randomized trials of screening). The NNI is larger than the number needed to screen because it is dependent on the uptake of screening; however, it may underestimate the effect of screening among individuals who participate fully in a program.
Observational Study (or Observational Study Design)	An observational study can be used to describe many designs that are not randomized trials (eg, cohort studies or case-control studies that have a goal of establishing causation, studies of prognosis, studies of diagnostic tests, and qualitative studies). The term is most often used in the context of cohort studies and case-control studies in which patient or caregiver preference, or happenstance, determines whether a person is exposed to an intervention or putative harmful agent or behavior (in contrast to the exposure being under the control of the investigator, as in a randomized trial).
Observer Bias	Occurs when an observer's observations differ systematically according to participant characteristics (eg, making systematically different observations in treatment and control groups). See also Bias.
Odds	The ratio of events to nonevents; the ratio of the number of study participants experiencing the outcome of interest to the number of study participants not experiencing the outcome of interest.
Odds Ratio (OR) (or Relative Odds)	A ratio of the odds of an event in an exposed group to the odds of the same event in a group that is not exposed.
Odds Reduction	The odds reduction expresses, for odds, what relative risk reduction expresses for risks. Just as the relative risk reduction is 1 − relative risk, the odds reduction is 1 − relative odds (the relative odds and odds ratio being synonymous). Thus, if a treatment results in an odds ratio of 0.6 for a particular outcome, the treatment reduces the odds for that outcome by 0.4.
One-Group Pretest-Posttest Design (or Before-After Design)	See Before-After Design.
Open-Ended Interviews/ Questions	Questions that offer no specific structure for the respondents' answers and allow the respondents to answer in their own words. In qualitative research, this is sometimes also referred to as "unstructured" interviews. Interviewers invite participants to narrate their stories or perspectives on a very general topic in their own terms, with as little prompting or steering from the interviewer as possible. Open-ended questions are used.
Opinion Leaders (or Local Opinion Leaders)	See Local Opinion Leaders.
Opportunity Costs	The value of (health or other) benefits forgone in alternative uses when a resource is used.

Term	Definition
Optimal Information Size (OIS)	When using a GRADE (Grading of Recommendations Assessment, Development and Evaluation) approach to interpreting precision, examining the 95% confidence intervals (CIs) provides the optimal primary approach. We are skeptical about early studies with large effects and apparently satisfactory CIs. The optimal information size (OIS) is a way of dealing with such situations. The OIS is the number of patients required for an adequately powered individual trial assuming a modest treatment effect. If the CIs appear satisfactory but the sample size is less than the OIS, we lose confidence in estimates because of imprecision.
Outcome Variable (or Dependent Variable or Target Variable)	The target variable of interest. The variable that is hypothesized to depend on or be caused by another variable (the independent variable).
Overdetection	The detection of inconsequential disease—that is, disease that meets pathologic criteria for disease but that would not cause symptoms or become life-threatening if left undetected and untreated.
Partial Verification Bias	Occurs when only a selected sample of patients who underwent the index test is verified by the reference standard, and that sample is dependent on the results of the test. For example, patients with suspected coronary artery disease whose exercise test results are positive may be more likely to undergo coronary angiography (the reference standard) than those whose exercise test results are negative. See also Bias.
Participant Observation	See Field Observation.
Patient-Important Outcomes	Outcomes that patients value directly. This is in contrast to surrogate, substitute, or physiologic outcomes that clinicians may consider important. One way of thinking about a patient-important outcome is that, were it to be the only thing that changed, patients would be willing to undergo an intervention with associated risk, cost, or inconvenience. This would be true of treatments that ameliorated symptoms or prevented morbidity or mortality. It would not be true of treatments that lowered blood pressure, improved cardiac output, improved bone density, or the like, without improving the quality or increasing the length of life.
Patient-Mediated Interventions	A strategy for changing clinician behavior. Any intervention aimed at changing the performance of health care professionals through interactions with, or information provided by or to, patients.
Patient Preferences	The relative value that patients place on various health states. Preferences are determined by values, beliefs, and attitudes that patients bring to bear in considering what they will gain—or lose—as a result of a management decision. Explicit enumeration and balancing of benefits and risks that are central to evidence-based clinical practice bring the underlying value judgments involved in making management decisions into bold relief.
Patient-Reported Outcomes	Any report of the status of a patient's health condition that comes directly from the patient without interpretation of the patient's response by a clinician or anyone else. Patient reported outcomes can be measured in absolute terms (eg, severity of a sign, symptom, or state of a disease) or as a change from a previous measure.
Pedigree	A diagram that depicts heritable traits across 2 or more generations of a family.
Pearson Correlation Coefficient	A statistical test of correlation between 2 groups of normally distributed data. The Pearson correlation provides a measure of association rather than measure of agreement. See also Correlation Coefficient.
Per-Protocol Analysis (Efficacy Analysis or Effectiveness Analysis)	Includes the subset of patients who complete the entire clinical trial according to the protocol. This approach compromises the prognostic balance that randomization achieves and is therefore likely to provide a biased estimate of treatment effect.

Term	Definition
Pharmacogenomics	The analysis of how genetic makeup affects an individual's response to drugs. Pharmacogenomics deals with the influence of genetic variation on drug response in patients by correlating gene expression or single-nucleotide polymorphisms with a drug's efficacy or toxicity. The goal is to optimize drug therapy according to a patient's genotype to ensure maximum efficacy with minimal adverse effects.
Phase 1 Studies	Studies, often conducted in healthy volunteers, that investigate a drug's physiologic effect and evaluate whether it manifests unacceptable early toxic effects.
Phase 2 Studies	Initial studies on patients that provide preliminary evidence of possible drug effectiveness.
Phase 3 Studies	Randomized clinical trials designed to test the magnitude of benefit and harm of a drug.
Phase 4 Studies (or Postmarketing Surveillance Studies)	Studies conducted after the effectiveness of a drug has been established and the drug marketed, typically to establish the frequency of uncommon or unanticipated toxic effects.
Phenomenology	In qualitative research, an approach to inquiry that emphasizes the complexity of human experience and the need to understand the experience holistically as it is actually lived.
Phenotype	The observable characteristics of a cell or organism, usually being the result of the product coded by a gene (genotype).
φ (or φ Statistic)	A measure of chance-independent agreement.
PICO (Patient, Intervention, Comparison, Outcome)	A method for answering clinical questions.
Placebo	A biologically inert substance (typically a pill or capsule) that is as similar as possible to the active intervention. Placebos are sometimes given to participants in the control arm of a drug trial to help ensure that the study is blinded.
Placebo Effect	The effect of an intervention independent of its biologic effect.
Point Estimate	The single value that best represents the value of the population parameter.
Polymorphism	The existence of 2 or more variants of a gene, occurring in a population, with at least 1% frequency of the less common variant. See also Mutation.
Pooled Estimate	A statistical summary measure representing the best estimate of a parameter that applies to all of the studies that contribute to addressing a similar question (such as a pooled relative risk and 95% confidence intervals from a set of randomized trials).
Positive Predictive Value (PPV)	See Predictive Value.
Positive Study (or Positive Trial)	A study with results that reveal a difference that investigators interpret as beyond the play of chance.
Posttest Odds	The odds of the target condition being present after the results of a diagnostic test are available.
Posttest Probability	The probability of the target condition being present after the results of a diagnostic test are available.
Power	The ability of a study to reject a null hypothesis when it is false (and should be rejected). Power is linked to the adequacy of the sample size: if a sample size is too small, the study will have insufficient power to detect differences between groups.
Practice Guidelines (or Clinical Practice Guidelines or Guidelines)	See Clinical Practice Guidelines.

Term	Definition
Prediction Rules (or Clinical Prediction Rules)	See Clinical Prediction Rules.
Predictive Value	There are 2 categories of predictive value. Positive predictive value is the proportion of people with a positive test result who have the disease; negative predictive value is the proportion of people with a negative test result and who are free of disease.
Preferences	See Values and Preferences.
Pretest Odds	The odds of the target condition being present before the results of a diagnostic test are available.
Pretest Probability	The probability of the target condition being present before the results of a diagnostic test are available.
Prevalence	Proportion of persons affected with a particular disease at a specified time. Prevalence rates obtained from high-quality studies can inform pretest probabilities.
Prevent (Prevention)	A preventive maneuver is an action that decreases the risk of a future event or the threatened onset of disease. Primary prevention is designed to stop a condition from developing. Secondary prevention is designed to stop or slow progression of a disease or disorder when patients have a disease and are at risk for developing something related to their current disease. Often, secondary prevention is indistinguishable from treatment. An example of primary prevention is vaccination for pertusis. An example of secondary prevention is administration of an antiosteoporosis intervention to women with low bone density and evidence of a vertebral fracture to prevent subsequent fractures. An example of tertiary prevention is a rehabilitation program for patients experiencing the adverse effects associated with a myocardial infarction.
Primary Studies	Studies that collect original data. Primary studies are differentiated from synopses that summarize the results of individual primary studies, and they are different from systematic reviews that summarize the results of a number of primary studies.
Principal Components Analysis	A series of microarray experiments that produces observations of differential expression for thousands of genes across multiple conditions. Principal components analysis is a statistical technique for determining the key variables in a multidimensional data set that explain the differences in the observations and can be used to simplify the analysis and visualization of multidimensional data sets.
Probabilistic Sensitivity Analysis	Related to economic analysis, this is an approach for dealing with uncertainty in economic models whereby distributions are defined for model variables and simulation techniques used to make random draws of the distributions to estimate the variability in estimated costs and outcomes.
Probability	Quantitative estimate of the likelihood of a condition existing (as in diagnosis) or of subsequent events (such as in an intervention study).
Prognosis	The possible consequences and outcomes of a disease and the frequency with which they can be expected to occur.
Prognostic Factors	Patient or participant characteristics that confer increased or decreased risk of a positive or adverse outcome.
Prognostic Study	A study that enrolls patients at a point in time and follows them forward to determine the frequency and timing of subsequent events.
Prospective Study (or Cohort Study or Longitudinal Study)	See Cohort Study.
Publication Bias	Occurs when the publication of research depends on the direction of the study results and whether they are statistically significant. See also Bias.

Term	Definition
Purposive Sampling (or Purposeful Sampling or Judgmental Sampling)	In qualitative research, a type of nonprobability sampling to select participants based on key characteristics relevant to the research question and on analytic questions as they arise during analysis. Specific sampling criteria may evolve during a project. Depending on the topic, examples include maximum variation sampling to document range or diversity; extreme case sampling, in which one selects cases that are opposite in some way; typical or representative case sampling to describe what is common in terms of the phenomenon of interest; critical sampling to make a point dramatically; and criterion sampling, in which all cases that meet some predetermined criteria of importance are studied.
P Value (or P)	The probability that results as extreme as or more extreme than those observed would occur if the null hypothesis were true and the experiment were repeated over and over. $P < .05$ means that there is a less than 1 in 20 probability that, on repeated performance of the experiment, results as extreme as or more extreme than those observed would occur if the null hypothesis were true.
Pyramid of EBM Resources	This term refers to the way evidence-based medicine resources can be viewed in 3 broad categories: summaries and guidelines, preappraised research, and non-preappraised research.
Qualitative Research	Qualitative research focuses on social and interpreted, rather than quantifiable, phenomena and aims to discover, interpret, and describe rather than to test and evaluate. Qualitative research makes inductive, descriptive inferences to theory concerning social experiences or settings, whereas quantitative research makes causal or correlational inferences to populations. Qualitative research is not a single method but a family of analytic approaches that rely on the description and interpretation of qualitative data. Specific methods include, for example, grounded theory, ethnography, phenomenology, case study, critical theory, and historiography.
Quality-Adjusted Life-Year (QALY)	A unit of measure for survival that accounts for the effects of suboptimal health status and the resulting limitations in quality of life. For example, if a patient lives for 10 years and his or her quality of life is decreased by 50% because of chronic lung disease, survival would be equivalent to 5 quality-adjusted life-years (QALYs).
Quality Improvement	An approach to defining, measuring, improving, and controlling practices to maintain or improve the appropriateness of health care services.
Quality of Care	The extent to which health care meets technical and humanistic standards of optimal care.
Quantitative Research	The investigation of phenomena that lend themselves to test well-specified hypotheses through precise measurement and quantification of predetermined variables that yield numbers suitable for statistical analysis.
Random	Governed by a formal chance process in which the occurrence of previous events is of no value in predicting future events. For example, the probability of assigning a participant to 1 of 2 specified groups is 50%.
Random Allocation (or Randomization)	See Randomization.
Random-Effects Model	A model used to give a summary estimate of the magnitude of effect in a meta-analysis that assumes that the studies included are a random sample of a population of studies that address the question posed in the meta-analysis. Each study estimates a different underlying true effect, and the distribution of these effects is assumed to be normal around a mean value. Because a random-effects model takes into account both within-study and between-study variability, the confidence interval around the point estimate is, when there is appreciable variability in results across studies, wider than it could be if a fixed-effects model were used.

Term	Definition
Random Error (or Chance)	We can never know with certainty the true value of an intervention effect because of random error. It is inherent in all measurement. The observations that are made in a study are only a sample of all possible observations that could be made from the population of relevant patients. Thus, the average or mean value of any sample of observations is subject to some variation from the true value for that entire population. When the level of random error associated with a measurement is high, the measurement is less precise, and we are less certain about the value of that measurement.
Randomization (or Random Allocation)	The allocation of participants to groups by chance, usually done with the aid of a table of random numbers. Not to be confused with systematic allocation or quasi-randomization (eg, on even and odd days of the month) or other allocation methods used at the discretion of the investigator.
Randomized Clinical Trial (RCT) or Randomized Trial	An experiment in which individuals are randomly allocated to receive or not receive an experimental diagnostic, preventive, therapeutic, or palliative procedure and then followed up to determine the effect of the intervention.
Random Sample	A sample derived by selecting sampling units (eg, individual patients) such that each unit has an independent and fixed (generally equal) chance of selection. Whether a given unit is selected is determined by chance (eg, by a table of randomly ordered numbers).
Recall Bias	Occurs when patients who experience an adverse outcome have a different likelihood of recalling an exposure than patients who do not experience the adverse outcome, independent of the true extent of exposure. See also Bias.
Receiver Operating Characteristic (ROC) Curve	A figure depicting the power of a diagnostic test. The receiver operating characteristic (ROC) curve presents the test's true-positive rate (ie, sensitivity) on the horizontal axis and the false-positive rate (ie, $1 -$ specificity) on the vertical axis for different cut points dividing a positive from a negative test result. An ROC curve for a perfect test has an area under the curve of 1.0, whereas a test that performs no better than chance has an area under the curve of only 0.5.
Recessive	Describes any trait that is expressed in a homozygote but not a heterozygote (ie, 2 copies of that allele are necessary to manifest its effect).
Recursive Partitioning Analysis	A technique for determining the optimal way of using a set of predictor variables to estimate the likelihood of an individual's experiencing a particular outcome. The technique repeatedly divides the population (eg, old vs young, among young and old) according to status on variables that discriminate between those who will have the outcome of interest and those who will not.
Reference Standard (or Criterion Standard or Gold Standard)	See Criterion Standard.
Referral Bias	Occurs when characteristics of patients differ between one setting (such as primary care) and another setting that includes only referred patients (such as secondary or tertiary care). See also Bias.
Reflexivity	In qualitative research using field observation, whichever of the 3 approaches used, the observer will always have some effect on what is being observed, small or large. This interaction of the observer with what is observed is called reflexivity. Whether it plays a positive or negative role in accessing social truths, the researcher must acknowledge and investigate reflexivity and account for it in data interpretation.
Regression (or Regression Analysis)	A technique that uses predictor or independent variables to build a statistical model that predicts an individual patient's status with respect to a dependent variable or target variable.

Term	Definition
Relative Diagnostic Odds Ratio	The diagnostic odds ratio is a single value that provides one way of representing the power of the diagnostic test. It is applicable when we have a single cut point for a test and classify test results as positive and negative. The diagnostic odds ratio is calculated as the product of the true-positive and true-negative results divided by the product of the false-positive and false-negative results. The relative diagnostic odds ratio is the ratio of one diagnostic odds ratio to another.
Relative Odds	See Odds Ratio. Just as relative risk and risk ratio are synonymous, relative odds and odds ratio are synonymous.
Relative Risk (RR) (or Risk Ratio)	The ratio of the risk of an event among an exposed population to the risk among the unexposed.
Relative Risk Increase (RRI)	The proportional increase in risk of harmful outcomes between experimental and control participants. It is calculated by dividing the risk of a harmful outcome in the experimental group (experimental group risk [EGR]) minus the risk of a harmful outcome in the control group (control group risk [CGR]) by the risk of a harmful outcome in the control group ([EGR − CGR]/CGR). Typically used with a harmful exposure.
Relative Risk Reduction (RRR)	The proportional reduction in risk of harmful outcomes between experimental and control participants. It is calculated by dividing the risk of a harmful outcome in the control group (control group risk [CGR]) minus the risk of a harmful outcome in the experimental group (experimental group risk [EGR]) by the risk of a harmful outcome in the control group ([CGR − EGR]/CGR). Used with a beneficial exposure or intervention. See also Relative Risk; Risk; Treatment Effect.
Reliability	A technical statistical term that refers to a measurement instrument's ability to differentiate among subjects, patients, or participants in some underlying trait. Reliability increases as the variability between subjects increases and decreases as the variability within subjects (over time or over raters) increases. Reliability is typically expressed as an intraclass correlation coefficient with between-subject variability in the numerator and total variability (between-subject and within-subject) in the denominator.
Reminding (or Reminders or Reminder Systems)	A strategy for changing clinician behavior. Manual or computerized reminders to prompt behavior change.
Reporting Bias (or Selective Outcome Reporting Bias)	The inclination of authors to differentially report research results according to the magnitude, direction, or statistical significance of the results. See also Bias.
Residual Confounding	Unknown, unmeasured, or suboptimally measured prognostic factors that remain unbalanced between groups after full covariable adjustment by statistical techniques. The remaining imbalance will lead to a biased assessment of the effect of any putatively causal exposure.
Responsiveness	The sensitivity or ability of an instrument to detect change over time.
Review	A general term for an article that systematically evaluates and summarizes the results of more than 1 primary study, as in a systematic review, or an article that summarizes a topic without an evidence-based approach, as in a narrative review. See also Systematic Review and Narrative Review.
Ribosome	The protein synthesis machinery of a cell where messenger RNA translation occurs.
Risk	A measure of the association between exposure and outcome (including incidence, adverse effects, or toxicity).
Risk Difference	The absolute difference in risk of a harmful outcome between experimental and control participants. It is calculated by subtracting the risk of a harmful outcome in the control group (control group risk [CGR]) minus the risk of a harmful outcome in the experimental group (experimental group risk [EGR]) (CGR − EGR).

Term	Definition
Risk Factors	Risk factors are patient characteristics associated with the development of a disease in the first place. Prognostic factors are patient characteristics that confer increased or decreased risk of a positive or adverse outcome from a given disease.
Risk of Bias	The extent to which study results are subject to systematic error.
Risk Ratio (or Relative Risk)	See Relative Risk.
Screening	Services designed to detect people at high risk of experiencing a condition associated with a modifiable adverse outcome, offered to persons who have neither symptoms of nor risk factors for a target condition.
Secondary Evidence-Based Journal	A secondary journal does not publish original research but rather includes synopses of published research studies that meet prespecified criteria of both clinical relevance and methodologic quality.
Secular Trends	Changes in the probability of events with time, independent of known predictors of outcome.
Semistructured Interview	In qualitative research, interviews that are structured in the sense of covering a specific list of issues relevant to the analysis but unstructured in the sense that both the way questions are asked and the way they are answered will vary from one interview to the next. Interviewers systematically touch on specific topics but pose questions in natural, conversational language and invite open-ended answers from participants.
Sensitivity	The proportion of people with a positive test result among those with the target condition. See also Specificity.
Sensitivity Analysis	Any test of the stability of the conclusions of a health care evaluation over a range of probability estimates, value judgments, and assumptions about the structure of the decisions to be made. This may involve the repeated evaluation of a decision model in which one or more of the parameters of interest are varied.
Sentinel Effect	The tendency for human performance to improve when participants are aware that their behavior is being evaluated, in contrast to the Hawthorne effect, which refers to behavior change as a result of being observed but not evaluated.
Sequential Sample (or Consecutive Sample)	See Consecutive Sample.
Sign	Any abnormality indicative of disease, discoverable by the clinician at an examination of the patient. It is an objective aspect of a disease.
Signal-to-Noise Ratio	Signal refers to the target of the measurement; noise, to random error that obscures the signal. When one is trying to discriminate among people at a single point in time (who is better off, who is worse off), the signal comes from differences in scores among patients. The noise comes from variability or differences in score within patients over time. The greater the noise, the more difficult it is to detect the signal. When one is trying to evaluate change over time, the signal comes from the difference in scores in patients whose status has improved or deteriorated. The noise comes from the variability in scores in patients whose status has not changed.
Sign Test	A nonparametric test for comparing 2 paired groups according to the relative ranking of values between the pairs.
Silo Effect	One of the main reasons for considering narrower viewpoints in conducting an economic analysis is to assess the effect of change on the main budget holders because budgets may need to be adjusted before a new intervention can be adopted (the silo effect).

Term	Definition
Single-Nucleotide Polymorphism (SNP)	A single base-pair change in the DNA sequence at a particular point compared with the common or wild-type sequence.
Social Desirability Bias	Occurs when participants answer according to social norms or socially desirable behavior rather than what is actually the case (eg, underreporting alcohol consumption). See also Bias.
Specificity	The proportion of people who are truly free of a designated disorder who are so identified by the test. The test may consist of, or include, clinical observations. See also Sensitivity.
Spectrum Bias	Ideally, diagnostic test properties will be assessed in a population in which the spectrum of disease in the target-positive patients includes all of those in whom clinicians might be uncertain about the diagnosis, and the target-negative patients include all of those with conditions easily confused with the target condition. Spectrum bias may occur when the accuracy of a diagnostic test is assessed in a population that differs from this ideal. Examples of spectrum bias would include a situation in which a substantial proportion of the target-positive population have advanced disease and target-negative participants are healthy or asymptomatic. Such situations typically occur in diagnostic case-control studies (for instance, comparing those with advanced disease to healthy individuals). Such studies are liable to yield an overly sanguine estimate of the usefulness of the test. See also Bias.
Stakeholder Analysis	A strategy that seeks to increase understanding of stakeholder behavior, plans, relationships, and interests and to generate information about stakeholders' levels of influence, support, and resources.
Standard Error	The standard deviation of an estimate of a population parameter. The standard error of the mean is the standard deviation of the estimate of the population mean value.
Standard Gamble	A direct preference or utility measure that effectively asks respondents to rate their quality of life on a scale from 0 to 1.0, where 0 is death and 1.0 is full health. Respondents choose between a specified time x in their current health state and a gamble in which they have probability P (anywhere from 0 to .99) of full health for time x and a probability $1 - P$ of immediate death.
Standardized Mean Difference (SMD)	A statistic used in meta-analysis when the studies all assess the same outcome but measure that outcome using different measurement instruments (eg, different instruments to measure anxiety or pain). Reported as d. See also Effect Size.
Statistical Process Control	A statistical method used for quality improvement based on understanding expected variation in process or outcomes. It involves measuring, plotting, and analyzing data over time to detect stable, improving, or declining performance, the last of which prompts controlling or corrective action.
Statistical Significance	A term that indicates that the results obtained in an analysis of study data are unlikely to have occurred by chance and the null hypothesis is rejected. When statistically significant, the probability of the observed results, given the null hypothesis, falls below a specified level of probability (most often $P < .05$). One-sided significance testing is conducted when only effects in one direction are considered. Note: P values do not provide an estimate of the magnitude of an effect or the precision of the estimate of magnitude. The results of specific statistical tests and measures of variance (eg, odds ratios and 95% confidence intervals, medians and interquartile ranges, means and standard deviations) should be provided.

Term	Definition
Stepped Wedge Design	The sequential rollout of a quality improvement (QI) intervention to study units (clinicians, organizations) during a number of periods so that by the end of the study all participants have received the intervention. The order in which participants receive the intervention may be randomized (similar rigor to cluster randomized designs). Data are collected and outcomes measured at each point at which a new group of participants ("step") receives the QI intervention. Observed differences in outcomes between the control section of the wedge with those in the intervention section are attributed to the intervention.
Stopped Early Trials (or Truncated Trials)	Truncated randomized clinical trials (RCTs) are trials stopped early due to apparent harm because the investigators have concluded that they will not be able to demonstrate a treatment effect (futility) or because of apparent benefit. Believing the treatment from RCTs stopped early for benefit will be misleading if the decision to stop the trial resulted from catching the apparent benefit of treatment at a random high.
Stopping Rules	These are methodologic and statistical guides that inform decisions to stop trials early. They can incorporate issues such as the planned sample size, planned and conducted interim analyses, presence and type of data monitoring including independent research oversight, statistical boundaries, and statistical adjustments for interim analyses and stopping.
Structured Abstract	A brief summary of the key elements of an article following prespecified headings. For example, the *ACP Journal Club* therapy abstracts include major headings of question, methods, setting, patients, intervention, main results, and conclusion. More highly structured abstracts include subheadings. For example, *ACP Journal Club* therapy abstracts methods sections include design, allocation, blinding, and follow-up period.
Subgroup Analysis	The separate analysis of data for subgroups of patients, such as those at different stages of their illness, those with different comorbid conditions, or those of different ages.
Substitute Outcomes or End Points (or Surrogate Outcomes or End Points)	See Surrogate End Points.
Summary-of-Findings Table	In a practice guideline developed according to the GRADE (Grading of Recommendations Assessment, Development and Evaluation) method, the summary-of-findings table provides the confidence ratings for all important outcomes and the associated estimates of relative and absolute effects. Summary-of-findings tables can facilitate shared decision making.
Superiority Trial	Superiority trials are designed to determine whether an experimental intervention is better than a control (typically a standard intervention or existing standard of care). Interpreting the results of superiority trials requires an a priori definition of the smallest difference in outcomes between the interventions that patients would consider large enough in favor of the experimental intervention to justify a preference for it given possible harms, burden, or cost.
Surrogate Outcomes or End Points (or Substitute Outcomes or End Points)	Outcomes that are not in themselves important to patients but are associated with outcomes that are important to patients (eg, bone density for fracture, cholesterol for myocardial infarction, and blood pressure for stroke). These outcomes would not influence patient behavior if they were the only outcomes that would change with an intervention.
Surveillance Bias	See Detection Bias.
Survey	An observational study that focuses on obtaining information about activities, beliefs, preferences, knowledge, or attitudes from respondents through interviewer-administered or self-administered methods.

Term	Definition
Survival Analysis	A statistical procedure used to compare the proportion of patients in each group who experience an outcome or end point at various intervals throughout the study (eg, death).
Survival Curve (or Kaplan-Meier Curve)	A curve that starts at 100% of the study population and shows the percentage of the population still surviving (or free of disease or some other outcome) at successive times for as long as information is available. See also Kaplan-Meier Curve.
Symptom	Any phenomenon or departure from the normal in function, appearance, or sensation reported by the patient and suggestive or indicative of disease.
Syndrome	A collection of signs or symptoms or physiologic abnormalities.
Synonymous single-nucleotide polymorphism	A single-nucleotide polymorphism (SNP) that does not lead to a change in the amino acid sequence compared with the common or wild-type sequence; in a nonsynonymous SNP, there is a change in the amino acid sequence as a result of the SNP.
Synopsis	A brief summary that encapsulates the key methodologic details and results of a single study or systematic review.
Systematic Error (or Bias)	See Bias.
Systematic Review	The identification, selection, appraisal, and summary of primary studies that address a focused clinical question using methods to reduce the likelihood of bias.
Systems	Systems include practice guidelines, clinical pathways, or evidence-based textbook summaries that integrate evidence-based information about specific clinical problems and provide regular updates to guide the care of individual patients.
Target Condition (or Target Disease)	In diagnostic test studies, the condition the investigators or clinicians are particularly interested in identifying (such as tuberculosis, lung cancer, or iron deficiency anemia).
Target Negative	In diagnostic test studies, patients who do not have the target condition.
Target Outcome (or Target End Points or Target Events)	In intervention studies, the condition the investigators or clinicians are particularly interested in identifying and in which it is anticipated the intervention will decrease (such as myocardial infarction, stroke, or death) or increase (such as ulcer healing).
Target Positive	In diagnostic test studies, patients who have the target condition.
Target Variable (or Dependent Variable or Outcome Variable)	See Dependent Variable.
Test Threshold	The probability below which the clinician decides a diagnosis warrants no further consideration.
Themes	A generic term for the elements of qualitative research findings. Researchers usually express themes in terms of labels and definitions for the phenomena they describe or interpret from patterns in their data.
Theoretical Saturation	In qualitative research, this is the point in the analysis at which themes are well organized into a coherent theory or conceptual framework; new data fit easily without requiring revision to the theory. This is considered an appropriate stopping point for data analysis, especially in grounded theory methods.
Theory	Theory consists of concepts and their relationships.
Theory Triangulation	See Triangulation.
Threshold Number Needed to Treat (or Threshold Number Needed to Harm)	The maximum number needed to treat or number needed to harm accepted as justifying the benefits and harms of therapy. See also Number Needed to Treat and Number Needed to Harm.

Term	Definition
Time Series Design (or Interrupted Time Series Design)	In this study design, data are collected at several points both before and after the intervention. Data collected before the intervention allow the underlying trend and cyclical (seasonal) effects to be estimated. Data collected after the intervention allow the intervention effect to be estimated while accounting for underlying secular trends. The intervention may be interrupted then reintroduced multiple times. The time series design monitors the occurrence of outcomes or end points during a number of cycles and determines whether the pattern changes coincident with the intervention.
Transferability	The extent to which knowledge based on research findings can reasonably be applied to situations that differ from the original research setting. This requires judgment and expertise and necessarily draws on information from other sources in addition to information provided by the research study.
Treatment Effect (or Intervention Effect)	The results of comparative clinical studies can be expressed using various intervention effect measures. Examples are absolute risk reduction (ARR), relative risk reduction (RRR), odds ratio (OR), number needed to treat (NNT), and effect size. The appropriateness of using these to express an intervention effect and whether probabilities, means, or medians are used to calculate them depend on the type of outcome variable used to measure health outcomes. For example, ARR, RRR, and NNT are used for dichotomous variables, and effect sizes are normally used for continuous variables.
Treatment Target	The manifestation of illness (a symptom, sign, or physiologic abnormality) toward which a treatment is directed.
Treatment Threshold (or Therapeutic Threshold)	Probability above which a clinician would consider a diagnosis confirmed and would stop testing and initiate treatment.
Trial of Therapy	In a trial of therapy, the physician offers the patient an intervention, reviews the effect of the intervention on that patient at some subsequent time, and, depending on the effect, recommends either continuation or discontinuation of the intervention.
Triangulation	In qualitative research, triangulation is an analytic approach in which key findings are corroborated using multiple sources of information. There are different types of triangulation. Investigator triangulation requires more than 1 investigator to collect and analyze the raw data, such that the findings emerge through consensus among a team of investigators. Theory triangulation is a process whereby emergent findings are corroborated with existing social science theories. Note that any discrepancies would not necessarily indicate that the research is biased or in error but rather that the next stage of empirical analysis should interpret and account for the discrepancies.
Trim-and-Fill Method	When publication bias is suspected in a systematic review, investigators may attempt to estimate the true intervention effect by removing, or trimming, small positive-result studies that do not have a negative-result study counterpart and then calculating a supposed true effect from the resulting symmetric funnel plot. The investigators then replace the positive-result studies they have removed and add hypothetical studies that mirror these positive-result studies to create a symmetric funnel plot that retains the new pooled effect estimate. This method allows the calculation of an adjusted confidence interval and an estimate of the number of missing trials.
True Negative	Those whom the test correctly identifies as not having the target disorder.
True Positive	Those whom the test correctly identifies as having the target disorder.
Truncated Trials (Stopped Early Trials)	See Stopped Early Trials.

Term	Definition
Trustworthiness (or Credibility)	See Credibility.
t Test	A parametric statistical test that examines the difference between the means of 2 groups of values.
Type I Error	An error created by rejecting the null hypothesis when it is true (ie, investigators conclude that an association exists among variables when it does not). See also α Level and Type II Error.
Type II Error	An error created by accepting the null hypothesis when it is false (ie, investigators conclude that no association exists among variables when, in fact, an association does exist). See also β Error and Type I Error.
Unblinded (or Unmasked)	Patients, clinicians, those monitoring outcomes, judicial assessors of outcomes, data analysts, and manuscript authors are aware of whether patients have been assigned to the experimental or control group.
Unit of Allocation	The unit or focus used for assignment to comparison groups (eg, individuals or clusters such as schools, health care teams, hospital wards, outpatient practices).
Unit of Analysis	The unit or focus of the analysis; although it is most often the individual study participant, in a study that uses cluster allocation, the unit of analysis is the cluster (eg, school, clinic).
Unit of Analysis Error	When investigators use any sort of cluster randomization (randomize by physician instead of patient, practice instead of physician or patient, or village instead of participant) and analyze as if they have randomized according to patient or participant, they have made a unit of analysis error. The appropriate analysis acknowledges the cluster randomization and takes into account the extent to which outcomes differ among clusters independent of treatment effect.
Univariate Regression (or Univariable Regression or Simple Regression)	This term is for simple descriptive analyses. It is often erroneously used for bivariable regression. See also Bivariable Regression.
Unmasked (or Unblinded)	See Unblinded.
Upfront Costs	Costs incurred to "produce" the treatment, such as the physician's time, nurse's time, and materials.
Utilitarian (or Consequentialist)	See Consequentialist.
Utility	Utility in the context of health economic modeling refers to the value of a health state, typically expressed from 0 (death) to 1.0 (full health).
Validity (or Credibility)	In terms of health status measurement, validity is the extent to which an instrument measures what it is intended to measure. In critical appraisal terms, validity reflects the extent to which the limitations in study design leave a study vulnerable to systematic error or spurious inferences. See also Credibility.
Values and Preferences	When used generically, as in "values and preferences," we refer to the collection of goals, expectations, predispositions, and beliefs that individuals have for certain decisions and their potential outcomes. The incorporation of patient values and preferences in decision making is central to evidence-based medicine. These terms also carry specific meaning in other settings. Measurement tools that require a choice under conditions of uncertainty to indirectly measure preference for an outcome in health economics (such as the standard gamble) quantify preferences. Measurement tools that evaluate the outcome on a scale with defined favorable and unfavorable ends (eg, visual analog scales, feeling thermometers) quantify values.

Term	Definition
Variance	The technical term for the statistical estimate of the variability in results.
Variant Allele	The allele at a particular single-nucleotide polymorphism that is the least frequent in a population.
Verification Bias	See Differential Verification Bias.
Visual Analog Scale	A scaling procedure that consists of a straight line anchored on each end with words or phrases that represent the extremes of some phenomenon (eg, "worst pain I have ever had" to "absolutely no pain"). Respondents are asked to make a mark on the line at the point that corresponds to their experience of the phenomenon.
Washout Period	In a crossover or n-of-1 trial, the period required for the treatment to cease to act once it has been discontinued.
Weighted Mean Difference	The weighted mean difference is the difference between initial and final values of a continuous measure in a group of patients in a study. The weighted mean difference is also a way of presenting the magnitude of effect in a meta-analysis in which all studies have used the same continuous variable (such as exercise capacity or a specific quality-of-life instrument). It presents the best estimate of the difference between 2 treatments using the units of the particular outcome used in all of the studies. It is calculated as the sum of the differences in the individual studies, weighted by the individual variances for each study.
Wild-Type Allele	The allele at a particular single-nucleotide polymorphism that is most frequent in a population, also called a common allele.
Willingness to Pay	In some economic analyses, it may be desirable to compare costs and outcomes using the same metric (ie, costs). In this case, an attempt is made to ask people how much they would pay to achieve an improvement in health or to avoid a negative health event/outcome.
Working Diagnosis (or Leading Hypothesis)	The clinician's single best explanation for the patient's clinical problem(s).
Workup Bias	See Differential Verification Bias.

INDEX

F

G